# Quick Find Guide

D1289317

# Patient Assessment Tutorials

## A STEP-BY-STEP GUIDE FOR THE DENTAL HYGIENIST

### THIRD EDITION

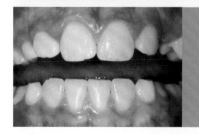

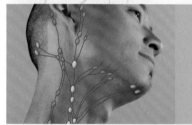

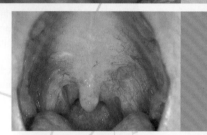

## Jill S. Nield-Gehrig, RDH, MA

Dean Emeritus, Division of Allied Health & Public Service Education
Asheville-Buncombe Technical Community College
Asheville, North Carolina

## Donald E. Wilmann, DDS, MS

University of Texas Health Science
Center at San Antonio Dental School
San Antonio, Texas

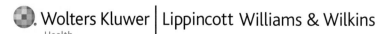

. Wolters Kluwer | Lippincott Williams & Wilkins
Health

Philadelphia • Baltimore • New York • London
Buenos Aires • Hong Kong • Sydney • Tokyo

*Acquisitions Editor:* Christopher Johnson
*Product Manager:* Kristin Royer
*Marketing Manager:* Shauna Kelley
*Production Project Manager:* Marian Bellus
*Senior Managing Editor:* Heather Rybacki
*Design Coordinator:* Stephen Druding
*Manufacturing Coordinator:* Margie Orzech
*Production Services / Compositor:* Absolute Service, Inc.

Third Edition

Copyright © 2013, 2010, 2007 Lippincott Williams & Wilkins, a Wolters Kluwer business.

351 West Camden Street
Baltimore, Maryland 21201

530 Walnut Street
Philadelphia, Pennsylvania 19106

Printed in China

All rights reserved. This book is protected by copyright. No part of this book may be reproduced or transmitted in any form or by any means, including as photocopies or scanned-in or other electronic copies, or utilized by any information storage and retrieval system without written permission from the copyright owner, except for brief quotations embodied in critical articles and reviews. Materials appearing in this book prepared by individuals as part of their official duties as U.S. government employees are not covered by the above-mentioned copyright. To request permission, please contact Lippincott Williams & Wilkins at 530 Walnut Street, Philadelphia, PA 19106, via email at permissions@lww.com, or via website at lww.com (products and services).

9 8 7 6 5 4 3 2 1

**Library of Congress Cataloging-in-Publication Data**

Nield-Gehrig, Jill S. (Jill Shiffer)
  Patient assessment tutorials: a step-by-step procedures guide for the dental hygienist / Jill S. Nield-Gehrig, Donald E. Willmann. – 3rd ed.
    p. ; cm.
  Includes bibliographical references and index.
  Summary: "The ability to accurately assess patients is vital to the practice of Dental Hygiene—a complete and accurate assessment is the starting point to providing thorough patient care. Patient Assessment Tutorials takes you through the process of patient assessment and provides you with information on both the actual physical assessment as well as effective patient communication. The highly visual, step-by-step style teaches you vital assessment processes quickly and thoroughly. Excellent features include detailed, full-color illustrations and photographs to visually guide you through procedures and techniques, case studies and personal accounts that bring the content to life, and more."–Provided by publisher.
  ISBN 978-1-4511-3148-2
  I. Willmann, Donald E. II. Title.
  [DNLM: 1. Diagnosis, Oral–methods–Programmed Instruction. 2. Dental Hygienists–Programmed Instruction. 3. Dental Records–Programmed Instruction. WU 18.2]

  617.6'01–dc23
                    2012035585

RRS1210

# PREFACE FOR COURSE INSTRUCTORS

*Patient Assessment Tutorials: A Step-by-Step Guide for the Dental Hygienist,* Third Edition is a detailed instructional guide to patient assessment procedures. *Tutorials* is unique in two regards: first, the Peak Procedures sections teach the "how to" of patient assessment procedures in a clear, step-by-step manner; second, *Tutorials* places a unique emphasis on the human element of patient assessment. Content on the human interaction aspect of patient assessment includes three chapters on communication, as well as the Human Element sections and communication role-plays throughout the book.

*Patient Assessment Tutorials* is designed for student use in two settings. Initially, the modules are designed to guide student practice of assessment and communication techniques in preclinical and clinical settings. Later, the Ready References from the modules—when laminated and assembled in a notebook—create a reference book that provides quick access to information during patient treatment.

## BOOK FEATURES

*Patient Assessment Tutorials: A Step-by-Step Guide for the Dental Hygienist* has many features designed to facilitate learning and teaching.

1. **Module Overview and Outline.** Each module begins with a concise overview of the module content. The module outline makes it easier to locate material within the chapter. The outline provides the reader with an organizational framework with which to approach new material. Learning objectives assist students in recognizing and studying important concepts in each chapter.

2. **Peak Procedures.** Step-by-step instructions are provided for each patient assessment procedure.
   - For students, the Peak Procedures section provides a straightforward, step-by-step guide for practicing and perfecting assessment techniques. The self-instructional format allows the learner to work independently—fostering student autonomy and decision-making skills.
   - For educators, the Peak Procedures section provides a reliable, evidence-based blueprint for the standardization of faculty members in the instruction and evaluation of patient assessment procedures.

3. **Ready References.** The Ready References provide rapid access to important information on each assessment topic. For example, there is a Ready Reference with the most commonly prescribed medications. The Ready Reference features are designed to be removed from the book, laminated or placed in plastic page protectors, and assembled in a notebook for use in the clinical setting.

4. **The Human Element.** This module feature focuses on the "people part" of patient assessment. Students, patients, and experienced clinicians were invited to share their experiences in this section of the modules. The features *Through the Eyes of a Student* and *Through the Eyes of a Patient* speak to the human element of the assessment process. In these real-life accounts, students share their struggles and triumphs with patient assessment procedures. Patient accounts evoke empathy and pride in the impact of caregiving.

5. **Internet Sites for Information Gathering.** A list of Internet sites in each module encourages students to develop skills in online information gathering. With the rapid explosion of knowledge in the dental and medical sciences, a student can no longer expect to learn everything that he or she needs to know, now and forever, in a few years of professional training. Reference books in print cannot be relied upon for the most up-to-date information. Therefore, students must learn how to quickly retrieve accurate information from reliable Internet sites, such as MEDLINE.

6. **English-to-Spanish Phrase Lists.** As the Spanish-speaking population increases, clinicians encounter growing numbers of Spanish-speaking patients in dental clinics and offices. Teaching students to pronounce and speak Spanish is well beyond the scope of this book and indeed, beyond the scope of most professional curriculums. For those times when a trained translator is not available, however, the modules include English-to-Spanish phrase lists with phrases pertinent to the assessment process. To use these phrase lists, the student clinician simply points to a specific phrase in the list to facilitate communication with a Spanish-speaking patient.

7. **Fictitious Patient Cases A–E.** Fictitious Patient Cases A–E promote the student's application of chapter information to patient care, much in the same way that he or she needs to do when caring for a real patient. With each module, more information is revealed about each patient's assessment findings. For example, Module 4 reveals the medical histories of fictitious Patients A–E. Module 9 provides the patients' blood pressure readings. This progressive disclosure of assessment findings parallels the manner in which students collect information on a patient in the clinical setting, gleaning new nuggets of information with each assessment procedure performed. In each module, the student is asked to interpret the assessment findings revealed in the module, relate it to information about the patient from previous chapters, and make decisions about patient care based upon these assessment findings.

8. **Skill Check.** The Module Skill Evaluation procedure checklists allow a student to self-evaluate his or her strengths and limitations in performing the assessment procedure and to identify additional learning needs. The checklists also provide benchmarks for instructor evaluation of student skill proficiency.
   **Suggestions for communication role-plays are available on the book's companion website, ThePoint. Refer to page viii for details on accessing online resources.** Communication checklists in the modules allow students to practice and self-evaluate their communication skills and to identify areas for improvement. The checklists also provide benchmarks for instructor evaluation of student skill proficiency in communicating with patients.

9. **Terminology and Glossary of Terms.** Terminology pertinent to patient assessment is highlighted in bold type and clearly defined within each module. The Glossary in the back of the book provides quick access to terminology.

10. **Comprehensive Fictitious Patient Cases F–K.** Module 17 of the book is composed of comprehensive patient cases. This module presents six entirely new comprehensive patient cases. Patient assessment data is presented for each patient, and the student is challenged to interpret and use this assessment information in care planning for the patient.

# ONLINE RESOURCES

*Patient Assessment Tutorials,* Third Edition includes additional resources for both instructors and students that are available on the book's companion website, thePoint.

## ONLINE INSTRUCTOR TEACHING RESOURCES

**Follow the steps below to access the online instructor resources.**

---

Accessing Online Instructor Resources

1. Open an Internet browser and select: **http://thePoint.lww.com/NieldGehrigPAT3e**

2. Existing users: log on. Skip to step 4 in this list.

3. New users: select "Register a New Account." Complete all required fields on the online access request form. Select **Submit Adoption Form** button. U.S. and Canadian educators, please allow three business days for a reply.

4. Locate **Patient Assessment Tutorials.** Select "Instructor Resources."

Note: Students can access resources by selecting "Student Resources." See the inside front cover of this text for more details.

---

## INSTRUCTORS

Approved adopting instructors will be given access to the following additional resources:

- Image Bank
- PowerPoint Presentations
- Test Bank Questions
- Video clip that allows students to hear the Korotkoff sounds and practice recording blood pressure readings
- Video clips showing proper head, neck, and oral examination techniques
- Morita CBCT Viewer
- Practical Focus Case Studies, Patient Case Studies, and Active Learning Cases
- Role-Playing Exercises
- Instructions on how to use the textbook and instructor resources
- WebCT- and Blackboard-ready cartridges

*thePoint is a trademark of Wolters Kluwer Health.

## STUDENTS

See the inside front cover of this text for more details, including the passcode needed to gain access to the website. Students who have purchased *Patient Assessment Tutorials,* Third Edition have access to the following additional resources:

- Video clip that allows students to hear the Korotkoff sounds and practice recording blood pressure readings.
- Video clips showing proper head, neck, and oral examination techniques
- Morita CBCT Viewer
- A searchable online version of the full text

# USER'S GUIDE

The ability to accurately assess patients is vital to the practice of Dental Hygiene—a complete and accurate assessment is the starting point to providing thorough patient care. *Patient Assessment Tutorials: A Step-by-Step Guide for the Dental Hygienist* takes you through the process of patient assessment and provides you with information on both the actual physical assessment as well as effective patient communication. The highly visual, step-by-step style teaches you vital assessment processes quickly and thoroughly.

## YOU'LL FIND THESE GREAT FEATURES IN THE TEXT:

### Module Overviews – Module Outlines – Skill Goals

Give an orientation to the information in the chapter and what you are expected to know after reading the chapter material. ▶

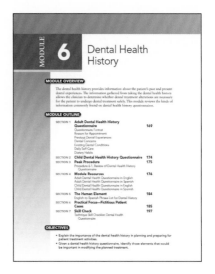

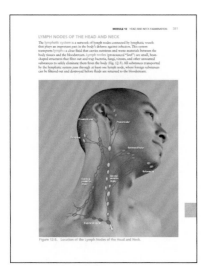

Figure 13-5. Location of the Lymph Nodes of the Head and Neck.

### ◀ Detailed Illustrations & Photographs

Bring the material in the book to life and help to visually guide you through the patient assessment process.

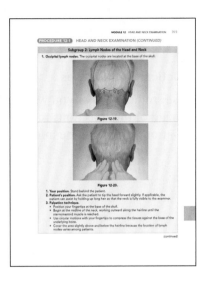

## Procedure Boxes

Outline procedures in an easy-to-follow, step-by-step format. Lists of necessary equipment and a rationale for each step are also provided. ▶

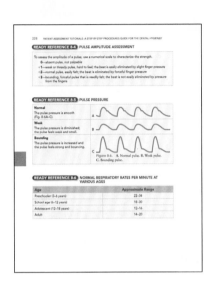

◀ **Ready References**

Provide vital information for use during the patient assessment process. Ready Reference pages can be removed from the book. Laminating or placing pages in plastic sleeves will make them ready to use in a clinical setting.

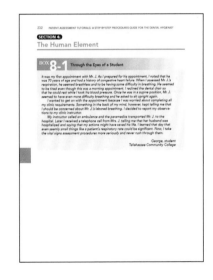

## The Human Element

Case studies and personal experiences of other students and hygienists relate to the chapter content and explain why each assessment procedure is clinically relevant to dental hygiene practice. ▶

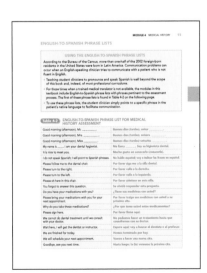

◀ **English-to-Spanish Phrase Lists**

These phrase lists facilitate communication with Spanish-speaking patients.

## Practical Focus Cases

Case studies present you with a clinical scenario. Questions at the end of these sections require you to think critically about the situation and apply the information you have learned. ▶

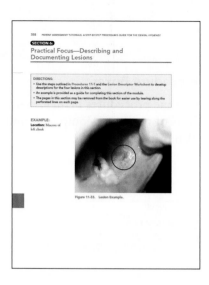

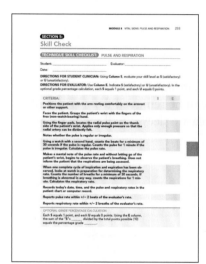

◀ **Skill Checks**

Assess your understanding and ability to perform the skills presented in the chapter.

## ONLINE FACULTY RESOURCES

Sharon Logue, RDH, MPH
Virginia Department of Health
Division of Dental Health
Richmond, Virginia
Rebecca Sroda, RDH, MA
Associate Dean, Allied Health
South Florida Community College
Avon Park, Florida

## MODULE 5: READY REFERENCES: MEDICAL HISTORY

Cynthia Biron Leiseca, RDH, EMT, MA
President, DH Meth-Ed, Inc.
Educational Consultant, Dental Hygiene Teaching Methodology
Fernandina Beach, Florida

## MODULE 6: DENTAL HEALTH HISTORY
## MODULE 16: DENTAL RADIOGRAPHS

John Preece, DDS, MS
Dental Diagnostic Science
University of Texas Health Science Center at San Antonio
San Antonio, Texas

## MODULE 10: TOBACCO CESSATION COUNSELING

Carol Southard, RN, MSN
Tobacco Cessation Specialist
Northwestern Memorial Hospital
Wellness Institute
Chicago, Illinois

## ENGLISH-TO-SPANISH TRANSLATIONS

Remberto (Ron) J. Leiseca, BBA, CSI, CCPR, MAI
DH Meth-Ed, Inc.
Consultant and Media Specialist
Fernandina Beach, Florida

## CLINICAL IMAGES

Richard Foster, DMD
Dental Director
Guilford Technical Community College
Jamestown, North Carolina
Informed Consent and Patient Scenarios

Robin B. Matloff, RDH, BSDH, JD
Associate Professor, Dental Hygiene Program
Mount Ida College
Newton, Massachusetts

# ACKNOWLEDGMENTS

We are extremely grateful to our many colleagues who have contributed to the completion of this project. Without their contributions, this textbook would not have been possible. Our thanks to all who generously gave their time, ideas, and resources, and we gratefully acknowledge the special contributions of the following individuals:

- **Holly R. Fischer**, MFA and **Charles D. Whitehead**, the highly skilled medical illustrators who created all the wonderful illustrations for the book.
- **Dee Robert Gehrig**, PE, Gehrig Photographic Studio, the talented individual who created the hundreds of photographs for this book.
- **Kevin Dietz**, colleague and friend, for his vision and guidance for this book.
- And finally, and with great thanks, my wonderful team at Lippincott Williams and Wilkins, without whose guidance and support this book would not have been possible: **Pete Sabatini, Kristin Royer**, and **Jennifer Clements**.

Jill S. Nield-Gehrig
Donald E. Willmann

# CONTENTS

**MODULE 11**   **Soft Tissue Lesions   336**

**MODULE 12**   **Head and Neck Examination   376**

**MODULE 13**   **Oral Examination   440**

**MODULE 14**   **Gingival Description   496**

**MODULE 15**   **Mixed Dentition and Occlusion   536**

## PART 3: COMPREHENSIVE PATIENT CASES

**The Point: Online Resources
(http://thePoint.lww.com/NieldGehrigPAT3e**

## MODULE 1

# Communication Skills for Assessment

MODULE

## MODULE OVERVIEW

Clear communication provides the foundation for patient assessment procedures from history taking to explaining assessment findings to the patient. Being able to communicate effectively—or participate in the exchange of information—is an essential skill for dental health care providers.

To a great extent, the patient's satisfaction with dental care is determined by the dental health care provider's ability and willingness to communicate and empathize with patient needs and expectations. Good communication during the assessment process sets the tone for quality care and loyal patients.

This module summarizes techniques for—as well as obstacles to—effective communication during the patient assessment process.

## MODULE OUTLINE

## OBJECTIVES

- Define communication and describe the communication process.
- Describe how ineffective communication hinders the provision of quality dental care.
- Describe the two major forms of communication and give examples of each.
- Discuss techniques that promote effective communication.
- Understand the role of effective communication in the provision of quality dental care.
- List and describe three ways in which people communicate nonverbally.
- Explain why appearance can often lead to incorrect assumptions about an individual.
- Define patient-centered care.
- List and describe five key elements of the RESPECT model for the patient-centered approach to communication.
- Discuss strategies for making health care words understandable to the patient.
- Demonstrate the use of communication strategies and questioning techniques that facilitate complete, accurate information gathering during patient assessment.

**SECTION 1:**

# The Communication Process

## WHAT IS COMMUNICATION?

Communication is the exchange of information between individuals. The word "exchange" is essential to understanding the act of communicating. The process of communication is an *exchange of information* that moves back and forth between two people. A dental health care provider must be a successful communicator, both as a sender and as a receiver of information. Communication with a patient not only involves telling the person something (sending information) but also is about listening to the patient's response—receiving information—in return. The understanding of how to convey and interpret meaning is essential for effective communication. In the context of dental care, communication's primary function is to establish understanding between the patient and the dental health care provider.

## INEFFECTIVE COMMUNICATION

There are always at least two parties involved in any communication. Communication blocks can occur when the clinician assumes that the patient knows what he or she is thinking (Fig. 1-1). (The patient **should know** that the health history is important; **shouldn't he**?) Box 1-1 shows examples of the impact of poor patient communication.

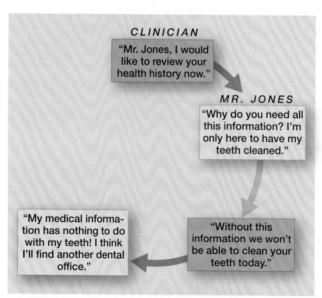

*CLINICIAN*
"Mr. Jones, I would like to review your health history now."

*MR. JONES*
"Why do you need all this information? I'm only here to have my teeth cleaned."

"Without this information we won't be able to clean your teeth today."

"My medical information has nothing to do with my teeth! I think I'll find another dental office."

**Figure 1-1.   Ineffective flow of communication.** The assumption that the patient knows what the clinician knows—such as why an accurate health history is important—presents a major roadblock to effective communication.

## BOX 1-1    The Impact of Poor Patient Communication

**POOR COMMUNICATION:**

- Decreases the patient's confidence and trust in dental care
- Deters the patient from revealing important information
- Leads to the patient not seeking further care
- Leads to misunderstandings
- Leads to the misinterpretation of advice
- Underlies most patient complaints

*These difficulties may lead to poor or suboptimal dental health for the patient.*

## EFFECTIVE COMMUNICATION

Being a good listener is key to interacting and responding to the patient in a manner that conveys empathy for, as well as interest in, his or her concerns. Successful communication begins by recognizing the patient's needs and concerns (Fig. 1-2). Box 1-2 shows examples of the benefits of effective communication.

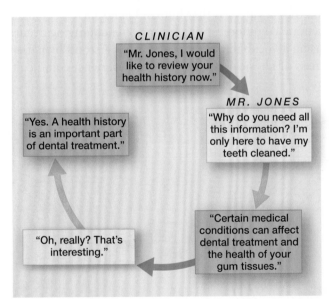

**Figure 1-2. Effective flow of communication.** Communication is most effective when the clinician uses words that the patient will understand and listens carefully to the patient's responses or questions.

## BOX 1-2    The Benefits of Good Patient Communication

**GOOD COMMUNICATION:**

- Builds trust between the patient and the health care provider
- May make it easier for the patient to disclose information
- Enhances patient satisfaction
- Allows the patient to participate more fully in health decision making
- Helps the patient to make better dental health decisions
- Leads to more realistic patient expectations

*The benefits of good communication may contribute to better dental health for the patient.*

## COMMUNICATION FILTERS

Each person involved in the act of communication interprets a message based on many factors such as his or her life experiences, age, gender, and cultural diversity. These factors act as **personal filters** that "distort" messages being sent and received (Fig. 1-3). *For this reason, the message received may not be the message sent. Normal human biases or personalized filters create major barriers to effective communication.* Communication is promoted by awareness that human beings have personalized filters that can impede accurate communication. Means of encouraging accurate communication include using a vocabulary that is easily understood by patients combined with an awareness of physical limitations, life experiences, and cultural differences.

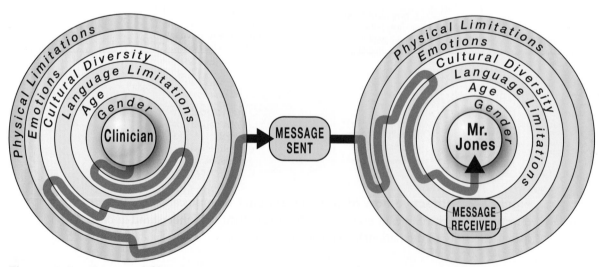

**Figure 1-3.    Personal filters.** Each individual interprets a messages based on his or her own filters such as life experiences, beliefs, physical limitations (e.g., hearing loss), and gender.

## NONVERBAL COMMUNICATION

There are two major forms of communication, verbal and nonverbal.[1] Dr. Albert Mehrabian, who pioneered the study of communication, found that only about 7% of the meaning of a message is communicated through verbal exchange (Fig. 1-4). About 38% is communicated by the use of the voice and tone. About 55% comes through gestures, facial expression, posture, and so forth. Dr. Mehrabian's communication model is useful in illustrating the importance of considering factors other than words when trying to convey meaning (as the speaker) or interpret meaning (as the listener). The understanding of how to convey and interpret meaning is essential for effective communication.

1. **Verbal communication** is the use of spoken, written, or sign language to exchange information between individuals. In the context of dental care, communication's primary function is to establish understanding between the patient and the clinician.
2. **Nonverbal communication** is the transfer of information between persons without using spoken, written, or sign language (Box 1-3).
   - In nonverbal communication, "wordless" messages are sent and received by means of facial expression, appearance, gaze, gestures, postures, tone of voice, hairstyle, grooming habits, and body positioning in space.
   - Each of us gives and responds to literally thousands of nonverbal messages daily in our personal and professional lives.
   - We all react to wordless nonverbal messages emotionally, often without consciously knowing why.

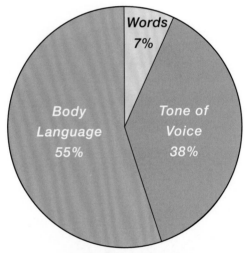

**Three Elements of Communication**

**Figure 1-4. Nonverbal communication.** Nonverbal communication is information that is communicated without using words.
- 7% of meaning is in spoken words
- 38% of meaning is paralinguistic (the way that words are said)
- 55% of meaning is in body language, such as facial expression

## BOX 1-3 Nonverbal Communication

*Nonverbal communication can include posture, facial expression, appearance, hairstyle, clothes, shaking hands, smiling, proximity to others, touch, color choice, and silence.*

## FIRST IMPRESSIONS

1. **Unconscious First Impressions.** Although health care providers prefer to be judged on their knowledge, skills, and the care they provide to patients, other factors such as first impressions often influence patients' judgments about clinicians.
   - It seems unfair, but first impressions count (Fig. 1-5).
   - When a person walks into a room, others make subconscious decisions about him or her. Within about 60 seconds, others have judged the person's educational background, likeability, and level of success.
   - After about 5 minutes, conclusions have been drawn about the person's trustworthiness, reliability, intelligence, and friendliness.
   - Impressions are based upon instinct and emotion, not on rational thought or careful investigation.
   - We all make associations between outward characteristics and the inner qualities we believe they reflect.
   - We filter everything we see and hear through our own experiences. We all have assumptions—**stereotypes**—regarding what it means to be: short or tall, heavy or thin, clean or dirty, native or foreign, young or old, male or female.
2. **Creating Positive First Impressions.** What can health care providers do to be in control a patient's first impression of us?
   - Each clinician has to determine his or her objectives and make choices in dress and behavior that convey competence and caring.
   - First impressions can open the lines of communication and build trust.

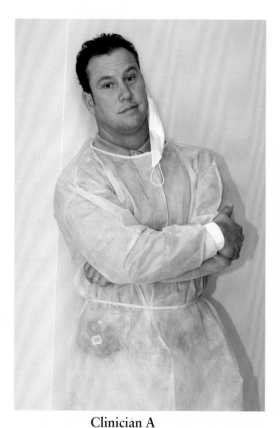
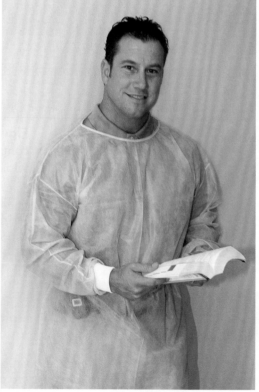

Clinician A                    Clinician B

**Figure 1-5   A,B. First impressions.** If you were a patient, what message would these two clinicians be sending to you?

# USE OF SPACE

1. **Proxemics** is the study of the distance an individual maintains from other people and how this separation relates to environmental and cultural factors.
   - Every person has around him or her an invisible "personal zone of comfort" defined as personal space. We have all felt uneasiness in an elevator or airplane when the stranger on either side inadvertently touches us.
   - When our personal zone of comfort has been invaded, we feel uncomfortable and resentful. **Personal space**—or distance from other persons—is a powerful concept that we use in determining the meaning of messages conveyed by another person (Table 1-1).
   - For example, an angry person is perceived as less threatening if the person is not standing nearby. If an angry person is close, however, the individual's anger is perceived as more threatening.
   - Personal space is a subtle but powerful part of nonverbal communication that health care providers must understand in order to relate better to the patient in the dental setting.
   - *Entering the personal or intimate zones of comfort is necessary in the dental health care setting and, if not carefully handled, may cause the patient to feel threatened or insecure.*

**Table 1-1** PERSONAL SPACE

| Territorial Zone | Body Space |
|---|---|
| Intimate | 1–18 in |
| Personal | 1.5–4 ft |
| Social | 4–12 ft |
| Public | More than 12 ft |

2. **Territory** is the space we consider as belonging to us.
   - The way that people handle space is largely determined by their culture.
   - Differences in culture can lead to different interpretations of personal space and touching.
   - North Americans and Latin Americans, for example, have fundamentally different proxemic systems.
   - Whereas North Americans usually remain at a distance from one another, Latin Americans stay very close to each other.
   - Remland and colleagues reported that in their sample of seven nations, the British sample showed on average the greatest distance between persons in a conversation (15.40 in). Southern European countries, such as Greece (13.86 in) and Italy (14.18 in), showed a closer distance between persons engaged in conversation.[2]
   - **Low-contact cultures** (North American, Northern Europeans, Asian) favor the social zone for interaction and little, if any, physical contact. (Box 1-4 shows examples of low-contact and high-contact cultures.)
   - **High-contact cultures** (Mediterranean, Arab, Latin) prefer the intimate and personal zones and much contact between people. In Saudi Arabia, persons engaged in conversation might be almost nose to nose with each other because their social space equates to a North American's intimate space.
   - Misunderstandings can occur when low-contact cultures interact with high-contact cultures and either invade or avoid personal space and physical contact.

> ## BOX 1-4   Low-Contact versus High-Contact Cultures
>
> **LOW-CONTACT CULTURES**
> **Asian:** *China, Indonesia, Japan, Philippines, Thailand*
> **Southern Asian:** *India and Pakistan*
> **Northern European:** *Australia, England, Germany, the Netherlands, Norway, Scotland*
> **North American**: *United States and Canada*
>
> **HIGH-CONTACT CULTURES**
> **Arab:** *Iraq, Kuwait, Saudi Arabia, Syria, United Arab Republic*
> **Latin American:** *Bolivia, Cuba, Ecuador, El Salvador, Mexico, Paraguay, Peru, Puerto Rico, Venezuela*
> **Southern European:** *France, Italy, Turkey*

## TOUCH AS NONVERBAL COMMUNICATION

1. **The Importance of Touch.** Touching is perhaps the most powerful nonverbal communication tool.
   - We can communicate a wide variety of emotions through touching, such as support, protection, anger, tenderness, or intimacy.
   - Touch is culturally determined. Each culture has a clear concept of what parts of the body one many not touch. Low-contact cultures—English, German, Scandinavian, Chinese, and Japanese—have little public touch. High-contact cultures—Latino, Middle Eastern, and Jewish—accept frequent touches.
2. **Touch is Universal.** Touch is perhaps the most universal of all forms of communication.
   - The comforting aspect of touch is significant in health care.
   - A comforting touch can say more than words (Fig. 1-6). A light pat on the shoulder or on the top of the hand is comforting and establishes a bond between the health care provider and the patient.
3. **Touch Taxonomy.** Richard Heslin has developed a taxonomy that classifies touch (Box 1-5).
   - Heslin's five categories are functional/professional, social/polite, friendship/warmth, love/intimacy, and sexual arousal.[3]
   - *Dental care involves being in close proximity to the patient—invading the patient's space—and touching the patient.*
   - A patient may be acutely aware of the clinician's touch, and some patients may question the appropriateness of touching.
   - Dental health care providers should recognize that the patient is entitled to know why and where he or she is to be touched.
   - Clinicians should respect, as much as possible, the patient's personal space.

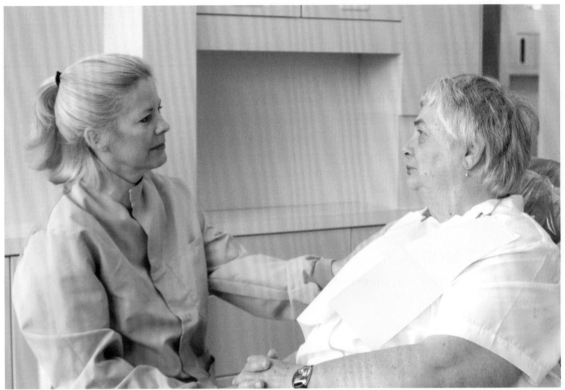

**Figure 1-6. The value of touch.** Of the many techniques for enhancing communication, nothing says, "I care about you and I want to help you" more effectively than a simple touch on a person's hand or shoulder.

---

BOX **1-5** Heslin's Categories of Touching Behavior

1. Functional/professional
2. Social/polite
3. Friendship/warmth
4. Love/intimacy
5. Sexual arousal

## SECTION 2:

# Communicating with Patients

## PATIENT-CENTERED COMMUNICATION

Effective communication involves **patient-centered care**—respecting the patient as a whole, unique individual. A patient-centered approach to patient care recognizes that there are two experts present during the interaction between a health care provider and a patient. One expert is the health care provider, who has clinical knowledge. The second expert is the patient, who brings experience, beliefs, and values to the dental treatment planning process. Both have rights and needs, and both have a role in decision making about care and implementation of treatment.

## THE RESPECT MODEL

The RESPECT model (Box 1-6) summarizes the patient-centered approach to communication.[4]

---

### BOX 1-6    The RESPECT Model for Patient-Centered Communication

*Rapport*
- Connect with a patient on a social level
- See the patient's point of view
- Consciously suspend judgment
- Recognize and avoid making assumptions

*Empathy*
- Remember that the patient has come to you for help
- Seek out and understand the patient's rationale for his or her behaviors or disease
- Verbally acknowledge and legitimize the patient's feelings

*Support*
- Ask about and understand the barriers to care and compliance
- Help the patient overcome barriers
- Involve family members if appropriate
- Reassure the patient that you are willing and able to help

*Partnership*
- Allow the patient to be an equal partner in the decision-making process
- Stress that you are working together to address dental problems

*Explanations*
- Check often for understanding
- Use verbal clarification techniques

*Cultural competence*
- Respect the patient's cultural beliefs
- Understand that the patient's interaction with you may be defined by ethnic or cultural stereotypes
- Be aware of your own cultural biases and preconceptions

*Trust*
- Recognize that self-disclosure may be difficult for some patients
- Consciously work to establish trust

## SKILLS FOR ESTABLISHING RAPPORT

In a dental setting, as in most other human interactions, first impressions count. Meeting and greeting a patient is the first step in the dental care process. Box 1-7 shows suggestions for actions when collaborating with patients.

1. **Get the Appointment off to a Good Start**
   - Review the chart before going to greet the patient.
   - Have an open, friendly expression; smile.
   - Greet an adult patient by last name and title (Mr., Mrs., Ms., Dr., etc.). Greet anyone accompanying the patient in a similar manner. Do not address the patient by his or her first name unless asked to. Ask how to pronounce unfamiliar names.
   - Introduce yourself. Escort the patient to the treatment room.
   - Use touch sparingly. Many people are not comfortable with strangers hugging, patting, or touching them.

2. **Monitor Your Body Language**
   - Sit facing the patient at eye level. Make eye contact; look directly at the patient. An exception to this suggestion occurs when the patient's culture may view direct eye contact as inappropriate. Koreans, Filipinos, certain Asian cultures, and Native Americans may find direct eye contact offensive.[5] Be guided by the patient's behavior; if he or she avoids eye contact, do likewise.
   - Maintain an appropriate distance from the patient.
   - Be aware of your own nonverbal behaviors. For example, glancing at your watch might convey that you are rushed. Use reassuring gestures, such as nodding your head, to encourage the patient to keep talking.
   - Be alert for nonverbal clues that indicate that the patient is uncomfortable or anxious. Some of these are fidgeting, rapid breathing, shakiness of hands, eyes wandering around the treatment room, or actual wringing of hands.

---

**BOX 1-7  Collaborating with Patients**

- Acknowledge that for care to be effective, the patient and the clinician must work together.
- Treat every patient as though he or she is the only expert on the problem—you are only a collaborator in producing solutions and/or providing advice regarding the problem.
- Interact with the patient as a peer; avoid a condescending approach.
- Inform the patient fully about treatment options and outcomes.
- Elicit the patient's opinion of the proposed treatment.
- Try to understand the patient's perspective.
- Avoid being defensive; state information clearly without a confrontational tone.
- Understand and respect patients' values, beliefs, and expectations.

## LISTENING SKILLS

The most effective dental health care providers are those who have developed good listening skills. When gathering information from the patient, not only is it important to know the right questions to ask but it is equally valuable to listen carefully to the patient's answers. The patient is the only person who knows the events of his or her life—such as medical conditions—and his or her expectations for dental care. Listed below are suggestions for becoming a better listener.

1. **General Tips for Attentive Listening**
   - Pay attention to what is being said; do not worry about what you are going to say next. Avoid interrupting the patient. Focus on the patient, who is telling you something that is important to him or her.
   - Use facial expressions and body language to confirm that you are listening to what the patient is saying. Make eye contact, lean forward, and nod your head at key points.
   - Be alert for language barriers. For example, does the patient speak and understand English? Can the patient hear you?
   - Respect each patient as an individual, taking care not to jump to assumptions about the patient.

2. **Reflective Listening**
   Reflection—or repeating something the patient has just said—can help the clinician to obtain more specific information. Reflection is a way of indicating that you are listening.
   - Repeat a key point of the patient's statement.
     **Patient:** *I get a sharp pain in this tooth.*
     **Clinician:** *The pain is sharp.*
     **Patient:** *Yes, I frequently feel a very sharp pain when chewing something hard.*
   - Offer confirmation that you hear what is being said. An "um-hmm," "go on," or "I see" may be all that is required.

3. **Empathic Listening**
   Be aware that patients are often anxious or concerned. Respond to patient concerns with genuine sympathy and support.
   - Reflect on what you think the patient is feeling.
     *You seem concerned.*
     *Most patients are anxious before having a root canal.*
     *Flossing is frustrating for you.*
   - Restate a question or summarize a statement.
     *You don't think that these x-rays are needed.*
   - Encourage the patient to talk about concerns rather than dismissing them.
     *Are you concerned that x-rays are not safe?*

4. **Clarify and Confirm Information**
   Clarify patient responses to questions. Restate what you heard using your own words and ask if your interpretation is correct. Use confirmation to ensure that both the clinician and the patient are on the same track and to clear up misconceptions.
   - Summarize what you heard the patient say.
     **Clinician:** *If I understand you correctly, you said . . .*
   - Clarify information. Ask a question, if you want to clarify the patient's statement.
     **Patient:** *This is too much for me to handle.*
     **Clinician:** *What is it that you cannot handle?* (Clinician gives the patient an opportunity to explain the statement.)
   - Rephrase the statement to clarify what the patient is saying.
     **Patient:** *I am worried that this is very serious.*
     **Clinician:** *So, are you worried that you might lose that molar tooth?*

## QUESTIONING SKILLS

Questioning skills are particularly important during the health history portion of the assessment process to gather complete and accurate information from the patient. Tips for effective questioning are summarized in Box 1-8.

---

**BOX 1-8** Tips for Effective Questioning

1. **General Tips for Gathering Information**
   - Use language that is understandable to the patient. Avoid medical/dental terminology if the patient does not have a medical or dental background. Most people have difficulty understanding the words used in health care. For example, rather than asking if the patient has ever experienced vertigo, ask if he or she felt dizzy.
   - Ask one question at a time. Keep questions brief and simple and give the patient plenty of time to answer.
   - Avoid leading questions. Avoid putting words in the patient's mouth.
   - Avoid interrupting the patient. If you need to ask a follow-up question, wait until the patient has completed his or her thought. Let the patient do the talking.
   - All questions should be asked in a positive way. Avoid accusing language in your questions (e.g., Why don't you floss every day?).

2. **Use of Closed Questions**
   Closed questions can be answered with a yes or no or a one- or two-word response and do not provide an opportunity for the patient to elaborate. Closed questions limit the development of rapport between the clinician and the patient. Use closed questions primarily to obtain facts and zero in on specific information. Examples of closed questions include:
   - *Are you allergic to latex?*
   - *How frequent are your seizures?*
   - *Did you check your blood sugar levels this morning?*

3. **Use of Open-Ended Questions**
   Open-ended questions require more than a one-word response and allow the patient to express ideas, feelings, and opinions. This type of questioning helps the clinician gather more information than can be obtained with closed questions. Open-ended questions facilitate good clinician–patient rapport because they show that the clinician is interested in what the patient has to say. Examples of such questions include:
   - *What happens to you if you are exposed to latex?*
   - *What things can trigger your seizures?*
   - *What were your blood sugar levels this morning?*

4. **Exploring Details with Open-Ended Questions**
   Focused, open-ended questions define a content area for the response but pose the question in a manner that cannot be answered in a simple word.
   - *Please describe the pain that you are feeling.*
   - *Please start from the beginning and tell me how this began and how it has progressed.*
   - *Do cold temperatures like an ice-cold drink cause the pain?*
   - *Which of your family members have diabetes?*

## COMMUNICATION TASKS DURING PATIENT ASSESSMENT

When performing assessment procedures, the dental health care provider should remember to communicate with the patient. It is easy for the clinician to concentrate so completely on the steps involved in a procedure that he or she forgets to explain the procedure to the patient or to keep the patient involved in what is happening.

Communication tasks during the patient assessment process include giving information to the patient, explaining a procedure to the patient, seeking the patient's cooperation, providing encouragement to the patient, reassuring the patient, and giving feedback to the patient. Box 1-9 shows a sample dialogue for communication during blood pressure assessment.

1. **Giving Information**

   Example: *We do this to make sure that your temperature, pulse, respiration, and blood pressure are OK before starting any treatment.* Other ways of phrasing this include:
   - *This is. . .*
   - *I need to. . .*
   - *This is important because. . .*

2. **Explaining a Procedure**

   Example: *I am going to wrap this cuff around your arm and pump some air into it so that I can read your blood pressure.* Other ways of phrasing this include:
   - *I just want to. . .*
   - *Now I would like to. . .*
   - *Now I am going to. . .*

3. **Seeking Cooperation from the Patient**

   Example: *Could you roll up your sleeve?* Other ways of phrasing this include:
   - *I would like you to. . .*
   - *If you would just. . .*
   - *Would you please. . .?*

4. **Offering Encouragement**

   Example: *Yes, that is fine.* Other ways of phrasing this include:
   - *That's good.*
   - *Well done.*

5. **Offering Reassurance**

   Example: *Do not worry; you will only feel the pressure of the cuff around your arm.* Other ways of phrasing this include:
   - *It won't take long.*
   - *This might feel a bit strange at first.*
   - *You've had this done before, haven't you?*

6. **Giving Feedback**

   Example: *Your readings are quite normal.* Other ways of phrasing this include:
   - *Everything is OK.*
   - *Your blood pressure is a bit high, so I'll let Dr. King know what your readings are.*

BOX **1-9** Sample Dialogue: Communication Tasks during Blood Pressure Assessment

**Clinician:** *Now, Mrs. Tanner, I need to take your blood pressure. We do this to make sure that your blood pressure readings are normal before beginning any dental treatment.* [Giving information to the patient]

**Patient:** *Oh . . . I see. I have been taking blood pressure pills; my doctor says that it is important to keep my blood pressure under control.*

**Clinician:** *I am going to wrap this cuff around your arm and pump some air into it so that I can read your blood pressure.* [Explaining the procedure to the patient] *Could you please roll up your sleeve a bit?* [Seeking cooperation from the patient]

**Patient:** *Yes.* (Rolls up sleeve.) *Is this far enough?*

**Clinician:** *Yes, that's just fine.* (Attaches the cuff and begins inflating the cuff.) [Giving feedback]

**Patient:** *It feels a bit funny.*

**Clinician:** *Yes, it does feel funny, but don't worry. I am almost done pumping up the cuff. Then, I will start releasing the air and you will feel less pressure against your arm.* [Offering reassurance to the patient]

**Patient:** *Is my blood pressure OK?*

**Clinician:** *Yes. It is quite normal. Your readings today are 110 over 70.* [Giving feedback to the patient]

## THE RIGHT WORDS

Empathy—identifying with the feelings or thoughts of another person—is an essential factor in communicating with patients. Communication between the dental health care provider and the patient is more complicated than a normal conversation. For many patients, being in a dental office is a high-stress situation. Pain, worry, and waiting can make a patient anxious or irritable. Many problems can be prevented by keeping patients informed about waiting times, billing or insurance charges, and other office policies that might trigger angry emotions. Diplomacy is the art of treating people with tact and genuine concern. Courtesy is based on sensitivity to the needs and feelings of others. As a health care professional, it is important to be aware of what you say and how you say it. Patient complaints about dental care often revolve around a seemingly innocent comment made by a dental team member. The wrong words can affect a patient's perceptions of the care that he or she receives. Table 1-2 presents some common situations encountered in a dental office and analyzes both effective and ineffective responses.

## Table 1-2 FINDING THE RIGHT WORDS

| Ineffective Response | Analysis | Effective Response | Analysis |
|---|---|---|---|
| **Situation A.** Mrs. Reman is a new patient. The health history form that she filled out in the reception area has many questions left blank and many things are crossed out. | | | |
| *Well, I can see that you had trouble filling this out. Here, why don't you start over with a new form?* | Dismisses the patient's efforts to fill out the form; she may not understand all the questions and may need help | *I know how difficult these forms are to fill out. Let's go over it together.* | Acknowledges the effort made by the patient and that the information is difficult to understand; provides assistance |
| **Situation B.** You notice Mr. Jones sitting alone in a treatment room. Two days ago, Mr. Jones learned that he has oral cancer. You can tell that he is very upset. | | | |
| *Cheer up! I am sure that everything will be OK after you see the oral surgeon.* | Insensitivity to the patient's feelings; provides false reassurance, you have no way of knowing the outcome of surgery | *I can't even begin to imagine how difficult this must be for you. Please let me know if there is anything that I can do to help.* | Demonstrates caring |
| **Situation C.** The woman approaching the reception desk is holding her cheek. She says that she is in a lot of pain and would like to see the dentist. | | | |
| *You don't have an appointment and there are three patients ahead of you. You will have to wait your turn.* | Ignores the patient's pain; punishes her for not making an appointment before she was in pain | *I can see you are in pain. Please sit down for a moment and I will get a treatment room ready for you.* | Recognizes that a patient in pain should have priority over routine dental care |
| **Situation D.** Mr. Daniels has not visited a dental office for many years. It is obvious that he is very nervous. | | | |
| *Just relax.* | This may seem like a good response, but actually it does nothing to put the patient at ease | *Tell me what is worrying you.* | Acknowledges the patient's concerns; elicits specific information about what is worrying the patient |

## SECTION 3:
# Ready References

**READY REFERENCE 1-1**   **INTERNET RESOURCES: HEALTH LITERACY**

**http://www.ama-assn.org/ama/pub/about-ama/ama-foundation/our-programs/**
**public-health/health-literacy-program/health-literacy-kit.page**
Information about the health literacy program of the American Medical Association.
Materials include a downloadable in-depth manual for health care providers.

## REFERENCES

1. Mehrabian A. *Nonverbal Communication*. Chicago, IL: Aldine-Atherton; 1972.
2. Remland MS, Jones TS, Brinkman H. Interpersonal distance, body orientation, and touch: effects of culture, gender, and age. *J Soc Psychol*. 1995;135(3):281–297.
3. Heslin R, Patterson ML. *Nonverbal Behavior and Social Psychology*. New York, NY: Plenum Press; 1982.
4. Mutha S, Allen C, Welch M. *Toward Culturally Competent Care: A Toolbox for Teaching Communication Strategies*. San Francisco, CA: Center for the Health Professions, University of California; 2002.
5. Desmond J, Copeland LR. *Communicating with Today's Patient: Essentials to Save Time, Decrease Risk, and Increase Patient Compliance*. San Francisco, CA: Jossey-Bass; 2000.

## SUGGESTED READINGS

Adubato S. Nonverbal communication. What message are you sending? *N Engl J Med*. 2004;101:40–41.

Allekian C. Intrusions of territory and personal space: an exploratory study of anxiety-inducing factors in hospitalized patients. *Int J Psychiatry Med*. 1974;5:27–39.

Ambady N, Koo J, Rosenthal R, et al. Physical therapists' nonverbal communication predicts geriatric patients' health outcomes. *Psychol Aging*. 2002;17:443–452.

Griffith CH III, Wilson JF, Langer S, et al. House staff nonverbal communication skills and standardized patient satisfaction. *J Gen Intern Med*. 2003;18:170–174.

Ihler E. MSJAMA. Patient-physician communication. *JAMA*. 2003;289:92.

Irving P, Dickson D. Empathy: towards a conceptual framework for health professionals. *Int J Health Care Qual Assur Inc Leadersh Health Serv*. 2004;17:212–220.

Mason L. Body language—nonverbal cues. *Br J Perioper Nurs*. 2000;10:512–518.

McCord RS, Floyd MR, Lang F, et al. Responding effectively to patient anger directed at the physician. *Fam Med*. 2002;34:331–336.

Miller G. Patient-centric discourse. *Hosp Health Netw*. 2004;78:8.

Nussbaum JF, Coupland J. *Handbook of Communication and Aging Research*. Mahwah, NJ: Lawrence Erlbaum Associates; 2004.

Roter D, Hall JA. *Doctors Talking with Patients/Patients Talking with Doctors: Improving Communication in Medical Visits*. Westport, CT: Auburn House; 1992.

Shannon C. As the patient voice grows louder, it is time to see who's listening. *Health Serv J*. 2004;114:121–123.

SECTION 4:

# The Human Element

Patient assessment procedures provide critical information for planning dental hygiene care. These complex procedures require practice and experience to master and methodical attention to detail to perform.

- Most textbook space, as well as classroom and laboratory time, is devoted to the technical aspects—the steps—that make up the patient assessment procedures.
- Yet, the nonprocedural human element of the assessment process is equally critical to the success of the assessment process.
- The Human Element section of each module of this book will reflect the struggles, fears, and triumphs of the students, clinicians, and patients who engage in the assessment process (Box 1-10).

---

BOX **1-10** Through the Eyes of a Patient

*I know that, as a student, you come into clinic today thinking about what you will accomplish during this appointment. Perhaps you wonder if you will remember to do all of the steps and if you will do them correctly. I am sure that you are worried about your clinic requirements and the instructor's comments about your performance today.*

*As the patient, I, too, come to this appointment with some needs and concerns. I am not simply a 60 year-old woman with bleeding gums who only has 20 teeth in her mouth. I wish that you would take a moment to consider what is important to me. Most of my needs are simple things that you can do each time that I have an appointment:*

- Do not keep me waiting.
- Ask me what I think.
- Really listen to me.
- Do not dismiss or ignore my concerns.
- Talk to me, not at me.
- Keep me informed about what you are doing.
- Do not treat me like a clinical requirement; treat me like a person.
- Do not tell me what I need to do without telling me why it is important and how to do it.
- Respect my privacy; do not talk about me to your classmates.
- Remember who I used to be. I was not always a 60 year-old woman; I used to be a young, enthusiastic research chemist.
- Let me know that you care about me.

*Mrs. G, dental patient,*
*South Florida Community College*

Used with permission and excerpted from a letter to the students of the Dental Hygiene Program, South Florida Community College.

## SECTION 5:
# Skill Check

**SKILL CHECKLIST:** COMMUNICATIONS ROLE-PLAY

Student: _____   Evaluator: _____

Date: _____

---

**Roles:**
- Student 1 = Plays the role of the patient.
- Student 2 = Plays the role of the clinician.

---

**DIRECTIONS FOR STUDENT CLINICIAN:** Use **Column S** to record your evaluation of your skill level as **S** (satisfactory) or **U** (unsatisfactory).

**DIRECTIONS FOR EVALUATOR:** Use **Column E** to record your evaluation of the student clinician's communication skills during the role-play. Indicate **S** (satisfactory) or **U** (unsatisfactory). In the optional grade percentage calculation, each **S** equals 1 point and each **U** equals 0 points.

| CRITERIA | S | E |
|---|---|---|
| **Uses appropriate nonverbal behavior such as maintaining eye contact, sitting at the same level as the patient, nodding head when listening to patient, etc.** | | |
| **Interacts with the patient as a peer and avoids a condescending approach. Collaborates with the patient and provides advice.** | | |
| **Communicates using common, everyday words. Avoids dental terminology.** | | |
| **Listens attentively to the patient's comments. Respects the patient's point of view.** | | |
| **Listens attentively to the patient's questions. Encourages patient questions. Clarifies for understanding when necessary.** | | |
| **Answers the patient's questions fully and accurately.** | | |
| **Checks for understanding by the patient. Clarifies information.** | | |

OPTIONAL GRADE PERCENTAGE CALCULATION

Each **S** equals 1 point, and each **U** equals 0 points. Using the **E** column, the sum of the "**S**"s _____ divided by the total points possible (7) equals the percentage grade _____.

**Note to Course Instructor:**
A series of role-play scenarios for this textbook can be found at http://thepoint.lww.com

the**Point**

**Note to the Course Instructor About the Skill Check Pages**
The Skill Check pages in the book are designed so that the forms can be removed from the book without loss of text content. They can be torn out and used for role-plays and exercises. If desired, they can be collected and retained for course grade determination.

# NOTES

# 2 Making Our Words Understandable

## MODULE OVERVIEW

Clear communication provides the foundation for the patient assessment procedures; yet, many people—even highly educated people—have trouble understanding words used in health care. In addition, health care terminology is filled with jargon—much of which can be difficult for patients to understand. This module explores strategies that dental health care providers can employ to help patients understand dental health information and advice.

## MODULE OUTLINE

## OBJECTIVES

- Discuss how effective communication improves health outcomes.
- Discuss strategies for making health care words understandable to the patient.
- Demonstrate the ability to gather relevant information for improving communication skills from the Internet.

## SECTION 1:
# Roadblocks to Effective Communication

### MEDICAL AND DENTAL TERMINOLOGY

1. **Unfamiliar Words**
   a. **Health literacy** in dentistry is "the degree to which individuals have the capacity to obtain, process, and understand basic health information and services needed to make appropriate oral health decisions."[1–3]
   b. Limited health literacy is a potential barrier to the diagnosis, treatment, and prevention of oral disease.[2] Clear, accurate, and effective communication is an essential skill for effective dental practice.
   c. The American Dental Association (ADA) developed a strategic action plan to provide guidance to dental professionals, policy makers, and others to improve health literacy. The plan, *Health Literacy in Dentistry Action Plan 2010–2015*, may be downloaded from the ADA's website in PDF format.
2. **Words in a New Context**
   a. Because health information can be complex and scientific, people often have difficulty reading and understanding written materials such as informational brochures about dental problems and treatments, medical history forms, consent forms, and directions on medication labels.
   b. In many cases, a word may be familiar, but the person may not understand it in a health care context.
      1. For example, "*you have a 6-mm pocket around this molar tooth*" might have no meaning to a patient. The patient might know what the words "deep" and "pocket" mean in everyday speech but have no idea what these words mean in terms of dental health.
      2. Even a patient who understands these dental terms may need more information than this sentence provides. He or she may need to know what constitutes normal bone support for the teeth.
   c. Box 2-1 provides suggestions for ways in which dental health care providers can improve communication with patients.
3. **Embarrassment.** Many patients, because they are embarrassed or intimidated, do not ask health care providers to explain difficult or complicated information. If patients do not understand treatment or self-care instructions, a crucial part of their dental care is missing, which may have an adverse effect on their dental health.

---

BOX **2-1**   **Best Practices for Promotion of Clear, Accurate Communication[1]**

- Create an environment that is respectful and "shame-free," where patients are offered assistance to better understand and use printed and written communications[9–11]
- Use clear and plain language in talking, writing, and printed education materials[12–19]
- Encourage question asking by patients and dialogue between clinicians and patients[20–24]
- Check for successful communication by asking patients to explain their interpretation of instructions and other information that has been provided[25–30]
- Offer patient education materials designed for easy use with clear directions[31–37]
- Periodically assess office/clinic for ways to improve communication[38,39]

## READING ABILITY

Reading ability can present another roadblock to effective communication.

1. **Reading Ability Correlates to Health Status.** According to a report published in the *Journal of the American Medical Association*, the ability to read is a stronger indication of health status than other variables, including race, age, ethnic group, and educational level.[4,5]

2. **Reading at Eighth to Ninth Grade Level.**

   a. One out of five American adults reads at the fifth grade level or below (Fig. 2-1).

   b. The average American reads at the eighth to ninth grade level, yet most health care materials are written about the 10th grade level.[6]

   c. Nearly nine out of ten U.S. adults have difficulty understanding and using everyday health information that is generally available in health care facilities.[7]

   d. Individuals with low health literacy are less likely to seek health care, comply with recommended treatment, and maintain self-care regimens.[1]

3. **Stigma of Illiteracy.** Patients often are embarrassed or ashamed to admit they have trouble understanding health information and instruction.

   a. There is a strong stigma attached to reading problems, and nearly all nonreaders or poor readers try to conceal the fact that they have trouble reading.[8]

   b. Many people with poor reading skills have developed coping skills that allow them to maneuver in the health care system with the least amount of embarrassment.

   c. Box 2-2 lists some clues that might indicate that the patient may need additional help with written material.

---

**BOX 2-2    Clues that a Patient May Have Reading Problems**

- Registration, health history, or other forms filled out incompletely or incorrectly
- Written materials handed to a relative or other person accompanying the patient
- *"Can you help me fill out this form, I forgot my glasses?"*
- *"I will take this with me and read it at home."*
- *"I can't read this now; I forgot my glasses."*

---

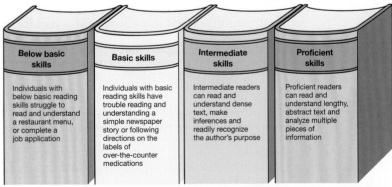

**Figure 2-1.  Reading ability.** The ability to read is a strong indication of an individual's health status. Many individuals have below basic or basic reading skills that make it difficult to read and understand most health care materials.

## SECTION 2:
# Making Health Care Words Understandable

## WORDS THAT MAY CONFUSE DENTAL PATIENTS

Many people, even highly literate people, have trouble understanding words used in health care. In some instances, a word may be totally unfamiliar. In other cases, a word may be familiar, but the person may not understand it in a health care context.

- Words with a Latin or Greek prefix present special problems. The health science field is full of such words. Here is a small sampling: pre-op, post-op, prenatal, premature, unsweetened, decontaminate, antibacterial. For example, the risk factor for poor readers with diabetes is that they may recognize one part of the word, such as the sweetened in unsweetened, and then skip the "un." This kind of guessing can lead to the opposite behavior.
- *The National Patient Safety Foundation believes that four kinds of words cause much of the misunderstanding:*
  - *Medical words*
  - *Concept words*
  - *Category words*
  - *Value judgment words*
- Tables 2-1 to 2-4 provide examples of common words and phrases that may be confusing to patients and suggestions for common words and phrases that can make health care information more understandable. Table 2-5 provides examples of dental terminology that could be confusing to patients.

### Table 2-1  "MEDICAL" WORDS TO WATCH[a]

| Problem Word | Consider Using |
| --- | --- |
| Ailment | Sickness; illness; problem with your health |
| Benign | Will not cause harm; is not cancer |
| Condition | How you feel; health problem |
| Dysfunction | Problem |
| Inhibitor | Treatment that stops something that is bad for you |
| Intermittent | Off and on, such as pain that comes and goes |
| Lesion | Wound; sore; infected patch of skin |
| Oral | By mouth |
| Procedure | Something done to treat your problem |
| Vertigo | Dizziness |

[a]Used with permission from the National Patient Safety Foundation.

**Table 2-2** "CONCEPT" WORDS TO WATCH[a]

| Problem Word | Consider Using |
| --- | --- |
| Active role | Taking part in |
| Avoid | Stay away from; do not use (or eat) |
| Collaborate | Work together |
| Factor | Other thing; thing involved in |
| Gauge | Measure; get a better idea of; test (dependent on the context) |
| Intake | What you eat or drink; what goes in your body |
| Option | Choice |
| Referral | Ask you to see another doctor; get a second opinion |
| Wellness | Good health; feeling good |

[a]Used with permission from the National Patient Safety Foundation.

**Table 2-3** "CATEGORY" WORDS TO WATCH[a]

| Problem Word | Consider Using |
| --- | --- |
| Activity | Something you do; something you do often, like snacking on candy |
| Adverse (reaction) | Bad |
| Cognitive | Learning; thinking |
| Hazardous | Not safe; dangerous |
| Generic | Product sold without a brand name, like ibuprofen (Advil is the brand name) |
| Noncancerous | Not cancer |
| Prosthesis | Replacement for a body part, such as a partial denture |
| Support | Help with your needs |

[a]Used with permission from the National Patient Safety Foundation.

## Table 2-4  "VALUE JUDGMENT" WORDS TO WATCH[a]

| Problem Word | Consider Using |
| --- | --- |
| Adequate | Enough (*Example: adequate water, 6–8 glasses a day*) |
| Adjust | Fine-tune; change |
| Cautiously | With care; slowly |
| Excessive | Too much (*Example: if blood soaks through the gauze later tonight*) |
| Increase gradually | Add to (*Example: increase the power level on the water irrigation device slightly over the next several weeks until it is on medium*) |
| Progressive | Gets worse (or better) |
| Routinely | Often (*Example: floss every day*) |
| Significantly | Enough to make a difference (*Example: quitting smoking greatly reduces your risk of lung cancer*) |
| Temporary | For a limited time (*Example: use the mouth rinse for 1 week*) |

[a]Used with permission from the National Patient Safety Foundation.

**Table 2-5** DENTAL TERMINOLOGY AND PHRASES TO WATCH

| Problem Word | Consider Using |
|---|---|
| Alveolar bone | Bone around the teeth; bone that supports the teeth in the mouth |
| Bleeding on probing | Bleeding from the gum tissue |
| Biofilm | Layer of bacteria attached to the teeth |
| Calculus | Hard deposits; tartar |
| Clean your teeth | Dental hygiene services; dental hygiene therapies |
| Diagnosis | Cause of problem |
| Discomfort | Pain; soreness |
| Edema | Swelling; swollen |
| Generalized | Most areas; widespread |
| Gingiva | Gum tissue; tissue that surrounds the teeth |
| Gingivitis | Gum disease; infection of the gum tissues |
| Health status | How healthy |
| Indicated | Used for |
| Inflammation | Swelling, redness, heat, and pain in an area; reaction to infection or injury |
| Infection | A disease caused by germs |
| Informed | Told in a way that is clear to you |
| Informed consent | Deciding what is the best choice for you, know what you are choosing, have the best information before choosing |
| Interproximal | Between the teeth |
| Localized | Limited to a small area |

*(continued)*

**Table 2-5** DENTAL TERMINOLOGY AND PHRASES TO WATCH *(CONTINUED)*

| Problem Word | Consider Using |
|---|---|
| Medical condition | Illness; disease; health problem |
| Medication | Medicine; drug |
| Motivated | To want to do something |
| Neglect | Lack of care; don't care for |
| Nonprescription (OTC) | Buy without a prescription; buy off the shelf |
| Normal range | Where it should be (*Example: blood pressure*) |
| Occlude | Bite your back teeth together |
| Periodontal disease | Infection of the tissue and bone surrounding the teeth; bone loss |
| Permanent | Lasting forever |
| Periodontal pocket | Space between the tooth root and the gum tissue caused by loss of bone support from around the tooth |
| Procedure | Something done to treat a problem |
| Progressive | Gets worse |
| Risk factor | Will increase your chance of getting |
| Side effect | Something caused by a medicine you take |
| Sulcus | Space normally found between the gum tissue and the tooth |
| Symptoms | Warning signs |
| Treatment plan | Treatment |

## ABBREVIATIONS THAT MAY CONFUSE DENTAL PATIENTS

Many abbreviations are used in medicine and dentistry. Some abbreviations are used so frequently that they can creep into a clinician's discussions with patients. Although the meaning of these abbreviations may be self-evident to the clinician, they may be quite confusing to a patient. Clinicians should be constantly alert to limit the use of medical and dental abbreviations with dental patients because of the high potential for confusion on the part of the patient. Table 2-6 lists abbreviations that frequently arise in a dental setting and provides suggestions for words to use instead when communicating with patients.

**Table 2-6** ABBREVIATIONS THAT MAY CONFUSE DENTAL PATIENTS

| Abbreviation | Meaning of Abbreviation | Words to Use Instead |
| --- | --- | --- |
| ADHD | attention deficit hyperactivity disorder | a behavioral disorder |
| AIDS | acquired immunodeficiency syndrome | infection caused by the human immunodeficiency virus |
| AMI | acute myocardial infarction | heart attack |
| AODM | adult onset diabetes mellitus | type 2 diabetes |
| BP | blood pressure | force of the blood pushing against the walls of the blood vessels |
| CBC | complete blood count | a blood test that measures properties of cells in your blood |
| CHD | congenital heart disease | heart disease you were born with |
| CHF | congestive heart failure | when the heart cannot pump enough blood throughout the body |
| CNS | central nervous system | brain and spinal cord |
| COPD | chronic obstructive lung disease | lung disease that makes it hard to breathe |
| CPR | cardiopulmonary resuscitation | emergency procedure for person who heart or breathing has stopped |
| CVA | cerebrovascular accident | stroke or brain attack |
| DM | diabetes mellitus | diabetes |
| ENT | ear, nose, and throat | physician who specializes in problems of the ear, nose, and throat |
| GERD | gastroesophageal reflux disease | condition in which stomach contents leak back into the throat |
| GI | gastrointestinal | the digestive system |
| HDL | high-density lipoprotein | type of cholesterol known as "good" cholesterol |

*(continued)*

**Table 2-6** ABBREVIATIONS THAT MAY CONFUSE DENTAL PATIENTS *(CONTINUED)*

| Abbreviation | Meaning of Abbreviation | Words to Use Instead |
| --- | --- | --- |
| HIV | *human immunodeficiency virus* | virus that causes AIDS |
| HPV | *human papilloma virus* | virus that can cause cervical cancer |
| IDDM | *insulin-dependent diabetes mellitus* | type 1 diabetes |
| IM | *intramuscular* | injection into a muscle |
| IV | *intravenous* | injection into a vein |
| LDL | *low-density lipoprotein* | type of cholesterol known as "bad" cholesterol |
| MRI | *magnetic resonance imaging* | type of imaging test |
| MRSA | *methicillin-resistant Staphylococcus aureus* | type of infection resistant to some antibiotics |
| NIDDM | *non–insulin-dependent diabetes mellitus* | type 2 diabetes |
| NSAID | *nonsteroidal anti-inflammatory drug* | drug that can help control pain and fever |
| PRN | *as needed* | as needed |
| RA | *rheumatoid arthritis* | type of joint disease |
| RBC | *red blood cell* | type of blood cell |
| SOB | *shortness of breath* | shortness of breath |
| STD | *sexually transmitted disease* | sexually transmitted disease |
| TIA | *transient ischemic attack* | a small stroke |
| TB | *tuberculosis* | an infection of the lungs |
| TMJ | *temporomandibular joint* | joint connecting jaw to skull |
| URI | *upper respiratory infection* | the common cold |
| WBC | *white blood cell* | type of blood cell |

**SECTION 3:**

# Using the Internet to Improve Communication Skills

One effective mechanism for health care providers to improve communications skills is through information gathering on the Internet. Procedure 2-1 provides guidelines for conducting Internet searches.

**PROCEDURE 2-1**  **PROCEDURE FOR SEARCHING THE INTERNET**

**Equipment:** Computer with Web browser software, a modem to connect to the Internet, and an active Internet connection

| Steps | Purpose |
|---|---|
| 1. Connect a computer to the Internet and open an Internet browser. Some of the most popular browsers are Internet Explorer, Safari, and Netscape. | The Internet browser is a software program used for searching and viewing various kinds of Internet resources such as information on a website. |
| 2. Locate a search engine. Most browsers have a built-in search engine. Popular search engines include Google, Lycos, AltaVista, Yahoo, and Excite. | The Internet has millions of pages of information. Search engines help you sift through all those pages to find the information that you need. |
| 3. Look at the search engine's Web page. Near the top of the page you will see a white box with the word SEARCH next to it. Click the search box and type a word or phrase that describes what you are looking for. Next, press the GO button next to the search box or hit the Return key on your keyboard. | The words that you type in the search box are called "keywords." Keywords tell the search engine what to look for. For best results, it is important to choose the keywords carefully. Use one to three words that are as specific as possible. |
| 4. View the results of your search. If you did not find what you are looking for, check spelling and retype or choose new keywords and try the search again. | If the keywords are misspelled or not specific enough, the search engine will not find the information that you need. |
| 5. From the search results page, select an appropriate site and double-click the address written in blue to open the website. | This allows you to view the information on the website. |
| 6. If the website information is helpful, either download the information or bookmark the page. If you need additional information, return to the results page or conduct another search. | Downloading the information or bookmarking the website gives you access to it in the future. |
| 7. Try to complete the search process within 10 or 15 minutes. | The ability to effectively search the Internet is a vital information-accessing tool for dental health care providers. |

## SECTION 4:

# Ready References

## USING THE READY REFERENCES SECTION

The Ready References may be removed from the book by tearing along the perforated lines on each page. Laminating or placing these pages in plastic protector sheets will allow them to be disinfected for use in a clinical setting.

### Internet Resources

The Ready References section of each module contains, among other things, Internet resources with websites that have information relevant to the module content. The Internet has a wealth of medical and dental health information; however, to access this information, each dental health care provider needs to be adept at searching the Internet. Ready Reference 2-1 provides some Internet resources related to health literacy. Ready Reference 2-2 points out a tool that can be used for health literacy assessment.

### General Suggestions for Using the Internet

1. Be careful to type the website address exactly as written.
   * Most website addresses will begin with "http://www" but there are some exceptions. Some addresses may not include "www" and others may include "www1" in the address.
   * Some addresses end in "html" and others in "htm." It makes all the difference in the world if you type "http:// www.umn.edu/perio/tobacco/tobhome.html" instead of "http://www1.umn.edu/perio/tobacco/ tobhome.html."
2. *The website addresses listed here were current at the time of publication. Website addresses change frequently, however, because the Internet is such a dynamic resource.*
   * If the listed website address is no longer valid, try using an Internet search engine (such as Google, Lycos, or Ask.com) to locate the new website for the organization.
   * Simply type the organization's name (such as "American Medical Association") or the name of the resource (such as "National Assessment of Adult Literacy" into the search box and click on "search." The search engine will find the new website address for you.

## READY REFERENCE 2-1    INTERNET RESOURCES: HEALTH LITERACY

**www.ada.org/sections/.../pdfs/topics_access_health_literacy_dentistry.pdf**
The **American Dental Association's** Health Literacy in Dentistry Strategic Action Plan 2010–2015 may be downloaded as a PDF document at this link.

**http://nces.ed.gov/naal**
The 2003 **National Assessment of Adult Literacy** is a nationally representative assessment of English literacy among American adults age 16 and older. Sponsored by the National Center for Education Statistics (NCES), NAAL is the nation's most comprehensive measure of adult literacy since the 1992 National Adult Literacy Survey (NALS).

*(continued)*

**READY REFERENCE 2-1** INTERNET RESOURCES: HEALTH LITERACY, *CONTINUED*

---

**http://www.health.gov/communication**
The **Department of Health and Human Services' (DHHS)** website on health communication, health literacy, and e-Health.

**http://www.npsf.org/pchc/index2.php**
**The Partnership for Clear Health Communication** is a coalition of national organizations that are working together to promote awareness and solutions around the issue of low health literacy and its effect on health outcomes.

**http://www.plainlanguage.gov/**
Plain language action and information network

**http://www.npsf.org/askme3**
The Partnership for Clear Health Communication has partnered with the **National Patient Safety Foundation** to promote health literacy. This link has information about the Ask Me 3 initiative.

**http://www.hsph.harvard.edu/healthliteracy**
The **Harvard School of Public Health, Health Literacy Studies** website is designed for professionals in health and education who are interested in health literacy. It contains many useful materials.

**http://www.ahrq.gov/questionsaretheanswer/**
**U.S. Department of Health & Human Services: Agency for Healthcare Research and Quality**. A site to help patients get more involved in their own health care.

**http://www.pfizerhealthliteracy.com/physicians-providers/Default.aspx**
The **Pfizer Clear Health Communication Initiative** is a compendium that highlights Pfizer's solutions and tools to address low health literacy.

**http://www.ama-assn.org/go/healthdisparities**
**American Medical Association Health Disparities** website includes information on AMA policy related to health disparities, resource links, and information on partnerships and activities that are part of the national effort to eliminate health disparities.

**http://minorityhealth.hhs.gov**
**The Office of Minority Health Resource Center** was established by the U.S. Department of Health and Human Services Office of Minority Health in 1987. OMH-RC serves as a national resource and referral service on minority health issues.

## READY REFERENCE 2-2  TOOL FOR HEALTH LITERACY ASSESSMENT

A free health literacy assessment tool is available at http://www.pfizerhealthliteracy.com/physicians-providers/NewestVitalSign.aspx

- The assessment tool—named the Newest Vital Sign (NVS)—is designed to quickly and effectively assess patients' health literacy skills.

- The NVS is a simple six-question assessment based on an ice cream nutrition label.

- It can be administered in about 3 minutes, and it will be available in both English and Spanish.

- The patient is given the label and asked a series of questions about it. Based on the number of correct answers given, health care providers can assess the patient's health literacy level and adjust their communication to ensure understanding.

- The assessment tool was tested with more than 1,000 patients.

## REFERENCES

1. ADA Council on Access P, and Interprofessional Relations. *Health Literacy in Dentistry Action Plan 2010–2015*. Chicago, IL: American Dental Association; 2009.
2. Association AD. *Transactions*. Chicago, IL: ADA; 2006.
3. U.S. Department of Health and Human Services. *Healthy People 2010*. 2nd ed. Washington, DC: U.S. Department of Health and Human Services: For sale by the U.S. G.P.O., Supt. of Docs.; 2000.
4. Ad Hoc Committee on Health Literacy for the Council on Scientific Affairs, American Medical Association. Health literacy: report of the Council on Scientific Affairs. *JAMA*. 1999;281(6):552–557.
5. Nielsen-Bohlman L, Panzer AM, Kindig DA; Institute of Medicine (U.S.), Committee on Health Literacy. *Health Literacy: A Prescription to End Confusion*. Washington, DC: National Academies Press; 2004.
6. Kirsch IS, U.S. Department of Education, Office of Educational Research and Improvement; Educational Testing Service, National Center for Education Statistics. *Adult Literacy in America: A First Look at the Results of the National Adult Literacy Survey*. 2nd ed. Washington, DC: Office of Educational Research and Improvement, U.S. Department of Education; 1993.
7. Kutner MA, National Center for Education Statistics. *The Health Literacy of America's Adults Results from the 2003 National Assessment of Adult Literacy*. Washington, DC: U.S. Department of Education, National Center for Education Statistics; 2006. http://purl.access.gpo.gov/GPO/LPS74550.
8. Center for Health Care Strategies I. *Strategies to improve patient education materials*. www.chcs.org/usr_doc/Health_Literacy_Fact_Sheets.pdf. Accessed
9. American Medical Association Foundation. *Health Literacy and Patient Safety: Help Patients Understand*. Chicago, IL: American Medical Association Foundation; 2009.
10. Howard DH, Gazmararian J, Parker RM. The impact of low health literacy on the medical costs of Medicare managed care enrollees. *Am J Med*. 2005;118(4):371–377.
11. Parikh NS, Parker RM, Nurss JR, et al. Shame and health literacy: the unspoken connection. *Patient Educ Couns*. 1996;27(1):33–39.
12. Plain Language Action and Information Network. http://www.plainlanguage.gov. Accessed July 18, 2011.
13. Baevsky R. Speaking in plain language. *Ann Emerg Med*. 2008;51(4):450–451.

14. Doak CC, Doak LG, Root JH. *Teaching Patients with Low Literacy Skills*. 2nd ed. Philadelphia, PA: J. B. Lippincott Company; 2007.
15. Friedman DB, Hoffman-Goetz L. An exploratory study of older adults' comprehension of printed cancer information: is readability a key factor? *J Health Commun*. 2007;12(5):423–437.
16. Jefford M, Moore R. Improvement of informed consent and the quality of consent documents. *Lancet Oncol*. 2008;9(5):485–493.
17. Ridpath JR, Wiese CJ, Greene SM. Looking at research consent forms through a participant-centered lens: the PRISM readability toolkit. *Am J Health Promot*. 2009;23(6):371–375.
18. Safeer RS, Keenan J. Health literacy: the gap between physicians and patients. *Am Fam Physician*. 2005;72(3):463–468.
19. Stableford S, Mettger W. Plain language: a strategic response to the health literacy challenge. *J Public Health Policy*. 2007;28(1):71–93.
20. Agency for Healthcare Research and Quality. *Questions are the answer*. http://www.ahrq.gov/questionsaretheanswer. Accessed July 18, 2011.
21. Mika VS, Wood PR, Weiss BD, et al. Ask Me 3: improving communication in a Hispanic pediatric outpatient practice. *Am J Health Behav*. 2007;31 Suppl 1:S115–S121.
22. Norlin C, Sharp AL, Firth SD. Unanswered questions prompted during pediatric primary care visits. *Ambul Pediatr*. 2007;7(5):396–400.
23. Roter DL, Hall JA. Communication and adherence: moving from prediction to understanding. *Med Care*. 2009;47(8):823–825.
24. Sleath B, Roter D, Chewning B, et al. Asking questions about medication: analysis of physician-patient interactions and physician perceptions. *Med Care*. 1999;37(11):1169–1173.
25. Baker DW. The meaning and the measure of health literacy. *J Gen Intern Med*. 2006;21(8):878–883.
26. Marcus EN. The silent epidemic—the health effects of illiteracy. *N Engl J Med*. 2006;355(4):339–341.
27. Parker RM, Ratzan SC, Lurie N. Health literacy: a policy challenge for advancing high-quality health care. *Health Aff (Millwood)*. 2003;22(4):147–153.
28. Rothman RL, DeWalt DA, Malone R, et al. Influence of patient literacy on the effectiveness of a primary care-based diabetes disease management program. *JAMA*. 2004;292(14):1711–1716.
29. Schillinger D, Piette J, Grumbach K, et al. Closing the loop: physician communication with diabetic patients who have low health literacy. *Arch Intern Med*. 2003;163(1):83–90.
30. Youmans SL, Schillinger D. Functional health literacy and medication use: the pharmacist's role. *Ann Pharmacother*. 2003;37(11):1726–1729.

31. Jacobson TA, Thomas DM, Morton FJ, et al. Use of a low-literacy patient education tool to enhance pneumococcal vaccination rates. A randomized controlled trial. *JAMA.* 1999;282(7):646–650.

32. Korhonen T, Huttunen JK, Aro A, et al. A controlled trial on the effects of patient education in the treatment of insulin-dependent diabetes. *Diabetes Care.* 1983;6(3):256–261.

33. Kreuter MW, Strecher VJ, Glassman B. One size does not fit all: the case for tailoring print materials. *Ann Behav Med.* 1999;21(4):276–283.

34. McGuckin M, Taylor A, Martin V, et al. Evaluation of a patient education model for increasing hand hygiene compliance in an inpatient rehabilitation unit. *Am J Infect Control.* 2004;32(4):235–238.

35. McGuckin M, Waterman R, Porten L, et al. Patient education model for increasing handwashing compliance. *Am J Infect Control.* 1999;27(4):309–314.

36. Meade CD, McKinney WP, Barnas GP. Educating patients with limited literacy skills: the effectiveness of printed and videotaped materials about colon cancer. *Am J Public Health.* 1994;84(1):119–121.

37. Soltner C, Lassalle V, Galienne-Bouygues S, et al. Written information that relatives of adult intensive care unit patients would like to receive—a comparison to published recommendations and opinion of staff members. *Crit Care Med.* 2009;37(7):2197–2202.

38. Detmar SB, Muller MJ, Wever LD, et al. The patient-physician relationship. Patient-physician communication during outpatient palliative treatment visits: an observational study. *JAMA.* 2001;285(10):1351–1357.

39. Fitzpatrick LA, Melnikas AJ, Weathers M, et al. Understanding communication capacity. Communication patterns and ICT usage in clinical settings. *J Healthc Inf Manag.* 2008;22(3):34–41.

**SECTION 5:**

# The Human Element

BOX **2-3**   **Through the Eyes of a Student**

*The first semester of school, I struggled to learn all the dental terminology. I had never worked in a dental office, and I felt that I was falling behind the others in my class. Each day brought new words for me to understand and learn to pronounce—words like armamentarium, line angle, and fossa. The dental terminology was like a whole new language.*

*Then, overnight, I found myself speaking a "new language." I felt so proud of all the new words I had learned. I even told my parents that one of the actresses on their favorite television show has a diastema.*

*Soon I was in clinic, explaining things to my patients using my dental terminology. I thought that I was giving my patients a lot of very important information. That is, until Mrs. M. was my patient. On our first appointment, I told Mrs. M. all about how I would be scaling her teeth in sextants. I asked her if she understood this treatment plan, and Mrs. M. gave me this big smile. She said, "I am sure that you are a very good dental hygienist, but my goodness, I have not understand one word you said in the past 10 minutes! If you want me to understand what you are saying, you are going to have to talk in everyday English."*

*Well, Mrs. M. was so nice and had that big grin on her face, and we both just started to laugh. So, right then and there, I told Mrs. M. just to interrupt me every single time that I used a word that she did not understand.*

*Now, I never talk to a patient without thinking of Mrs. M. Of all the things that I have learned, I think that she taught me one of the most important things. Now, I talk with patients in everyday words.*

*Kim, student,*
*South Florida Community College*

## SECTION 6:

# Skill Check

**SKILL CHECKLIST:   COMMUNICATIONS ROLE-PLAY**

Student: _____   Evaluator: _____

Date: _____

> **Roles:**
> - Student 1 = Plays the role of the patient.
> - Student 2 = Plays the role of the clinician.

**DIRECTIONS FOR STUDENT CLINICIAN:** Use **Column S** to record your evaluation of your skill level as **S** (satisfactory) or **U** (unsatisfactory).

**DIRECTIONS FOR EVALUATOR:** Use **Column E** to record your evaluation of the student clinician's communication skills during the role-play. Indicate **S** (satisfactory) or **U** (unsatisfactory). In the optional grade percentage calculation, each **S** equals 1 point, and each **U** equals 0 points.

| CRITERIA | S | E |
| --- | --- | --- |
| **Uses appropriate nonverbal behavior such as maintaining eye contact, sitting at the same level as the patient, nodding head when listening to patient, etc.** | | |
| **Interacts with the patient as a peer and avoids a condescending approach. Collaborates with the patient and provides advice.** | | |
| **Communicates using common, everyday words. Avoids dental terminology.** | | |
| **Listens attentively to the patient's comments. Respects the patient's point of view.** | | |
| **Listens attentively to the patient's questions. Encourages patient questions. Clarifies for understanding, when necessary.** | | |
| **Answers the patient's questions fully and accurately.** | | |
| **Checks for understanding by the patient. Clarifies information.** | | |

OPTIONAL GRADE PERCENTAGE CALCULATION

Each **S** equals 1 point, and each **U** equals 0 points. Using the **E** column, total the sum of the "**S**"s _____ divided by the total points possible (7) equals the percentage grade _____.

**Note to Course Instructor:**
A series of role-play scenarios for this textbook can be found at http://thepoint.lww.com

**thePoint**

# NOTES

# Overcoming Communication Barriers

## MODULE OVERVIEW

Being able to communicate effectively—or to participate in the exchange of information—is an essential skill for dental health care providers. For many dental health care providers in the United States today, providing patient-centered care involves learning to communicate effectively with patients even when various barriers to communication are present.

This module presents strategies for effectively communicating with:

- Patients who speak a different language than that of the dental health care provider
- Patients with culturally influenced health behaviors that differ from the health care beliefs of the dental clinician
- Young and school-age children
- Adolescents
- Older adults
- Children with attention deficit hyperactivity disorder (ADHD)
- Vision-, hearing-, or speech-impaired individuals

## MODULE OUTLINE

**OBJECTIVES**

- Describe some of the changes in the population of North America during the last few decades and explain how these changes can affect dental health care.
- Give an example of how cultural differences could affect communication.
- Define cultural competence.
- Discuss effective communication techniques for interacting with patients from different cultures.
- Explore how cultural variables impact the delivery of health care services.
- Discuss strategies that health care providers can use to improve communication with children.
- Discuss strategies that health care providers can use to improve communication with adolescents.
- Discuss strategies that health care providers can use to improve communication with older adults.
- Discuss strategies that health care providers can use to improve communication with children with attention deficit hyperactivity disorder (ADHD).
- Discuss strategies that health care providers can use to improve communication with hearing-, vision-, and speech-impaired patients.

## SECTION 1:
# Language Barriers

## CROSS-CULTURAL COMMUNICATION

### Multiculturalism

1. **Ethnic and Cultural Diversity.** North American communities are becoming increasingly diverse in their ethnic and cultural makeup. This increasingly diverse cultural makeup means that strategies need to be developed to ensure that all segments of the population are receiving the oral health care that they need.[1–5]

   a. Findings from the "Unequal Treatment" report in the United States indicated that health care providers might contribute to ethnic health disparities because of prejudice, stereotyping, and lack of knowledge regarding how to provide care to diverse ethnic populations.[6–8]

   b. In Canada, the report, "Building on Values: The Future of Health Care in Canada" identifies ethnic minorities as populations whose health is at greatest risk.[9]

   c. Factors that contribute to health disparities are ethnicity, socioeconomic status, gender, level of education, and age.[1,5] These same factors contribute to oral health disparities in dental caries rates, periodontal disease, tooth loss, oral cancer, and tobacco use.[1]

2. **Non-English Speaking Communities.** For many dental health care providers in North America today, providing patient-centered care involves learning to communicate effectively with patients from non–English-speaking communities and with cultural backgrounds that may be unfamiliar.

   a. The United States has always had a significant foreign-born population, but the number of foreign born reached an all-time high of 32.5 million in 2002—equal to 11.5% of the U.S. population—according to the Current Population Survey (CPS).[10] By the year 2030, the Census Bureau predicts that 60% of the U.S. population will self-identify as White, non-Hispanic, and 40% will self-identify as members of other diverse racial and ethnic groups.

   b. The Canadian 2001 population census indicates that 18.5% of the population in Canada is foreign born.

   c. More than one-half of the 2002 foreign-born residents in the United States were born in Latin America—with 30% from Mexico alone. Among foreign-born residents in the United States, 26% were born in Asia, 14% in Europe, and 8% from Africa and other regions.

   d. Data from the 2000 Census show that over 47 million persons speak a language other than English at home, up nearly 48% since 1990. Although the majority are able to speak English, over 21 million speak English less than "very well," up 52% from 14 million in 1990.[11,12]

   e. Communication problems can easily occur if a patient is not fluent in English. An individual who is just learning the language may communicate well in everyday situations, but in the dental setting, the same person may not fully understand what is being discussed.

   f. Being competent to meet the communication challenge created by a multicultural population requires a set of skills, knowledge, and attitudes that enable the clinician to understand and respect patients' values, beliefs, and expectations.

**Table 3-1** U.S.-BORN AND FOREIGN-BORN POPULATION, 1980–2000[11,12]

|  | U.S. Born | Foreign Born |
|---|---|---|
| Number in millions |  |  |
| 1980 | 226.5 | 14.1 |
| 1990 | 248.7 | 19.8 |
| 2000 | 281.4 | 31.1 |
| Percent change |  |  |
| 1980–1990 | 9.8 | 40.4 |
| 1990–2000 | 13.1 | 57.1 |

## Minority Populations in the United States

According to the Census Bureau,[10,11] the proportion of the overall population in the United States considered to be minority will increase from 26.4% in 1995 to 47.2% in 2050. Figure 3-1 shows the racial distribution of the current U.S. population. Figure 3-2 shows the percentage increases in each racial minority group that occurred between 2000 and 2010 in the United States.

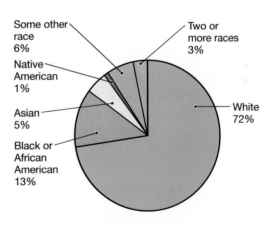

**Figure 3-1. Current U.S. population reported by race.** This pie chart shows the approximate current U.S. population reported by race as summarized from the 2010 United States Census.[13]

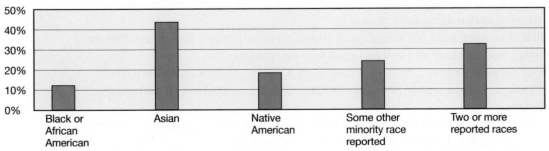

**Figure 3-2. Percentage increases of minorities reported by race in U.S. national population between 2000 and 2010.** The chart shows the approximate percentage increases of racial minority populations in the U.S. population as summarized from the 2010 United States Census.[13]

## The Hispanic Population in the United States

- Hispanics are the largest minority ethnic group in the United States, and this group continues to grow in number; as reported in the 2010 U.S. Census, the Hispanic population increased by 43.0% between 2000 and 2010 (Fig. 3-3).
- Among all Hispanics living in this country, 62% are native born and 38% are foreign born.
- Currently in the United States, the Hispanic population makes up 16.3% of the overall population (Fig. 3-4). Geographically, there are a number of areas—particularly in the South and West—that have much larger Hispanic populations.
- English language skills vary throughout the U.S. Hispanic population, and developing strategies for communicating with Hispanics who have limited skills in English is an important goal for all health care providers in the United States.

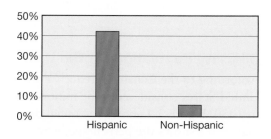

**Figure 3-3.   Percentage increase in Hispanic and non-Hispanic populations in the United States between 2000 and 2010.** This chart shows the approximate percentage increases in the Hispanic and non-Hispanic populations in the United States from 2000 to 2010 as summarized from the 2010 U.S. Census.[14]

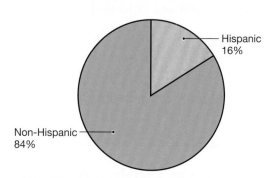

**Figure 3-4.   Current distribution between Hispanic and non-Hispanic populations in the United States.** The pie chart depicts the approximate current U.S. population—Hispanic versus non-Hispanic—as reported from the 2010 U.S. Census.[14]

## CULTURAL COMPETENCE

**Cultural competency** is the application of cultural knowledge, behaviors, interpersonal skills, and clinical skills to enhance a dental health care provider's effectiveness in managing patient care.

- Cultural competence indicates an understanding of important differences that exist among various ethnic and cultural groups in our country.
- Understanding patients' diverse cultures—their values, traditions, history, and institutions—is not simply political correctness. It is essential in providing quality patient care.
- Culture shapes individuals' experiences, perceptions, decisions, and how they relate to others. It influences the way patients respond to dental services and preventive interventions and impacts the way dental health care providers deliver dental care.
- In a culturally diverse society, dental professionals need to increase their awareness of and sensitivity toward diverse patient populations and work to understand culturally influenced health behaviors. Box 3-1 outlines actions to develop cultural competence.

## BOX 3-1  Ways to Develop Cultural Competence

- Recognize your own assumptions.
- Value diversity. Demonstrate an appreciation for the customs, values, and beliefs of people from different cultural and language backgrounds.
- Demonstrate flexibility. Carry out changes to meet the needs of your diverse patients.
- Communicate respect. Do not judge. Show empathy.

## Cultural Differences

Dental professionals interact with people from varied ethnic backgrounds and cultural origins who bring with them beliefs and values that may differ from the care provider's own.

- Understanding cultural differences can aid communication and thereby improve patient care.
- Preconceived ideas about a given culture can hinder a clinician from providing good care.
- Each patient is unique, and his or her dental care needs differ. Some cultures may be offended by the intensely personal questions necessary for a health history and may perceive them as an inexcusable invasion of privacy.
- People of various backgrounds also perceive the desirability of making direct eye contact differently.
- To help avoid miscommunication and offending patients, dental health care providers must be sensitive to these cultural differences.

## Tips for Improving Cross-cultural Communication

Cross-cultural communication is about dealing with people from other cultures in a way that minimizes misunderstandings and maximizes trust between patients and health care providers. The following simple tips will improve cross cultural communication.

1. **Speak slowly, not loudly.** Slow down and be careful to pronounce words clearly. Do not speak loudly. A loud voice implies anger in many cultures. Speaking loudly might cause the patient to become nervous. Use a caring tone of voice and facial expressions to convey your message.
2. **Separate questions.** Try not to ask double questions. Let the patient answer one question at a time.
3. **Repeat the message in different ways.** If the patient does not understand a statement, try repeating the message using different words. Be alert to words that the patient understands and use them frequently.
4. **Avoid idiomatic expressions or slang.** American English is full of idioms. An idiom is a distinctive, often colorful expression whose meaning cannot be understood from the combined meaning of its individual words, for example, the phrase "to kill two birds with one stone."
5. **Avoid difficult words and unnecessary information.** Use short, simple sentences. Do not overwhelm the patient with too many facts and lengthy, complicated explanations.
6. **Check meanings.** When communicating across cultures, never assume that the other person has understood. Be an active listener. Summarize what has been said in order to verify it. This is a very effective way of ensuring that accurate cross-cultural communication has taken place.

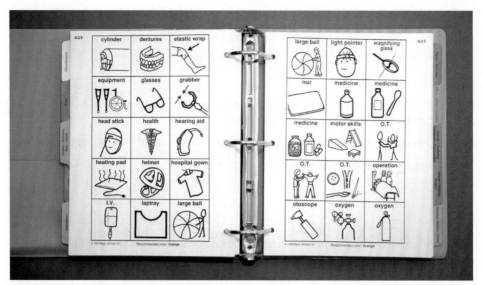

**Figure 3-5.   Picture board.** A picture board can be used to communicate when pictures are more effective than words. (From Carter PJ, Lewsen S. Communication skills. In: *Lippincott's Textbook for Nursing Assistants*. Philadelphia, PA: Lippincott Williams & Wilkins; 2005:65.

7. **Use visuals where possible.** A picture really is worth a thousand words; the universal language of pictures can make communication easier. Picture boards (Fig. 3-5) with medical/dental images are helpful in getting your message across.

8. **Avoid negative questions.** For example, "So then, you don't want an appointment on Monday?" A better question would be "What day of the week is best for you?" Questions with negative verbs such as "don't" or "can't" are particularly confusing to Asian patients.

9. **Take turns.** Give the patient time to answer and explain his or her response.

10. **Be supportive.** Giving encouragement to those with weak English skills gives them confidence and a trust in you.

11. **Use humor with caution.** In many cultures, health care is taken very seriously. Some foreign-born patients may not appreciate the use of humor or jokes in the dental office setting.

12. **Watch for nonverbal cues.** Be attentive for signs of fear, anxiety, or confusion in the patient.

13. **Use interpreters to improve communication.** If the patient speaks no English or has limited understanding, use a trained clinical interpreter who is fluent in the patient's native language as well as in medical and dental terminology. When using an interpreter, speak directly to the patient rather than to the interpreter.

14. **Don't use family members as translators.** A family member who is not knowledgeable in medical and dental terminology is likely to translate your message incorrectly. The presence of a family member or a friend may also constitute a serious breach of patient confidentiality.

15. **Ask permission to touch the patient.** Ask permission to examine the patient and do not touch the patient until permission is granted.

16. **Check for understanding.** Ask the patient to repeat instructions. Correct any misunderstandings. This can be done diplomatically by saying something like, "Will you repeat the instructions that I gave you to make sure that I did not forget anything?"

17. **Provide written material.** When possible, provide simple, illustrated materials for the patient to take home.

**SECTION 2:**

# Age Barriers

Young children, adolescents, and older patients present unique communication concerns.

- Even experienced health care providers can find it challenging to communicate effectively with individuals who are much younger or older in age. It can be difficult to relate to the life experiences or health problems of someone who is 30 or 40 years older.
- Some health care providers with limited experience with young children find it difficult to know what to say and what not to say when speaking with young children.
- Children and adolescents frequently are accompanied to the office by a parent. An adult child or caregiver may accompany older adults. Parents, adult children, and caregivers add a unique aspect to the communication process. The patient should always be the focus of the clinician's attention and, whenever possible, information is exchanged directly with the patient.
- Suggestions for communicating with children, adolescents, and older adults are outlined in Box 3-2, Box 3-3, and Box 3-4.

## COMMUNICATING WITH CHILDREN

BOX **3-2**   **Strategies for Communicating with Children**

- Introduce yourself to the child. Speak softly; use simple words and the child's name.
- Adjust your height to that of the child.
- Treat children with respect—over the age of 4, they can understand a lot.
- Describe actions before carrying them out.
- Make contact with the child (e.g., "*I promise to tell you everything I'm going to do if you'll help me by cooperating.*").
- Talk to young children throughout the assessment procedure.
- Give praise during each stage of the assessment, such as, "*that's good,*" "*well done,*" etc.
- Be aware of needs and concerns that are unique to children. For example, children may avoid wearing orthodontic headgear due to pressures and comments from peers.
- Do not ask the child's permission to perform a procedure if it will be performed in any case.
- Do not talk about procedures that will be done later in the appointment to children who are younger than 5 years of age. Very young children have no clear concept of future events and will imagine the worst about what could happen.
- Communicate all information directly to the child or to both child and parent, ensuring that the child remains the center of your attention. If complex information must be communicated to the parent, arrange to speak to the parent alone (without the child's presence).

## COMMUNICATING WITH ADOLESCENTS

BOX **3-3**  Strategies for Communicating with Teens

- Speak in a respectful, friendly manner, as to an adult.
- Respect independence; address the teenager directly rather than the parent.
- Obtain health history information directly from the teenager rather than the parent, if possible.
- Recognize that a teenager may be reluctant to answer certain questions honestly in the parent's presence.
- Ask questions about tobacco, drug, or alcohol use privately.
- Some teenagers may be intensely shy or self-conscious; others may be overconfident and boastful. Allow silence so that the teenager can express opinions and concerns.

## COMMUNICATING WITH OLDER ADULTS

* The U.S. population is aging at a dramatic rate.
* The U.S. population of persons aged 65 and older will increase by 76% from 2010 to 2030.
* The numbers of persons aged 85 and older in the United States will increase by 116% from 2010 to 2030.
* This tremendous demographic shift will have a profound effect on the health care sector. Over the next 50 years or so, there will most likely be an increased demand for dental health care providers skilled in caring for the geriatric population.
* Communicating with older people often requires extra time and patience because of physical, psychological, and social changes of normal aging.
* Even more effort is needed when an elderly person has a communication disorder.
* Communicating with older adults requires many of the same rules as for children—the patient should always be the focus of the dental health care provider's attention.

---

## BOX 3-4  Strategies for Communicating with Older Adults

* Before you begin your conversation, reduce background noises that may be distracting (close the treatment room door; move from a noisy reception area to a quieter place).
* Begin the conversation with casual topics such as the weather or special interests of the person.
* Keep your sentences and questions short. Avoid quick shifts from topic to topic.
* Allow extra time for responding. As people age, they function better at a slower pace; do not hurry them.
* Take time to understand the patient's true concerns. Some older people will hold back information feeling that nothing can be done or not wanting to "waste your time."
* Take time to explain in easy-to-understand language the findings of your examination.
* Look for hints from eye gaze and gestures that your message is being understood.
* Speak plainly and make sure that the patient understands by having him or her repeat instructions. For example, say, *"I may have forgotten to tell you something important. Would you please repeat what I told you?"*

# COMMUNICATING WITH CHILDREN WITH ATTENTION DEFICIT HYPERACTIVITY DISORDER

**Attention deficit hyperactivity disorder (ADHD)** is a developmental disorder believed to be caused primarily by genetic factors. Although this disorder occurs mainly in boys, it can also occur in girls. Currently, many researchers think certain neurotransmitters in the brain may be deficient in patients with this disorder. ADHD is a chronic condition with 30% to 50% of those individuals diagnosed in childhood continuing to display some symptoms into adulthood. Because adolescents and adults with ADHD tend to develop coping mechanisms for some or all of their behavioral impairments, management of children with this condition is the greatest challenge in a dental setting. Children with ADHD can display an inability to regulate their behavior to such a degree that it can have significant effects on their daily lives. These patients can display a variety of problems that can make the delivery of dental care difficult. Examples of these types of problems include the following:

- Difficulties with sustained attention
- Difficulties with impulse control
- Excessive activity
- Increased distractibility
- Difficulty following rules or instructions

Treatment for patients with this disorder can involve some combination of medications, behavior modifications, lifestyle changes, and counseling. Box 3-5 outlines strategies that can aid in communicating with children with ADHD during an appointment in a dental setting.

---

**BOX 3-5** Strategies for Improving Communication with Children with Attention Deficit Hyperactivity Disorder

- If the child is on medications for ADHD, remind the parents to have the child take the medications (as prescribed by the patient's physician) on the day of the appointment.
- Schedule the child for the time of the day when the child will best tolerate the appointment—this is usually a morning appointment, but the child's parents can guide you as to what is best for the individual patient.
- Explain to the child what is expected of him or her during the appointment; during the explanation to the child, always use clear and concise words.
- When giving instructions to the child during the appointment, give only one direction or command at a time.
- Sincerely praise the child who is doing well during the appointment.
- Consider using small rewards for reinforcement as you might with other children.
- Focus on the task and ignore minor inappropriate behaviors in the child.

**SECTION 3:**

# Vision and Hearing Barriers

## COMMUNICATION WITH THE VISUALLY IMPAIRED

Although estimates vary, there are approximately 10 million blind and visually impaired people in the United States. Approximately 1.3 million Americans are legally blind. There are approximately 5.5 million elderly individuals who are either blind or visually impaired. There are approximately 55,200 legally blind children. Box 3-6 presents suggestions for effective communication with a person who is blind or who is visually impaired.

---

**BOX 3-6   Strategies for Communicating with a Person Who Is Blind or Visually Impaired**

- As soon as you enter the room, be sure to greet the person. This alerts the person to your presence, avoids startling him or her, and eliminates uncomfortable silences. Address the person by name so he or she will immediately know that you are talking to him or her rather than someone who happens to be nearby. When greeting a person who is blind or visually impaired, do not forget to identify yourself. For example, "*Hello, Mrs. Jones. I am Robin Shiffer, the dental hygienist here in Dr. Rolfs' office.*"

- Speak directly to the person who is visually impaired, not through an intermediary such as a relative or a caregiver.

- Speak distinctly, using a natural conversational tone and speed. Unless the person has a hearing impairment, you do not need to raise your voice.

- Explain the reason for touching the person before doing so.

- Be an active listener. Give the person opportunities to talk. Respond with questions and comments to keep the conversation going. A person who is visually impaired cannot necessarily see the look of interest on your face, so give verbal cues to let him or her know that you are actively listening.

- Always answer questions and be specific or descriptive in your responses.

- Orient the person to sounds in the environment. For example, explain and demonstrate the sound that an ultrasonic instrument makes before using it in the patient's mouth.

- Tell the patient when you are leaving the room and where you are going (e.g., *I am going to develop the x-rays that we just took*).

- Be precise and thorough when you describe people, places, or things to someone who is blind. Do not leave out things or change a description because you think it is unimportant or unpleasant.

- Feel free to use words that refer to vision during the course of a conversation. Vision-oriented words such as look, see, and watching TV are a part of everyday verbal communication. Making reference to colors, patterns, designs, and shapes is perfectly acceptable. The words *blind* and *visually impaired* are also acceptable in conversation.

- Indicate the end of a conversation with a person who is blind or severely visually impaired to avoid the embarrassment of leaving the person speaking when no one is actually there.

- When you speak about someone with a disability, refer to the person and then to the disability. For example, refer to "a person who is blind" rather than to "a blind person."

## Providing Directions to a Blind or Visually Impaired Individual

When giving directions from one place to another, people who are not visually impaired tend to use gestures—pointing, looking in the direction referred to, etc.—at least as much as they use verbal cues. That is not helpful to a person who is blind or has a visual impairment. And often, even verbal directions are not precise enough for a person who cannot see—for example, "*It's right over there*" or "*It's just around the next corner.*" Where is "there"? Where is "the next corner"? In the dental office, you might say something like: "Walk along the wall to your left past three doorways. The room that we want is at the fourth doorway; make a sharp turn to the right to enter the room."

The Americans with Disabilities Act (ADA) prohibits businesses that serve the public from banning service animals. A service animal is defined as any guide dog or other animal that is trained to provide assistance to a person with a disability. The animal does not have to be licensed or certified by the state as a service animal. The service animal should not be separated from its owner and must be allowed to enter the treatment room with the patient. The ADA law supersedes local health department regulations that ban animals in health care facilities. Box 3-7 provides suggestions for useful techniques when acting as a sighted guide for a blind or visually impaired individual.

---

## BOX 3-7 Acting as a Sighted Guide

*Sighted guide technique enables a person who is blind to use a person with sight as a guide. The technique follows a specific form and has specific applications.*

- Offer to guide a person who is blind or visually impaired by asking if he or she would like assistance. Be aware that the person may not need or want guided help; in some instances, it can be disorienting and disruptive. Respect the wishes of the person you are with.

- If your help is accepted, offer the person your arm. To do so, tap the back of your hand against the palm of his or her hand. The person will then grasp your arm directly above the elbow. Never grab the person's arm or try to direct him or her by pushing or pulling.

- Relax and walk at a comfortable normal pace. Stay one step ahead of the person you are guiding, except at the top and bottom of stairs. At these places, pause and stand alongside the person. Then resume travel, walking one step ahead. Always pause when you change directions, step up, or step down.

- It is helpful, but not necessary, to tell the person you are guiding about stairs, narrow spaces, elevators, and escalators.

- The standard form of sighted guide technique may have to be modified because of other disabilities or for someone who is exceptionally tall or short. Be sure to ask the person you are guiding what, if any, modifications he or she would like you to use.

- When acting as a guide, never leave the person in "free space." When walking, always be sure that the person has a firm grasp on your arm. If you have to be separated briefly, be sure the person is in contact with a wall, railing, or some other stable object until you return.

- To guide a person to a seat, place the hand of your guiding arm on the seat. The person you are guiding will find the seat by following along your arm.

## COMMUNICATION WITH THE HEARING IMPAIRED

Approximately 1 out of every 10 people has a significant hearing loss. Within the population of individuals who are hearing impaired, most are hard of hearing. Only a small proportion of this group is deaf. In describing hearing loss, people who are hard of hearing may say that they can hear sounds but cannot understand what is being said. For many people who are hard of hearing, low-frequency speech sounds such as "*a*," "*o*," and "*u*" may be clearly heard, while other high-frequency sounds such as "*s*," "*th*," and "*sh*" may be much less distinct. In this situation, speech is heard but often misunderstood. "*Watch*" may be mistaken for "*wash*" and "*pen*" for "*spent*." A clearer comprehension of speech may be gained with a hearing aid or a cochlear implant. However, use of these devices does not restore normal hearing.

Presbycusis (presby = elder, cusis = hearing) is the loss of hearing that gradually occurs in most individuals as they grow old. Everyone who lives long enough will develop some degree of presbycusis, some sooner than others. Those who damage their ears from loud noise exposure will develop it sooner. It is estimated that 40% to 50% of people aged 75 and older have some degree of hearing loss. It involves a progressive loss of hearing, beginning with high-frequency sounds such as speech. The loss associated with presbycusis is usually greater for high-pitched sounds. It may be difficult for someone to hear the nearby chirping of a bird or the ringing of a telephone, whereas they would be able to hear low-pitched voices.

Box 3-8 provides suggestions for actions that can promote effective communication with a person who is hearing impaired.

---

**BOX 3-8**   **Strategies for Communicating with a Person who is Hearing Impaired**

- Move closer to the person. Shortening the distance between the speaker and the listener will increase the loudness of sound. This approach is much more effective than raising your voice. Never shout at a person who is hard of hearing.

- Reduce background noise. Many noises that we take for granted are amplified by a hearing aid or a cochlear implant.

- Talk face to face. Speak at eye level. Do not cover your mouth with a mask when you are asking the patient questions or giving instructions.

- Try rewording a message. At times, a person with a hearing loss may be partially dependent on speech reading (lip reading) because some sounds may not be easily heard even with a hearing aid. Because some words are easier to speech read than others, rephrasing a message may make it easier for the person to understand.

- Use a notepad to write down important questions or directions so that the person can read them. This helps eliminate misunderstandings. If the person cannot read or reads in a language that is unfamiliar to you, a picture board (see Fig. 3-5) may be quite helpful.

- Make sure that the person fully understands what you said. Some people, especially if the hearing loss is recent, are reluctant to ask others to repeat themselves. They feel embarrassed by their hearing loss. Simply ask the person to repeat what you said. For example, say, "*If you could please repeat back to me what I said, I can make sure I told you everything that I need to.*"

- Show special awareness of the hearing problem. Call the person with a hearing loss by name to initiate a communication. Give a frame of reference for the discussion by mentioning the topic at the outset ("*I would like to review your medications.*").

- Be patient, particularly when the person is tired or ill and may be less able to hear.

## SECTION 4:

# Speech Barriers

## COMMUNICATION WITH THE SPEECH IMPAIRED

It is important to remember that problems with speech or language do not necessarily mean that the person has an intellectual impairment. For example, people who have suffered a stroke are often frustrated when others think that their intellect has been impaired because of their problems with communication. Difficulty with speech does not have anything to do with intelligence. If understanding is difficult, it may be useful to ask the person to write a word or phrase.

### Dysarthria

**Dysarthria** refers to speech problems that are caused by the muscles involved with speaking or the nerves controlling them. Individuals with dysarthria have difficulty expressing certain words or sounds. Speech problems experienced include:
- Slurred speech
- Speaking softly or barely able to whisper
- Slow rate of speech
- Rapid rate of speech with a "mumbling" quality
- Limited tongue, lip, and jaw movement
- Abnormal rhythm when speaking
- Changes in vocal quality ("nasal" speech or sounding "stuffy")
- Drooling or poor control of saliva
- Chewing and swallowing difficulty
- Common causes of dysarthria are poorly fitting dentures, stroke, any degenerative neurological disorder, and alcohol intoxication.
- After a stroke or other brain injury, the muscles of the mouth, face, and respiratory system may become weak, move slowly, or not move at all.
- Some former severe alcoholics who have developed brain damage due to drinking may have continued problems with language, even after years of sobriety.

### Aphasia

**Aphasia** is a disorder that results from damage to language centers of the brain.
- It can result in a reduced ability to understand what others are saying, to express ideas, or to be understood.
- Some individuals with this disorder may have no speech, whereas others may have only mild difficulties recalling names or words.
- Others may have problems putting words in their proper order in a sentence.
- The ability to understand oral directions, to read, to write, and to deal with numbers may also be disturbed.
- For almost all right-handers and for about half of left-handers, damage to the left side of the brain causes aphasia. As a result, individuals who were previously able to communicate through speaking, listening, reading, and writing become more limited in their ability to do so.
- The most common cause of aphasia is stroke, but gunshot wounds, blows to the head, other traumatic brain injury, brain tumor, Alzheimer disease, and transient ischemic attack (TIA) can also cause aphasia.

Box 3-9 provides suggestions for useful actions when communicating with patients with speech impairment.

| BOX **3-9** | **Strategies for Communicating with Persons with Speech Impairment** |
|---|---|

- Book longer appointment times to allow for the longer time needed for communication.
- Whenever possible, speak directly to the patient; even if comprehension is limited, the patient will be more responsive if he or she is an active participant.
- Develop a tolerance for silences. Many patients require extra time to process your questions and/or to formulate a response.
- Do not talk while the patient is formulating a response—this is very distracting.
- Try not to panic when communicating with a person who has impaired speech. If you feel nervous, do not let it show.
- Never finish a sentence for someone who is struggling with his or her speech—be patient and wait for him or her to finish.
- Find out if the patient has his or her own way of indicating "yes" or "no" (e.g., looking up for yes).
- If you are having problems understanding the person, say so. Do not pretend you understand if you do not as this will inevitably create problems later on. Simply apologize and ask if the patient would mind writing down what it is he or she wants to say.
- If you are having difficulties communicating with the patient, ask permission to direct your questions to the support person. Remember to look directly at the patient from time to time so that he or she still feels part of the conversation.
- Use gestures and pictures to help the patient understand. For example, wave hello and goodbye, point to a tooth, or show simple pictures to clarify procedures.

# COMMUNICATION WITH THE VOICE IMPAIRED

## Laryngectomy

**Laryngectomy**—the surgical removal of the voice box due to cancer—affects approximately 9,000 individuals each year; most are older adults. People who have undergone laryngectomy have several options for communication:

- **The artificial larynx.** Held against the neck, the artificial larynx transmits an electronic sound through the tissues, which is then shaped into speech sounds by the lips and tongue. The user articulates in the normal way.
- **Esophageal voice.** Esophageal voice is achieved by learning to pump air from the mouth into the upper esophagus. The air is then released, causing the pharyngo-esophageal segment to vibrate to produce a hoarse low-pitched voice.
- **Surgical voice restoration.** Fitting a prosthesis or valve into a puncture hole between the trachea and esophagus either at the time of surgery or at a later date may restore voice. The individual occludes the stoma when he or she wishes to speak. Air then passes through the valve into the esophagus, producing voice in the same way as for esophageal voice.
- **Silent mouthing/writing/gesture.** A small percentage of patients never acquire a voice and are unable to use an electronic larynx. They communicate by silently articulating words or a mixture of writing and gesture.

Box 3-10 provides suggestions for actions that can promote effective communication with a person with a laryngectomy.

---

BOX **3-10**  **Strategies for Communicating with a Person with a Laryngectomy**

- Give the patient plenty of time to speak. Do not hurry the person; if the patient feels pressured, it can affect his or her ability to communicate.
- Ask the patient to repeat if you do not understand. Do not pretend you understand if you do not—it will be obvious to the patient that you do not understand.
- Watch a person's lips if you are finding it hard to understand.
- Do not assume it is a hoax call or that someone playing is a joke if you hear an electronic-sounding voice or someone struggling to communicate over the telephone.

## SECTION 5:
# Ready References

**READY REFERENCE 3-1** ENGLISH–SPANISH MEDICAL DICTIONARIES

McElroy OH, Grabb LL. *Spanish-English, English-Spanish Medical Dictionary.* 4th ed. Philadelphia, PA: Lippincott Williams & Wilkins; 2010.

Springhouse. *English & Spanish Medical Words & Phrases.* 4th ed. Philadelphia, PA: Lippincott Williams & Wilkins; 2007.

Springhouse. *Medical Spanish Made Incredibly Easy.* 3rd ed. Philadelphia, PA: Lippincott Williams & Wilkins; 2008.

Wilber CJ, Lister S. *Medical Spanish: The Instant Survival Guide.* 4th ed. Boston, MA: Butterworth-Heinemann; 2004.

**READY REFERENCE 3-2** INTERNET RESOURCES: CULTURAL COMPETENCE

**http://gucchd.georgetown.edu/nccc/index.html**
Website of the **National Center for Cultural Competence (NCCC)**. The mission of the NCCC is to increase the capacity of health care and mental health care programs to design, implement, and evaluate culturally and linguistically competent service delivery systems to address growing diversity, persistent disparities, and to promote health and mental equity.

**http://gucchd.georgetown.edu/nccc/topic3.html**
Information on **disparities in oral health** on the **National Center for Cultural Competence** website.

**http://www.diversityrx.org/HTML/DIVRX.htm**
Promoting language and cultural competence to improve the quality of health care for minority, immigrant, and ethnically diverse communities.

**READY REFERENCE 3-3**    INTERNET RESOURCES: HEARING AND VISION IMPAIRMENT

**http://www.asha.org**
The **American Speech-Language-Hearing Association (ASHA)** website has resources on communication and communication disorders.

**http://www.nidcd.nih.gov/health/voice/index.asp**
The **National Institute on Deafness and other Communication Disorders (NIDCD)** index of resources on voice, speech, and language.

**http://www.nidcd.nih.gov/health/hearing/index.asp**
The **National Institute on Deafness and other Communication Disorders (NIDCD)** resources on hearing and deafness.

**http://medlineplus.gov/**
The **MedlinePlus** website provides health information from the world's largest medical library, the National Library of Medicine. MedlinePlus has extensive information from the National Institutes of Health and other trusted sources on over 650 diseases and conditions. The **Health Topics** section has information on hearing problems and disorders, speech communication disorders, vision impairment, and blindness.

**http://www.agbell.org/**
The **Alexander Graham Bell Association for the Deaf and Hard of Hearing** is dedicated to the mission of promoting communication for people with hearing loss. The **Information and Resources** section offers up-to-date statistics, fact sheets, and information on communication options.

**http://www.audiology.org/consumer/guides/**
The **American Academy of Audiology** offers consumer guides, including "Getting Through: Talking to a Person Who is Hard of Hearing."

**http://www.raisingdeafkids.org/communicating/tips/adult.jsp**
Website of the **Deafness and Family Communication Center (DFCC) at the Children's Hospital of Philadelphia**: tips on communicating with a person who is deaf.

**http://www.afb.org/Section.asp?SectionID=&DocumentID=2104**
Instructions on how to guide a person who is blind on the website of the **American Foundation for the Blind**.

**READY REFERENCE 3-4**  **INTERNET RESOURCES: VOICE AND SPEECH IMPAIRMENT**

**http://www.nidcd.nih.gov/health/voice/aphasia.asp**
The **National Institute on Deafness and other Communication Disorders (NIDCD)** resources on aphasia.

**http://www.nidcd.nih.gov/health/voice/dysph.asp**
The **National Institute on Deafness and other Communication Disorders (NIDCD)** resources on dysarthria.

**http://www.aphasia.org/**
The website of the **National Aphasia Association** has links to a wealth of information on aphasia. It includes links to information about aphasia in different languages, including Spanish.

**http://www.americanheart.org**
Enter "aphasia" in the SEARCH box on the **American Heart Association** website for many resources on this topic.

**www.aphasia.org/NAAfactsheet.html**
**National Aphasia Association** website: aphasia fact sheet.

## REFERENCES

1. Dong M, Loignon C, Levine A, Bedos C. Perceptions of oral illness among Chinese immigrants in Montreal: a qualitative study. *J Dent Educ*. 2007;71(10):1340–1347.

2. Fitch P. Cultural competence and dental hygiene care delivery: integrating cultural care into the dental hygiene process of care. *J Dent Hyg*. 2004;78(1):11–21.

3. Formicola AJ, Klyvert M, McIntosh J, Thompson A, Davis M, Cangialosi T. Creating an environment for diversity in dental schools: one school's approach. *J Dent Educ*. 2003;67(5):491–499.

4. Formicola AJ, Stavisky J, Lewy R. Cultural competency: dentistry and medicine learning from one another. *J Dent Educ*. 2003;67(8):869–875.

5. Mertz E, O'Neil E. The growing challenge of providing oral health care services to all Americans. *Health Aff (Millwood)*. 2002;21(5):65–77.

6. Betancourt JR, Maina AW, Soni SM. The IOM report unequal treatment: lessons for clinical practice. *Del Med J*. 2005;77(9):339–348.

7. Betancourt JR, Maina AW. The Institute of Medicine report "Unequal Treatment": implications for academic health centers. *Mt Sinai J Med*. 2004;71(5):314–321.

8. Betancourt JR, King RK. Unequal treatment: the Institute of Medicine report and its public health implications. *Public Health Rep*. 2003;118(4):287–292.

9. Commission on the Future of Health Care in Canada, Romanow RJ. *Building on Values: The Future of Health Care in Canada*. Saskatoon, Sask.: Commission on the Future of Health Care in Canada; 2002.

10. U.S. Census Bureau, Ethnic and Hispanic Statistics Branch. *The Foreign-born Population in the United States, March 2001*. Washington DC: U.S. Bureau of the Census; 2003.

11. Hobbs F, Stoops N, U.S. Census Bureau. *Census 2000 Special Reports, Series CENSR-4: Demographic Trends in the 20th Century*. Washington, DC: U.S. Census Bureau, U.S. Government Printing Office; 2002.

12. U.S. Department of Commerce, Economics and Statistics Administration. Census 2000. *Modified Race Data Summary File Census of Population and Housing [Numeric Data]*. Washington DC: U.S. Department of Commerce, Economics and Statistics Administration, U.S. Census Bureau; 2002. Available at: http://purl.access.gpo.gov/GPO/LPS32088.

13. Mackun P, Wilson S. *Population Distribution and Change: 2000 to 2010*. Washington DC: U.S. Department of Commerce, Economics and Statistics Administration, U.S. Bureau of the Census; 2011.

14. Humes KR, Jones NA, Ramirez RR; United States Bureau of the Census. *Overview of Race and Hispanic Origin: 2010*. Washington DC: U.S. Department of Commerce, Economics and Statistics Administration, U.S. Census Bureau; 2011.

# SUGGESTED READINGS

## Cultural Competency

Gebru K, Willman A. A research-based didactic model for education to promote culturally competent nursing care in Sweden. *J Transcult Nurs.* 2003;14(1):55–61.

Narayan MC. Cultural assessment in home healthcare. *Home Healthc Nurse.* 1997;15(10):663–670; quiz 71–72.

Purnell L. A description of the Purnell Model for Cultural Competence. *J Transcult Nurs.* 2000;11(1):40–46.

Watts RJ. Race consciousness and the health of African Americans. *Online J Issues Nurs.* 2003;8(1):4.

## Attention Deficit Hyperactivity Disorder

Blomqvist M, Holmberg K, Fernell E, Ek U, Dahllof G. Oral health, dental anxiety, and behavior management problems in children with attention deficit hyperactivity disorder. *Eur J Oral Sci.* 2006;114(5):385–390.

Clinical practice guideline: diagnosis and evaluation of the child with attention-deficit/hyperactivity disorder. American Academy of Pediatrics. *Pediatrics.* 2000;105(5):1158–1170.

## Hearing Impaired

Nattinger AB. Communicating with deaf patients. *JAMA.* 1995;274(10):795.

**SECTION 6:**

# The Human Element

BOX **3-11**    **Through the Eyes of a Student:**
**Helping Patients with Special Needs**

*I have this 92-year-old patient, Mrs. W, who always comes with her daughter. Mrs. W. lives in an assisted living facility. I saw Mrs. W. in the dental clinic last year, too, and she always has a heavy amount of plaque when she comes in. I talked to her daughter about this in the past. The daughter lives an hour away from her mother and so cannot be there to brush her mother's teeth every day. Today, the daughter said that she asked the staff at the assisted living facility to assist her mother in brushing her teeth, but she doesn't think that they have been helping her. I felt sorry for Mrs. W. because I know assisted living facilities commonly are understaffed and oral hygiene care is not a priority.*

*The daughter said that there is a problem getting the staff to do things for her mother because they are so busy. She said that her mother has low blood sugar and is supposed to have a protein snack each afternoon. Her mother didn't get her needed snack until her physician wrote it as a "prescription" to the staff.*

*For me, her story about the snack was like a lightbulb going off in my head! What a great idea! So I talked with our clinic's dentist, and he wrote "brush teeth after evening meal" on a prescription and signed it. Mrs. M's daughter was very pleased that we cared enough about her mother to write this "prescription."*

*Melissa, recent graduate*
*East Tennessee State University*

## SECTION 7:
# Skill Check

**SKILL CHECKLIST:**  COMMUNICATIONS ROLE-PLAY

Student: _____    Evaluator: _____

Date:    _____

> **Roles:**
> - Student 1 = Plays the role of the patient.
> - Student 2 = Plays the role of the clinician.

DIRECTIONS FOR STUDENT CLINICIAN: Use **Column S** to record your evaluation of your skill level as **S** (satisfactory) or **U** (unsatisfactory).

DIRECTIONS FOR EVALUATOR: Use **Column E** to record your evaluation of the student clinician's communication skills during the role-play. Indicate **S** (satisfactory) or **U** (unsatisfactory). In the optional grade percentage calculation, each **S** equals 1 point, and each **U** equals 0 points.

| CRITERIA | S | E |
|---|---|---|
| **Uses appropriate nonverbal behavior such as maintaining eye contact, sitting at the same level as the patient, nodding head when listening to patient, etc.** | | |
| **Interacts with the patient as a peer, and avoids a condescending approach. Collaborates with the patient and provides advice.** | | |
| **Communicates using common, everyday words. Avoids dental terminology.** | | |
| **Listens attentively to the patient's comments. Respects the patient's point of view.** | | |
| **Listens attentively to the patient's questions. Encourages patient questions. Clarifies for understanding when necessary.** | | |
| **Answers the patient's questions fully and accurately.** | | |
| **Checks for understanding by the patient. Clarifies information.** | | |

OPTIONAL GRADE PERCENTAGE CALCULATION

Each **S** equals 1 point, and each **U** equals 0 points. Using the **E** column, total the sum of the "**S**"s _____ divided by the total points possible (7) equals the percentage grade _____.

**Note to Course Instructor:**
A series of role-play scenarios for this textbook can be found at http://thepoint.lww.com

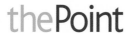

# NOTES

MODULE

4

# Medical History

## MODULE OVERVIEW

The medical history is a critical step in the care for every dental patient. The medical history provides important information related to the patient's physical and psychological condition. The information gathered during the medical history is ultimately used during the planning of dental care when determining how a patient's medical condition may be impacted by the planned dental care. This information allows the clinician to determine whether dental treatment alterations are necessary for the patient to safely undergo each specific dental procedure.

In addition, a thorough understanding of the implications of the findings from the medical history is a critical component in interprofessional collaboration. One of the key foundations of the concept of interprofessional practice is for all health care providers to share a common vocabulary and common understanding of caring for the patient as a whole. A thorough health history is the first step for a dental hygienist or dentist to participate in collaborating with other health care providers about the overall welfare of a patient.

This module covers taking and interpreting the medical history, including:

- Gathering information regarding a patient's medical conditions and diseases
- Gathering information regarding a patient's medications and supplements
- Informed consent and the medical history
- Determining how a patient's medical conditions and/or medications impact dental care

## MODULE OUTLINE

## OBJECTIVES

- Demonstrate skills in conducting online research on medical conditions/diseases and medications.
- Describe how various systemic conditions/diseases and medications can impact dental care.
- Discuss the ways in which a clinician's choice of words can facilitate or hinder communication with patients regarding patient assessment procedures.
- Define and discuss the terms *informed consent*, *capacity for consent*, and *informed refusal* as these terms apply to patient assessment procedures.
- Demonstrate skills necessary to obtain a complete and thorough medical history.
- Describe the types of information that should be entered in the medical alert box on the medical history form.
- List the information that should be indicated on a medical consultation form.
- Describe contraindications and complications for dental care presented by various medical conditions/diseases and medications.
- Identify findings that have implications in planning dental treatment.
- Provide appropriate referral to a physician or dental specialist when findings indicate the need for further evaluation.
- Demonstrate the ability to apply information learned in the classroom and clinical activities to the fictitious patient cases A–E in this module, including reviewing completed health history forms, conducting research, formulating follow-up questions, conducting a patient interview, and determining the medical risk of dental treatment to the patient.

**SECTION 1:**

# The Medical History Assessment

## RELATIONSHIP BETWEEN SYSTEMIC AND ORAL HEALTH

There are many reasons for conducting a thorough assessment of the patient's past and current health status. The most important reason is to protect the health of the patient. There is a strong, two-way relationship between systemic health and oral conditions.

- Systemic diseases and conditions may have oral implications. For example, patients with poorly controlled diabetes do not respond well to therapy for periodontal diseases.
- Medications used to treat systemic diseases and conditions can produce changes in oral health. For example, certain medications can result in gingival hyperplasia (overgrowth of the gingiva).
- Systemic conditions, diseases, or medications may necessitate precautions to ensure that planned dental treatment will not be harmful to the patient's systemic health. For example, a patient who has a history of well-controlled congestive heart failure may need certain treatment modifications such as short appointments and supplemental oxygen by nasal cannula.
- Oral manifestations may identify conditions that should be evaluated by a primary care physician. For example, periodontal disease that does not respond to treatment may be an indication of uncontrolled diabetes because this condition increases susceptibility to infection and results in slower healing rates.
- Substances, materials, or drugs used in dental treatment may produce an adverse reaction in certain patients. For example, a patient with allergies may be allergic to latex.

## HEALTH HISTORY FORMS

A health history form is used to gather subjective data about the patient and explore past and present problems. This form assists patients in providing an account of their health history.

- Health history forms are available in many different formats and lengths.
- Many health history forms include a list of diseases and medical conditions that aid patients in recalling their medical history.
- Most forms ask the patient to check or circle "yes" or "no" for each question or item on the form. Some health history forms have space that allows patients to provide additional information in response to questions and to list their medications.
- It is common for dental offices and clinics to design history forms to meet the unique needs of the office or clinic and its patient population.
- Regardless of the format or length, the health history form should provide the health care professional with complete information regarding the past and present health of each patient.

## CARING FOR PATIENTS IN A MULTICULTURAL SOCIETY

The United States and Canada are multicultural societies where many of the residents report being born in a foreign country. This diversity in ethnicity, culture, and language enriches these countries, but it also complicates efforts to provide safe dental care.

- For many dental health care providers in the United States and Canada, assessing a patient's history involves finding a way to communicate with patients who speak another language.
- Ideally, an interpreter who is specially trained to conduct translations involving medical and dental terminology, conditions, and procedures would be a member of every dental staff. Employing a trained medical/dental interpreter who is fluent in many different languages is an unrealistic option for most dental offices and clinics.
- Using a health history form that has been translated into different languages is a more practical solution to the problem of obtaining history information from non-English speaking patients. Today, more than half of the foreign-born residents in the United States were born in Latin America. The American Dental Association has adult and child history forms in Spanish to meet the needs of patients whose language of origin is Spanish.

## MULTI-LANGUAGE HEALTH HISTORY PROJECT

The **Multi-Language Health History Project** began as an initiative of the University of the Pacific (UOP) Arthur A. Dugoni School of Dentistry to address the needs of patients and dental health care providers who do not speak the same language. With the assistance of the California Dental Association and MetLife Inc., the history form has been translated into over 25 different languages. Transcend, a California company specializing in translations services, certifies that the translations are correct.

## OBTAINING AND USING THE UNIVERSITY OF THE PACIFIC MULTI-LANGUAGE FORMS

- Directions for downloading copies of the UOP multi-language health history forms are found in Box 4-1.
- The English version of the UOP health history form was translated into over 25 different languages, keeping the same question numbering sequence. Using a translated form, a dental health care provider who speaks English and is caring for a patient who doesn't, can ask the patient to complete the health history in his or her own language.
- The clinician then compares the English health history to the patient's translated health history, scanning the translated version for "yes" responses. When a "yes" is found, the dental health care provider is able to look at the question number and match it to the question number on the English version. For example, question 34 on the Japanese version is the same as question 34 on the English version and relates to high blood pressure.
- In the same manner, a dental health care provider who speaks Spanish could use the multi-language health history form with a patient who speaks French. A few examples of the UOP health history form are shown in Figures 4-1 to 4-4.
- The UOP multi-language health history form is used in each of the fictitious patient activities that appear at the end of this module.

## BOX 4-1 Instructions for Downloading the University of the Pacific Multi-Language Forms

The multi-language health history forms can be downloaded at no cost on the Internet.

1. Connect a computer to the internet and open an Internet browser.

2. On the Internet browser, enter the website address in the rectangular box near the top of the browser:
   - http://www.dental.pacific.edu/Professional_Services_and_ Resources/Dental_Practice_Documents.html

3. Click on "GO" or hit the "return key" on the keyboard. The selected web page should open.

NOTE:  A software application—Adobe Acrobat Reader—is needed to open and view a PDF document and can be downloaded at http://get.adobe.com/reader

| MetLife | **HEALTH HISTORY**<br>English | University of the Pacific |
|---|---|---|

Patient Name:_____    Patient Identification Number:_____

Birth Date:_____

**I. CIRCLE APPROPRIATE ANSWER** (leave Blank if you do not understand question):

1. Yes No Is your general health good?
2. Yes No Has there been a change in your health within the last year?
3. Yes No Have you been hospitalized or had a serious illness in the last three years?
   If YES, why?_____
4. Yes No Are you being treated by a physician now? For what?    _____
   Date of last medical exam?_____Date of last Dental exam_____
5. Yes No Have you had problems with prior dental treatment?
6. Yes No Are you in pain now?

**II. HAVE YOU EXPERIENCED:**

| 7. | Yes | No | Chest pain (angina)? | 18. | Yes | No | Dizziness? |
|---|---|---|---|---|---|---|---|
| 8. | Yes | No | Swollen ankles? | 19. | Yes | No | Ringing in ears? |
| 9. | Yes | No | Shortness of breath? | 20. | Yes | No | Headaches? |
| 10. | Yes | No | Recent weight loss, fever, night sweats? | 21. | Yes | No | Fainting spells? |
| 11. | Yes | No | Persistent cough, coughing up blood? | 22. | Yes | No | Blurred vision? |
| 12. | Yes | No | Bleeding problems, bruising easily? | 23. | Yes | No | Seizures? |
| 13. | Yes | No | Sinus problems? | 24. | Yes | No | Excessive thirst? |
| 14. | Yes | No | Difficulty swallowing? | 25. | Yes | No | Frequent urination? |
| 15. | Yes | No | Diarrhea, constipation, blood in stools? | 26. | Yes | No | Dry mouth? |
| 16. | Yes | No | Frequent vomiting, nausea? | 27. | Yes | No | Jaundice? |
| 17. | Yes | No | Difficulty urinating, blood in urine? | 28. | Yes | No | Joint pain, stiffness? |

**III. DO YOU HAVE OR HAVE YOU HAD:**

| 29. | Yes | No | Heart disease? | 40. | Yes | No | AIDS |
|---|---|---|---|---|---|---|---|
| 30. | Yes | No | Heart attack, heart defects? | 41. | Yes | No | Tumors, cancer? |
| 31. | Yes | No | Heart murmurs? | 42. | Yes | No | Arthritis, rheumatism? |
| 32. | Yes | No | Rheumatic fever? | 43. | Yes | No | Eye diseases? |
| 33. | Yes | No | Stroke, hardening of arteries? | 44. | Yes | No | Skin diseases? |
| 34. | Yes | No | High blood pressure? | 45. | Yes | No | Anemia? |
| 35. | Yes | No | Asthma, TB, emphysema, other lung diseases? | 46. | Yes | No | VD (syphilis or gonorrhea)? |
| 36. | Yes | No | Hepatitis, other liver disease? | 47. | Yes | No | Herpes? |
| 37. | Yes | No | Stomach problems, ulcers? | 48. | Yes | No | Kidney, bladder disease? |
| 38. | Yes | No | Allergies to: drugs, foods, medications, latex? | 49. | Yes | No | Thyroid, adrenal disease? |
| 39. | Yes | No | Family history of diabetes, heart problems, tumors? | 50. | Yes | No | Diabetes? |

**IV. DO YOU HAVE OR HAVE YOU HAD:**

| 51. | Yes | No | Psychiatric care? | 56. | Yes | No | Hospitalization? |
|---|---|---|---|---|---|---|---|
| 52. | Yes | No | Radiation treatments? | 57. | Yes | No | Blood transfusions? |
| 53. | Yes | No | Chemotherapy? | 58. | Yes | No | Surgeries? |
| 54. | Yes | No | Prosthetic heart valve? | 59. | Yes | No | Pacemaker? |
| 55. | Yes | No | Artificial joint? | 60. | Yes | No | Contact lenses? |

**V. ARE YOU TAKING:**

| 61. | Yes | No | Recreational drugs? | 63. | Yes | No | Tobacco in any form? |
|---|---|---|---|---|---|---|---|
| 62. | Yes | No | Drugs, medications, over-the-counter medicines<br>(including Aspirin), natural remedies? | 64. | Yes | No | Alcohol? |

Please list:_____
_____

**VI. WOMEN ONLY:**

| 65. | Yes | No | Are you or could you be pregnant or nursing? | 66. | Yes | No | Taking birth control pills? |
|---|---|---|---|---|---|---|---|

**VII. ALL PATIENTS:**

67. Yes No Do you have or have you had any other diseases or medical problems NOT listed on this form?
If so, please explain:_____
_____

*To the best of my knowledge, I have answered every question completely and accurately. I will inform my dentist of any change in my health and/or medication.*

Patient's signature:_____Date:_____

**RECALL REVIEW:**

1. Patient's signature_____Date:_____

2. Patient's signature_____Date:_____

3. Patient's signature_____Date:_____

The Health History is created and maintained by the University of the Pacific School of Dentistry, San Francisco, California.
Support for the translation and dissemination of the Health Histories comes from MetLife Dental Care.

**Figure 4-1. History form in English.** Shown here is the University of the Pacific Arthur A. Dugoni School of Dentistry's health history form in English.

**MetLife**

# DOSSIER MÉDICAL
French

**University of the Pacific**

Nom du patient/de la patiente : _____    No d'identification du patient : _____

Date de naissance : _____

## I. ENTOURER LA MENTION CORRESPONDANTE (laisser en blanc si la question n'est pas comprise) :

| | | | |
|---|---|---|---|
| 1. | Oui | Non | Êtes-vous en général en bonne santé ? |
| 2. | Oui | Non | Votre état de santé a-t-il changé depuis l'année dernière ? |
| 3. | Oui | Non | Avez-vous été hospitalisé(e) ou avez-vous été gravement malade au cours des trois dernières années ? |
| | | | Si vous avez répondu OUI, pour quelle raison/maladie ? _____ |
| 4. | Oui | Non | Êtes-vous actuellement en traitement médical sur ordre d'un médecin ? Pour quelle maladie ? _____ |
| | | | Date du dernier examen médical _____    Date du dernier examen dentaire _____ |
| 5. | Oui | Non | Avez-vous eu des problèmes avec un traitement dentaire précédent ? |
| 6. | Oui | Non | Souffrez-vous actuellement ? |

## II. AVEZ-VOUS DÉJÀ EU :

| | | | | | | | |
|---|---|---|---|---|---|---|---|
| 7. | Oui | Non | Douleurs thoraciques (angine de poitrine) ? | 18. | Oui | Non | Vertiges ? |
| 8. | Oui | Non | Chevilles enflées ? | 19. | Oui | Non | Bourdonnement d'oreilles ? |
| 9. | Oui | Non | Essoufflement ? | 20. | Oui | Non | Maux de tête ? |
| 10. | Oui | Non | Perte de poids, fièvre, sueurs nocturnes, récemment ? | 21. | Oui | Non | Pertes de connaissance ? |
| 11. | Oui | Non | Toux persistante, toux sanglante ? | 22. | Oui | Non | Troubles de la vision ? |
| 12. | Oui | Non | Problèmes de saignements, contusions fréquentes ? | 23. | Oui | Non | Crises d'épilepsie ? |
| 13. | Oui | Non | Problèmes de sinus ? | 24. | Oui | Non | Soif excessive ? |
| 14. | Oui | Non | Difficultés à avaler ? | 25. | Oui | Non | Urination fréquente ? |
| 15. | Oui | Non | Diarrhées, constipation, sang dans les selles ? | 26. | Oui | Non | Xérostomie (bouche sèche) ? |
| 16. | Oui | Non | Vomissements fréquents, nausées ? | 27. | Oui | Non | Jaunisse ? |
| 17. | Oui | Non | Difficultés à uriner, sang dans les urines ? | 28. | Oui | Non | Douleurs articulaires, raideur articulaire ? |

## III. AVEZ-VOUS ACTUELLEMENT OU AVEZ-VOUS EU :

| | | | | | | | |
|---|---|---|---|---|---|---|---|
| 29. | Oui | Non | Maladie du cœur ? | 40. | Oui | Non | SIDA? |
| 30. | Oui | Non | Crise cardiaque, malformations cardiaques ? | 41. | Oui | Non | Tumeurs, cancer ? |
| 31. | Oui | Non | Souffles au cœur ? | 42. | Oui | Non | Arthrite, rhumatismes ? |
| 32. | Oui | Non | Rhumatisme articulaire aigu ? | 43. | Oui | Non | Maladies oculaires ? |
| 33. | Oui | Non | Accident vasculaire cérébral, durcissement des artères ? | 44. | Oui | Non | Maladies de peau ? |
| 34. | Oui | Non | Hypertension ? | 45. | Oui | Non | Anémie ? |
| 35. | Oui | Non | Asthme, tuberculose, emphysème pulmonaire, autres maladies pulmonaires ? | 46. | Oui | Non | MST (syphilis ou blennorragie) ? |
| | | | | 47. | Oui | Non | Herpès ? |
| 36. | Oui | Non | Hépatite, autres maladies du foie ? | 48. | Oui | Non | Maladies rénales, de la vessie ? |
| 37. | Oui | Non | Problèmes d'estomac, ulcères ? | 49. | Oui | Non | Maladies thyroïdiennes, surrénales ? |
| 38. | Oui | Non | Allergies : médicaments, aliments, produits médicaux, latex ? | 50. | Oui | Non | Diabète ? |
| 39. | Oui | Non | Antécédents familiaux de diabète, problèmes cardiaques, tumeurs ? | | | | |

## IV. AVEZ-VOUS ACTUELLEMENT OU AVEZ-VOUS EU :

| | | | | | | | |
|---|---|---|---|---|---|---|---|
| 51. | Oui | Non | Soins psychiatriques ? | 56. | Oui | Non | Hospitalisation ? |
| 52. | Oui | Non | Radiothérapie ? | 57. | Oui | Non | Transfusions sanguines ? |
| 53. | Oui | Non | Chimiothérapie ? | 58. | Oui | Non | Opérations chirurgicales ? |
| 54. | Oui | Non | Valvule prothétique ? | 59. | Oui | Non | Stimulateur cardiaque (Pacemaker) ? |
| 55. | Oui | Non | Articulation artificielle ? | 60. | Oui | Non | Lentilles de contact ? |

## V. CONSOMMEZ-VOUS ACTUELLEMENT :

| | | | | | | | |
|---|---|---|---|---|---|---|---|
| 61. | Oui | Non | Drogues à usage récréatif ? | 63. | Oui | Non | Tabac (sous toutes ses formes) ? |
| 62. | Oui | Non | Médicaments sur prescription, des médicaments obtenus sans ordonnance médicale (dont l'Aspirine), des remèdes naturels ? | 64. | Oui | Non | Alcool ? |

Veuillez indiquer : _____

## VI. POUR LES FEMMES UNIQUEMENT :

| | | | | | | | |
|---|---|---|---|---|---|---|---|
| 65. | Oui | Non | Êtes-vous actuellement ou pourriez-vous être enceinte ou allaitez-vous ? | 66. | Oui | Non | Prenez-vous actuellement des pilules contraceptives ? |

## VII. TOUS PATIENTS :

| | | | |
|---|---|---|---|
| 67. | Oui | Non | Avez-vous actuellement ou avez-vous eu toute autre maladie ou tout autre problème médical NON indiqué sur ce formulaire ? |

Si tel est le cas, veuillez expliquer : _____

*Je soussigné(e), déclare avoir répondu à chaque question le plus complètement et précisément possible, dans la mesure de mes connaissances. Je m'engage à informer mon dentiste de tout changement dans mon état de santé et (ou) de toute prise de médicaments.*

Signature du patient/de la patiente : _____    Date : _____

## REVUE DE RAPPEL :

1. Signature du patient/de la patiente _____    Date : _____

2. Signature du patient/de la patiente _____    Date : _____

3. Signature du patient/de la patiente _____    Date : _____

The Health History is created and maintained by the University of the Pacific School of Dentistry, San Francisco, California.
Support for the translation and dissemination of the Health Histories comes from MetLife Dental Care.

**Figure 4-2. History form in French.** Shown here is the University of the Pacific Arthur A. Dugoni School of Dentistry's health history form in French. The UOP health history form in English was translated, keeping the same question numbering sequence so that a clinician can compare the English health history to the patient's translated health history.

**MetLife**                     健康記錄                     **University of the Pacific**
                               Chinese

姓名: _____         病人身份號碼: _____
                                        出生日期: _____

**I. 選擇適當答案**（若不知道請留空）:
1.  是  否  您的健康是否良好?
2.  是  否  過去一年您的健康有沒有改變?
3.  是  否  過去三年有沒有住院或患重病?
            如果有，什麼原因? _____
4.  是  否  您現在是否在接受醫生治療?  什麼原因? _____
            上次全身檢查是何時: _____ 上次牙科檢查是何時: _____
5.  是  否  牙齒治療之後是否有過問題?
6.  是  否  您現在有無痛楚?

**II. 您曾否有下列症狀或疾病:**

| | | | | | | |
|---|---|---|---|---|---|---|
| 7. | 是 | 否 | 胸痛（狹心病）? | 18. | 是 否 | 頭暈? |
| 8. | 是 | 否 | 腳踝腫? | 19. | 是 否 | 耳鳴? |
| 9. | 是 | 否 | 呼吸急促? | 20. | 是 否 | 頭痛? |
| 10. | 是 | 否 | 最近體重減輕，發燒，夜汗? | 21. | 是 否 | 暈眩? |
| 11. | 是 | 否 | 咳嗽，咳血? | 22. | 是 否 | 眼花? |
| 12. | 是 | 否 | 流血問題，容易發瘀? | 23. | 是 否 | 癲癇（羊癲瘋）? |
| 13. | 是 | 否 | 鼻竇問題? | 24. | 是 否 | 極度口渴? |
| 14. | 是 | 否 | 吞食問題? | 25. | 是 否 | 尿頻? |
| 15. | 是 | 否 | 腹瀉，便秘，便血? | 26. | 是 否 | 口乾? |
| 16. | 是 | 否 | 嘔吐，噁心? | 27. | 是 否 | 黃膽? |
| 17. | 是 | 否 | 小便困難，尿血? | 28. | 是 否 | 關節疼痛，僵硬? |

**III. 您現在或過去是否有下列疾病:**

| | | | | | | |
|---|---|---|---|---|---|---|
| 29. | 是 | 否 | 心臟衰弱? | 40. | 是 否 | 愛滋病? |
| 30. | 是 | 否 | 心臟病發作，心臟有缺陷? | 41. | 是 否 | 腫瘤? 癌症? |
| 31. | 是 | 否 | 心雜音? | 42. | 是 否 | 風濕性關節炎? |
| 32. | 是 | 否 | 風濕熱? | 43. | 是 否 | 眼病? |
| 33. | 是 | 否 | 中風，血管硬化? | 44. | 是 否 | 皮膚病? |
| 34. | 是 | 否 | 高血壓? | 45. | 是 否 | 貧血? |
| 35. | 是 | 否 | 哮喘、肺結核、肺氣腫或其他肺疾病? | 46. | 是 否 | 性病（梅毒、淋病）? |
| 36. | 是 | 否 | 肝炎或其他肝病? | 47. | 是 否 | 皰疹? |
| 37. | 是 | 否 | 胃病（潰瘍）? | 48. | 是 否 | 腎病、膀胱病? |
| 38. | 是 | 否 | 食物、藥物或橡膠製品過敏? | 49. | 是 否 | 甲狀腺、腎上腺病? |
| 39. | 是 | 否 | 家族中有無糖尿病、心臟病、腫瘤病史? | 50. | 是 否 | 糖尿病? |

**IV. 您現在或過去是否有下列的疾病或治療:**

| | | | | | | |
|---|---|---|---|---|---|---|
| 51. | 是 | 否 | 精神病治療? | 56. | 是 否 | 住院? |
| 52. | 是 | 否 | 放射性治療? | 57. | 是 否 | 輸血? |
| 53. | 是 | 否 | 化學治療? | 58. | 是 否 | 手術? |
| 54. | 是 | 否 | 人工心臟瓣膜? | 59. | 是 否 | 心律調節器? |
| 55. | 是 | 否 | 人工關節? | 60. | 是 否 | 隱形眼鏡? |

**V. 您現在是否服用:**

| | | | | | | |
|---|---|---|---|---|---|---|
| 61. | 是 | 否 | 迷幻藥? | 63. | 是 否 | 香煙、雪茄或其他煙草製品? |
| 62. | 是 | 否 | 處方藥品、一般藥品（包括：阿司匹林）或天然藥材? | 64. | 是 否 | 飲酒? |

請説明: _____

**VI. 只限女士們;**

65.  是  否  您是否現在懷孕或哺乳，或可能懷孕?      66.  是  否  服避孕藥?

**VII. 所有病者:**

67.  是  否  您現在或以前是否有任何本表格中**沒有**列出的病症?
請説明: _____
我已經盡我所知完整及準確地回答上述每一個問題。 若有任何身體狀況或服藥方面的變化，我將通知我的牙科醫生。
簽名: _____                     日期: _____

**覆診:**
1. 簽名: _____                  日期: _____
2. 簽名: _____                  日期: _____
3. 簽名: _____                  日期: _____

The Health History is created and maintained by the University of the Pacific School of Dentistry, San Francisco, California.
Support for the translation and dissemination of the Health Histories comes from MetLife Dental Care.

**Figure 4-3.   History form in Chinese.** Shown here is the University of the Pacific Arthur A. Dugoni School of Dentistry's health history form in Chinese. The UOP health history form in English was translated, keeping the same question numbering sequence so that a clinician can compare the English health history to the patient's translated health history.

**MetLife**                                      تاریخچه تندرستی                                      **University of the Pacific**
Farsi

نام بیمار: _____

شماره شناسائی بیمار: _____

تاریخ تولد: _____

**I. دور جواب درست دایره بکشید.( اگر سئوالی را متوجه نمیشوید جایش را خالی بگذارید):**

1. بله    خیر    آیا از سلامت کامل برخوردارید؟
2. بله    خیر    آیا در یک سال اخیر تغییری در سلامتی شما حاصل شده است؟
3. بله    خیر    آیا در سه سال اخیر به علت بیماری مهمی در بیمارستان بستری شده اید؟
چرا؟ _____
4. بله    خیر    آیا در حال حاضر تحت نظر پزشکی هستید؟ به چه عنوان؟ _____
تاریخ آخرین معاینه پزشکی _____ تاریخ آخرین معاینه دندانپزشکی _____
5. بله    خیر    آیا با معالجات گذشته دندانپزشکی مشکل داشته اید؟
6. بله    خیر    آیا در حال حاضر درد دارید؟

**II. آیا تجربه کرده اید:**

| | | |
|---|---|---|
| 18. بله خیر   سرگیجه؟ | 7. بله خیر   درد سینه (آژین)؟ |
| 19. بله خیر   صدای زنگ در گوشها؟ | 8. بله خیر   تورم مچ پا؟ |
| 20. بله خیر   سردرد؟ | 9. بله خیر   نفس تنگی؟ |
| 21. بله خیر   احساس غش؟ | 10. بله خیر   کاهش وزن ، تب ، عرق کردن هنگام شب؟ |
| 22. بله خیر   تیرگی بینائی ؟ | 11. بله خیر   سرفه پی در پی، سرفه توام با خون؟ |
| 23. بله خیر   حمله ناگهانی؟ | 12. بله خیر   خونریزی، کبود شدن سریع؟ |
| 24. بله خیر   تشنگی بیش از حد؟ | 13. بله خیر   بیماری سینوس؟ |
| 25. بله خیر   ادرار مکرر؟ | 14. بله خیر   اشکال در بلعیدن؟ |
| 26. بله خیر   خشکی دهان؟ | 15. بله خیر   اسهال، یبوست، خون در مدفوع؟ |
| 27. بله خیر   زردی؟ | 16. بله خیر   استفراغ مکرر، حالت تهوع؟ |
| 28. بله خیر   درد مفاصل، سفتی مفاصل؟ | 17. بله خیر   به سختی ادرار کردن، خون در ادرار؟ |

**III. آیا شما دارید یا داشته اید:**

| | | |
|---|---|---|
| 40. بله خیر   ایدز؟ | 29. بله خیر   بیماری قلبی؟ |
| 41. بله خیر   غده، سرطان؟ | 30. بله خیر   سکته قلبی، نقص قلبی؟ |
| 42. بله خیر   التهاب مفاصل ، روماتیسم؟ | 31. بله خیر   صدا های غیر طبیعی قلب؟ |
| 43. بله خیر   بیماری چشم؟ | 32. بله خیر   تب روماتیسم؟ |
| 44. بله خیر   بیماری پوست؟ | 33. بله خیر   حمله قلبی، سفت شدن سرخ رگها؟ |
| 45. بله خیر   کم خونی؟ | 34. بله خیر   فشار خون بالا؟ |
| 46. بله خیر   بیماریهای جنسی  (سفلیس سوزاک)؟ | 35. بله خیر   آسم، سل، آمفیزم، دیگر بیماریهای ریه؟ |
| 47. بله خیر   تبخال؟ | 36. بله خیر   هپاتیت، دیگر بیماریهای کبد؟ |
| 48. بله خیر   بیماریهای کلیه ، مثانه؟ | 37. بله خیر   مشکلات معده ، زخم معده؟ |
| 49. بله خیر   بیماریهای تیروئید ، غده فوق کلیوی؟ | 38. بله خیر   آلرژی (حساسیت)  به دوا، غذا، دارو، شیرگیاهی؟ |
| 50. بله خیر   مرض قند؟ | 39. بله خیر   تاریخچه خانوادگی از نظر مرض قند، قلب ، غده؟ |

**IV. آیا شما دارید یا داشته اید:**

| | | |
|---|---|---|
| 56. بله خیر   بستری شدن در بیمارستان؟ | 51. بله خیر   معالجه روانپزشکی؟ |
| 57. بله خیر   انتقال خون؟ | 52. بله خیر   معالجات اشعه ای؟ |
| 58. بله خیر   جراحی؟ | 53. بله خیر   شیمی درمانی؟ |
| 59. بله خیر   دستگاه تنظیم کننده  ضربان قلب؟ | 54. بله خیر   دریچه مصنوعی قلب؟ |
| 60. بله خیر   عدسی تماسی؟ (کانتکت لنز) | 55. بله خیر   مفصل مصنوعی؟ |

**V. آیا شما استفاده می کنید:**

| | | |
|---|---|---|
| 63. بله خیر   تنباکو (از هر نوع)؟ | 61. بله خیر   مواد تفریحی (مواد مخدر)؟ |
| 64. بله خیر   الکل؟ | 62. بله خیر   دارو با نسخه ، بدون نسخه  از قبیل (آسپرین، مواد مخدر، دارو های  طبیعی |

لطفاً موارد بالا را  لیست کنید _____

**VI. خانمها فقط:**

| | |
|---|---|
| 66. بله خیر   آیا شما قرص جلوگیری از حاملگی استفاده میکنید؟ | 65. بله خیر   آیا شما باردار هستید یا میتوانید باردار باشید و یا کودکی را شیر میدهید؟ |

**VII. برای تمام بیماران:**

67. بله خیر   آیا شما هرنوع بیماری یا مشکلات دیگر پزشکی که در این فرم ذکر نشده است دارید یا داشته اید؟
اگر چنین است  لطفا توضیح بدهید: _____

من تمام سئوالات را کاملا و دقیقا جواب داده ام . من دندانپزشکم را از هر گونه تغییراتی در سلامتی خویش یا مصرف دارو مطلع خواهم کرد.

امضاء بیمار: _____ تاریخ: _____

مراجع مجدد:

1. امضاء بیمار: _____ تاریخ: _____
2. امضاء بیمار: _____ تاریخ: _____
3. امضاء بیمار: _____ تاریخ: _____

The Health History is created and maintained by the University of the Pacific School of Dentistry, San Francisco, California.
Support for the translation and dissemination of the Health Histories comes from MetLife Dental Care.

**Figure 4-4.   History form in Farsi.** Shown here is the University of the Pacific Arthur A. Dugoni School of Dentistry's health history form in Farsi. The UOP health history form in English was translated, keeping the same question numbering sequence so that a clinician can compare the English health history to the patient's translated health history.

SECTION 2:
# Informed Consent and the Medical History

The core value of "Individual Autonomy and Respect for Human Beings" within the Code of Ethics for the American Dental Hygienists' Association (ADHA) discusses informed consent.[1] According to this core value, "People . . . have the right to full disclosure of all relevant information so they can make informed choices about their care."

1. **Informed Consent for Patient Assessment**
   a. It is the responsibility of the dental hygienist to provide complete and comprehensive information about patient assessment procedures and planned dental hygiene treatments so that the patient can make a well-informed decision about either accepting or rejecting the proposed treatment.
   b. Informed consent not only involves informing the patient about the expected successful outcomes of assessment procedures but the possible risks, unanticipated outcomes, and alternative treatments as well. The patient also should be made aware of the costs for each of the options involved, which may influence the patient's ultimate decision.
2. **Capacity for Consent.** A patient must also have the capacity to consent.
   a. Capacity for consent—the ability of a patient to fully understand the proposed treatment, possible risks, unanticipated outcomes, and alternative treatments—takes into account the patient's age, mental capacity, and language comprehension.
   b. A dialogue between the patient and the hygienist is the best way to initiate the informed consent process.
3. **Informed Refusal.** Despite being informed of the proposed treatments, risks, and alternatives, the patient may decide to refuse one or more of the recommended assessment procedures. This is called "informed refusal."
   a. Autonomy, as defined by the ADHA Code of Ethics, guarantees "self-determination" of the patient and is linked to informed consent.[1]
   b. Only after the patient has received informed consent can a decision be made to either accept or reject the proposed treatment. Radiographs, fluoride treatments, and sealants are a few of the dental services for which patients have exercised informed refusal.
   c. Although refusal may not be the optimal choice of the treating hygienist, the patient has a right to make any decision about his or her treatments that only affects him or her personally and does not pose a threat to others.
   d. In the case of *Erickson v. Dilgard*, the patient's right of refusal of a blood transfusion was upheld by the court despite the possibility of causing the patient's death (*Erickson v. Dilgard*, 44 Misc. 2d 27, 252 N.Y.S. 2d 705 [Sup. Ct., 1962]). Patients may refuse treatment for a number of reasons, including religious beliefs, fear, or simply impulse. Proceeding with a treatment that has been refused by a patient can subject the clinician to liability for assault (causing fear) and/or battery (unconsented touching).

4. **Patient Responsibilities**

   a. The patient also has responsibilities and duties when receiving oral health care. One duty is to provide accurate responses on the medical history assessment regarding his or her current health status.

      1. In a case in Newfoundland, Canada, the judge stated that "... a patient has a duty to herself to do everything reasonably necessary to ensure she is properly diagnosed ... As part of that duty, the patient must disclose all relevant and pertinent information in order to permit ... a proper diagnosis of her medical condition."[2]

      2. Simply stated, the practitioner and patient relationship is a "two-way street." A practitioner should attempt to put the patient at ease when filling out a medical history so the patient is comfortable revealing the most private of medical details.

   b. For some patients, the obstacles of comprehending the medical history questions prevent them from filling out the forms completely. For others, there may be embarrassment in being truthful and fear of being judged or refused treatment.

   c. Other patients may ask about the necessity of filling out such a comprehensive medical history assessment when "I only want my teeth cleaned." All patients must be made aware of the link between systemic and oral health, as noted in the text, and the importance of an accurate medical history in order for the practitioner to provide optimal treatment. Box 4-2 provides an example of how a clinician might respond to a patient's questions about why it is necessary to fill out a comprehensive medical history in the dental office.

---

BOX **4-2**    **Sample Explanation on the Importance of a Medical History**

It is extremely important for you to fill out a complete and accurate medical history today. The decision about what treatments are best for you cannot be decided unless Dr. _____ is aware of all of your medical conditions and medications/supplements that you take. This information is needed to protect your health and, in turn, not cause you harm.

Some medical conditions require premedication, such as an antibiotic, before dental treatment. Some medical conditions may cause you to have a poor outcome of a proposed dental treatment. Some materials/drugs used in dentistry may conflict with medications you are presently taking and/or cause an adverse reaction. It is impossible to know how you are going to react to a given dental treatment if we are unaware of your total physical, mental, and dental heath. By taking the time to fill out comprehensive medical history, you can help Dr. _____ decide which dental treatments are optimal and designed specifically for you, without the possible risks of medical or dental complications.

It is also important that your medical history be reviewed at each appointment to account for any changes since your last visit. Even if you were in a week before, you could have started a new medication or had a medical procedure that could influence your dental treatment.

You and the dental team assume equal roles in your overall dental care. Your role is to provide correct medical information so that the dental team can, in turn, provide dental treatment individually designed for your dental care needs.

# Conducting a Medical History Assessment

To conduct a thorough medical history assessment, the dental health care provider must have a methodical plan for information gathering and review. The plan should prevent oversights or omissions of important information about the patient's medical history. This section describes a methodical plan for conducting the thorough medical history assessment required for safe patient treatment. The main steps in conducting a medical history assessment are (1) information gathering and (2) determination of medical risk.

The goal of the medical history assessment is to obtain complete information about the patient's past and present history of medical conditions and diseases, including prescription and over-the-counter (OTC) medications. One successful approach for obtaining information is to combine the use of a written questionnaire (such as the UOP form) completed by the patient with an interview of the patient. The interview provides an opportunity to clarify information and ask follow-up questions about information on the written questionnaire.

## INFORMATION GATHERING

The **information-gathering phase** of patient's medical history involves:

- **Reading thoroughly.** Carefully read every line and every check box on the history form completed by the patient.
- **Prioritizing.** Determine if the patient is in pain. If the patient is in pain, remember that alleviating pain takes precedence over other dental treatment.
- **Researching conditions.** Research medical conditions and diseases.
- **Researching drugs.** Research medications—prescription or OTC.
- **Formulating questions.** Formulate questions to ask the patient during the medical history interview.
- **Interviewing.** After a thorough review of the health history form, the clinician should interview the patient. In order to acquire a comprehensive picture of the patient's health and medications, the clinician asks questions to clarify information on the form and to obtain additional information.
- **Consulting.** Determine the need for a physician consultation.

## MEDICAL ALERT BOX

Medical conditions/diseases or medications that necessitate modifications or special precautions should be clearly marked in a **medical alert box** on the patient record (Box 4-3).

BOX 4-3  **Contents of Medical Alert Box**

- Any medical condition or disease that will alter dental treatment
- Any medical condition or disease that will alter drugs used during dental treatment or prescribed for the patient to treat dental conditions
- Any medical condition or disease that places the patient at risk for medical emergency during dental treatment
- Any medical condition or disease that could result in a postoperative complication

## RISK ASSESSMENT: PHYSICAL STATUS

At this stage in the health history assessment process, the dental health care provider should consider the patient's medical risk for undergoing dental treatment. Modification of dental treatment may be necessary in certain medically complex patients.[3] Today, many patients seen in the dental office have multiple medical conditions and are taking many medications. It is more difficult to manage these types of patients and thorough assessment of their physical status is an important part of clinical practice.

The American Society of Anesthesiologists, one of the pioneers in the field of patient safety in medical and dental care, developed a physical status system for assessing the risk to the patient of medical or dental treatment. The American Society of Anesthesiologists Physical Status Classification System (ASA-PS) serves an integral part of risk assessment in determining how the dental team should manage a patient.[3,4] The ASA physical status classification system is described in Table 4-1. This table outlines how a patient's physical status can affect the planning of dental care.

**Table 4-1** PHYSICAL STATUS IMPLICATIONS FOR DENTAL TREATMENT

|  | ASA-PS Classification | Modifications for Safe Patient Care |
|---|---|---|
| ASA 1 | • A normal healthy patient with little or no anxiety about dental treatment | • Green flag for dental treatment<br>• No treatment modifications |
| ASA 2 | • A patient with mild systemic disease<br>• ASA 1 patients who are anxious or fearful of dental treatment<br>• Examples: well-controlled diabetes, epilepsy, asthma | • Yellow flag for dental treatment<br>• Employ stress-reduction strategies |
| ASA 3 | • A patient with severe systemic disease that limits activity<br>• Examples: angina, stroke, heart attack, congestive heart failure | • Yellow flag for dental treatment<br>• Employ stress-reduction strategies<br>• Treatment modifications needed, such as antibiotic premedication |
| ASA 4 | • A patient with severe systemic disease that is a constant threat to life<br>• Examples: heart attack or stroke within the last 6 months | • Red flag for dental treatment<br>• Elective dental care should be postponed until patient's medical condition has improved to at least an ASA 3 classification. |

## BLOOD GLUCOSE LEVELS

Another example of how risk assessment for a patient can affect planned dental care is the blood glucose level for patients. Ready Reference 4-3 outlines common measures for a patient's blood glucose levels and how these findings relate to the risk of infection for planned treatment.

## CONSULTATION WITH A PHYSICIAN

If all health questions are not completely answered through research and the patient interview, or if there is any question or doubt in making the best decisions, consulting with the patient's physician is necessary. A consultation is simply a request for additional information and/or advice about the medical implications of oral health care treatment. A written request and reply referral is ideal because there is no doubt about either the question or the answer. Figures 4-5A and 4-5B provide an example of a written request form for consultation with a physician.

1. **Request in writing.** A consultation request may be faxed to the physician to expedite the process. The request should be specific, concise, and directly to the point; therefore, a consultation form may be used to standardize and simplify the written request and the physician's reply. All consultation requests should clearly indicate the following:
   a. Medical condition or disease of concern
   b. An explanation of the planned dental treatment and the likely systemic consequences
   c. A request for additional information and/or the physician's professional opinion
   d. The patient's signature authorizing the release of information; the dentist's signature; and the dental office's address, phone number, and fax number
   e. *Preferably, the consult form should be in triplicate.* One copy of the form is kept in the patient's chart, one copy is given to the patient for his or her records, and one is sent or faxed to the physician.
2. **Explain planned treatment.** When consulting with a physician, it is important to remember that the physician is a medical expert who may have little or no knowledge regarding dental treatment procedures and how these procedures may relate to the patient's medical health. The use of dental terminology or jargon should be avoided when explaining the planned dental treatment.
3. **Outline procedures.** When explaining the planned dental treatment to the physician, it is important to outline the procedures planned, length of time for each appointment, what surgical procedures will be done—including periodontal instrumentation; the amount of anticipated blood loss; possible complications, if any; and medications or anesthetics that will be used.
4. **Obtain patient consent.** Before contacting a patient's physician, the *patient must grant written consent* for the physician to release information about the patient's medical findings.
5. **Meet legal requirements.** Telephone consultations are not acceptable from a legal standpoint. If a consultation is conducted by telephone, request that the physician provide the information in writing by mail or fax.

# Medical Consultation Request

To Dr: **SAMUEL SNEED**
**620 MARKET STREET**
**ASHEVILLE, NC 28801**

RE: **MR. ALAN ASCARI**
**46 MAILSTRUM DRIVE**
**ARDEN, NC 28751**

Date of Birth: _____

Date **2/05/XX**

Please complete the form below and return to:
Dr: **MARK STEWART, DMD**
**1625 POPLAR DRIVE, SUITE 10**
**ASHEVILLE, NC 28801**
Phone: **(828) 555-9856**
Fax #: **(828) 555-9854**

**Dear Dr:** **SNEED** _____

The above named patient has presented with the following medical problem(s): _____

_____

| | | |
|---|---|---|
| _____ Adrenal insufficiency or steroid therapy | _____ Leukemia |
| _____ Anemia | _____ Mitral valve prolapse |
| _____ Anticoagulant therapy | _____ Pacemaker |
| _____ Bleeding disorder | _____ Prescription diet drugs |
| _____ Cardiovascular disease | _____ Prosthetic heart valve |
| _____ Chemotherapy | _____ Prosthetic joint |
| **X** Diabetes | _____ Pulmonary disease |
| _____ Drug allergies | _____ Radiation therapy to head/neck |
| _____ Endocarditis | _____ Renal dialysis with shunts |
| _____ Heart murmur | _____ Renal disease |
| _____ Hepatitis | _____ Rheumatic heart disease |
| _____ HIV | _____ Systemic lupus erythematosus |
| _____ Hypertension | _____ Systemic-pulmonary artery shunt |
| _____ Liver disease | _____ Other:_____ |

**Treatment to be performed on this patient includes:**

**X** Oral surgical procedures
_____ Extractions
_____ Endodontic treatment (root canal)
_____ Deep scaling (with some removal of epithelial tissue)
_____ Dental radiographs (x-rays)
_____ Use of magnetostrictive ultrasonic devices

_____ Local anesthesia obtained with 2% Lidocaine, 1:100,000 epinephrine
**X** Local anesthesia epinephrine concentration may be increased to 1:50,0000 for hemostasis, but will NOT exceed 0.2mg total

**Most patients experience the following with the above planned procedures:**

_____ Minimal bleeding with transient bacteria
**X** Prolonged bleeding
_____ Stress and anxiety: ___ Low **X** Moderate ___ High
_____ Other: _____

**X** Appointment length: **2 HOURS**
**X** Number and frequency of appointments: _____
**2 APPOINTMENTS AT**
**1 WEEK INTERVALS**

*Dr. Mark Stewart*
Dentist's Signature

**2/05/XX**
Date

**Figure 4-5A.** **Sample medical consultation request, page 1.** This form shows an example of page 1 of a completed medical consultant request for a fictitious patient, Mr. Alan Ascari. Page 2 of this request form is shown on the next page.

# Medical Consultation Request, page 2

I agree to the release of my medical information to: ___DR. MARK STEWART___

___Alan Ascari___                    ___2/05/XX___
Patient's Signature                    Date

## PHYSICIAN'S RESPONSE

**Please provide any information regarding the above patient's:**
- **Need for antibiotic prophylaxis**
- **Current cardiovascular condition**
- **Coagulation therapy**
- **History and status of infectious disease**

## CHECK ALL THAT APPLY:

_____ OK to **PROCEED** with dental treatment with **NO** special precautions and **NO** prophylactic antibiotics.

_____ Antibiotic prophylaxis **IS** required for dental treatment according to the American Heart Association and/or the American Academy of Orthopedic Surgeons guidelines.

_____ **OTHER PRECAUTIONS** are required (please list): _____

_____

_____

_____ **DO NOT PROCEED** with dental treatment (please provide reason):_____

_____

_____

_____ **DELAY** treatment until this date: _____ (please provide reason): _____

_____

_____

_____ Patient **HAS** infectious disease (please circle):

      AIDS (please provide current lab results)

      TB (PPD+/active)

      Hepatitis, Type _____ (acute / carrier)

      Other (explain): _____

_____

_____ Relevant medical and/or laboratory information is attached.

_____          _____
Physician's Signature              Date

**Figure 4-5B.   Sample medical consultation request, page 2.** Page 2 of a sample medical consultation form shows the patient's signature, giving his physician permission to release medical information to the dental office. The remainder of the form is for the physician's response.

## STRESS REDUCTION PROTOCOL FOR ANXIOUS PATIENTS

An upcoming dental appointment causes considerable anxiety and stress for some patients. For anxious patients, stress reduction strategies are recommended (Box 4-4).

---

### BOX 4-4   Strategies for Stress Reduction

- **Good Communication.** Use empathy and effective communication to establish trust and determine the cause(s) of the patient's anxiety.
- **Reduce Anxiety.** Premedicate as needed with an antianxiety medication for use (a) the night before the appointment to aid the patient in getting a good night's sleep and (b) the day of the appointment.
- **Scheduling.** Schedule appointments early in the day so that patient will not have all day to worry about the upcoming treatment.
- **Suggestions for Patient.** Suggest that the patient eat a normal meal before the appointment and allow ample travel time to get to the dental office or clinic.
- **Length of Treatment.** Keep appointments short.
- **Pain Control.** Ensure good pain control before, during, and after the appointment as appropriate, including the use of pain medications and local anesthesia.

## SECTION 4:
# Peak Procedure

**PROCEDURE 4-1**  REVIEW OF WRITTEN QUESTIONNAIRE AND PATIENT INTERVIEW

| Action | Rationale |
|---|---|
| **1.** Read through every line and check box. Are all the questions answered? | • Complete information is important to protect the patient's health. |
| **2.** Can you understand what is written? | • Make a note to ask the patient about anything that is not clear. |
| **3.** Did the patient sign and date the form? | • The history must be signed and dated. |
| **4.** Circle **YES** responses in red pencil. | • YES answers should be discussed during the interview. |
| **5.** Read through handwritten responses made by the patient. Circle concerns in red pencil. | • Discuss concerns during the interview. |
| **6.** Research medical conditions and diseases including:<br>a. Definition<br>b. Symptoms or manifestations<br>c. Treatments and medications<br>d. Systemic side effects that may necessitate treatment modifications<br>e. Oral manifestations<br>f. Impact on dental care | • This is basic data that will be used to formulate questions for the patient and to determine if dental care involves any risks for the patient.<br><br>Common medical conditions and diseases may be researched by using the Ready References found in Module 5. |
| **7.** Identify risks to the patient's overall health such as poorly controlled diabetes, obesity, periodontal disease, and tobacco use.<br><br>Identify systemic factors that increase the risk of periodontal disease, such as tobacco use, poorly controlled diabetes, hormone alterations, psychosocial stress, and medications.<br><br>**Circle concerns in red pencil.** | • Dental health care providers should identify systemic health risks and promote wellness.<br>• There is a connection between periodontitis and overall systemic health. Periodontal infection may contribute to the development of heart disease, premature/underweight babies, poorly controlled diabetes, and respiratory diseases.<br>• Dental health care providers should be alert for systemic factors that may increase the risk of developing periodontal disease. |

*(continued)*

**PROCEDURE 4-1**     **REVIEW OF WRITTEN QUESTIONNAIRE AND PATIENT INTERVIEW** *(CONTINUED)*

| Action | Rationale |
|---|---|
| **8.** Research the patient's medications, prescribed and nonprescription, including:<br>a. Drug use<br>b. Systemic side effects<br>c. Oral side effects<br>d. Dental treatment modifications or concerns<br><br>Medications can be researched on the Internet, in drug reference books, and using the Ready References found in Module 5 of this book. | • It is important to determine why each medication is being taken.<br>• Some patients are not knowledgeable about their medical conditions. In such cases, medications can be a valuable clue to the patient's health status.<br>• Many medications have systemic side effects that may necessitate modifications to dental treatment. For example, many medications cause dizziness or orthostatic hypotension, thus, indicating that the clinician should adjust the chair position slowly.<br>• Other medications have side effects that can alter a patient's dental health. Xerostomia, gingival overgrowth, and gingival bleeding are examples of oral side effects.<br>• Some medications dictate modifications or precautions before, during, or after dental treatment. For example, Coumadin reduces the ability of the blood to clot. |
| **9.** Ask the patient questions about his or her medical conditions or diseases.<br>a. **Duration**—When was the condition first diagnosed?<br>b. **Treatments and Procedures**—What is being done to treat the condition?<br>c. **Episodes**—What brings on the condition? What changes the severity? | • This factual information is important in determining whether the patient can be treated safely.<br>• Certain medical conditions and diseases have oral manifestations.<br>• Certain medical conditions affect the health of the periodontium. |
| **10.** Ask the patient questions about the medications, prescription and OTC, as well as any supplements that he or she is taking.<br>a. How long? Date started and ended<br>b. How much? Dosage | • This factual information is important in determining whether the patient can be treated safely.<br>• Certain medical conditions and diseases have oral manifestations. |

## SECTION 5:
# Ready References

NOTE: The Ready References in this book may be removed from the book by tearing along the perforated lines on each page. Laminating or placing these pages in plastic protector sheets will allow them to be disinfected for use in a clinical setting.

**READY REFERENCE 4-1** INTERNET RESOURCES: CONDITIONS/DISEASES

The surest way to obtain the most current information on a medical condition, disease, or drug is by using the Internet.

- **Restricted Access Sites.** Some college libraries subscribe to websites requiring a password. The password allows access to reference books and scientific journals.

- **Public Access Sites.** There is a wealth of information on the Internet, however, that is free to the public. All the websites listed below allow public access without a password.

- **Help.** Refer to Peak Procedure 2-1 in Module 2 for directions on how to search the Internet.

**http://medlineplus.gov/**
**MedlinePlus** provides health information from the National Library of Medicine, including information on diseases and conditions, drug information, and a medical encyclopedia.

**http://www.nlm.nih.gov/medlineplus/tutorials/**
MedlinePlus presents interactive health tutorials from the Patient Education Institute. The tutorials explain the symptoms, diagnosis, and treatment for a variety of diseases and conditions. Other tutorials explain surgeries, prevention, and wellness. Each tutorial includes animated graphics, audio, and easy-to-read language.

**http://www.ncbi.nlm.nih.gov/entrez/query.fcgi**
**PubMed** is the National Library of Medicine's free search service, which includes over 15 million citations for biomedical articles dating back to the 1950s. PubMed includes links to many sites providing full-text articles and other related resources.

**http://www.healthfinder.gov/library/**
The **Healthfinder** website, a service of the National Health Information Center, has a library of reliable health information. Information includes a guide to diseases and conditions, medical dictionaries, and prescription drug information.

**http://www.mercksource.com**
The **Merck Source** website has health information on medical conditions and diseases.

**http://my.webmd.com/webmd_today/home/default**
The **WebMD Health** website has information on diseases and conditions plus a medical library.

**http://www.mayoclinic.com/index.cfm**
The **Mayo Clinic** website has information on diseases and conditions. This site also includes information on drugs and supplements.

## READY REFERENCE 4-2   INTERNET RESOURCES: DRUG REFERENCES

**http://www.nlm.nih.gov/medlineplus/druginformation.html**
MedlinePlus has information on thousands of prescription and OTC medications.

**http://www.accessdata.fda.gov/scripts/cder/drugsatfda/**
**U.S. Food and Drug Administration** website provides a drug database and a glossary.

**http://www.medicinenet.com/**
The **MedicineNet** website has information on medical conditions and medications.

**http://www.pdrhealth.com/drug_info/rxdrugprofiles/alphaindexa.shtm**l
This site includes a Family Guide to Prescription Drugs.

**http://www.drugs.com/**
**Drugs.com** provides drug information resources online. Fast, easy searching of over 24,000 approved medications.

**http://www.rxlist.com/top200a.htm**
**RxList** provides an Internet drug index.

## READY REFERENCE 4-3   GLUCOSE BLOOD LEVELS IN DIABETES

| Test | Glucose Levels |
|------|----------------|
| Hemoglobin $A_{1c}$ | Goal for most people with diabetes = less than 7% |
| | High susceptibility to infection = above 8% |
| Finger-stick test | Glucose level at appointment time: |
| | • Acceptable = 80–120 mg/dl |
| | • Risk of infection = 180–300 mg/dl |
| | • Unacceptable = greater than 300 mg/dl |

> **NOTE:** The next module, **Module 5: Ready References: Medical History**, contains two Ready References designed to provide fast access to commonly encountered medical conditions and medications.
>
> * Ready Reference 5-1: Common Conditions of Concern in Dentistry
> * Ready Reference 5-2: Commonly Prescribed Drugs

## REFERENCES

1. American Dental Hygienists' Association. *Bylaws and Code of Ethics*. Chicago, IL: American Dental Hygienists' Association; 2009.
2. Malik P. The perils of omission. *Can J Cardiol*. 2006;22(12):1011.
3. Maloney WJ, Weinberg MA. Implementation of the American Society of Anesthesiologists Physical Status classification system in periodontal practice. *J Periodontol*. 2008;79(7): 1124–1126.
4. Malamed SF, Robbins KS. *Medical Emergencies in the Dental Office*. 5th ed. St. Louis, MO: Mosby; 2000.

## SUGGESTED READINGS

American Dental Association. *ADA Guide to Dental Therapeutics*. 3rd ed. Chicago, IL: American Dental Association Pub.; 2003.

Beemsterboer P. *Ethics and Law in Dental Hygiene*. 2nd ed. St. Louis, MO: Saunders/ Elsevier; 2010.

Dexter F, Thompson E. Relative value guide basic units in operating room scheduling to ensure compliance with anesthesia group policies for surgical procedures performed at each anesthetizing location. *AANA J*. 2001;69(2):120–123.

Fremgen BF. *Medical Law and Ethics*. 4th ed. Upper Saddle River, NJ: Pearson/Prentice Hall; 2010.

Garcia-Miguel FJ, Serrano-Aguilar PG, Lopez-Bastida J. Preoperative assessment. *Lancet*. 2003;362(9397):1749–1757.

Kimbrough-Walls V, Jautar C. *Ethics, Jurisprudence & Practice Management in Dental Hygiene*. 3rd ed. Upper Saddle River, NJ: Pearson; 2012.

Moore VA. Make the connection: the exceptional new patient interview. *J Calif Dent Assoc*. 1997;25(4):305–311.

Rule JT, Veatch RM. *Ethical Questions in Dentistry*. 2nd ed. Chicago, IL: Quintessence Pub.; 2004.

## SECTION 6:

# The Human Element

---

**BOX 4-5    Through the Eyes of a Student**

*It was my third week of clinic, and I was feeling quite confident about medical history assessments. I started thinking that the lecture we had in clinic theory on assessing medical histories was very unrealistic. The example the instructor gave us was a patient on seven different drugs and who had three different diseases.*

*Well today was the day! The health history form seemed to have as many questions checked in the "Yes" column as the "No" column. I started to panic, thinking that it was going to take me all day to review the medical history and that the patient would be upset with me for taking so long. The patient was overweight and had diabetes, high blood pressure, and high cholesterol. She checked "yes" to chest pain on exertion, sleep disorder, and being out of breath. Her medications included several cardiac drugs as well as insulin.*

*I began looking things up in a reference book when my instructor looked over my shoulder and asked me if I had ever heard of "metabolic syndrome." I looked it up in a reference book. Suddenly, all the "Yes" questions made sense. I felt I had a handle on the patient's overall condition. That confidence allowed me to readily gather the rest of the information, link it together, and conduct the patient interview. It turned out to be a great appointment. My patient was so nice, and I learned a lot about her and her health history.*

*Stephanie, student*
*Tallahassee Community College*

---

**PATIENT SCENARIO**

Your last patient of the morning is Sandy L., a 17-year-old who is new to the dental practice. Her mother is sitting with Sandy in the waiting room, helping her fill out her medical history assessment. You call Sandy into your operatory. Her mother tells you that she will wait for Sandy and would like to speak to the dentist before she is discharged today.

You begin reviewing Sandy's medical history with her, which appears uneventful. After you complete her extraoral and intraoral exams, you discuss with Sandy the office policy of taking radiographs on new patients. Sandy states that she has not had any x-rays in a few years and agrees. As you are about to place the first radiograph in her mouth, Sandy begins to cry. Assuming she has fear of the dental office, you stop and try to comfort her. Sandy states that she has no fear but suspects that she may be pregnant and has heard that radiation "could harm the baby." Sandy pleads with you not to tell anyone, especially her mother.

1. What is the best way for you to handle this ethical dilemma?
2. Can a 17-year-old consent to treatment, or must you receive parental consent?
3. Under the ethical principle of confidentiality, can you discuss this with your employer dentist, without violating Sandy's confidentiality?
4. Do you have the right to divulge Sandy's pregnancy to her mother?

## ENGLISH-TO-SPANISH PHRASE LISTS

### USING THE ENGLISH-TO-SPANISH PHRASE LISTS

According to the Bureau of the Census, more than one-half of the 2002 foreign-born residents in the United States were born in Latin America. Communication problems can occur when an English-speaking clinician tries to communicate with a patient who is not fluent in English.

- Teaching student clinicians to pronounce and speak Spanish is well beyond the scope of this book and, indeed, of most professional curriculums.

- For those times when a trained medical translator is not available, the modules in this textbook include English-to-Spanish phrase lists with phrases pertinent to the assessment process. The first of these phrase lists is found in Table 4-2 on the following page.

- To use these phrase lists, the student clinician simply points to a specific phrase in the patient's native language to facilitate communication.

**Table 4-2**   ENGLISH-TO-SPANISH PHRASE LIST FOR MEDICAL HISTORY ASSESSMENT

| | |
|---|---|
| Good morning (afternoon), Mr. _____. | Buenos días (tardes), señor _____. |
| Good morning (afternoon), Mrs. _____. | Buenos días (tardes), señora _____. |
| Good morning (afternoon), Miss _____. | Buenos días (tardes) señorita _____. |
| My name is ____. I am your dental hygienist. | Me llama _____. Soy su higienista dental. |
| It is nice to meet you. | Mucho gusto en conocerlo (conocerla). |
| I do not speak Spanish; I will point to Spanish phrases. | No hablo español; voy a indicar las frases en español. |
| Please follow me to the dental chair. | Por favor siga me a la silla dental. |
| Please turn to the right. | Por favor valla a la derecha. |
| Please turn to the left. | Por favor valla a la izquierda. |
| Please sit here in this chair. | Por favor siéntese en esta silla. |
| You forgot to answer this question. | Se olvidó responder esta pregunta. |
| Do you have your medications with you? | ¿Tiene sus medicinas con usted? |
| Please bring your medications with you for your next appointment. | Por favor traiga sus medicinas con usted a su próximo cita. |
| Why do you take these medications? | ¿Por que tome usted estos medicamentos? |
| Please sign here. | Por favor firme aquí. |
| We cannot do dental treatment until we consult with your doctor. | No podemos hacer un tratamiento hasta que consultemos con su doctor. |
| Wait here, I will get the dentist or instructor. | Espere aquí; voy a buscar el dentista o el profesor. |
| We are finished for today. | Hemos terminado por hoy. |
| We will schedule your next appointment. | Vamos a hacer una nueva cita. |
| Goodbye, see you next time. | Hasta luego; la (lo) veremos la próxima cita. |

## SECTION 7:

# Practical Focus—Fictitious Patient Cases

This section contains the medical history and medication list for five fictitious patients, Patients A–E. In addition, Health History Interview and Medical Consultation Request forms are provided for Patients A–E (Figs. 4-6 to 4-25).

> **DIRECTIONS:**
>
> • Remove the forms for Patients A–E from the book for ease of use.
>
> • For each patient, follow the steps outlined below to conduct an assessment of the medical history and medications.

1. **Review Medical History**
   • Carefully read the patient's completed medical history form.
   • Circle all "Yes" answers in red.
   • Circle any unanswered questions.
2. **Research Medical Conditions and Diseases**
   • Research all medical conditions and diseases. Start by locating the Ready Reference 5-1: Medical Conditions and Diseases, found in **Module 5** of this book.
   • As needed, conduct additional research. If a computer connected to the Internet is available, go online to locate additional information. If you do not have a computer, use oral medicine books to do additional research.
3. **Research Medications—Prescription and OTC**
   • Research all medications.
   • Start by using Ready Reference 5-2: Common Prescription Medications, found in **Module 5** of this book.
   • As needed, conduct additional research either on the Internet or using drug reference books.
4. **Summarize Information and Formulate Questions**
   • Complete the Health History Interview form for each patient.
   • At this point—after reviewing the patient's medical history, medications, and doing your research—do you have concerns about treating the patient?
   • Do you think any modifications will need to be made in order to treat this patient safely?
   • Make a list of follow-up questions that you should ask during the patient interview. Write your questions on page 2 of the health history interview form.
5. **Determine if a Medical Consultation is Needed**
   • For each patient, assess the need for a medical consultation. If needed, complete page 1 of the Medical Consultation Request.

MetLife                                                                                          University of the Pacific

### HEALTH HISTORY · English

Patient Name: _Ascari,    Alan    A._          Patient Identification Number: _A-546390_

Birth Date: _70 years_

### I. CIRCLE APPROPRIATE ANSWER (leave BLANK if you do not understand question):

1. (Yes)  No     Is your general health good?
2. Yes  (No)    Has there been a change in your health within the last year?
3. (Yes)  No     Have you been hospitalized or had a serious illness in the last three years?
   If YES, why? _too little insulin_
4. (Yes)  No     Are you being treated by a physician now? For what? _diabetes_
   Date of last medical exam? _6 months_          Date of last dental exam? _about 5 years ago_
5. Yes  (No)    Have you had problems with prior dental treatment?
6. Yes  (No)    Are you in pain now?

### II. HAVE YOU EXPERIENCED:

| | | |
|---|---|---|
| 7. Yes (No) | Chest pain (angina)? | 18. Yes (No) Dizziness? |
| 8. Yes (No) | Swollen ankles? | 19. Yes (No) Ringing in ears? |
| 9. Yes (No) | Shortness of breath? | 20. Yes (No) Headaches? |
| 10. (Yes) No | Recent weight loss, fever, night sweats? | 21. Yes (No) Fainting spells? |
| 11. Yes (No) | Persistent cough, coughing up blood? | 22. Yes (No) Blurred vision? |
| 12. Yes (No) | Bleeding problems, bruising easily? | 23. Yes (No) Seizures? |
| 13. Yes (No) | Sinus problems? | 24. Yes (No) Excessive thirst? |
| 14. Yes (No) | Difficulty swallowing? | 25. Yes (No) Frequent urination? |
| 15. Yes (No) | Diarrhea, constipation, blood in stools? | 26. (Yes) No Dry mouth? |
| 16. Yes (No) | Frequent vomiting, nausea? | 27. Yes (No) Jaundice? |
| 17. Yes (No) | Difficulty urinating, blood in urine? | 28. (Yes) No Joint pain? |

### III. DO YOU HAVE OR HAVE YOU HAD:

| | | |
|---|---|---|
| 29. Yes (No) | Heart disease? | 40. Yes (No) AIDS? |
| 30. Yes (No) | Heart attack, heart defects? | 41. Yes (No) Tumors, cancer? |
| 31. Yes (No) | Heart murmurs? | 42. Yes (No) Arthritis, rheumatism? |
| 32. Yes (No) | Rheumatic fever? | 43. Yes (No) Eye diseases? |
| 33. Yes (No) | Stroke, hardening of arteries? | 44. Yes (No) Skin deases? |
| 34. Yes (No) | High blood pressure? | 45. Yes (No) Anemia? |
| 35. Yes (No) | Asthma, TB, emphysema, other lung disease? | 46. Yes (No) VD (syphilis or gonorrhea)? |
| 36. Yes (No) | Hepatitis, other liver disease? | 47. Yes (No) Herpes? |
| 37. Yes (No) | Stomach problems, ulcers? | 48. Yes (No) Kidney, bladder disease? |
| 38. Yes (No) | Allergies to: drugs, foods, medications, latex? | 49. Yes (No) Thyroid, adrenal disease? |
| 39. Yes (No) | Family history of diabetes, heart problems, tumors? | 50. (Yes) No Diabetes? |

### IV. DO YOU HAVE OR HAVE YOU HAD:

| | | |
|---|---|---|
| 51. Yes (No) | Psychiatric care? | 56. Yes (No) Hospitalization? |
| 52. Yes (No) | Radiation treatments? | 57. Yes (No) Blood transfusions? |
| 53. Yes (No) | Chemotherapy? | 58. Yes (No) Surgeries? |
| 54. Yes (No) | Prosthetic heart valve? | 59. Yes (No) Pacemaker? |
| 55. Yes (No) | Artificial joint? | 60. Yes (No) Contact lenses? |

### V. ARE YOU TAKING:

| | | |
|---|---|---|
| 61. Yes (No) | Recreational drugs? | 63. (Yes) No Tobacco in any form? _Smoke 2 packs a day_ |
| 62. (Yes) No | Drugs, medications, over-the-counter medicines (including Aspirin), natural remedies? | 64. Yes (No) Alcohol? |

Please list: _See Medication List_

### VI. WOMEN ONLY:

65. Yes (No)    Are you or could you be pregnant or nursing?          63. Yes (No)    Taking birth control pills?

### VII. ALL PATIENTS:

64. (Yes)  No     Do you have or have you had anyother diseases or medical problems NOT listed on this form?
If so, please explain: _teeth very sensitive to cold drinks and ice cream; dry mouth_

To the best of my knowledge, I have answered every question completely and accurately. I will inform my dentist of any change in my health and/or medication.

Patient's signature: _Alan A. Ascari_                                           Date: _1-15-20XX_

### RECALL REVIEW:

1. Patient's signature: _____          Date: _____
2. Patient's signature: _____          Date: _____
3. Patient's signature: _____          Date: _____

The Health History is created and maintained by the University of Pacific School of Dentistry, San Francisco, California.
Support for the translation and dissemination of the Health Histories comes from MetLife Dental Care.

**Figure 4-6.** The health history form for fictitious patient Mr. Ascari.

# Medication List

Patient _____ALAN ASCARI_____          Date _____1/15/XX_____

| PRESCRIBED |
| --- |
| HUMULIN R: ONE INJECTION TWICE A DAY |

| OVER-THE-COUNTER |
| --- |
| DAYQUIL LIQUICAP |
| NYQUIL |

| VITAMINS, HERBS, DIET SUPPLEMENTS |
| --- |
| CHROMIUM 100 MCG PER D |
| ALPHA LIPOIC ACID 200 MG PER DAY |

**Figure 4-7.** Medication list for fictitious patient Mr. Ascari.

## Health History Interview: PART 1

Patient Name: _Ascari, Alan A._

Directions: Record the number and details of any YES answer noted on the Health History.

| Number | Significant Medical Findings | Dental Management Considerations |
|---|---|---|
| | | |
| | | |
| | | |
| | | |
| | | |
| | | |
| | | |
| | | |
| | | |
| | | |
| | | |
| | | |
| | | |

| Medications | Dental Management Considerations |
|---|---|
| | |
| | |
| | |
| | |
| | |
| | |
| | |
| | |
| | |
| | |
| | |

_____     _____     _____

Date               Student Clinician Signature                    Instructor Signature

Figure 4-8A.  Mr. Ascari: Health history synopsis part 1.

## Health History Interview: PART 2

Patient Name:    _Ascari, Alan A._

### Additional Information or Consultations
**Directions:** List any additional information that should be obtained before dental treatment begins.

### Questions for Patient Interview
**Directions:** Formulate a list of questions for the patient interview.

**Figure 4-8B.**    Mr. Ascari: Health history synopsis part 2.

# Medical Consultation Request

To Dr: _____

_____

_____

RE: _____

_____

_____

Date of Birth: _____

Date _____

**Please complete the form below and return to:**

Dr: _____

_____

_____

Phone: _____

Fax #: _____

**Dear Dr:** _____

The above named patient has presented with the following medical problem(s): _____

_____

| | |
|---|---|
| _____ Adrenal insufficiency or steroid therapy | _____ Leukemia |
| _____ Anemia | _____ Mitral valve prolapse |
| _____ Anticoagulant therapy | _____ Pacemaker |
| _____ Bleeding disorder | _____ Prescription diet drugs |
| _____ Cardiovascular disease | _____ Prosthetic heart valve |
| _____ Chemotherapy | _____ Prosthetic joint |
| _____ Diabetes | _____ Pulmonary disease |
| _____ Drug allergies | _____ Radiation therapy to head/neck |
| _____ Endocarditis | _____ Renal dialysis with shunts |
| _____ Heart murmur | _____ Renal disease |
| _____ Hepatitis | _____ Rheumatic heart disease |
| _____ HIV | _____ Systemic lupus erythematosus |
| _____ Hypertension | _____ Systemic-pulmonary artery shunt |
| _____ Liver disease | _____ Other: _____ |

## Treatment to be performed on this patient includes:

_____ Oral surgical procedures

_____ Extractions

_____ Endodontic treatment (root canal)

_____ Deep scaling (with some removal of epithelial tissue)

_____ Dental radiographs (x-rays)

_____ Use of magnetostrictive ultrasonic devices

_____ Local anesthesia obtained with 2% Lidocaine, 1:100,000 epinephrine

_____ Local anesthesia epinephrine concentration may be increased to 1:50,0000 for hemostasis, but will NOT exceed 0.2mg total

## Most patients experience the following with the above planned procedures:

_____ Minimal bleeding with transient bacteria

_____ Prolonged bleeding

_____ Stress and anxiety: ___ Low ___ Moderate ___ High

_____ Other: _____

_____ Appointment length: _____

_____ Number and frequency of appointments: _____

_____

_____

_____ 
Dentist's Signature

_____ 
Date

**Figure 4-9.** Page 1 of medical consultation request for Mr. Ascari (if needed).

HEALTH HISTORY - Children's

Name of Child: _Biddle,_____ _Bethany_____ _B._____
                   Last                        First                      Middle

Birth Date: _Age 9_____    Child's Gender:  M  (F)

Custodial Parent's or Guardian's Name: _Brenda Biddle_____    Relationship to Child: _Mother_____

Address: _311 First Avenue, Hendersonville_____ _NC_____ _28777_____
             City:                                  State:                Zip Code:

Phone Numbers: __(828) 555-6153_____   __(828) 555-4367_____   __(828) 555-8707_____
                   Home:                       Work:                       Cell:

Name and Phone Number for the Child's Physician: _Dr. Mary Mercer___ _(828) 555-2345_____

### I. DOES THE CHILD HAVE OR HAS THE CHILD HAD ANY OF THE CONDITIONS/DISEASES BELOW?

1.  Yes  (No)   Anemia?
2.  (Yes) No    Asthma or Breathing Problems? _Asthma_
3.  Yes  (No)   Arthritis or Joint Problems?
4.  Yes  (No)   Attention Disorder?
5.  Yes  (No)   Bleeding or Clotting Disorder?
6.  Yes  (No)   Cancer or Chemotherapy?
7.  Yes  (No)   Diabetes?
8.  Yes  (No)   Fainting Spells?
9.  Yes  (No)   Ear or Hearing Problems?
10. Yes  (No)   Heart Defect or Problems?

11. Yes  (No)   Hepatits?
12. Yes  (No)   HIV/AIDS?
13. Yes  (No)   Hyperactivity Disorder?
14. Yes  (No)   Kidney or Liver Problems?
15. Yes  (No)   Mononucleosis?
16. Yes  (No)   Persistent Cough or Coughing up Blood?
17. Yes  (No)   Rheumatic Fever?
18. Yes  (No)   Seizures or Epilpsy?
19. Yes  (No)   Tuberculosis?

### II. FOR EACH ITEM BELOW LIST THE INFORMATION REQUESTED FOR THE CHILD:

Allergies/Sensitivities to Medications, Food, or other Substances:
Please list: _latex (hives and breathing difficulty); penicillin, bananas, seafood_____

Concerns about Social or Developmental needs:
Please list: _none_____

Current Immunizations:
Please list: _meningitis; pneumonia, hepatitis A and B; polio, measles, mumps, rubella, varicella, flu_

Hopsitalizations:
Please list: _6 months ago for severe asthma attacks_____

Inherited Problems:
Please list: _none_____

Serious Injuries:
Please list: _none_____

Over-the-Counter Medications or Supplements being taken:
Please list: _See Medication List_____

Prescription Medications being taken:
Please list: _See Medication List_____

Vitamins, Herbs, or Diet Supplements being taken:
Please list: _See Medication List_____

Has the Child had or does the Child have any diseases or conditions not already listed on this form?     Yes     (No)

If yes, please explain: _____

_To the best of my knowledge, I have answered every question completely and accurately. I will inform my dentist of any change in my health and/or medication._

Parent's or Guardian's signature: _Brenda Biddle_____    Date: _1-10-20XX_____

**Figure 4-10.**  Health history form for fictitious patient Bethany Biddle.

# Medication List

Patient ___BETHANY BIDDLE___          Date ___1/10/XX___

| PRESCRIBED |
| --- |

FLOVENT ROTADISK 50MCG: 1 INHALATION TWICE A DAY
SEREVENT DISCUS: 1 INHALATION TWICE A DAY
ZYRTEC CHEWABLE TABLETS: 5MG THREE TIMES A DAY
VENTOLIN INHALER, WHEN NEEDED FOR ATTACK

| OVER-THE-COUNTER |
| --- |

| VITAMINS, HERBS, DIET SUPPLEMENTS |
| --- |

FLINTSTONES MULTIVITAMINS

**Figure 4-11.**  Medication list for fictitious patient Bethany Biddle.

## Health History Interview: PART 1

Patient Name: _Biddle, Bethany B._

Directions:    Record the number and details of any YES answer noted on the Health History.

| Number | Significant Medical Findings | Dental Management Considerations |
|---|---|---|
|  |  |  |
|  |  |  |
|  |  |  |
|  |  |  |
|  |  |  |
|  |  |  |
|  |  |  |
|  |  |  |
|  |  |  |
|  |  |  |
|  |  |  |
|  |  |  |
|  |  |  |
|  |  |  |

| Medications | Dental Management Considerations |
|---|---|
|  |  |
|  |  |
|  |  |
|  |  |
|  |  |
|  |  |
|  |  |
|  |  |
|  |  |
|  |  |
|  |  |

_____    _____    _____

Date          Student Clinician Signature                  Instructor Signature

Figure 4-12A.    Bethany Biddle: Health history synopsis part 1.

## Health History Interview: PART 2

Patient Name: _Biddle, Bethany B._

**Additional Information or Consultations**
**Directions:** List any additional information that should be obtained before dental treatment begins.

**Questions for Patient Interview**
**Directions:** Formulate a list of questions for the patient interview.

**Figure 4-12B.** Bethany Biddle: Health history synopsis part 2.

# Medical Consultation Request

To Dr: _____

_____

_____

RE: _____

_____

_____

Date of Birth: _____

Date _____

**Please complete the form below and return to:**

Dr: _____

_____

Phone: _____

Fax #: _____

**Dear Dr:**_____

The above named patient has presented with the following medical problem(s): _____

_____

_____ Adrenal insufficiency or steroid therapy

_____ Anemia

_____ Anticoagulant therapy

_____ Bleeding disorder

_____ Cardiovascular disease

_____ Chemotherapy

_____ Diabetes

_____ Drug allergies

_____ Endocarditis

_____ Heart murmur

_____ Hepatitis

_____ HIV

_____ Hypertension

_____ Liver disease

_____ Leukemia

_____ Mitral valve prolapse

_____ Pacemaker

_____ Prescription diet drugs

_____ Prosthetic heart valve

_____ Prosthetic joint

_____ Pulmonary disease

_____ Radiation therapy to head/neck

_____ Renal dialysis with shunts

_____ Renal disease

_____ Rheumatic heart disease

_____ Systemic lupus erythematosus

_____ Systemic-pulmonary artery shunt

_____ Other:_____

## Treatment to be performed on this patient includes:

_____ Oral surgical procedures

_____ Extractions

_____ Endodontic treatment (root canal)

_____ Deep scaling (with some removal of epithelial tissue)

_____ Dental radiographs (x-rays)

_____ Use of magnetostrictive ultrasonic devices

_____ Local anesthesia obtained with 2% Lidocaine, 1:100,000 epinephrine

_____ Local anesthesia epinephrine concentration may be increased to 1:50,0000 for hemostasis, but will NOT exceed 0.2mg total

## Most patients experience the following with the above planned procedures:

_____ Minimal bleeding with transient bacteria

_____ Prolonged bleeding

_____ Stress and anxiety: ___ Low ___ Moderate ___ High

_____ Other: _____

_____ Appointment length:_____

_____ Number and frequency of appointments:_____

_____

_____

Dentist's Signature _____      Date _____

**Figure 4-13.** Page 1 of medical consultation request for Bethany Biddle (if needed).

MetLife                                                                University of the Pacific

## HISTORIA MÉDICA - Spanish

Nombre del paciente: *Chavez, Carlos C.*     No. de Ident. del Paciente: *C-093841*

Fecha de nacimiento: *25 años (25 years)*

### I. MARQUE CON UN CÍRCULO LA RESPUESTA CORRECTA (Deje en BLANCO si no entiende la pregunta):

1. (Sí) No — ¿Está en buena salud general?
2. Sí (No) — ¿Han habido cambios en su salud durante el último año?
3. Sí (No) — ¿Ha estado hospitalizado/a o ha tenido de una enfermedad grave en los últimos tres años?
   ¿Si Sí, por qué? _____
4. (Sí) No — ¿Se encuentra actualmente bajo tratamiento médico? ¿Para qué? *Epilepsía (epilepsy)*

   Fecha de su último examen médico: *Hace un año (1 year ago)* Fecha de su última cita dental: *Hace dos años (2 years ago)*
5. Sí (No) — ¿Ha tenido problemas con algún tratamiento dental en el pasado?
6. Sí (No) — ¿Tiene algún dolor ahora?

### II. HA NOTADO:

7. Sí (No) — ¿Dolor de pecho (angina)?
8. Sí (No) — ¿Los tobillos hinchados?
9. Sí (No) — ¿Falta de aliento?
10. Sí (No) — ¿Reciente pérdida de peso, fiebre, sudor en la noche?
11. Sí (No) — ¿Tos persistente o tos con sangre?
12. Sí (No) — ¿Problemas de sangramiento, moretes?
13. Sí (No) — ¿Problemas nasales (sinusitis)?
14. Sí (No) — ¿Dificultad al tragar?
15. Sí (No) — ¿Diarrea, estreñimiento, sangre en las heces?
16. Sí (No) — ¿Vómitos con frecuencia, náuseas?
17. Sí (No) — ¿Dificltad al orinar, sangre en la orina?

18. Sí (No) — ¿Mareos?
19. Sí (No) — ¿Ruidos o zumbidos en los oídos?
20. (Sí) No — ¿Dolores de cabeza? *migranas*
21. Sí (No) — ¿Desmayos?
22. Sí (No) — ¿Vista borrosa?
23. (Sí) No — ¿Convulsiones?
24. Sí (No) — ¿Sed excesiva?
25. Sí (No) — ¿Orina con frecuencia?
26. Sí (No) — ¿Boca seca?
27. Sí (No) — ¿Ictericia?
28. Sí (No) — ¿Dolor o rigidez en las articulaciones?

### III. TIENE O HA TENIDO:

29. Sí (No) — ¿Enfermedades del corazón?
30. Sí (No) — ¿Infarto de corazón, defectos en el corazón?
31. Sí (No) — ¿Soplos en la corazón?
32. Sí (No) — ¿Fiebre reumática?
33. Sí (No) — ¿Apoplejía, endurecimiento de las arterias?
34. Sí (No) — ¿Presión sanguínea alta?
35. Sí (No) — ¿Asma, tuberculosis, enfisema, otras enfermedades pulmonares?
36. Sí (No) — ¿Hepatitis, otras enfermedades del hígado?
37. Sí (No) — ¿Problemas del estómago, úlceras?
38. Sí (No) — ¿Alergias a remedios, comidas, medicamentos látex?
39. Sí (No) — ¿Familiares con diabetes, problemas de corazón, tumores?

40. Sí (No) — ¿SIDA?
41. Sí (No) — ¿Tumores, cáncer?
42. Sí (No) — ¿Artritis, reuma?
43. Sí (No) — ¿Enfermedades de los ojos?
44. Sí (No) — ¿Enfermedades de la piel?
45. Sí (No) — ¿Anemia?
46. Sí (No) — ¿Enfermedades venéreas (sífilis o gonorrea)?
47. Sí (No) — ¿Herpes?
48. Sí (No) — ¿Enfermedades renales (riñión), vejiga?
49. Sí (No) — ¿Enfermedades de tiroides o glándulas suprarrenales?
50. Sí (No) — ¿Diabetes?

### IV. TIENE O HA TENIDO:

51. Sí (No) — ¿Tratamiento psiquiátrico?
52. Sí (No) — ¿Tratamientos de radiación?
53. Sí (No) — ¿Quimioterapia?
54. Sí (No) — ¿Válvula artificial del corazón?
55. Sí (No) — ¿Articulación articial?

56. Sí (No) — ¿Hospitalizaciones?
57. Sí (No) — ¿Transfusiones de sangre?
58. Sí (No) — ¿Circugías?
59. Sí (No) — ¿Marcapasos?
60. Sí (No) — ¿Lentes de contacto?

### V. ESTÁ TOMANDO:

61. Sí (No) — ¿Drogas de uso recreativo?
62. (Sí) No — ¿Remedios, medicamentos, medicamentos sin receta (incluyendo aspirina)?

63. (Sí) No — ¿Tabaco de cualquier tipo?
64. (Sí) No — ¿Alcohol (bebidas alcohólicas)? *4 Cervesas (4 beers per week)*

Liste por favor: *Ver lista adjunta (see attached list)*

### VI. SÓLO PARA MUJERES:

65. Sí (No) — ¿Está o podría estar embarazada o dando pecho?

63. Sí No — ¿Está tomando pastillas anticonceptivas?

### VII. PARA TODOS LOS PACIENTES:

64. Sí (No) — ¿Tiene o ha tenido alguna otra enfermedad o problema médico que NO está en este cuestionario?
Si la respuesta es afirmativa, explique: *Ulceas en la boca (ulcers in mouth)*

*Que yo sepa, he respondido completamente y correctamente todas las preguntas. Informaré a mi dentista si hay algún cambio en mi salud y/o en los medicamentos que tomo.*

Firma del Paciente: *Carlos C. Chavez*     Fecha: *1-15-20XX*

### REVISIÓN SUPLEMENTARIA:

1. Firma del Paciente: _____ Fecha: _____
2. Firma del Paciente: _____ Fecha: _____
3. Firma del Paciente: _____ Fecha: _____

**The Health History is created and maintained by the University of Pacific School of Dentistry, San Francisco, California.
Support for the translation and dissemination of the Health Histories comes from MetLife Dental Care.**

**Figure 4-14.** The health history form for fictitious patient Mr. Chavez.

# Medication List

Patient __CARLOS CHAVEZ__          Date __1/05/XX__

## PRESCRIBED

PHENYTOIN 100MG THREE TIMES A DAY

## OVER-THE-COUNTER

ASPIRIN FOR STRAINED MUSCLE IN BACK

## VITAMINS, HERBS, DIET SUPPLEMENTS

**Figure 4-15.**  Medication list for fictitious patient Mr. Chavez.

## Health History Interview: PART 1

Patient Name: _Chavez, Carlos C._

Directions: Record the number and details of any YES answer noted on the Health History.

| Number | Significant Medical Findings | Dental Management Considerations |
|---|---|---|
| | | |
| | | |
| | | |
| | | |
| | | |
| | | |
| | | |
| | | |
| | | |
| | | |
| | | |
| | | |
| | | |
| | | |

| Medications | Dental Management Considerations |
|---|---|
| | |
| | |
| | |
| | |
| | |
| | |
| | |
| | |
| | |
| | |
| | |

| | | |
|---|---|---|
| _____ | _____ | _____ |
| Date | Student Clinician Signature | Instructor Signature |

Figure 4-16A. Mr. Chavez: Health history synopsis part 1.

## Health History Interview: PART 2

Patient Name: _Chavez, Carlos C._

### Additional Information or Consultations
**Directions:** List any additional information that should be obtained before dental treatment begins.

### Questions for Patient Interview
**Directions:** Formulate a list of questions for the patient interview.

**Figure 4-16B.**    Mr. Chavez: Health history synopsis part 2.

# Medical Consultation Request

To Dr: _____

_____

_____

RE: _____

_____

_____

Date of Birth: _____

Date _____

**Please complete the form below and return to:**

Dr: _____

_____

_____

Phone: _____

Fax #: _____

**Dear Dr:**_____

The above named patient has presented with the following medical problem(s): _____

_____

_____ Adrenal insufficiency or steroid therapy

_____ Anemia

_____ Anticoagulant therapy

_____ Bleeding disorder

_____ Cardiovascular disease

_____ Chemotherapy

_____ Diabetes

_____ Drug allergies

_____ Endocarditis

_____ Heart murmur

_____ Hepatitis

_____ HIV

_____ Hypertension

_____ Liver disease

_____ Leukemia

_____ Mitral valve prolapse

_____ Pacemaker

_____ Prescription diet drugs

_____ Prosthetic heart valve

_____ Prosthetic joint

_____ Pulmonary disease

_____ Radiation therapy to head/neck

_____ Renal dialysis with shunts

_____ Renal disease

_____ Rheumatic heart disease

_____ Systemic lupus erythematosus

_____ Systemic-pulmonary artery shunt

_____ Other:_____

## Treatment to be performed on this patient includes:

_____ Oral surgical procedures

_____ Extractions

_____ Endodontic treatment (root canal)

_____ Deep scaling (with some removal of epithelial tissue)

_____ Dental radiographs (x-rays)

_____ Use of magnetostrictive ultrasonic devices

_____ Local anesthesia obtained with 2% Lidocaine, 1:100,000 epinephrine

_____ Local anesthesia epinephrine concentration may be increased to 1:50,0000 for hemostasis, but will NOT exceed 0.2mg total

## Most patients experience the following with the above planned procedures:

_____ Minimal bleeding with transient bacteria

_____ Prolonged bleeding

_____ Stress and anxiety: ___ Low ___ Moderate ___ High

_____ Other: _____

_____ Appointment length:_____

_____ Number and frequency of appointments:_____

_____

_____

Dentist's Signature _____          Date _____

**Figure 4-17.** Page 1 of medical consultation request for Mr. Chavez (if needed).

MetLife                                                                                                    University of the Pacific

### HEALTH HISTORY - English

Patient Name: _Doi,  Donna  D._                    Patient Identification Number: _D-912540_

Birth Date: _27 years_

### I. CIRCLE APPROPRIATE ANSWER (leave BLANK if you do not understand question):

1. (Yes)  No    Is your general health good?
2. Yes  (No)    Has there been a change in your health within the last year?
3. Yes  (No)    Have you been hospitalized or had a serious illness in the last three years?
          If YES, why? _____
4. (Yes)  No    Are you being treated by a physician now? For what? _5 months pregnant with first child_
          Date of last medical exam? _last week_          Date of last dental exam? _6 months ago_
5. Yes  (No)    Have you had problems with prior dental treatment?
6. Yes  (No)    Are you in pain now? _Bleeding gums_

### II. HAVE YOU EXPERIENCED:

| | | |
|---|---|---|
| 7. Yes (No) | Chest pain (angina)? | 18. Yes (No) Dizziness? |
| 8. Yes (No) | Swollen ankles? | 19. Yes (No) Ringing in ears? |
| 9. Yes (No) | Shortness of breath? | 20. (Yes) No Headaches? _migraines_ |
| 10. Yes (No) | Recent weight loss, fever, night sweats? | 21. Yes (No) Fainting spells? |
| 11. Yes (No) | Persistent cough, coughing up blood? | 22. Yes (No) Blurred vision? |
| 12. Yes (No) | Bleeding problems, bruising easily? | 23. Yes (No) Seizures? |
| 13. (Yes) No | Sinus problems? | 24. Yes (No) Excessive thirst? |
| 14. Yes (No) | Difficulty swallowing? | 25. Yes (No) Frequent urination? |
| 15. Yes (No) | Diarrhea, constipation, blood in stools? | 26. Yes (No) Dry mouth? |
| 16. Yes (No) | Frequent vomiting, nausea? | 27. Yes (No) Jaundice? |
| 17. Yes (No) | Difficulty urinating, blood in urine? | 28. Yes (No) Joint pain? |

### III. DO YOU HAVE OR HAVE YOU HAD:

| | | |
|---|---|---|
| 29. Yes (No) | Heart disease? | 40. Yes (No) AIDS? |
| 30. Yes (No) | Heart attack, heart defects? | 41. Yes (No) Tumors, cancer? |
| 31. Yes (No) | Heart murmurs? | 42. Yes (No) Arthritis, rheumatism? |
| 32. Yes (No) | Rheumatic fever? | 43. Yes (No) Eye diseases? |
| 33. Yes (No) | Stroke, hardening of arteries? | 44. Yes (No) Skin deases? |
| 34. Yes (No) | High blood pressure? | 45. Yes (No) Anemia? |
| 35. Yes (No) | Asthma, TB, emphysema, other lung disease? | 46. Yes (No) VD (syphilis or gonorrhea)? |
| 36. Yes (No) | Hepatitis, other liver disease? | 47. Yes (No) Herpes? |
| 37. Yes (No) | Stomach problems, ulcers? | 48. Yes (No) Kidney, bladder disease? |
| 38. (Yes) No | Allergies to: drugs, foods, medications, latex? _Aspirin, cats_ 49. Yes (No) Thyroid, adrenal disease? |
| 39. Yes (No) | Family history of diabetes, heart problems, tumors? | 50. Yes (No) Diabetes? |

### IV. DO YOU HAVE OR HAVE YOU HAD:

| | | |
|---|---|---|
| 51. Yes (No) | Psychiatric care? | 56. (Yes) No Hospitalization? _for knee replacement_ |
| 52. Yes (No) | Radiation treatments? | 57. Yes (No) Blood transfusions? |
| 53. Yes (No) | Chemotherapy? | 58. Yes (No) Surgeries? |
| 54. Yes (No) | Prosthetic heart valve? | 59. Yes (No) Pacemaker? |
| 55. (Yes) No | Artificial joint? _knee replacement, 3 years ago_ | 60. Yes (No) Contact lenses? |

### V. ARE YOU TAKING:

| | | |
|---|---|---|
| 61. Yes (No) | Recreational drugs? | 63. Yes (No) Tobacco in any form? |
| 62. (Yes) No | Drugs, medications, over-the-counter medicines (including Aspirin), natural remedies? | 64. Yes (No) Alcohol? |

Please list: _See Medication List_ _____

### VI. WOMEN ONLY:

65. (Yes)  No    Are you or could you be pregnant or nursing?          63. Yes  (No)    Taking birth control pills?

### VII. ALL PATIENTS:

64. (Yes)  No    Do you have or have you had anyother diseases or medical problems NOT listed on this form?
If so, please explain: _frequent heartburn during pregnancy; hay fever_

To the best of my knowledge, I have answered every question completely and accurately. I will inform my dentist of any change in my health and/or medication.

Patient's signature: _Donna Doi_                                        Date: _1-15-20XX_

### RECALL REVIEW:

1. Patient's signature: _____    Date: _____

2. Patient's signature: _____    Date: _____

3. Patient's signature: _____    Date: _____

The Health History is created and maintained by the University of Pacific School of Dentistry, San Francisco, California.
Support for the translation and dissemination of the Health Histories comes from MetLife Dental Care.

**Figure 4-18.**  The health history form for fictitious patient Mrs. Doi.

# Medication List

Patient _____ DONNA DOI _____          Date _____ 1/30/XX _____

| PRESCRIBED |
|---|
| PRENATAL VITAMINS |

| OVER-THE-COUNTER |
|---|
| SALINE NASAL SPRAY FOR DRY NOSE |

| VITAMINS, HERBS, DIET SUPPLEMENTS |
|---|
| METAMUCIL 1 TSP. PER DAY |

**Figure 4-19.**   Medication list for fictitious patient Mrs. Doi.

## Health History Interview: PART 1

Patient Name: _Doi, Donna D._

**Directions:**    Record the number and details of any YES answer noted on the Health History.

| Number | Significant Medical Findings | Dental Management Considerations |
|---|---|---|
|  |  |  |
|  |  |  |
|  |  |  |
|  |  |  |
|  |  |  |
|  |  |  |
|  |  |  |
|  |  |  |
|  |  |  |
|  |  |  |
|  |  |  |
|  |  |  |
|  |  |  |

| Medications | Dental Management Considerations |
|---|---|
|  |  |
|  |  |
|  |  |
|  |  |
|  |  |
|  |  |
|  |  |
|  |  |
|  |  |
|  |  |
|  |  |

Date            Student Clinician Signature                    Instructor Signature

**Figure 4-20A.**    Mrs. Doi: Health history synopsis part 1.

## Health History Interview: PART 2

Patient Name: _Doi, Donna D._

### Additional Information or Consultations
**Directions:** List any additional information that should be obtained before dental treatment begins.

### Questions for Patient Interview
**Directions:** Formulate a list of questions for the patient interview.

**Figure 4-20B.** Mrs. Doi: Health history synopsis part 2.

# Medical Consultation Request

To Dr: _____

RE: _____

Date of Birth: _____

Date _____

**Please complete the form below and return to:**

Dr: _____

Phone: _____

Fax #: _____

**Dear Dr:**_____

**The above named patient has presented with the following medical problem(s):**_____

_____

_____ Adrenal insufficiency or steroid therapy

_____ Anemia

_____ Anticoagulant therapy

_____ Bleeding disorder

_____ Cardiovascular disease

_____ Chemotherapy

_____ Diabetes

_____ Drug allergies

_____ Endocarditis

_____ Heart murmur

_____ Hepatitis

_____ HIV

_____ Hypertension

_____ Liver disease

_____ Leukemia

_____ Mitral valve prolapse

_____ Pacemaker

_____ Prescription diet drugs

_____ Prosthetic heart valve

_____ Prosthetic joint

_____ Pulmonary disease

_____ Radiation therapy to head/neck

_____ Renal dialysis with shunts

_____ Renal disease

_____ Rheumatic heart disease

_____ Systemic lupus erythematosus

_____ Systemic-pulmonary artery shunt

_____ Other:_____

**Treatment to be performed on this patient includes:**

_____ Oral surgical procedures

_____ Extractions

_____ Endodontic treatment (root canal)

_____ Deep scaling (with some removal of epithelial tissue)

_____ Dental radiographs (x-rays)

_____ Use of magnetostrictive ultrasonic devices

_____ Local anesthesia obtained with 2% Lidocaine, 1:100,000 epinephrine

_____ Local anesthesia epinephrine concentration may be increased to 1:50,0000 for hemostasis, but will NOT exceed 0.2mg total

**Most patients experience the following with the above planned procedures:**

_____ Minimal bleeding with transient bacteria

_____ Prolonged bleeding

_____ Stress and anxiety: __ Low __ Moderate __High

_____ Other: _____

_____ Appointment length:_____

_____ Number and frequency of appointments:_____

_____

_____

Dentist's Signature

Date

**Figure 4-21.**    Page 1 of medical consultation request for Mrs. Doi (if needed).

MetLife                                                                                    University of the Pacific

**HEALTH HISTORY - English**

Patient Name: _Eads, Esther  E._          Patient Identification Number: _E-073218_

Birth Date: _79 years_

**I. CIRCLE APPROPRIATE ANSWER (leave BLANK if you do not understand question):**

1. Yes (No)   Is your general health good?
2. Yes No     Has there been a change in your health within the last year?
3. (Yes) No   Have you been hospitalized or had a serious illness in the last three years?
   If YES, why? _heart valve replaced and bypass surgery_
4. (Yes) No   Are you being treated by a physician now? For what? _Heart problems_
   Date of last medical exam? _6 weeks ago_          Date of last dental exam? _2 years ago_
5. Yes (No)   Have you had problems with prior dental treatment?
6. Yes (No)   Are you in pain now?

**II. HAVE YOU EXPERIENCED:**

| | | | | | | |
|---|---|---|---|---|---|---|
| 7. | Yes (No) | Chest pain (angina)? | 18. | Yes (No) | Dizziness? |
| 8. | (Yes) No | Swollen ankles? | 19. | Yes (No) | Ringing in ears? |
| 9. | (Yes) No | Shortness of breath? | 20. | Yes (No) | Headaches? |
| 10. | Yes (No) | Recent weight loss, fever, night sweats? | 21. | Yes (No) | Fainting spells? |
| 11. | Yes (No) | Persistent cough, coughing up blood? | 22. | Yes (No) | Blurred vision? |
| 12. | Yes (No) | Bleeding problems, bruising easily? | 23. | Yes (No) | Seizures? |
| 13. | (Yes) No | Sinus problems? | 24. | Yes (No) | Excessive thirst? |
| 14. | Yes (No) | Difficulty swallowing? | 25. | Yes (No) | Frequent urination? |
| 15. | Yes (No) | Diarrhea, constipation, blood in stools? | 26. | Yes (No) | Dry mouth? |
| 16. | Yes (No) | Frequent vomiting, nausea? | 27. | Yes (No) | Jaundice? |
| 17. | Yes (No) | Difficulty urinating, blood in urine? | 28. | Yes (No) | Joint pain? |

**III. DO YOU HAVE OR HAVE YOU HAD:**

| | | | | | | |
|---|---|---|---|---|---|---|
| 29. | (Yes) No | Heart disease? | 40. | Yes (No) | AIDS? |
| 30. | (Yes) No | Heart attack, heart defects? _6 months ago_ | 41. | Yes (No) | Tumors, cancer? |
| 31. | Yes (No) | Heart murmurs? | 42. | Yes (No) | Arthritis, rheumatism? |
| 32. | Yes (No) | Rheumatic fever? | 43. | Yes (No) | Eye diseases? |
| 33. | Yes (No) | Stroke, hardening of arteries? | 44. | Yes (No) | Skin deases? |
| 34. | (Yes) No | High blood pressure? | 45. | Yes (No) | Anemia? |
| 35. | Yes (No) | Asthma, TB, emphysema, other lung disease? | 46. | Yes (No) | VD (syphilis or gonorrhea)? |
| 36. | Yes (No) | Hepatitis, other liver disease? | 47. | Yes (No) | Herpes? |
| 37. | Yes (No) | Stomach problems, ulcers? | 48. | Yes (No) | Kidney, bladder disease? |
| 38. | (Yes) No | Allergies to: drugs, foods, medications, latex? _Aspirin, Penicillin_ | 49. | Yes (No) | Thyroid, adrenal disease? |
| 39. | Yes (No) | Family history of diabetes, heart problems, tumors? | 50. | Yes (No) | Diabetes? |

**IV. DO YOU HAVE OR HAVE YOU HAD:**

| | | | | | | |
|---|---|---|---|---|---|---|
| 51. | Yes (No) | Psychiatric care? | 56. | (Yes) No | Hospitalization? |
| 52. | Yes (No) | Radiation treatments? | 57. | (Yes) No | Blood transfusions? |
| 53. | Yes (No) | Chemotherapy? | 58. | (Yes) No | Surgeries? |
| 54. | (Yes) No | Prosthetic heart valve? | 59. | Yes (No) | Pacemaker? |
| 55. | Yes (No) | Artificial joint? | 60. | Yes (No) | Contact lenses? |

**V. ARE YOU TAKING:**

| | | | | | | |
|---|---|---|---|---|---|---|
| 61. | Yes (No) | Recreational drugs? | 63. | Yes (No) | Tobacco in any form? |
| 62. | (Yes) No | Drugs, medications, over-the-counter medicines (including Aspirin), natural remedies? | 64. | Yes (No) | Alcohol? |

Please list: _See Medication List_

**VI. WOMEN ONLY:**

| | | | | | | |
|---|---|---|---|---|---|---|
| 65. | Yes (No) | Are you or could you be pregnant or nursing? | 63. | Yes (No) | Taking birth control pills? |

**VII. ALL PATIENTS:**

64. (Yes) No   Do you have or have you had anyother diseases or medical problems NOT listed on this form?
If so, please explain: _osteoporosis; frequent infections of my legs_

_To the best of my knowledge, I have answered every question completely and accurately. I will inform my dentist of any change in my health and/or medication._

Patient's signature: _Esther E. Eads_                                    Date: _1-15-20XX_

**RECALL REVIEW:**

1. Patient's signature: _____   Date: _____

2. Patient's signature: _____   Date: _____

3. Patient's signature: _____   Date: _____

The Health History is created and maintained by the University of Pacific School of Dentistry, San Francisco, California.
Support for the translation and dissemination of the Health Histories comes from MetLife Dental Care.

**Figure 4-22.**   The health history form for fictitious patient Ms. Eads.

# Medication List

**Patient** ESTHER EADS          **Date** 1/24/XX

| PRESCRIBED |
| --- |
| WARFARIN 5MG ONCE A DAY |
| CALAN SR (VERAPAMIL) 240MG EACH MORNING |
| ENALAPRIL 5MG TWICE A DAY |
| SIMVASTATIN 5MG ONCE A DAY IN PM |

| OVER-THE-COUNTER |
| --- |

| VITAMINS, HERBS, DIET SUPPLEMENTS |
| --- |
| MELATONIN ONE TABLET EACH EVENING |

**Figure 4-23.**    Medication list for fictitious patient Ms. Eads.

## Health History Interview: PART 1

Patient Name: _Eads, Esther E._

**Directions:** Record the number and details of any YES answer noted on the Health History.

| Number | Significant Medical Findings | Dental Management Considerations |
|--------|------------------------------|----------------------------------|
|        |                              |                                  |
|        |                              |                                  |
|        |                              |                                  |
|        |                              |                                  |
|        |                              |                                  |
|        |                              |                                  |
|        |                              |                                  |
|        |                              |                                  |
|        |                              |                                  |
|        |                              |                                  |
|        |                              |                                  |
|        |                              |                                  |
|        |                              |                                  |

| Medications | Dental Management Considerations |
|-------------|----------------------------------|
|             |                                  |
|             |                                  |
|             |                                  |
|             |                                  |
|             |                                  |
|             |                                  |
|             |                                  |
|             |                                  |
|             |                                  |
|             |                                  |
|             |                                  |

Date        Student Clinician Signature        Instructor Signature

**Figure 4-24A.** Ms. Eads: Health history synopsis part 1.

## Health History Interview: PART 2

Patient Name: _Eads, Esther E._

**Additional Information or Consultations**
**Directions:** List any additional information that should be obtained before dental treatment begins.

**Questions for Patient Interview**
**Directions:** Formulate a list of questions for the patient interview.

**Figure 4-24B.**    Ms. Eads: Health history synopsis part 2.

# Medical Consultation Request

To Dr: _____

_____

_____

RE: _____

_____

_____

Date of Birth: _____

Date _____

**Please complete the form below and return to:**

Dr: _____

_____

_____

Phone: _____

Fax #: _____

**Dear Dr:**_____

The above named patient has presented with the following medical problem(s): _____

_____

_____ Adrenal insufficiency or steroid therapy

_____ Anemia

_____ Anticoagulant therapy

_____ Bleeding disorder

_____ Cardiovascular disease

_____ Chemotherapy

_____ Diabetes

_____ Drug allergies

_____ Endocarditis

_____ Heart murmur

_____ Hepatitis

_____ HIV

_____ Hypertension

_____ Liver disease

_____ Leukemia

_____ Mitral valve prolapse

_____ Pacemaker

_____ Prescription diet drugs

_____ Prosthetic heart valve

_____ Prosthetic joint

_____ Pulmonary disease

_____ Radiation therapy to head/neck

_____ Renal dialysis with shunts

_____ Renal disease

_____ Rheumatic heart disease

_____ Systemic lupus erythematosus

_____ Systemic-pulmonary artery shunt

_____ Other:_____

## Treatment to be performed on this patient includes:

_____ Oral surgical procedures

_____ Extractions

_____ Endodontic treatment (root canal)

_____ Deep scaling (with some removal of epithelial tissue)

_____ Dental radiographs (x-rays)

_____ Use of magnetostrictive ultrasonic devices

_____ Local anesthesia obtained with 2% Lidocaine, 1:100,000 epinephrine

_____ Local anesthesia epinephrine concentration may be increased to 1:50,0000 for hemostasis, but will NOT exceed 0.2mg total

## Most patients experience the following with the above planned procedures:

_____ Minimal bleeding with transient bacteria

_____ Prolonged bleeding

_____ Stress and anxiety: ___ Low ___ Moderate ___ High

_____ Other: _____

_____ Appointment length:_____

_____ Number and frequency of appointments:_____

_____

_____

_____

Dentist's Signature

_____

Date

**Figure 4-25.**   Page 1 of medical consultation request for Ms. Eads (if needed).

## SECTION 8:
# Skill Check

**TECHNIQUE SKILL CHECKLIST:**     MEDICAL HISTORY QUESTIONNAIRE

Student: _____     Evaluator: _____

Date: _____

**DIRECTIONS FOR STUDENT:** Use **Column S**, evaluate your skill level as **S** (satisfactory) or **U** (unsatisfactory).

**DIRECTIONS FOR EVALUATOR:** Use **Column E**. Indicate **S** (satisfactory) or **U** (unsatisfactory). In the optional grade percentage calculation, each **S** equals 1 point, each **U** equals 0 points.

| CRITERIA | S | E |
|---|---|---|
| **Reads through every line and "Yes/No" answer on the completed health history form. Identifies any unanswered questions on the health history form and follows up to obtain complete information.** | | |
| **Makes notes about any information that is not clear or difficult to read. Confirms that the patient has signed and dated the form.** | | |
| **Circles YES responses in red. Reads through all handwritten responses and circles concerns in red.** | | |
| **Researches medical conditions and diseases including definition, symptoms, and manifestations. Lists potential impact on oral health and any treatment concerns or needed modifications for dental treatment.** | | |
| **Researches all prescription and OTC medications. Lists potential impact on oral health and any concerns or needed modifications for dental treatment.** | | |
| **Formulates a list of follow-up questions for the patient interview.** | | |
| **Formulates a preliminary opinion of the medical risk to the patient of dental treatment and whether a medical consult will be needed. (After completing the patient interview, discusses medical risk and need for medical consultation with a clinical instructor.)** | | |

OPTIONAL GRADE PERCENTAGE CALCULATION

Each **S** equals 1 point and each **U** equals 0 points. Using the **E** column, total the sum of the "**S**"s _____ divided by the total points possible (7) to calculate the percentage grade.

## COMMUNICATION SKILL CHECKLIST: ROLE-PLAY FOR MEDICAL HISTORY

Student: _____    Evaluator: _____

Date: _____

---

**Roles:**

- Student 1 = Plays the role of a fictitious patient.
- Student 2 = Plays the role of the clinician.
- Student 3 or Instructor = Plays the role of the clinic instructor near the end of the role-play.

---

**DIRECTIONS FOR STUDENT CLINICIAN:** Use **Column S**, evaluate your skill level as **S** (satisfactory) or **U** (unsatisfactory).

**DIRECTIONS FOR EVALUATOR:** Use **Column E** to record your evaluation of the student clinician's communication skills during the role-play. Indicate **S** (satisfactory) or **U** (unsatisfactory). In the optional grade percentage calculation, each **S** equals 1 point, each **U** equals 0 points.

| CRITERIA | S | E |
|---|---|---|
| Explains the purpose of the medical history assessment to the patient. | | |
| After researching medical conditions and medications, asks appropriate follow-up questions to gain complete information from the patient. | | |
| Encourages patient questions before and during the medical history assessment. | | |
| Answers the patient's questions fully and accurately. | | |
| Communicates with the patient at an appropriate level and avoids dental/medical terminology or jargon. | | |
| Accurately communicates the findings to the clinical instructor. Discusses the implications of the medical history findings for dental treatment. Uses correct medical and dental terminology. | | |

**OPTIONAL GRADE PERCENTAGE CALCULATION**

Each **S** equals 1 point and each **U** equals 0 points. Using the **E** column, total the sum of the "**S**"s _____ divided by the total points possible (6) to calculate the percentage grade.

# 5 Ready References: Medical History

## MODULE OVERVIEW

This module contains two ready references designed to provide fast access to commonly encountered medical conditions and prescription medications.

- Ready Reference 5-1: Common Conditions of Concern in Dentistry
- Ready Reference 5-2: Commonly Prescribed Drugs

## MODULE OUTLINE

## OBJECTIVES

- Demonstrate skills in using the "Ready References" in this module to research patient medical conditions/diseases and prescription medications.
- Describe contraindications and complications for dental care presented by various medical conditions/diseases and medications.

### Introduction to Ready References

In a dental office or clinic, using the Internet or reference books to research medical conditions and medications may not be practical within minutes of seeing a newly appointed patient. This module contains two Ready References designed to provide fast access to dentally relevant information on medical conditions/diseases and prescription medications commonly encountered in dental offices and clinics.

- These Ready References may be removed from the book by tearing along the perforated lines on each page.
- Laminating or placing these pages in plastic protector sheets will allow them to be disinfected for use in a clinical setting.

## SECTION 1

# Medical Conditions and Diseases

**READY REFERENCE 5-1** **COMMON CONDITIONS OF CONCERN IN DENTISTRY**[a]

| Medical Condition or Disease | Treatment Considerations<br>Red font = Potential Medical Emergency Alert |
|---|---|
| **Addison disease (Adrenal insufficiency)**—endocrine or hormonal disorder characterized by weight loss, muscle weakness, fatigue, low blood pressure, and sometimes darkening of the skin; Addison disease occurs when the adrenal glands do not produce enough of the hormone cortisol and, in some cases, the hormone aldosterone | Body less able to respond to stress<br>Increased susceptibility to infection<br>**Acute adrenal insufficiency** |
| **AIDS**: See HIV | |
| **Alcoholism**—addiction to alcohol | Avoid mouthwashes or other products containing alcohol<br>Bleeding tendency<br>Caution when using conscious sedation or central nervous system (CNS) depressant drugs<br>Patient may lack interest in dental health |
| **Allergy**—a sensitivity to a normally harmless substance that provokes a strong reaction from the person's body | Possible allergy to latex or other products or materials used in dentistry<br>Possible xerostomia due to medications<br>**Anaphylaxis** |
| **Amyotrophic lateral sclerosis (ALS)**: See Lou Gehrig disease | |
| **Alzheimer disease**—progressive deterioration of intellectual functions such as memory | Communication and patient management |
| **Anemia**—a blood condition in which there are too few red blood cells or the red blood cells are deficient in hemoglobin | Gingival inflammation<br>Bleeding tendency |
| **Angina**—a medical condition in which lack of blood to the heart causes severe chest pains | If taking aspirin therapy, clotting may be reduced<br>Reduce stress by scheduling shorter, early morning appointments; minimize stress<br>**Anginal attack** |
| **Anticoagulant therapy**—used to prevent blood clots from forming in the deep veins of the body for prevention of stroke and heart attack | Anticoagulants work by increasing the time it takes for the blood to clot; increased bleeding from invasive dental treatment, including periodontal debridement (scaling and root planing) |

*(continued)*

[a] Ready Reference 5-1 adapted with permission from Cynthia Biron Leisica, DH Meth-Ed.

**READY REFERENCE 5-1**    COMMON CONDITIONS OF CONCERN IN DENTISTRY[a]
(CONTINUED)

| Medical Condition or Disease | Treatment Considerations<br>Red font = Potential Medical Emergency Alert |
|---|---|
| **Arthritis**—inflammation of the joints causing pain, swelling, enlargement, and redness; also see Rheumatoid arthritis | Daily plaque control may be difficult, suggest alternatives to hand brushing and flossing<br>If taking prednisone or other corticosteroid, increased susceptibility to infection (see Corticosteroid therapy)<br>If taking aspirin, bleeding (see Aspirin) |
| **Aspirin/antiplatelet therapy**—used to prevent platelet clumping and formation of blood clots | Control of bleeding after periodontal debridement (scaling) or surgical procedures |
| **Asthma**—a respiratory disease that causes blockage and narrowing of the airways, making it difficult to breathe | If taking prednisone: increased risk for infection, poor wound healing, and adrenal insufficiency<br>**Asthma attack** |
| **Bell palsy**—a paralysis or weakness of the muscles on one side of the face; it causes one side of the face to droop and affects taste sensation and tear and saliva production | Protect the eye on the affected side due to the absence of blinking |
| **Bipolar affective disorder**—a condition that causes extreme shifts in mood, energy, and functioning | If taking Lithium, this drug can interact with non-steroidal anti-inflammatory agents used for pain control |
| **Cerebral palsy**—a group of motor problems and physical disorders that result from a brain injury or abnormal brain development; results in uncontrolled reflex movements and muscle tightness (spasticity) | Patient management<br>Dental problems |
| **Cerebrovascular accident (stroke)**—a sudden blockage or rupture of a blood vessel in the brain resulting in loss of speech, movement, or sensation for a period of 24 hours or longer | Patient positioning during treatment<br>If taking anticoagulants, bleeding tendency<br>If taking corticosteroids, increased susceptibility to infection and less able to withstand stress |
| **Chemotherapy**—the use of chemical agents to treat diseases, infections, or other disorders, especially cancer | Immune suppression results in increased risk of infection and poor wound healing |
| **Chronic bronchitis**—a long-term inflammation and irritation of the airways of the lungs; symptoms include a cough that produces too much sputum, mild wheezing, and chest pain; common in smokers | Patient positioning<br>**Respiratory difficulty** |
| **Congenital heart defects**—structural heart problems or abnormalities that have been present since birth | Consult physician to determine need for antibiotic premedication<br>Susceptibility to bacterial endocarditis |

(continued)

**READY REFERENCE 5-1** COMMON CONDITIONS OF CONCERN IN DENTISTRY[a]
*(CONTINUED)*

| Medical Condition or Disease | Treatment Considerations<br>Red font = Potential Medical Emergency Alert |
| --- | --- |
| **Congestive heart failure (CHF)**—a condition in which the heart pumps ineffectively, leading to a buildup of fluid in the lungs, legs, and elsewhere; people with CHF often experience shortness of breath and/or ankle or leg swelling related to this excess fluid | May have breathing problems, may prefer semi-upright position in dental chair<br>Minimize stress<br>If taking diuretic, possible xerostomia<br>**Respiratory difficulty** |
| **Corticosteroid therapy**—corticosteroids are anti-inflammatory drugs widely used for treating a variety of conditions in which tissues become inflamed; an example is prednisone | Immune suppression with increased risk of infection and poor wound healing; lowered tolerance for stress |
| **Crohn disease**—an inflammatory bowel disease (IBD) thought to be an autoimmune response to bacterial flora in intestines | Immune suppression with increased risk of infection and poor wound healing |
| **Cushing syndrome**—a rare disorder that develops when the body is exposed to too much of the hormone cortisol; may cause weight gain, skin changes, and fatigue and lead to such serious conditions as diabetes, high blood pressure, depression, and osteoporosis | Immune suppression with increased risk of infection and poor wound healing |
| **Cystic fibrosis (CF)**—a genetically inherited disease; in the lungs, CF causes thicker-than-normal mucus to form in the airways and lungs, leading to respiratory problems and infections | Increased susceptibility to infection<br>Patient positioning |
| **Diabetes (Type I)**—a lifelong disease that develops when the pancreas stops producing insulin; insulin injections must be taken daily | Increased susceptibility to infection and poor wound healing<br>Appropriate appointment time in regard to insulin therapy and meals<br>Frequent maintenance appointments<br>**Insulin reaction** if using insulin |
| **Diabetes (Type II)**—a chronic disease that develops when the pancreas cannot produce enough insulin, or the body cannot use it properly; it can often be treated without insulin injections | Increased risk of infection<br>Poor wound healing<br>Frequent maintenance appointments<br>**Insulin reaction** if taking oral hypoglycemic drugs or using insulin |
| **Down syndrome**—people with Down syndrome have an extra or irregular chromosome in some or all of their body's cells; the chromosomal abnormalities impair physical and mental development with mild to moderate below-normal intelligence | Increased risk of infection, leukemia, and hypothyroidism<br>May need caregiver's assistance with daily plaque control self-care |

*(continued)*

**READY REFERENCE 5-1** COMMON CONDITIONS OF CONCERN IN DENTISTRY[a]
*(CONTINUED)*

| Medical Condition or Disease | Treatment Considerations<br>Red font = Potential Medical Emergency Alert |
|---|---|
| **Emphysema**—a chronic lung disease in which the alveoli of the lungs are damaged; air is trapped in the lungs, leading to shortness of breath | Breathing problems, may prefer semi-upright position in dental chair<br>If emergency situation, no high concentrations of supplemental oxygen |
| **Endocarditis**—an infection of the endocardium (inner lining of the heart) | History of endocarditis indicated high risk for recurrence from dental procedures |
| **Epilepsy**—a brain disorder involving recurrent seizures; a seizure can be a sudden, violent, uncontrollable contraction of a group of muscles or consist of only a brief "loss of contact" or what appears to be daydreaming | Dilantin: gingival hyperplasia<br>Minimize stress<br>Document type, frequency, and precipitating factors<br>Seizures |
| **Fibromyalgia**—a syndrome distinguished by chronic pain in the muscles, ligaments, tendons, or bursae around joints | One-third of fibromyalgia patients have temporomandibular joint (TMJ) disorders<br>May appreciate shorter appointments |
| **Gastroesophageal reflux disease (GERD)**—the abnormal backflow of stomach acid and juices into the esophagus—the tube that leads from the throat to the stomach; results in heartburn and damage to the esophagus | Erosion of teeth<br>Drugs for GERD may interact with antibiotics, analgesics |
| **Glaucoma**—damage to the optic nerve, accompanied by an abnormally high pressure inside the eyeball that can lead to blindness if untreated | Avoid drugs that increase ocular pressure (i.e., atropine) |
| **Glomerulonephritis**—a kidney disease caused by inflammation or scarring of the small blood vessels (glomeruli); if chronic, leads to kidney failure; also see Kidney disease | Medical consultation<br>Toxic accumulation of drugs, including local anesthesia, due to poor drug elimination<br>Increased susceptibility to infection<br>Less able to withstand stress |
| **Graves disease**—the most common cause of hyperthyroidism in which the thyroid gland produces too much thyroid hormone | Epinephrine given to hyperthyroid patient could cause the medical emergency thyroid storm |
| **Heart attack**—see Myocardial infarction | |
| **Hemophilia**—a rare genetic bleeding disorder caused by a shortage of certain clotting factors that are needed to help stop bleeding after a cut or injury and to prevent spontaneous bleeding | Hemorrhage from dental procedures, including periodontal debridement (scaling and root planning) |
| **Hepatitis B**—a serious liver infection from hepatitis B virus (HBV); infection may become chronic, leading to liver failure, cancer, or cirrhosis | Laboratory clearance (ensure that infection has been successfully treated)<br>Infection, bleeding, delayed wound healing<br>Universal precautions |

*(continued)*

**READY REFERENCE 5-1**    **COMMON CONDITIONS OF CONCERN IN DENTISTRY[a]**
*(CONTINUED)*

| Medical Condition or Disease | Treatment Considerations<br>Red font = Potential Medical Emergency Alert |
|---|---|
| **Hepatitis C**—the most serious of all hepatitis viruses; usually leads to liver failure, liver cancer, or cirrhosis | Laboratory clearance (ensure that infection has been successfully treated)<br>Infection, bleeding, delayed wound healing<br>Universal precautions |
| **High blood pressure**—see Hypertension | |
| **HIV/AIDS**—the HIV (human immunodeficiency virus) is a virus that attacks the immune system, making it difficult for the body to fight off infection and some diseases; HIV eventually causes acquired immunodeficiency syndrome (AIDS) | Oral lesions and infections<br>Risk of infection from dental procedures<br>Severe periodontal disease<br>Universal precautions |
| **Hypertension**—high blood pressure; a resting blood pressure that is consistently 140/90 mm Hg or higher | Epinephrine contraindication<br>If taking diuretic, possible xerostomia<br>If taking calcium blocker, possible gingival enlargement<br>**Cerebrovascular accident (CVA; stroke), Myocardial infarction (MI; heart attack)** |
| **Hyperthyroidism**—an overproduction of thyroid hormone | Epinephrine given to hyperthyroid patient could cause medical emergency **thyroid storm** |
| **Hypothyroidism**—an insufficient production of thyroid hormone | In severe hypothyroidism, CNS depressant drugs can pose a risk for **myxedema coma** |
| **Kidney disease, chronic**—develops when the kidneys permanently lose most of their ability to remove waste and maintain fluid and chemical balances in the body; in chronic kidney disease, the kidneys have not stopped working altogether but are not working as well as they should. Dialysis or kidney transplantation is required when kidney function drops to about 15% of normal | Medical consultation<br>Toxic accumulation of drugs, including local anesthesia, due to poor elimination<br>Increased susceptibility to infection<br>Less able to withstand stress<br>Salt restriction<br>Bleeding tendency |
| **Implantable cardioverter defibrillator**—a device that delivers an electrical shock to prevent potentially dangerous heart rhythm abnormalities | Medical consultation |
| **Kidney dialysis**—a mechanical process that performs part of the work that healthy kidneys normally do by removing wastes and extra fluid from the blood | Medical consultation<br>Toxic accumulation of drugs, including local anesthesia, due to poor drug elimination<br>Increased susceptibility to infection<br>Less able to withstand stress<br>Salt restriction<br>Bleeding tendency |

*(continued)*

**READY REFERENCE 5-1** COMMON CONDITIONS OF CONCERN IN DENTISTRY[a]
*(CONTINUED)*

| Medical Condition or Disease | Treatment Considerations<br>Red font = Potential Medical Emergency Alert |
|---|---|
| **Latex allergy**—an unusual sensitivity to latex that varies from a mild allergic reaction to an anaphylactic response | Avoid latex products; in a clinical setting, all clinicians should avoid "snapping" gloves, which creates airborne latex particles |
| **Leukemia**—cancer of the blood cells in which the bone marrow produces abnormal white blood cells that over time crowd out the normal white blood cells, red blood cells, and platelets | Bleeding tendency<br>Periodontal disease; need for excellent self-care<br>Immune compromised<br>Medical consultation recommended |
| **Liver disorder**—impaired function of the liver due to cirrhosis, hepatitis, cancer, alcoholism | Infection, bleeding, delayed wound healing |
| **Lou Gehrig disease (Amyotrophic lateral sclerosis)**—a progressive wasting away of certain nerve cells of the brain and spinal column; walking, speaking, eating, swallowing, breathing, and other basic functions become more difficult as the disease progresses | Swallowing difficulties; physical disabilities make patient positioning a challenge<br>Daily plaque control may be difficult, suggest alternatives to hand brushing and flossing or educate caregiver |
| **Lupus erythematosus**—an autoimmune disease in which a person's immune system attacks its own tissues as though they were foreign substances; may cause problems with kidneys, heart, lungs, or blood cells | Increased susceptibility to infection due to compromised immune system<br>Adrenal crisis |
| **Meniere disease**—a problem in the inner ear that affects hearing and balance, characterized by repeated attacks of dizziness that occur suddenly and without warning; the vertigo experienced during an attack can be intense, leading to nausea and vomiting, and can last anywhere from several minutes to many hours | Medications may cause xerostomia<br>Hearing loss in affected ear<br>Dizziness; raise chair slowly from supine position<br>Might need assistance in walking due to dizziness |
| **Mental disorder**—any disease or condition affecting the brain that influences the way a person thinks, feels, behaves, and/or relates to others and to his or her surroundings | Reduced stress tolerance<br>Xerostomia<br>Avoid mouth rinse containing alcohol |
| **Metabolic syndrome**—a group of abnormal findings related to the body's metabolism including excess body fat, high triglycerides and blood pressure, and high cholesterol; causes increased risk of diabetes, heart disease, or stroke | Monitor blood pressure at every appointment |
| **Mitral valve prolapse**—an improper closing of the leaflets of the mitral valve; may cause back flow of blood into the left atrium | Medical consult and probable preoperative antibiotic premedication |

*(continued)*

**READY REFERENCE 5-1** COMMON CONDITIONS OF CONCERN IN DENTISTRY[a]
(CONTINUED)

| Medical Condition or Disease | Treatment Considerations<br>Red font = Potential Medical Emergency Alert |
|---|---|
| **Mitral valve stenosis**—a heart condition in which the mitral valve fails to open as wide as it should; can cause irregular heartbeats and possibly heart failure or other complications, including stroke, heart infection, pulmonary edema, and blood clots | Medical consult and probable antibiotic premedication |
| **Mononucleosis**—a viral illness usually caused by the Epstein-Barr virus (EBV); most common symptoms of mononucleosis include high fever, severe sore throat, swollen glands (especially the tonsils), and fatigue; once infected with EBV, the body may periodically shed (or give off) the virus throughout a person's lifetime, possibly spreading the virus | Universal precautions as the usual route of transmission is through saliva |
| **Multiple myeloma**—a rare form of cancer characterized by excessive production and improper function of the plasma cells found in the bone marrow; symptoms may include bone pain, anemia, weakness, fatigue, lack of color, and kidney abnormalities; affected individuals are more susceptible to bacterial infections such as pneumonia | Antibiotics may be indicated to control or reduce the incidence of infection |
| **Multiple sclerosis (MS)**—a chronic neurological disease involving the brain, spinal cord, and optic nerves; causes problems with muscle control and strength, vision, balance, sensation, and mental functions | Adverse reactions to drugs may include risks for infection, difficulties keeping mouth open during long appointments<br>Daily plaque control may be difficult, suggest alternatives to hand brushing and flossing or educate caregiver |
| **Muscular dystrophy (MD)**—a group of inherited diseases in which the muscles that control movement progressively weaken | Daily plaque control may be difficult; suggest alternatives to hand brushing and flossing or educate caregiver<br>Muscle weakness and range of motion decrease as the disease progresses will eventually require oral hygiene assistance for patient |
| **Myasthenia gravis**—a neuromuscular disorder primarily characterized by muscle weakness and muscle fatigue; most individuals develop weakness and drooping of the eyelids, double vision, and excessive muscle fatigue; additional features commonly include weakness of facial muscles, impaired articulation of speech, difficulties chewing and swallowing, and weakness of the arms/legs | Patients may have difficulty in chewing, swallowing, and talking<br>Daily plaque control may be difficult; suggest alternatives to hand brushing and flossing or educate caregiver |

(continued)

**READY REFERENCE 5-1**  **COMMON CONDITIONS OF CONCERN IN DENTISTRY**[a]
*(CONTINUED)*

| Medical Condition or Disease | Treatment Considerations<br>Red font = Potential Medical Emergency Alert |
| --- | --- |
| **Myocardial infarction (MI)**—a heart attack; caused by a lack of blood supply to the heart for an extended time period, results in permanent damage to the heart muscle | No elective dental treatment for 6 months<br>Bleeding tendency if taking anticoagulant or aspirin<br>Monitor vital signs<br>Minimize stress with shorter appointments, early morning appointments |
| **Narcolepsy**—a chronic sleep disorder mainly characterized by an excessive daytime drowsiness with episodes of suddenly falling asleep | Be alert for sudden episodes of sleeping<br>Stress may cause cataplexy resulting in slurred speech or total physical collapse |
| **Non-Hodgkin lymphoma**—cancer of the lymphatic system resulting in painless, swollen lymph nodes; symptoms include fever, drowsiness, weight loss | Swollen lymph nodes may be the only sign of condition in early phase |
| **Oral/Head and neck cancer**—cancerous lesions of the oral cavity and/or head and neck region | Radiation therapy<br>Medical consultation recommended; may need antibiotic premedication<br>Xerostomia may be present<br>Increased susceptibility to infection<br>Risk of dental caries due to radiation<br>Prevention: early detection of lesions |
| **Organ transplant**—a surgical procedure to remove a damaged or diseased organ and replace it with a healthy donor organ; heart, intestine, kidney, liver, lung, pancreas replacement | Extra precautions to avoid infections<br>**Adrenal insufficiency** |
| **Pacemaker**—a small device that sends electrical impulses to the heart muscle to maintain a suitable heart rate and rhythm; it is implanted just under the skin of the chest during a minor surgical procedure | Avoid use of ultrasonic devices |
| **Parkinson disease**—a chronic, progressive motor system disorder; the four primary symptoms are tremor or trembling in hands, arms, legs, jaw, and face; rigidity or stiffness of the limbs and trunk; slowness of movement; and impaired balance and coordination; patients may have difficulty walking, talking, or completing other simple tasks | Assist patient with positioning in dental chair and when walking to and from treatment area<br>Swallowing difficulties<br>Poor motor control; daily plaque control may be difficult; suggest alternatives to hand brushing and flossing or educate caregiver |

*(continued)*

**READY REFERENCE 5-1** COMMON CONDITIONS OF CONCERN IN DENTISTRY[a] (CONTINUED)

| Medical Condition or Disease | Treatment Considerations — Red font = Potential Medical Emergency Alert |
|---|---|
| **Panic disorder**—consists of several, unexpected panic attacks, which usually begin with a sudden feeling of extreme anxiety; an attack can be triggered by a stressful event or occur for no apparent reason and can last several minutes; symptoms may include a feeling of intense fear or terror, difficulty breathing, chest pain or tightness, heartbeat changes, dizziness, sweating, and shaking; patients can mistake a panic attack for a heart attack | Provide a stress reduction protocol if the patient is apprehensive about dental treatment |
| **Peripheral arterial disease (PAD)**—poor circulation to limbs, especially the legs; occurs when arteries supplying blood to limbs become clogged or partially blocked | Patient may not be able to tolerate long appointments without frequent walking breaks |
| **Polymyalgia rheumatica**—an inflammatory disorder that causes widespread muscle aching and stiffness, especially in the neck, shoulders, thighs, and hips | If on long-term corticosteroid therapy, increased susceptibility to infection |
| **Rheumatic heart disease**—a condition that can result from rheumatic fever; usually a thickening and constriction of one or more of the heart valves that often requires surgery to repair or replace the involved valve(s) | Medical consultation<br>Antibiotic premedication<br>Minimize stress<br>Monitor vital signs |
| **Rheumatic fever**—a rare but potentially life-threatening disease, rheumatic fever is a complication of untreated strep throat | If patient is taking prednisone or another corticosteroid, increased susceptibility to infection<br>**Adrenal crisis** |
| **Rheumatoid arthritis**—a relatively common disease of the joints; the tissues lining the joints become inflamed; over time, the inflammation may destroy the joint tissues, leading to disability. Rheumatoid arthritis affects women twice as often as men and frequently begins between the ages of 40 and 60. | If patient is taking corticosteroids, susceptibility to infection<br>**Adrenal crisis** |
| **Schizophrenia**—a severe brain disease that interferes with normal brain and mental function—it can trigger hallucinations, delusions, paranoia, and significant lack of motivation; without treatment, schizophrenia affects the ability to think clearly, manage emotions, and interact appropriately with other people | Personality problems; may be paranoid, feel threatened, apprehensive<br>If taking medications faithfully, most problems will be well controlled; may be drowsy or react slowly to requests or questions |

(continued)

**READY REFERENCE 5-1** **COMMON CONDITIONS OF CONCERN IN DENTISTRY**[a] *(CONTINUED)*

| Medical Condition or Disease | Treatment Considerations<br>Red font = Potential Medical Emergency Alert |
|---|---|
| **Scleroderma**—a connective tissue disorder characterized by abnormal thickening of the skin; some types affect specific parts of the body, whereas other types can affect the whole body and internal organs | Cardiac, circulatory, pulmonary, and kidney complications |
| **Sexually transmitted diseases (STDs)**—those diseases that are spread by sexual contact; STDs can also be spread from a pregnant woman to her fetus before or during delivery | Refer to physician and postpone treatment when oral lesions or other signs suggest infection |
| **Sickle cell anemia**—an inherited disease in which the red blood cells, normally disc shaped, become crescent shaped; these cells function abnormally and cause small blood clots; these clots give rise to recurrent painful episodes called "sickle cell pain crises" | Patients have episodes of pain in the chest, abdomen, and joints<br>At greater risk for infection due to sickle cell damage to the spleen |
| **Sjögren's syndrome** (pronounced "showgrins")—is a disorder in which the immune system attacks the body's moisture-producing glands, such as the tear and salivary glands; these glands may become scarred and damaged, and exceptional dryness in the eyes and mouth may develop | Xerostomia predisposes patients to dental caries<br>If major organs are involved, there is greater risk for infection |
| **Splenectomy**—the removal of a spleen that is enlarged or injured; patients without a spleen are termed *asplenic* | Increased susceptibility to infection |
| **Stroke**—see Cerebrovascular accident | |
| **Thrombophlebitis**—a blood clot and inflammation in one or more veins, typically in the legs; cause is inactivity due to travel or convalescence | Consult with physician regarding anticoagulant therapy and risks for hemorrhage |
| **Tourette syndrome**—a condition that causes patients to exhibit uncontrolled behaviors known as tics; tics range from bouts of lip smacking, blinking, shrugging, repetitive phrases, or shouting obscenities | Patient management if tics are not controlled |
| **Tuberculosis (TB)**—a bacterial infection that usually affects the lungs but can affect other parts of the body; is classified as latent or active; active TB can be spread to others | Active TB may spread through aerosols in clinic (patient should not receive elective dental care)<br>Consult with physician if patient presents with history of TB |

## SECTION 2

# Common Prescription Medications

Key: Brand Names are printed in: **Bold letters**
Generic names are printed in: *Italics*

## READY REFERENCE 5-2 COMMONLY PRESCRIBED DRUGS[a]

| Drug | Use | Concerns/Oral Manifestations |
|---|---|---|
| **Abilify**, *aripiprazole* | Antipsychotic drug used to treat various psychoses (such as hallucinations, delusional beliefs, disorganized thinking) | Involuntary muscle contractions and tremor that can present problems with patient management during the appointment. |
| **Abstral**, *fentanyl* (sublingual) | Sublingual administration of fentanyl, a powerful opioid pain reliever | Dizziness, nausea, fainting |
| **Accupril**, *quinapril* | Medication used to treat high blood pressure and heart failure and for preventing kidney failure due to high blood pressure and diabetes | Altered taste, dizziness, nausea, vomiting; use of epinephrine or levonordefrin in local anesthetic should be minimized; angioedema, hypotension |
| **Accutane, Amnesteem, Claravis, Sotret**, *isotretinoin* | A strong vitamin A oral medication used to treat acne when other medications are not effective | Causes serious and fatal birth defects; frequently causes depression |
| *Acetaminophen/ codeine*, **Tylenol 3** | Acetaminophen is used for the relief of pain and fever | Nausea, vomiting |
| **Aciphex**, *rabeprazole* | Acid blocker for treatment of heartburn and gastroesophageal reflux disease (acid reflux) | Xerostomia, altered taste, nausea, dizziness, nervousness |
| **Actiq**, *fentanyl citrate* (lozenge) | Narcotic oral lozenge for pain | Dental caries, respiratory depression |
| **Actonel**, *risedronate* | Medication for the treatment of Paget disease (a disease in which the formation of bone is abnormal) and in persons with osteoporosis | Nausea, osteonecrosis of the jaw |
| **Actos**, *pioglitazone* | Oral medication used to treat type II diabetes | Respiratory tract infection, headache, sinusitis, low blood sugar, sore throat; if diabetes is poorly controlled, increased risk of periodontitis |

*(continued)*

[a] Ready Reference 5-2 adapted with permission from Cynthia Biron Leisica, DH Meth-Ed.

**READY REFERENCE 5-2**   **COMMONLY PRESCRIBED DRUGS**[a] *(CONTINUED)*

| Drug | Use | Concerns/Oral Manifestations |
|---|---|---|
| *Acyclovir,* **Zovirax** | Antiviral: herpes I, II, herpes zoster (shingles) | Lightheadedness, dry lips |
| **Adderall,** *amphetamine/ dextroamphetamine* mixed salts | Medication to treat attention deficit hyperactivity disorder (ADHD) and narcolepsy (CNS disease causing excessive daytime sleepiness) | Xerostomia, nervousness, anxiety, restlessness, excitability, dizziness, tremor; blood pressure and heart rate may increase |
| **Advair,** *salmeterol/ fluticasone* | Inhaled drug that is used to treat asthma, chronic bronchitis, or emphysema | Xerostomia, upper respiratory infections |
| **Advil,** *ibuprofen* | Nonsteroidal anti-inflammatory drug (NSAID) for relief of mild to moderate pain | Xerostomia, ulcerations, lichen planus on buccal mucosa/lateral border of tongue, dizziness, drowsiness, nausea, heartburn, increased bleeding tendency |
| **Aggrenox,** *aspirin/ dipyridamole* | A medication that reduces the clumping of platelets in the blood; used to prevent blood clots and stroke | Hemorrhage, headaches |
| *Albuterol,* **Ventolin, Alupent,** *Metaproternol sulfate* | Inhaler for asthma | Xerostomia, sore throat |
| **Aldara,** *imiquimod* (topical) | Medication for warts in sexually transmitted diseases (STDs), also used to treat some cancers | Treatment for oral warts |
| *Alendronate,* **Fosamex** | Used for the treatment of persons with osteoporosis | Osteonecrosis of the jaw |
| **Aleve,** *naproxen* | NSAID for relief of mild to moderate pain | Xerostomia, dizziness, drowsiness, nausea, heartburn, increased bleeding tendency |
| **Allegra,** *Fexofenadine HCl,* **Allegra-D,** *Fexofenadine HCl and Pseudoephedrine HCl.* | An antihistamine used to treat the signs and symptoms of allergy. Allegra-D has a decongestant to reduce mucus and running nose. | Xerostomia, dizziness, headache, anxiety, tremor |
| *Allopurinol,* **Alloprin, Zyloprim** | Reduces uric acid production for the treatment of gouty arthritis | Salty taste |
| **Alphagan,** *brimonidine* | Medication for the treatment of glaucoma | Xerostomia |
| *Alprazolam,* **Xanax** | Used to treat anxiety associated with situations such as dental appointments, or in general anxiety disorders | Xerostomia, lightheadedness |

*(continued)*

**READY REFERENCE 5-2** COMMONLY PRESCRIBED DRUGS[a] (CONTINUED)

| Drug | Use | Concerns/Oral Manifestations |
|------|-----|------------------------------|
| **Altace**, *Ramipril* | Medication used to treat high blood pressure, heart failure, and for preventing kidney failure due to high blood pressure and diabetes | Altered taste, dizziness, nausea, vomiting; use of epinephrine or levonordefrin in local anesthetic should be minimized; angioedema, hypotension |
| **Alupent inhaler**, *Metaproternol sulfate* | Inhaled bronchodilator | Xerostomia |
| **Amaryl**, *Glimepiride* | Oral drug for the control of diabetes | Hypoglycemia, dizziness, nausea; if diabetes is poorly controlled, increased risk of periodontitis |
| **Ambien**, *Zolpidem* | Insomnia treatment (sleep aid) | Xerostomia |
| **Ambien CR**, *Zolpidem* | Controlled release formula for insomnia | Xerostomia |
| *Amiodarone HCl*, **Cordarone** | Medication for irregular heartbeat | Altered saliva flow and taste |
| *Amitriptyline*, **Elavil** | Tricyclic antidepressant with pain-relieving effects. Also used to treat TMJ pain | Xerostomia, orthostatic hypotension, altered taste |
| *Amlodipine*, **Norvasc** | Calcium channel blocker used to treat angina | Gingival hyperplasia; involuntary muscle contractions, tremors, changes in breathing and heart rate |
| *Amoxicillin*, **Amoxil** | An antibiotic used to treat infections and for the prevention of bacterial endocarditis | Oral candidiasis, black hairy tongue, dizziness, nausea |
| **AndroGel**, *testosterone* | Hormone medication for low testosterone levels in men | Ankle swelling |
| **Apri**, *Desogestrel/ Ethinyl estradiol* | Birth control | Antibiotics taken for dental infections can decrease the effectiveness of oral contraceptives |
| **Aranesp**, *Darbepoetin alfa* | A medication to treat anemia in patients undergoing chemotherapy | Hypertension/hypotension in 20% of patients |
| **Aricept**, *Donepezil* | Treatment for Alzheimer disease | Slow heartbeat, fainting |
| **Armour thyroid**, *thyroid hormone* | Thyroid hormone supplement or replacement | No precautions if controlled |
| **Arthrotec**, *Diclofenac/ Misoprostol* | NSAID effective in treating fever, pain, and inflammation | Bleeding |

*(continued)*

**READY REFERENCE 5-2**   COMMONLY PRESCRIBED DRUGS[a] *(CONTINUED)*

| Drug | Use | Concerns/Oral Manifestations |
|------|-----|------------------------------|
| **Asacol**, *Mesalamine* | Treatment for ulcerative colitis in inflammatory bowel disease or Crohn disease | Pharyngitis |
| *Aspirin*, **Bayer, Bufferin** | NSAID effective in treating fever, pain, and inflammation | Bleeding |
| **Astelin**, *Azelastine* | Nasal spray for swelling and inflammation of the mucous membranes inside the nose | Xerostomia, aphthous ulcers, altered taste |
| **Atacand**, *Candesartan* | Medication for lowering high blood pressure | Runny nose, sore throat, cough, back pain, headache, dizziness |
| **Atelvia**, *Risedronate sodium* | Used for the treatment of persons with osteoporosis | Osteonecrosis of the jaw |
| *Atenolol* **Tenormin** | Beta blocker used to treat angina and high blood pressure | None |
| **Ativan**, *Lorazepam* | Antianxiety medication for depression; also a sleep aid | Dizziness; xerostomia |
| *Atorvastatin*, **Lipitor** | Treatment to lower high cholesterol to prevent coronary artery disease | Muscle pain, tenderness, or weakness with fever or flu symptoms; or nausea, stomach pain, low fever, loss of appetite |
| **Atrovent**, *Ipratropium* | Inhaled bronchodilator used for chronic bronchitis and emphysema | Xerostomia, tremor, nervousness |
| **Augmentin ES-600**, *Amoxicillin/Clavulanate potassium* | Antibiotic used to treat bacterial infections | Black hairy tongue, coated tongue, oral candidiasis, nausea, vomiting |
| **Avalide**, *Irbesartan/ Hydrochlorothiazide* | Used to treat high blood pressure, also contains diuretic | Dizziness, nausea |
| **Avandamet**, *Rosiglitazone maleate/ Metformin HCl* | Oral medication used to treat type II diabetes | If patient is experiencing increased stress, there is a risk of hypoglycemia |
| **Avandia**, *Rosiglitazone maleate* | Oral medication used to treat type II diabetes | If patient is experiencing increased stress, there is a risk of hypoglycemia |
| **Avapro**, *Irbesartan* | Medication used to treat high blood pressure, congestive heart failure | Dizziness; use of epinephrine or levonordefrin in local anesthetic should be minimized |
| **Avelox**, *Moxifloxacin* | Antibiotic used to treat pneumonia and eye and skin infections | None |

*(continued)*

**READY REFERENCE 5-2** COMMONLY PRESCRIBED DRUGS[a] *(CONTINUED)*

| Drug | Use | Concerns/Oral Manifestations |
|---|---|---|
| **Aviane**, *Levonorgestrel/ Ethinyl estradiol* | Birth control | Antibiotics taken for dental infections can decrease the effectiveness of oral contraceptives |
| **Avinza**, *Morphine sulfate* | Narcotic for moderate to severe pain | Dizziness, nausea |
| **Avodart**, *Dutasteride* | Medication for benign prostate enlargement | None |
| **Avonex**, *Interferon beta-1a* | Medication for relapsing forms of multiple sclerosis | Headache, nausea |
| **Axiron**, *topical testosterone* | Testosterone for hypogonadism in men | Nausea |
| *Azathioprine*, **Azasan, Imuran** | Immunosuppressant for lichen planus, erythema multiforme, pemphigus | Fever, malaise, rash, gastrointestinal effects |
| *Azithromycin*, **Z-Pak, Zithromax** | Antibiotic, alternative for prevention of endocarditis | Caution in liver disorders |
| **Azor**, *Amlodipine/ Olmesartan* | Combined medications to lower high blood pressure | Hypotension, xerostomia |
| *Baclofen*, **Lioresal** | Muscle relaxant for multiple sclerosis | Drowsiness |
| **Bactroban**, *Mupirocin* | Topical antibiotic used for the treatment of impetigo, infected eczema, also used as a nasal ointment | None |
| *Benazepril*, **Lotensin** | Medication used to treat high blood pressure and heart failure and for preventing kidney failure due to high blood pressure and diabetes | Altered taste, dizziness, nausea, vomiting; use of epinephrine or levonordefrin in local anesthetic should be minimized; angioedema, hypotension |
| **Benicar**, *Olmesartan* **Benicar HCT**, *Olmesartan medoxomil- hydrochlorothiazide* | Medication for high blood pressure with diuretic; hydrochlorothiazide for high blood pressure | Altered taste, dizziness, nausea, vomiting; use of epinephrine or levonordefrin in local anesthetic should be minimized; angioedema, hypotension |
| **Betaseron**, *Interferon beta-1b* | Medication for treatment of multiple sclerosis | Flu-like syndrome |
| **Beyaz**, *drospirenone/ ethinyl estradiol/ levomefolate calcium* | Combination of drugs for birth control, premenstrual disorders, and acne | Antibiotics taken for dental infections can decrease the effectiveness of oral contraceptives |
| *Benzonatate*, **Tessalon** | Cough medicine, topical anesthetic | None |

*(continued)*

**READY REFERENCE 5-2**  COMMONLY PRESCRIBED DRUGS[a] *(CONTINUED)*

| Drug | Use | Concerns/Oral Manifestations |
|---|---|---|
| **Biaxin XL**, *Clarithromycin* | Antibiotic used to treat bacterial infections | Oral candidiasis, altered taste, cough, dizziness, nausea |
| *Bisoprolol fumarate/ Hydrochlorothiazide,* **Ziac** | Medication for treatment of high blood pressure | Abnormal taste, hypotension |
| **Bonine**, *meclizine* | Used for the treatment of nausea, vomiting, and dizziness | Xerostomia, drowsiness |
| **Boniva**, *Ibandronate* | Oral medication used to treat osteoporosis | New research shows that only IV administration increases the risk of osteonecrosis of the jaw |
| *Bupropion,* **Budeprion SR, Wellbutrin SR** (sustained release), **Wellbutrin XL** (extended release) | Antidepressant | Xerostomia, altered taste |
| *Buspirone,* **Buspar** | Medication for the management of anxiety | Dizziness, nausea, xerostomia |
| *Butalbital/ Acetaminophen/ Caffeine,* **Fioricet** | Combination of drugs for pain relief | Dizziness, lightheadedness |
| **Byetta**, *Exenatide* | Oral medication for type II diabetes | Hypoglycemia, nausea |
| *Cabergoline,* **Dostinex** | Treatment of hyperprolactinemia | Xerostomia, toothache, throat irritation |
| **Caduet**, *Amlodipine/ Atorvastatin* | Combination of drugs used to lower blood pressure and high cholesterol to prevent coronary artery disease | Muscle pain, tenderness, or weakness with fever or flu symptoms; or nausea, stomach pain, low fever, loss of appetite |
| *Calcitonin (salmon),* **Calcimar** | Hormone that stops bone resorption | None |
| *Calcitriol,* **Calcijex, Rocaltrol** | A form of vitamin D used to treat and prevent low levels of calcium in the blood | Metallic taste, xerostomia |
| *Captopril,* **Capoten** | Medication used to treat high blood pressure, heart failure, and for preventing kidney failure due to high blood pressure and diabetes | Altered taste, dizziness, nausea, vomiting; use of epinephrine or levonordefrin in local anesthetic should be minimized; angioedema, hypotension |
| *Carbamazepine,* **Carbatrol, Epitol, Tegretol** | Anticonvulsant; also for trigeminal or glossopharyngeal neuralgia | Xerostomia |

*(continued)*

**READY REFERENCE 5-2** COMMONLY PRESCRIBED DRUGS[a] *(CONTINUED)*

| Drug | Use | Concerns/Oral Manifestations |
|---|---|---|
| *Carbidopa,* **Lodosyn**; *carbidopa/levodopa,* **Sinemet** | Medication used to treat Parkinson disease | Hypotension, fainting, anxiety |
| *Carisoprodol,* **Soma** | Medication used for muscle relaxant and TMJ pain | Hypotension, fainting |
| **Cartia XT**, *Diltiazem* | Medication for chest pain from angina | Gingival hyperplasia |
| *Carvedilol,* **Coreg CR** | Medication to lower blood pressure | Xerostomia, hypotension |
| **Casodex**, *Bicalutamide* | Chemotherapy for prostate cancer | Xerostomia |
| **Catapres**, *Clonidine HCl* | Medication for the treatment of hypertension; also used to manage the symptoms of narcotic withdrawal and nicotine withdrawal | Drowsiness, xerostomia, salivary gland enlargement, dizziness; vasoconstrictors in local anesthetic should be minimized |
| *Cefadroxil,* **Duricef** | Antibiotic: alternative to penicillin for prevention of infective endocarditis | None |
| *Cefdinir,* **Omnicef** | Antibiotic medication for pneumonia, ear infection, sinusitis, pharyngitis, tonsillitis, and skin infections | Nausea, headache |
| *Cefprozil,* **Cefzil** | Antibiotic: ear, respiratory, and skin infections | Nausea, headache |
| **Ceftin**, *Cefuroxime* | Antibiotic: lower respiratory, skin, bone, full body infection (sepsis) | Nausea, headache |
| **Celebrex**, *Celecoxib* | NSAID for relief of mild to moderate pain of arthritis | Possible increased risk of heart attack, xerostomia, altered taste, vomiting, aphthous ulcers, stomatitis |
| **Celexa**, *Citalopram* | Antidepressant for treatment of depression, obsessive-compulsive disorders, panic disorders | Xerostomia, altered taste, nausea, oral candidiasis, dizziness |
| **CellCept**, *Mycophenolate* | Immunosuppressant agent: prevent rejection of organ transplant | Oral ulcers, oral candidiasis, sore mouth, gingival hyperplasia |
| *Cephalexin,* **Keflex** | Antibiotic: alternative to penicillin for prevention of infective endocarditis | Nausea, headache |
| *Cetirizine,* **Zyrtec** | Antihistamine: for allergy, hay fever | Xerostomia |

*(continued)*

**READY REFERENCE 5-2**   **COMMONLY PRESCRIBED DRUGS**[a] *(CONTINUED)*

| Drug | Use | Concerns/Oral Manifestations |
|---|---|---|
| **Chantix**, *varenicline* | Non-nicotine medication designed to help smokers quit more easily than without the drug | Bad taste in mouth; suicidal thoughts while using medication; suicidal thoughts following withdrawal from medication; nausea, heartburn, depression, agitation, drowsiness, headache; changes in mood or behavior |
| **Cialis**, *Tadalafil* | Erectile dysfunction | **If chest pain – No nitroglycerine** |
| *Cilostazol*, **Pletal** | Antiplatelet agent: used to prevent platelets from clumping and forming clots | Headache in 27%–34% |
| **Cipro**, *Ciprofloxacin* | Antibiotic for treatment of bacterial infections: also used for periodontitis associated with *Actinobacillus actinomycetemcomitans* | Oral candidiasis, nausea |
| **Ciprodex**, *Ciprofloxacin/ Dexamethasone* | Combination of ciprofloxacin and cortisone for ear infections | None |
| **Clarinex**, *Desloratadine* | Nasal spray for runny nose and nasal congestion | Xerostomia |
| *Clarithromycin*, **Biaxin** | Antibiotic used to treat bacterial infections | Oral candidiasis, altered taste, cough, dizziness, nausea |
| **Claritin**, *Loratadine*, **Claritin-D**, *Loratadine/ Pseudoephedrine* | Antihistamine used to treat the symptoms of allergy | Xerostomia, tachycardia, palpitations |
| *Clindamycin*, **Cleocin** | Antibiotic for treatment of infections, prevention of bacterial endocarditis | Oral candidiasis, dizziness |
| *Clindamycin* (topical), **Cleocin T** | Antibacterial agent for acne | None |
| *Clobetasol Propionate* **Clobevate** | Topical cortisone: erosive disorders | Use: lichen planus, aphthae |
| *Clonazepam*, **Klonopin** | Medication for certain types of seizures in the treatment of epilepsy and for the treatment of panic disorders | Dizziness, hypotension, fainting |
| *Clonidine*, **Catapres** | Medication for the treatment of hypertension; also used to manage the symptoms of narcotic withdrawal and nicotine withdrawal | Drowsiness, xerostomia, salivary gland enlargement, dizziness; vasoconstrictors in local anesthetic should be minimized. |

*(continued)*

**READY REFERENCE 5-2**  COMMONLY PRESCRIBED DRUGS[a] *(CONTINUED)*

| Drug | Use | Concerns/Oral Manifestations |
|---|---|---|
| *Clopidogrel,* **Plavix** | A medication that reduces the clumping of platelets in the blood; reduces risks for heart attack and stroke | Increased bleeding |
| *Clorazepate,* **Tranxene** | Medication used to treat general anxiety disorder, partial seizures | Xerostomia, drowsiness, hypotension, fainting |
| *Clotrimazole,* **Lotrimin** | Topical antifungal medication in the form of a lozenge (troche) used to treat oral candidiasis | None |
| *Clotrimazole/ Betamethasone,* **Lotrisone** | Antifungal with cortisone: topical dental use: oral lesions | None |
| *Co-trimoxazole,* **Bactrim** | Antibiotic for infections of the urinary tract, ear, lower respiratory system | Nausea, vomiting |
| **Colchicine/Probenecid**, *colchicine/probenecid* | Medication for the treatment for gout | Dizziness, headache, sore gums, nausea |
| **Combivent**, *Ipratropium/Albuterol* | Inhaler for chronic obstructive pulmonary disease (COPD) | Xerostomia |
| **Combivir**, *Zidovudine/ Lamivudine* | Two antiretroviral drugs combined for treatment of HIV infection | Headache, joint or muscle pain, nausea, nervousness, tiredness, vomiting, weakness |
| **Concerta**, *Methylphenidate HCl (XR)* | Medication for treatment of ADHD | Hypertension |
| *Conjugated estrogens,* **Premarin** | Hormone replacement therapy | None |
| **Copaxone**, *Glatiramer acetate* | Medication for relapsing multiple sclerosis | Anxiety, back pain, flushing, headache, nausea, vomiting, weakness |
| **Coreg**, *Carvedilol* | Used to treat high blood pressure and congestive heart failure | Hypotension, dizziness; use of epinephrine or levonordefrin in local anesthetic should be minimized |
| **Cosopt**, *Dorzolamide/ Timolol* | Used to decrease intraocular pressure (pressure within the eyeball) | Altered taste |
| **Cotrim**, *Co-trimoxazole* | Antibiotic used for urinary tract infections, respiratory tract infections, middle ear infections | Oral candidiasis, dizziness, nausea |

*(continued)*

**READY REFERENCE 5-2** COMMONLY PRESCRIBED DRUGS[a] *(CONTINUED)*

| Drug | Use | Concerns/Oral Manifestations |
|---|---|---|
| **Coumadin**, *Warfarin* | Anticoagulant that is helpful in preventing blood clot formation in patients with atrial fibrillation and artificial heart valves to reduce the risk of strokes | Ulcerations; increased bleeding tendency, medical consult |
| **Cozaar**, *Losartan* | Used to treat high blood pressure, congestive heart failure | Xerostomia, dizziness; use of epinephrine or levonordefrin in local anesthetic should be minimized |
| **Crestor**, *Rosuvastatin* | Treatment to lower high cholesterol to prevent coronary artery disease | Muscle pain, tenderness, or weakness with fever or flu symptoms; or nausea, stomach pain, low fever, loss of appetite |
| *Cyclobenzaprine,* **Flexeril** | Muscle relaxant; also used for TMJ dysfunction | Dizziness, syncope, edema |
| *Cyclosporine,* **Sandimmune** | Immunosuppressant in organ transplant | Gingival hyperplasia, oral lesions |
| **Cymbalta**, *Duloxetine* | Medication for depression | Xerostomia |
| **Deltasone**, *Prednisone* | An oral corticosteroid used to treat arthritis, colitis, asthma, and bronchitis | Oral candidiasis<br>With long-term use: increased susceptibility to infection, adrenal insufficiency |
| **Depakote**, *Divalproex* | Medication for the treatment of seizures, bipolar disorder, and prevention of migraines | Dizziness, nausea, tremor, periodontal abscess, taste abnormality |
| *Desogestrel/Ethinyl estradiol,* **Apri** | Birth control | Antibiotics taken for dental infections can decrease the effectiveness of oral contraceptives |
| *Desoximetasone,* **Topicort** | Topical corticosteroid used to treat inflammation of the skin | None |
| **Detrol LA**, *Tolterodine tartrate* | Used to treat uncontrollable urination due to what is often referred to as an "overactive" bladder | Xerostomia |
| *Dextroamphetamine sulfate,* **Dexedrine** | Stimulant used to treat narcolepsy and ADHD<br>Stimulant for obesity, depression | Nervousness; interacts with vasoconstrictors in local anesthesia Xerostomia, taste perversion |
| *Diazepam,* **Valium** | Used for treatment of general anxiety disorder | Nausea |
| *Diclofenac,* **Voltaren** | NSAID for treatment of rheumatoid arthritis | Dizziness, drowsiness, headache, heartburn, nausea |

*(continued)*

## READY REFERENCE 5-2   COMMONLY PRESCRIBED DRUGS[a] (CONTINUED)

| Drug | Use | Concerns/Oral Manifestations |
|---|---|---|
| *Didanosine*, **Videx** | Medication for the treatment of HIV+ | Headache, joint or muscle pain, nausea, nervousness, tiredness, vomiting, weakness |
| **Differin**, *Adapalene* | Topical treatment for acne | Erythema, scaling, dryness |
| **Diflucan**, *Fluconazole* | Antifungal used to treat oral, esophageal, urinary, and vaginal infections caused by the fungus *Candida* | Dizziness, nausea |
| **Digitek**, *Digoxin* | Used to treat heart failure and abnormal heart rhythms | Hypotension, gagging |
| **Dilantin**, *Phenytoin* | An anticonvulsant medication used to prevent seizures | Gingival hyperplasia, dizziness |
| *Diltiazem*, **Cardizem, Cartia XT** | Medication for chest pain from angina | Gingival hyperplasia |
| **Diovan**, *Valsartan* | Medication to lower high blood pressure and treat congestive heart failure | Dizziness; use of epinephrine or levonordefrin in local anesthetic should be minimized |
| **Diovan HCT**, *Valsartan/Hydrochlorothiazide* | Medication to lower high blood pressure and treat congestive heart failure | Hypotension |
| *Diphenoxylate/Atropine*, **Lomotil** | Medication for adults with symptoms of diarrhea and intestinal spasms | Xerostomia |
| **Ditropan XL**, *Oxybutynin* | Used for adults with symptoms of overactive bladder | Xerostomia |
| *Divalproex*, **Depakote** | Used for the treatment of seizures, bipolar disorder, and prevention of migraines | Dizziness, nausea, tremor, periodontal abscess, taste abnormality |
| *Docusate sodium*, **Colace** | Stool softener to treat constipation | None |
| **Dovonex**, *Calcipotriene* (topical) | Treatment for psoriasis (a skin disease with red, scaly patches) | None |
| *Doxazosin*, **Cardura XL** | For the treatment of high blood pressure and benign enlargement of the prostate | Xerostomia, orthostatic hypotension |
| *Doxepin HCl*, **Prudoxin** | Antidepressant | Xerostomia, altered taste |
| *Doxycycline*, **Vibramycin** | Antibiotic for treatment of numerous infections, including periodontitis | Glossitis, tooth staining, and opportunistic candidiasis |

*(continued)*

**READY REFERENCE 5-2**  COMMONLY PRESCRIBED DRUGS[a] *(CONTINUED)*

| Drug | Use | Concerns/Oral Manifestations |
|---|---|---|
| **Duexis**, *Ibuprofen/ Famotidine* | For the relief of signs and symptoms of rheumatoid arthritis and osteoarthritis | Bleeding |
| **Dulera**, *Formoterol/ Mometasone* | Inhaler for the treatment of asthma | Can lower patient immune system and increase chances of infection |
| **Duragesic**, *Fentanyl* | Transdermal patch used for patients with severe chronic pain, for example, the pain of cancer | Hypotension |
| *Econazole nitrate,* **Spectazole** | Antifungal agent: topical | None |
| **Edarbi**, *Azilsartan medoxomil* | For the treatment of high blood pressure | Hypotension |
| **Edluar**, *Zolpidem* | Sublingual tablet for treatment of insomnia | Dizziness, xerostomia; not to be used with other CNS depressants |
| **Elidel**, *Pimecrolimus* (topical) | Used for the treatment of mild to moderate dermatitis | Respiratory tract and viral infections |
| **Elocon**, *Mometasone furoate* | Corticosteroid lotion used for the relief of itching and skin conditions | Increased glucose concentration in blood, adrenal insufficiency |
| **Enbrel**, *Etanercept* | Medication for treatment of rheumatoid arthritis | Increased risk for infection |
| *Enalapril,* **Vasotec** | Used to treat high blood pressure and heart failure and for preventing kidney failure due to high blood pressure and diabetes | Altered taste, persistent cough, dizziness, nausea, vomiting; use of epinephrine or levonordefrin in local anesthetic should be minimized; angioedema, hypotension |
| **Endocet**, *Oxycodone/ Acetaminophen* | Narcotic analgesics used to relieve pain | Nausea, dizziness |
| **Epzicom**, *Abacavir sulfate/Lamivudine,* **Trizivir**, *Abacavir sulfate/ Lamivudine/Zidovudine* | Three antiretroviral drugs combined for treatment of HIV+ | Headache, joint or muscle pain, nausea, nervousness, tiredness, vomiting, weakness |
| *Erythromycin* | Antibiotic | Oral candidiasis |
| **Esidrix**, *Hydrochlorothiazide* | Diuretic commonly used to lower high blood pressure | Hypotension |
| **Eskalith**, *Lithium carbonate* | Medication used most frequently for bipolar affective disorder (manic-depressive illness) | Fine hand tremor, dry mouth, altered taste, salivary gland enlargement |
| *Esomeprazole,* magnesium **Nexium** | Decreases the amount of acid produced in the stomach, treatment for GERD | Nausea |

*(continued)*

**READY REFERENCE 5-2**   COMMONLY PRESCRIBED DRUGS[a] *(CONTINUED)*

| Drug | Use | Concerns/Oral Manifestations |
|---|---|---|
| *Estradiol*, **Alora** | Estrogen replacement therapy by transdermal patch | Headache |
| *Ethinyl estradiol and norethindrone,* **Ortho-Novum** | Birth control | Antibiotics taken for dental infections can decrease the effectiveness of oral contraceptives |
| Etodolac, **Lodine** | NSAID medication for pain, arthritis | Abnormal taste |
| **Evista**, *Raloxifene HCl* | Medication to treat or prevent osteoporosis | Hot flashes |
| **Evoclin**, *clindamycin phosphate* (topical) | Alternative antibiotic for amoxicillin for infective endocarditis | – |
| *Famotidine*, **Pepcid** | Decreases the amount of acid produced in the stomach, treatment of GERD | Dizziness, headache |
| **Famvir**, *Famciclovir* | Antiviral medication for herpes zoster (shingles), herpes labialis, genital herpes | Headache in 17%–39% of patients, nausea in 7%–13% of patients, diarrhea |
| *Felodipine*, **Plendil** | For the management of high blood pressure and congestive heart failure | Gingival hyperplasia headache in 11%–15% of patients |
| **Femara**, *Letrozole* | Chemotherapy for breast cancer | Numerous adverse effects |
| *Fenofibrate*, **Lipidil** | Medication that lowers cholesterol and triglycerides | Xerostomia, tooth disorder |
| *Ferrous sulfate* $(FeSO_4)$, **Feosol** | Supplement for iron deficiency anemia | Liquid $FeSO_4$ stains teeth |
| *Fexofenadine HCl,* **Allegra**, *Fexofenadine HCl/ Pseudoephedrine HCl,* **Allegra-D** | An antihistamine used to treat the signs and symptoms of allergy | Xerostomia, dizziness, headache, anxiety, tremor |
| *Flecainide acetate,* **Tambocor** | Medication used to treat irregular heartbeat | Dizziness in 19%–30% of patients |
| **Flomax**, *tamsulosin* | Treatment of men who are having difficulty urinating due to enlarged prostate | Orthostatic hypotension |
| **Flonase, Flovent**, *Fluticasone* | Topical corticosteroid used for the control of the symptoms of allergic rhinitis (stuffy nose) | Oral candidiasis |
| *Fluconazole*, **Diflucan** | Antifungal used to treat oral, esophageal, urinary, vaginal infections caused by the fungus *Candida* | Dizziness, nausea |

*(continued)*

**READY REFERENCE 5-2** COMMONLY PRESCRIBED DRUGS[a] (CONTINUED)

| Drug | Use | Concerns/Oral Manifestations |
|---|---|---|
| *Fluocinonide,* **Lidex** (topical) | Treatment for psoriasis (a skin disease with red, scaly patches) | None |
| *Fluoxetine,* **Prozac** | Medication for treatment of depression | Oral candidiasis, xerostomia, hypotension, nausea; can initiate bruxism |
| *Fluticasone/Salmeterol,* **Advair** | Inhaled drug that is used to treat asthma, chronic bronchitis, or emphysema | Xerostomia, upper respiratory infections |
| *Fluvastatin,* **Lescol** | Treatment to lower high cholesterol to prevent coronary artery disease | Muscle pain, tenderness, or weakness with fever or flu symptoms; or nausea, stomach pain, low fever, loss of appetite |
| *Fluvoxamine,* **Luvox** | Medication for treatment of depression and obsessive-compulsive disorder | Xerostomia, bruxism |
| **Focalin XR,** *Dexmethylphenidate* | For treatment of ADHD | Xerostomia, headache |
| **Folvite,** *Folic acid* | Vitamin: water soluble | None |
| **Forteo,** *Teriparatide* | Parathyroid hormone for osteoporosis | Tooth disorder |
| **Fortesta,** *testosterone* (topical) | Testosterone gel for topical treatment of hypogonadism in men | Ankle swelling |
| **Fosamax,** *Alendronate* | Used for the treatment of persons with osteoporosis | Osteonecrosis of the jaws |
| **Fosamax Plus D,** *Alendronate/ cholecalciferol* | Used for the treatment of persons with osteoporosis | Osteonecrosis of the jaws |
| *Fosinopril,* **Monopril** | Used to treat high blood pressure and heart failure and for preventing kidney failure due to high blood pressure and diabetes | Altered taste, dizziness, nausea, vomiting; use of epinephrine or levonordefrin in local anesthetic should be minimized; angioedema, hypotension |
| *Furosemide,* **Lasix** | Diuretic used to treat high blood pressure and congestive heart failure | Orthostatic hypotension |
| **Fuzeon,** *Enfuvirtide* | Antiretroviral agent: HIV-1 | Xerostomia, altered taste |
| *Gabapentin,* **Neurontin** | Anticonvulsant (used to prevent seizures) | Xerostomia, dizziness |
| *Gatifloxacin,* **Tequin, Zymar** | Antibiotic for the bacterial infections | Oral candidiasis |

*(continued)*

**READY REFERENCE 5-2** COMMONLY PRESCRIBED DRUGS[a] (CONTINUED)

| Drug | Use | Concerns/Oral Manifestations |
|---|---|---|
| *Gemfibrozil*, **Lopid** | Medication used to lower triglycerides | None known |
| **Geodon**, *Ziprasidone hydrochloride* | Antipsychotic used to treat schizophrenia and bipolar disorder with or without psychosis | Xerostomia, hypotension, tooth disorder, tongue edema |
| **Gleevec**, *Imatinib* | Chemotherapy for sarcomas, leukemia | Numerous adverse effects |
| *Glimepiride*, **Amaryl** | Oral drug for the control of diabetes | Hypoglycemia, dizziness, nausea; if diabetes is poorly controlled, increased risk of periodontitis |
| *Glipizide*, **Glucotrol** | Oral drug for the control of diabetes | Hypoglycemia, dizziness, nausea; if diabetes is poorly controlled, increased risk of periodontitis |
| *Glucagon*, **GlucaGen** | Emergency treatment for unconscious diabetic patients in insulin shock | Available for injection; there is a paste for oral administration in patients who are conscious |
| **Glucophage XR**, *Metformin* | Oral drug for the control of type II diabetes | Oral candidiasis, altered taste, hypoglycemia, dizziness, nausea; if diabetes is poorly controlled, increased risk of periodontitis |
| **Glucotrol**, *Glipizide* | Oral drug for the control of type II diabetes | Hypoglycemia, dizziness, nausea; if diabetes is poorly controlled, increased risk of periodontitis |
| **Glucovance**, *Glyburide/Metformin* | Oral drug for the control of type II diabetes | Hypoglycemia, dizziness, nausea; if diabetes is poorly controlled, increased risk of periodontitis |
| *Glyburide*, **DiaBeta** | Oral drug for the control of type II diabetes | Hypoglycemia, dizziness, nausea; if diabetes is poorly controlled, increased risk of periodontitis |
| *Glyburide/Metformin* **Glucovance** | Oral drug for the control of type II diabetes | Hypoglycemia, dizziness, nausea; if diabetes is poorly controlled, increased risk of periodontitis |
| *Griseofulvin*, **Gris-PEG** | Antifungal drug for infections of the skin or nails caused by fungi | Mouth/tongue irritation, thrush |
| *Guaifenesin*, **Robitussin, Fenesin** | Cough medicine and expectorant that loosens phlegm | None |
| *Guanethidine*, **Ismelin** | Medication to lower high blood pressure | Hypotension |

*(continued)*

**READY REFERENCE 5-2** COMMONLY PRESCRIBED DRUGS[a] *(CONTINUED)*

| Drug | Use | Concerns/Oral Manifestations |
|------|-----|------------------------------|
| *Haloperidol,* **Haldol** | Used for treating psychotic disorders and for tics and vocal utterances of Tourette syndrome | Gingival bleeding; xerostomia; ulcerations; sudden motions of the head, neck, and arms; involuntary movements of mouth/tongue; dizziness; orthostatic hypotension |
| **Humalog,** *Insulin lispro* | Injectable insulin for type I diabetes | Respiratory tract infection, hypoglycemia, sore throat; if diabetes is poorly controlled, increased risk of periodontitis |
| **Humira,** *Adalimumab* | Medication for treatment of rheumatoid arthritis and Crohn disease | Nausea; runny or stuff nose |
| **Humulin 70/30,** *Insulin* | Injectable insulin for type I diabetes | Oral candidiasis, respiratory tract infection, hypoglycemia, sore throat; if diabetes is poorly controlled, increased risk of periodontitis |
| *Hydralazine,* **Apresoline** | Medication for treatment of severe high blood pressure | Hypotension |
| *Hydrochlorothiazide,* **Esidrix** | Diuretic for lowering high blood pressure and treating congestive heart failure | Hypokalemia (below normal levels of potassium in the blood), hypotension |
| *Hydrocodone/ Ibuprofen,* **Reprexain, Vicoprofen** | Narcotic combined with NSAID for moderate to severe pain | Xerostomia, dizziness, nausea, vomiting |
| *Hydrocodone with acetaminophen,* **Vicodin, Lortab** | Narcotic combined with Acetaminophen for pain | Xerostomia, dizziness, nausea, vomiting |
| *Hydrocortisone,* **Solu-Cortef** | Corticosteroid: anti-inflammatory agent | Infection, adrenal crisis if taken long term |
| *Hydromorphone HCl,* **Dilaudid** | Narcotic medication for severe pain | Hypotension, nausea, vomiting |
| *Hydroxychloroquine sulfate,* **Plaquenil** | Used to treat acute attacks of malaria; also used to treat lupus erythematosus and rheumatoid arthritis in patients whose symptoms have not improved with other treatments | Nausea, dizziness, headache, eyesight problems |
| *Hydroxyzine,* **Atarax, Vistaril** | Antihistamine used to treat allergic reactions; antianxiety agent used as a preoperative sedative | Xerostomia |

*(continued)*

**READY REFERENCE 5-2** COMMONLY PRESCRIBED DRUGS[a] (CONTINUED)

| Drug | Use | Concerns/Oral Manifestations |
|---|---|---|
| Hyoscyamine, **Anaspaz** | Medication to stop spasms of the intestines associated with diarrhea with irritable bowel syndrome | Xerostomia |
| **Hyzaar**, Losartan/Hydrochlorothiazide | Combination of two medications to lower high blood pressure | Hypotension |
| Ibuprofen, **Motrin, Advil** | NSAID for relief of mild to moderate pain | Xerostomia, dizziness, drowsiness, nausea, heartburn, bleeding |
| Imipramine HCL, **Tofranil-PM** | Treatment for depression | Xerostomia, hypotension |
| **Imitrex**, sumatriptan | Medication for relief of migraine headaches | Bad taste, dysphagia, mouth/tongue discomfort |
| Indapamide, **Lozol** | Diuretic used to lower blood pressure and treat congestive heart failure | Xerostomia, hypotension, palpitations, rhinorrhea |
| **Inderal LA**, Propranolol | Medication used to lower high blood pressure and prevent angina, tremor, arrhythmias | Hypotension |
| Indinavir, **Crixivan** | Antiviral agent for treatment of HIV+ | Headache, joint or muscle pain, nausea, nervousness, tiredness, vomiting, weakness |
| Indomethacin, **Indocin** | NSAID for relief of mild to moderate pain | Xerostomia, ulcerations, dizziness, drowsiness, nausea, heartburn, increased bleeding tendency |
| Insulin lispro, **Humalog** | Injectable insulin for type I diabetes | Respiratory tract infection, hypoglycemia, sore throat; if diabetes is poorly controlled, increased risk of periodontitis |
| Ipratropium/Albuterol, **Combivent** | Inhaler for respiratory diseases | Xerostomia |
| Ipratropium bromide, **Atrovent** | Inhaler used for chronic bronchitis and emphysema | Xerostomia, tremor, nervousness |
| Irbesartan, **Avapro** | Medication used to lower high blood pressure and relieve symptoms of congestive heart failure | Dizziness; use of epinephrine or levonordefrin in local anesthetic should be minimized |
| Isocarboxazid, **Marplan** | Medication for generalized depression that does not respond to other antidepressants | Dizziness, drowsiness, hypotension; this drug interacts with most drugs and cannot be used with local anesthesia that has epinephrine or levonordefrin |

*(continued)*

**READY REFERENCE 5-2**   COMMONLY PRESCRIBED DRUGS[a] (CONTINUED)

| Drug | Use | Concerns/Oral Manifestations |
|------|-----|------------------------------|
| *Isosorbide dinitrate,* **Isordil** | Calcium channel blocker for angina, high blood pressure, rapid heart rhythm | Gingival hyperplasia, dizziness |
| *Isosorbide mononitrate,* **Imdur** | Medication to prevent angina attacks | Headache |
| Isotretinoin, **Accutane** | A strong vitamin A oral medication used to treat acne when other medications are not effective | Causes serious and fatal birth defects; frequently causes depression |
| Itraconazole, **Sporanox** | Antifungal agent used in immunocompromised patients with oropharyngeal candidiasis | None |
| **Januvia**, *Sitagliptin* | Treatment of type II diabetes | Stress-induced hypoglycemia |
| **Kadian**, *Morphine sulfate* | Narcotic medication for severe pain | Hypotension, nausea, vomiting |
| **Kaletra**, *Lopinavir/ Ritonavir* | Antiretroviral drug for treatment of HIV+ | Headache, joint or muscle pain, nausea, nervousness, tiredness, vomiting, weakness |
| **Kapidex**, *dexlansoprazole* | Medication for erosive esophagitis and GERD | Dwelling of lips, tongue, cheeks (angioedema), fainting, chest tightness |
| **Kapvay**, *Clonidine HCl* | Medication for treatment of ADHD | Dizziness, fainting, xerostomia, headache. Severe reaction: angioedema |
| **K-Dur, Klor-Con**, *Potassium chloride* | Electrolyte supplement to prevent potassium depletion (hypokalemia) | Xerostomia |
| **Keppra**, *Levetiracetam* | An antiseizure medication (anticonvulsant) used to prevent seizures | Gingival hyperplasia, dizziness |
| *Ketoconazole*, **Nizoral** | Antifungal agent used to treat fungal infections such as oral candidiasis | Numerous drug interactions |
| **Kombiglyze XR**, *Metformin/Saxagliptin* | Extended release medication for type II diabetes | Stress-induced hypoglycemia |
| *Labetalol HCl,* **Trandate** | Treatment for high blood pressure | Hypertensive crisis, low heart rate (bradycardia) |
| **Lamictal**, *Lamotrigine* | Anticonvulsant medication to prevent seizures | Xerostomia |
| **Lamisil**, *Terbinafine* | Antifungal drug for ringworm/ athlete's foot | Taste disturbance |

*(continued)*

**READY REFERENCE 5-2** COMMONLY PRESCRIBED DRUGS[a] *(CONTINUED)*

| Drug | Use | Concerns/Oral Manifestations |
|---|---|---|
| **Lanoxin**, *Digoxin* | Used to treat congestive heart failure | Hypotension, gagging |
| *Lansoprazole*, **Prevacid** | Reduces stomach acid production | Xerostomia, oral candidiasis, altered taste, aphthous ulcers, stomatitis |
| **Lantus**, *Insulin glargine* | Insulin for type I diabetes | Hypoglycemia |
| **Lasix**, *Furosemide* | Diuretic used to treat high blood pressure and congestive heart failure | Orthostatic hypotension |
| *Latanoprost*, **Xalatan** | Ophthalmic agent (eye preparation) for treatment of glaucoma | None |
| *Leflunomide*, **Arava** | Medication for rheumatoid arthritis | Sore mouth (stomatitis) candidasis, abnormal taste, tooth disorder, gingivitis |
| **Lexcol**, *Fluvastatin* | Medication to lower high cholesterol to prevent coronary artery disease | Muscle pain, tenderness, or weakness with fever or flu symptoms; or nausea, stomach pain, low fever, loss of appetite |
| **Levaquin**, *Levofloxacin* | Antibiotic for treatment of sinusitis and urinary tract infections | Oral candidiasis |
| **Levitra**, *Vardenafil* | Medication for erectile dysfunction | **If patient has chest pain – No nitroglycerine should be given** |
| *Levonorgestrel/Ethinyl estradiol*, **Aviane** | Birth control | Antibiotics taken for dental infections can decrease the effectiveness of oral contraceptives |
| **Levothroid**, **Levoxyl** Levothyroxine | Thyroid replacement hormone | High blood pressure |
| **Lexapro**, *Escitalopram* | Treatment for depression and generalized anxiety | Xerostomia, nausea |
| **Lipitor**, *Atorvastin calcium* | Medication to lower high cholesterol to prevent coronary artery disease | Muscle pain, tenderness, or weakness with fever or flu symptoms; or nausea, stomach pain, low fever, loss of appetite |
| *Lisinopril*, **Prinivil, Zestril** | Used to treat high blood pressure and heart failure and for preventing kidney failure due to high blood pressure and diabetes | Altered taste, dizziness, nausea, vomiting; use of epinephrine or levonordefrin in local anesthetic should be minimized; angioedema, hypotension |
| *Lisinopril/ Hydrochlorothiazide combination*, **Zestoretic** | Used to treat high blood pressure and heart failure and for preventing kidney failure due to high blood pressure and diabetes | Altered taste, dizziness, nausea, vomiting; use of epinephrine or levonordefrin in local anesthetic should be minimized; angioedema, hypotension |

*(continued)*

**READY REFERENCE 5-2** COMMONLY PRESCRIBED DRUGS[a] *(CONTINUED)*

| Drug | Use | Concerns/Oral Manifestations |
|---|---|---|
| *Lithium*, **Eskalith, Lithobid** | Used most frequently for bipolar affective disorder (manic-depressive illness) | Fine hand tremor, dry mouth, altered taste, salivary gland enlargement |
| **Livalo**, *Pitavastatin* | Treatment to lower high cholesterol to prevent coronary artery disease | Muscle pain, tenderness, or weakness with fever or flu symptoms; or nausea, stomach pain, low fever, loss of appetite |
| *L-Norgestrel/Ethinyl estradiol* | Birth control | Antibiotics taken for dental infections can decrease the effectiveness of oral contraceptives |
| **Loestrin Fe**, *Ethinyl estradiol/ Norethindrone* | Birth control | Antibiotics taken for dental infections can decrease the effectiveness of oral contraceptives |
| *Loratadine*, **Claritin,** *Loratadine/ Pseudoephedrine*, **Claritin-D** | Antihistamine for allergies | Xerostomia, stomatitis, tachycardia, palpitations |
| *Lorazepam*, **Ativan** | Medication for treatment of anxiety | Xerostomia |
| *Losartan*, **Cozaar** | Used to treat high blood pressure and congestive heart failure | Xerostomia, dizziness; use of epinephrine or levonordefrin in local anesthetic should be minimized |
| *Losartan/ Hydrochlorothiazide*, **Hyzaar** | Used to treat high blood pressure and congestive heart failure | Xerostomia, dizziness; use of epinephrine or levonordefrin in local anesthetic should be minimized |
| **Lotensin**, *Benazepril* | Used to treat high blood pressure and congestive heart failure | Altered taste, dizziness, nausea, vomiting; use of epinephrine or levonordefrin in local anesthetic should be minimized; angioedema, hypotension |
| **Lotrel**, *Amlodipine/ Benazepril* | Medication used to lower high blood pressure | Altered taste, orthostatic hypotension, dizziness, fatigue, headache, nausea, vomiting; use of epinephrine or levonordefrin in local anesthetic should be minimized |
| *Lovastatin*, **Altoprev, Mevacor** | Treatment to lower high cholesterol to prevent coronary artery disease | Muscle pain, tenderness, or weakness with fever or flu symptoms; or nausea, stomach pain, low fever, loss of appetite |

*(continued)*

**READY REFERENCE 5-2**    COMMONLY PRESCRIBED DRUGS[a] *(CONTINUED)*

| Drug | Use | Concerns/Oral Manifestations |
|---|---|---|
| **Lovaza**, *Omega-3-acid ethyl esters* | Prescription level of omega-3 fish oil for the treatment of high triglyceride blood levels | Burping, indigestion |
| **Low-Ogestrel**, *Norgestrel/Ethinyl estradiol* | Birth control | Antibiotics taken for dental infections can decrease the effectiveness of oral contraceptives |
| **Lumigan**, *Bimatoprost* | Ophthalmic agent (eye preparation) for treatment of glaucoma | None |
| **Lunesta**, *Eszopiclone* | Sleep aid for insomnia | Bad taste, xerostomia |
| **Lyrica**, *Pregabalin* | Medication for either fibromyalgia or prevention of seizures in epilepsy | Xerostomia |
| **Macrobid**, *Nitrofurantoin* | Antibiotic | Nausea |
| **Maxalt-MLT**, *Rizatriptan* | Medication for migraine headaches and symptoms | Xerostomia |
| *Meclizine*, **Antivert, Maxalt-MLT, Bonine** | Used for the treatment of nausea, vomiting, and dizziness | Xerostomia, drowsiness |
| *Medroxyprogesterone*, **Provera** | Birth control | May cause gingival bleeding |
| *Meloxicam*, **Mobic** | NSAID for relief of mild to moderate pain | Oral ulcers, xerostomia |
| *Mercaptopurine*, **Purinethol** | Chemotherapy for leukemia | Stomatitis, mucositis |
| *Metaxalone*, **Skelaxin** | Skeletal muscle relaxant | Dizziness |
| *Metformin*, **Glucophage** | Medication for type II diabetes | Stress-induced hypoglycemia |
| *Methadone HCl*, **Dolophine** | Narcotic for moderate to severe pain | Xerostomia, glossitis |
| *Methocarbamol*, **Robaxin** | Skeletal muscle relaxant | Metallic taste |
| *Methotrexate*, **Rheumatrex** | Used to treat rheumatoid arthritis, severe psoriasis, and also some cancers | Ulcerative stomatitis, glossitis, dry cough |
| *Methylphenidate HCl*, **Ritalin** | A stimulant to treat ADHD and narcolepsy | Fast, uneven heartbeat; headache; sore throat; restlessness |
| *Methylprednisolone*, **Medrol**, *Methylprednisolone sodium succinate*, **Solu-Medrol** | Corticosteroid, systemic: anti-inflammatory, immunosuppressant | Ulcerative esophagitis; adrenal insufficiency if taken long term |

*(continued)*

**READY REFERENCE 5-2** COMMONLY PRESCRIBED DRUGS[a] *(CONTINUED)*

| Drug | Use | Concerns/Oral Manifestations |
|---|---|---|
| *Metoclopramide,* **Reglan** | Used short term for persistent heartburn | Xerostomia |
| *Metolazone,* **Zaroxolyn** | Diuretic for lowering high blood pressure | Hypotension, xerostomia |
| *Metoprolol,* **Lopressor** | For lowering high blood pressure | Hypotension |
| *Metronidazole,* **Flagyl** | Amebicide (a substance used to kill or capable of killing amebas); antibiotic | Xerostomia; avoid mouthwash containing alcohol |
| **Miacalcin,** *Calcitonin* | A hormone that prevents bone resorption | Nasal inflammation in 12% of patients |
| **Microgestin FE,** *Norethindrone/Ethinyl estradiol* | Birth control | Antibiotics taken for dental infections can decrease the effectiveness of oral contraceptives |
| *Midodrine,* **Amatine** | Medication for treatment of fainting spells | Xerostomia |
| *Minocycline,* **Dynacin** | Broad-spectrum antibiotic, also used to treat periodontitis associated with *Actinobacillus actinomycetemcomitans* | Dizziness, oral candidiasis, discoloration of teeth if used in patients below 8 years of age |
| **MiraLAX,** *polyethylene glycol 3350* | Laxative | Nausea, weakness, stomach cramping |
| **Mirapex,** *Pramipexole* | Medication for Parkinson disease | Xerostomia, dysphagia |
| **Mircette,** *Ethinyl estradiol/Desogestrel* | Birth control | Antibiotics taken for dental infections can decrease the effectiveness of oral contraceptives |
| *Mirtazapine,* **Remeron** | For treatment of depression | Xerostomia |
| **Mobic,** *Meloxicam* | NSAID for relief of mild to moderate pain | Oral ulcers, xerostomia |
| *Mometasone,* **Elocon, Nasonex** | Topical corticosteroid: two types (topical, inhaled) | Xerostomia |
| **Monopril,** *Fosinopril* | Used to treat high blood pressure and heart failure and for preventing kidney failure due to high blood pressure and diabetes | Altered taste, dizziness, nausea, vomiting; use of epinephrine or levonordefrin in local anesthetic should be minimized; angioedema, hypotension |
| *Montelukast,* **Singulair** | Oral medication used for the treatment of asthma and seasonal allergic rhinitis | Dizziness, sore throat |
| *Morphine sulfate,* **Astramorph/PF** | Opioid medication for pain relief | Xerostomia |

*(continued)*

**READY REFERENCE 5-2** **COMMONLY PRESCRIBED DRUGS**[a] *(CONTINUED)*

| Drug | Use | Concerns/Oral Manifestations |
|---|---|---|
| *Multivitamins with fluoride* | Vitamin supplement | Refer to individual vitamins |
| *Mupirocin*, **Bactroban** | Topical antibiotic | Xerostomia |
| *Nabumetone*, **Relafen** | NSAID pain medication for rheumatoid arthritis and osteoarthritis | Xerostomia, stomatitis |
| *Nadolol*, **Corgard** | Medication for lowering high blood pressure | NSAIDS increase hypotensive effects |
| **Namenda**, *Memantine* | Medication for Alzheimer disease | Dizziness, fainting |
| *Naproxen*, **Aleve, Anaprox** | NSAID; analgesic used mostly for arthritis | Bleeding |
| **Nasacort AQ**, *Triamcinolone* | Corticosteroid: anti-inflammatory nasal, oral topical, inhalation administration. Use: lichen planus, aphthous, stomatitis | None |
| **Nasonex**, *Mometasone* | Corticosteroid: topical, inhaled | None |
| **Necon**, *Ethinyl estradiol/Norethindrone* | Birth control | Antibiotics taken for dental infections can decrease the effectiveness of oral contraceptives |
| *Nefazodone*, **Serzone** | Medication for depression | Xerostomia, hypotension |
| **Neupogen**, *Filgrastim* | For treatment of leukemia | |
| **Neurontin**, *Gabapentin* | Anticonvulsant to prevent seizures | Xerostomia, dental problems |
| **Nexium**, *Esomeprazole* | Medication to lower acid production in the stomach for treatment of GERD | Xerostomia |
| **Niaspan**, *Niacin* | Cholesterol-lowering medication | Flushing of the skin |
| *Nicotine transdermal*, **Nicorette** | Smoking cessation aid, patch or gum | Numerous effects from gum |
| **Nifediac CC**, *Nifedipine* (**NOT** for emergencies) | For the treatment of angina and high blood pressure | Gingival hyperplasia |
| **Nifedical XL**, *Nifedipine* (**NOT** for emergencies) | For the treatment of angina and high blood pressure | Gingival hyperplasia |
| *Nitrofurantoin*, **Macrobid** | Antibiotic | None known |
| *Nitroglycerin*, **Nitrostat, NitroQuick** (**EMERGENCY DRUG**) | Medication that is placed under the tongue for angina attacks | Xerostomia, hypotension; call emergency medical services (EMS) if no relief in 2 minutes |

*(continued)*

**READY REFERENCE 5-2**  COMMONLY PRESCRIBED DRUGS[a] *(CONTINUED)*

| Drug | Use | Concerns/Oral Manifestations |
|---|---|---|
| *Norethindrone,* **Aygestin** | Birth control | Antibiotics taken for dental infections can decrease the effectiveness of oral contraceptives |
| **Norpramin,** *Desipramine HCl* | Medication for treatment of depression | Hypotension, xerostomia |
| **Norvasc,** *Amlodipine* | For treatment of high blood pressure and congestive heart failure | Gingival hyperplasia; involuntary muscle contractions, tremors, changes in breathing and heart rate |
| **Norvir,** *Ritonavir* | Antiretroviral agent for HIV+ | Xerostomia, taste perversion |
| **NovoLog,** *Insulin aspart* | Insulin for type I diabetes | Hypoglycemia, morning apts. |
| **NovoLog Mix 70/30** | Insulin for type I diabetes | Hypoglycemia, morning apts. |
| **NPH Human Insulin,** *Insulin* | Injectable insulin for type I diabetes | Respiratory tract infection, hypoglycemia, sore throat; if diabetes is poorly controlled, increased risk of periodontitis |
| **NuvaRing,** *Etonogestrel/Ethinyl estradiol* | Birth control | Antibiotics taken for dental infections can decrease the effectiveness of oral contraceptives |
| *Nystatin,* **Mycostatin** | Antifungal agent: candidiasis | Avoid occlusal dressings |
| *Nystatin-triamcinolone,* **Mycolog-II** | Antifungal with corticosteroid for cheilitis, cutaneous candidiasis | Avoid occlusal dressings |
| *Olanzapine,* **Zyprexa** | Antidepressant/antipsychotic for depression with bipolar episodes | Xerostomia, tooth disorder, abnormal taste |
| **Oleptro,** *Trazodone* (XR) | Medication for treatment of depression | Xerostomia, headache, nausea, hypotension |
| *Omeprazole,* **Prilosec** | Reduces stomach acid production for treatment of GERD | Xerostomia, esophageal candidiasis, mucosal atrophy |
| **Omnicef,** *Cefdinir* | Antibiotic for sinusitis and ear infections | Nausea, vomiting, headache |
| **Oravig,** *Miconazole* (buccal) | Buccal adhesive for oropharyngeal candidiasis | Dizziness, hypotension, xerostomia, headache |
| **Ortho Evra,** *Norelgestromin/Ethinyl estradiol* | Birth control | Antibiotics taken for dental infections can decrease the effectiveness of oral contraceptives |
| **Ortho-Novum,** *Norethindrone/Ethinyl estradiol* | Birth control | Antibiotics taken for dental infections can decrease the effectiveness of oral contraceptives |

*(continued)*

**READY REFERENCE 5-2**   COMMONLY PRESCRIBED DRUGS[a] *(CONTINUED)*

| Drug | Use | Concerns/Oral Manifestations |
|---|---|---|
| **Ortho Tri-Cyclen Lo**, *Norgestimate/Ethinyl estradiol* | Birth control | Antibiotics taken for dental infections can decrease effectiveness of oral contraceptives |
| **Oxandrin**, *Oxandrolone* | Medication to help underweight patients to gain weight | Also for pain with osteoporosis |
| *Oxybutynin chloride*, **Ditropan** | Bladder control medication for adults with symptoms of overactive bladder | Xerostomia, sedation, nausea |
| **OxyContin**, *Oxycodone* | Narcotic for moderate to severe pain | Xerostomia, sedation, nausea |
| *Pantoprazole*, **Protonix** | Reduces stomach acid production for treatment of GERD | Headache |
| *Paroxetine*, **Paxil, Paxil CR** | Medication for depression and general anxiety disorder | Xerostomia, hypotension |
| **Patanol**, *Olopatadine* | Medication for allergic conjunctivitis of the eye | Xerostomia |
| **Pagasys**, *Peginterferon Alfa-2a* | For treatment of hepatitis C | Fatigue, headache, muscle and joint pain, nausea |
| *Penicillin V potassium*, **Pen VK** | Antibiotic, penicillin: not for prevention of infectious endocarditis | Oral candidiasis |
| **Percocet**, *Oxycodone/ Acetaminophen* | Narcotic with Acetaminophen for moderate to severe pain | Xerostomia, sedation, nausea |
| *Phenazopyridine*, **Pyridium** | Medication for pain relief from urinary tract infections | Temporarily turns urine an orange color |
| **Phenergan**, *Promethazine* | Medication for treatment of nausea and motion sickness | Hypotension, xerostomia |
| *Phenobarbital*, **Lumina** | An antiseizure medication (anticonvulsant) used to prevent seizures | Bradycardia, syncope |
| *Phenytoin*, **Dilantin** | An antiseizure medication (anticonvulsant) used to prevent seizures | Gingival hyperplasia |
| *Pioglitazone*, **Actos** | Oral medication used to treat type II diabetes | Stress-induced hypoglycemia |
| **Plavix**, *Clopidogrel* | A medication that reduces the clumping of platelets in the blood; reduces risk of heart attack and stroke | Bleeding |

*(continued)*

**READY REFERENCE 5-2**  COMMONLY PRESCRIBED DRUGS[a] *(CONTINUED)*

| Drug | Use | Concerns/Oral Manifestations |
| --- | --- | --- |
| **Plendil,** *Felodipine* | For the management of high blood pressure and congestive heart failure | Gingival hyperplasia headache |
| *Polyethylene glycol,* **GlycoLax 3350** | Laxative | Nausea |
| *Potassium chloride,* **K-Dur** | Electrolyte supplement to prevent potassium depletion (hypokalemia) | Xerostomia |
| **Pravachol,** *Pravastatin* | Medication to lower high cholesterol to prevent coronary artery disease | Muscle pain, tenderness, or weakness with fever or flu symptoms; or nausea, stomach pain, low fever, loss of appetite |
| *Prednisone,* **Deltasone** | Corticosteroid to treat a variety of diseases, inflammation | Infection, adrenal insufficiency if taken long term |
| **Premarin,** *Conjugated estrogens* | Hormone replacement therapy | Nausea, sinus irritation |
| **Prempro,** *Conjugated estrogens/ Medroxyprogesterone* | Hormone replacement therapy | Nausea, sinus irritation |
| **Prevacid,** *Lansoprazole* | Reduces stomach acid production for treatment of GERD | Xerostomia, oral candidiasis, altered taste, aphthous ulcers, stomatitis |
| *Primidone,* **Mysoline** | Anticonvulsant for the prevention of seizure and benign familial tremor | Overexcitement, nausea, vomiting |
| **Prinivil,** *Lisinopril* | Used to treat high blood pressure and congestive heart failure | Altered taste, orthostatic hypotension, dizziness, fatigue, headache, nausea, vomiting; use of epinephrine or levonordefrin in local anesthetic should be minimized |
| **ProAir HFA,** *Albuterol* | Inhaler for prevention of asthma | Xerostomia, sore throat, inflammation of the nose |
| **Procrit,** *Epoetin alfa* | Used to treat anemia in chemotherapy and HIV+ | High blood pressure, water retention, headache, rapid heart rate, nausea |
| **Prograf,** *Tacrolimus* (topical) | Ointment for skin rash | Headache, acne |
| *Promethazine/Codeine,* **Prothazine DC** | Antihistamine/decongestion for upper respiratory cold, flu | Fast heart rate, loss of muscle control, twitching, xerostomia |

*(continued)*

**READY REFERENCE 5-2**    COMMONLY PRESCRIBED DRUGS[a] *(CONTINUED)*

| Drug | Use | Concerns/Oral Manifestations |
|---|---|---|
| *Promethazine,* **Phenergan** | Medication for treatment of nausea and motion sickness | Hypotension, xerostomia |
| **Prometrium**, *Progesterone* | Hormone replacement therapy for menopause | Gingival bleeding |
| *Propafenone,* **Rythmol** | Medication for treatment of irregular heartbeat | Xerostomia |
| *Propranolol,* **Inderal** | Medication for treatment of high blood pressure, angina, tremor, arrhythmias | Hypotension |
| **Proscar, Propecia**, *Finasteride* | Medication for treatment of male pattern baldness | Hypotension |
| **Protonix**, *Pantoprazole* | Reduces stomach acid production for treatment of GERD | Headache |
| **Provigil**, *Modafinil* | Medication for treatment of daily drowsiness (narcolepsy) | Xerostomia, ulcers, gingivitis |
| **Prozac**, *Fluoxetine* | Medication for treatment of depression | Oral candidiasis, xerostomia, hypotension, nausea; can initiate bruxism |
| **Pulmicort**, *Budesonide* | Inhaler for prevention of asthma | Oropharyngeal candidiasis |
| **Pulmozyme**, *Dornase alfa* | Enzyme for treatment of cystic fibrosis | Sore throat, nasal inflammation |
| *Quinapril,* **Accupril** | Used to treat high blood pressure and heart failure and for preventing kidney failure due to high blood pressure and diabetes | Altered taste, dizziness, nausea, vomiting; use of epinephrine or levonordefrin in local anesthetic should be minimized; angioedema, hypotension |
| *Rabeprazole,* **Aciphex** | Acid blocker for treatment of heartburn and GERD | Xerostomia, altered taste, nausea, dizziness, nervousness |
| *Raloxifene,* **Evista** | Prevention of osteoporosis | None known |
| *Ramipril,* **Altace** | Used to treat high blood pressure and heart failure and for preventing kidney failure due to high blood pressure and diabetes | Altered taste, dizziness, nausea, vomiting; use of epinephrine or levonordefrin in local anesthetic should be minimized; angioedema, hypotension |
| *Ranitidine HCl,* **Zantac** | Stomach acid blocker for GERD | Drowsiness, headache, nausea |
| **Relpax**, *Eletriptan* | Medication for relief of migraine headaches and symptoms | Headache; xerostomia; pain in jaw, neck, or throat |
| **Remeron**, *Mirtazapine* | Medication for treatment of depression | Xerostomia |

*(continued)*

**READY REFERENCE 5-2**   COMMONLY PRESCRIBED DRUGS[a] *(CONTINUED)*

| Drug | Use | Concerns/Oral Manifestations |
|---|---|---|
| **Renagel,** *Sevelamer* | Prevents calcium depletion in patients with kidney disease and undergoing hemodialysis | Nausea, vomiting, stomach pain |
| **Requip,** *Ropinirole* | Medication for treatment of Parkinson disease | Xerostomia, dysphagia |
| **Restasis, Sandimmune,** *Cyclosporine* | Immunosuppressant in organ transplant | Gingival hyperplasia, oral lesions |
| **Reyataz,** *Atazanavir* | Antiretroviral drug for HIV infection | Feeling faint, back pain, sore throat, headache, flu-like symptoms |
| **Rhinocort Aqua,** *Budesonide* | Corticosteroid inhaler/spray: asthma | Oropharyngeal candidiasis |
| *Ribavirin,* **Copegus** | Medication that controls symptoms by reducing the number of viruses in hepatitis C patients | Xerostomia, taste perversion, sore throat, headache, flu-like symptoms |
| **Risperdal,** *Risperidone* | Antipsychotic medication for schizophrenia, mania | Hypotension, xerostomia |
| *Rosiglitazone maleate,* **Avandia** | Oral medication for type II diabetes | Stress-induced hypoglycemia |
| **Roxicet,** *Oxycodone/ Acetaminophen* | Narcotic pain reliever combined with Acetaminophen | Nausea, sedation, xerostomia |
| *Salmeterol,* **Serevent** | Inhaler for asthma | Xerostomia, dental pain, oropharyngeal candidiasis |
| *Salmeterol/Fluticasone propionate oral inhaler,* **Advair Diskus** | Inhaler that includes cortisone for treatment of asthma | Xerostomia, dental pain, oropharyngeal candidiasis |
| **Savella,** *Milnacipran* | Medication for the management of fibromyalgia | Dizziness, xerostomia, headache, hot flush, sweating, nausea, vomiting |
| **Sensipar,** *Cinacalcet* | Medication used to treat hypoparathyroidism (decreased functioning of the parathyroid glands) in people who are on long-term dialysis for kidney disease | Numbness or tingling around the mouth, irregular heart rate, dizziness, muscle pain |
| **Serevent Diskus,** *Salmeterol* | Inhaler for asthma and other respiratory conditions | Xerostomia, dental pain, oropharyngeal candidiasis |
| **Seroquel,** *Quetiapine* | Antipsychotic medication for the treatment of schizophrenia manic episodes in bipolar disorder | Xerostomia, white patches or sores on lips and inside the mouth, sore throat |

*(continued)*

**READY REFERENCE 5-2**    COMMONLY PRESCRIBED DRUGS[a] *(CONTINUED)*

| Drug | Use | Concerns/Oral Manifestations |
|---|---|---|
| *Sertraline,* **Zoloft** | Treatment for depression | Anxiety, mood change |
| *Sildenafil citrate,* **Viagra** | Treatment for erectile dysfunction | **If chest pain: No nitroglycerine** |
| **Silenor,** *Doxepin* | Sleep aid medication for the treatment of insomnia | Dizziness, drowsiness, nausea |
| **Simcor,** *Niacin/ Simvastatin* | Treatment used to lower high cholesterol to prevent coronary artery disease | Muscle pain, tenderness, or weakness with fever or flu symptoms; or nausea, stomach pain, low fever, loss of appetite |
| *Simvastatin,* **Zocor** | Treatment to lower high cholesterol to prevent coronary artery disease | Muscle pain, tenderness, or weakness with fever or flu symptoms; or nausea, stomach pain, low fever, loss of appetite |
| **Singulair,** *Montelukast* | Medication for maintenance therapy to prevent asthma attacks | Dizziness, dental pain |
| **Skelaxin,** *Metaxalone* | Skeletal muscle relaxant | Dizziness |
| **SMZ-TMP, Bactrim, Septra,** *Sulfamethoxazole/ Trimethoprim* | Antibiotic: urinary tract infection | Stomatitis |
| *Sotalol,* **Betapace** | Medication for irregular heartbeat | Minimize use of epinephrine in local anesthesia |
| **Spiriva,** *Tiotropium* | Treatment of bronchospasm in respiratory diseases | Xerostomia, ulcerative stomatitis |
| *Spironolactone/ Hydrochlorothiazide,* **Aldactazide** | Diuretic to reduce edema in congestive heart failure | Hypotension |
| **Strattera,** *Atomoxetine* | Medication for ADHD | Xerostomia |
| **Suboxone,** *Buprenorphine/ Naloxone* | Medication for drug withdrawal | Headache, dizziness, nausea |
| *Sucralfate,* **Carafate** | Liquid for coating duodenal ulcers to help with healing | None |
| *Sumatriptan,* **Imitrex** | Medication for relief of migraine headaches | Bad taste, dysphagia, mouth or tongue discomfort |
| **Sustiva,** *Efavirenz* | Antiviral agent for HIV-1 | Abnormal taste |
| **Symbyax,** *Fluoxetine/ Olanzapine* | Combined drugs for the treatment of resistant depression | Dizziness, drowsiness, xerostomia, sore throat, weakness |

*(continued)*

## READY REFERENCE 5-2   COMMONLY PRESCRIBED DRUGS[a] (CONTINUED)

| Drug | Use | Concerns/Oral Manifestations |
|------|-----|------------------------------|
| **Synthroid**, *Levothyroxine* | Thyroid replacement | High blood pressure |
| *Tamoxifen*, **Nolvadex** | Chemotherapy for and to prevent breast cancer | Nausea, vomiting, hot flashes |
| *Tamsulosin*, **Flomax** | Improves urinary flow in men with enlarged prostate | Hypotension |
| **Tarceva**, *Erlotinib* | Chemotherapy for lung and pancreatic cancer | Nausea, vomiting |
| *Temazepam*, **Restoril** | Sleep aid for insomnia | Xerostomia, hypotension |
| **Tequin**, *Gatifloxacin* | Antibiotic | Taste disturbance |
| *Terazosin*, **Hytrin** | Medication to lower high blood pressure | Xerostomia |
| *Terconazole*, **Terazol** | Antifungal agent: vaginal candidiasis | None |
| *Tetracycline*, **Achromycin, Sumycin** | Antibiotic for many infections | Candidiasis, intrinsic tooth stain |
| **Thalomid**, *Thalidomide* | Medication for multiple myeloma, erythema nodosum leprosum | Xerostomia moniliasis, stomatitis |
| *Theophylline*, **Slo-Bid** | For asthma, bronchitis | Nausea, vomiting |
| **Tiazac, Cardizem**, *Diltiazem* | To lower blood pressure and prevent angina attack | Gingival hyperplasia |
| *Timolol*, **Timoptic** | To lower blood pressure; ophthalmic agent: glaucoma | Xerostomia |
| *Tizanidine HCl*, **Zanaflex** | Muscle relaxant | Hypotension |
| **TobraDex**, *Tobramycin/ Dexamethasone* | Antibiotic/cortisone ophthalmic (eye) drops | None |
| *Tolterodine*, **Detrol** | Medication for overactive bladder | Xerostomia |
| **Topamax**, *Topiramate* | Medication to prevent seizures and migraine headaches | Gingival hyperplasia; not to be taken by pregnant women as it can cause cleft palate birth defect |
| **Toprol-XL**, *Metoprolol* | To lower high blood pressure | Hypotension |
| *Torsemide*, **Demadex** | Diuretic for edema | Hypotension |
| **Tradjenta**, *Linagliptin* | Oral medication for type II diabetes | Headache, joint pain, runny or stuffy nose, sore throat |
| *Tramadol*, **Ultram** | Narcotic for moderate to severe pain | Xerostomia |

*(continued)*

**READY REFERENCE 5-2**   COMMONLY PRESCRIBED DRUGS[a] *(CONTINUED)*

| Drug | Use | Concerns/Oral Manifestations |
|---|---|---|
| **Travatan**, *Travoprost* | Ophthalmic agent: glaucoma | None |
| *Trazodone*, **Desyrel** | Medication for depression | Xerostomia |
| *Tretinoin*, **Retin-A** topical cream | Treatment for acne, wrinkles | None |
| *Triamcinolone acetonide*, **Orabase** | Corticosteroid: anti-inflammatory for lichen planus, aphthous, stomatitis; nasal, oral topical, inhalation | None |
| *Triamterene/ Hydrochlorothiazide*, **Dyrenium** | Antihypertensive and diuretic for lowering blood pressure | Hypotension |
| **Tribenzor**, *Amlodipine /Hydrochlorothiazide/ Olmesartan* | Combination of three drugs for lowering high blood pressure | Hypotension, xerostomia, hypocalcemia |
| **Tricor, Lipidil**, *Fenofibrate* | Medication to lower high cholesterol to prevent coronary artery disease | Muscle pain, tenderness, or weakness with fever or flu symptoms; or nausea, stomach pain, low fever, loss of appetite |
| **Trileptal**, *Oxcarbazepine* | Medication for prevention of seizures | None known |
| **Trimox**, *Amoxicillin* | Antibiotic for many infections, also to prevent infective endocarditis | Prolonged use: candidiasis |
| **TriNessa**, *Norgestimate/Ethinyl estradiol* | Birth control | Antibiotics taken for dental infections can decrease the effectiveness of oral contraceptives |
| **Triphasil 21**, *Levonorgestrel/Ethinyl estradiol* | Birth control | Antibiotics taken for dental infections can decrease the effectiveness of oral contraceptives |
| **TRI-Sprintec**, *Ethinyl estradiol/Norgestimate* | Birth control | Antibiotics taken for dental infections can decrease the effectiveness of oral contraceptives |
| **Trivora-28**, *Levonorgestrel/ethinyl estradiol* | Birth control | Antibiotics taken for dental infections can decrease the effectiveness of oral contraceptives |
| **Trizivir**, *Abacavir, Lamivudine, Zidovudine* | Three antiretroviral drugs combined for treatment of HIV+ | Headache, joint or muscle pain, nausea, nervousness, tiredness, vomiting, weakness |
| **Truvada**, *Emtricitabine/ Tenofovir* | Antiretroviral drug for HIV+ | Headache, joint or muscle pain, nausea, nervousness, tiredness, vomiting, weakness |

*(continued)*

**READY REFERENCE 5-2** COMMONLY PRESCRIBED DRUGS[a] *(CONTINUED)*

| Drug | Use | Concerns/Oral Manifestations |
|------|-----|------------------------------|
| **Tussionex,** *Hydrocodone/ Chlorpheniramine* | Antihistamine/antitussive: cough medicine | Xerostomia |
| **Ultram,** *Tramadol* | Narcotic for moderate to severe pain | Xerostomia |
| *Ursodiol,* **Actigall** | Gallstone dissolution agent | None |
| *Valacyclovir,* **Valtrex** | Antiviral agent: herpes I, II, herpes zoster (shingles) | Xerostomia, headache |
| *Valsartan,* **Diovan** | For lowering high blood pressure | Hypotension |
| **Valturna,** *Aliskiren/ Valsartan* | For lowering high blood pressure | Hypotension, dizziness, headache, sore throat, joint pain, runny nose |
| **Veetids,** *Penicillin V Potassium* | Antibiotic, penicillin—**not** for prevention of infective endocarditis | Oral candidiasis |
| *Venlafaxine,* **Effexor** | For depression | Xerostomia, altered taste |
| *Verapamil,* **Calan, Isoptin** | For lowering blood pressure and preventing angina attack | Gingival hyperplasia |
| **Viagra,** *Sildenafil citrate* | Erectile dysfunction | **If chest pain: NO nitroglycerine** |
| **Vicoprofen,** *Hydrocodone/ Ibuprofen* | Narcotic and NSAID combination for pain relief | Xerostomia, nausea |
| **Vigamox,** *Moxifloxacin* | Antibiotic eye drops | Xerostomia, glossitis, stomatitis |
| **Viibryd,** *Vilazodone* | Medication for depression; adjunct therapy to lithium for bipolar I | Dizziness, fast heartbeat, insomnia, muscle twitching |
| **Vimovo,** *Naproxen/ Esomeprazole* | Combination of medications to treat pain while preventing gastroesophageal reflux | Bleeding |
| **Viramune XR,** *Nevirapine* | Combination of antiviral agents for HIV+ | Liver problems, bleeding, nausea, dry cough |
| **Viread,** *Tenofovir* | Antiretroviral agent for HIV+ | Headache, joint or muscle pain, nausea, nervousness, tiredness, vomiting, weakness |
| **Vivelle-DOT,** *estradiol transdermal patch* | Hormone replacement therapy (skin patch) | None |
| **Vytorin,** *Ezetimibe/ Simvastatin* | Treatment to lower high cholesterol to prevent coronary artery disease | Muscle pain, tenderness, or weakness with fever or flu symptoms; or nausea, stomach pain, low fever, loss of appetite |

*(continued)*

**READY REFERENCE 5-2** COMMONLY PRESCRIBED DRUGS[a] *(CONTINUED)*

| Drug | Use | Concerns/Oral Manifestations |
|------|-----|------------------------------|
| **Vyvanse**, *Lisdexamfetamine* | For treatment of ADHD in adolescents | Fast-pounding, irregular heartbeat; tremors; nervousness; insomnia |
| *Warfarin*, **Coumadin, Coumarin** | Anticoagulant helpful in preventing blood clot formation in patients with atrial fibrillation and artificial heart valves to reduce the risk of strokes | Ulcerations; increased bleeding tendency, medical consult |
| **Wellbutrin**, *Bupropion HCl* | Medication for depression | Hypotension, xerostomia |
| **Xalatan**, *Latanoprost* | Ophthalmic agent: glaucoma | None |
| **Xeloda**, *Capecitabine* | Chemotherapy for colon/breast cancer | Stomatitis, abnormal taste |
| **Xopenex**, *Levalbuterol* | Inhaler for asthma | Sore throat |
| **Yasmin 28, YAZ,** *drospirenone/ethinyl estradiol* | Birth control | Antibiotics taken for dental infections can decrease the effectiveness of oral contraceptives |
| **Zegerid OTC**, *Omeprazole/Sodium bicarbonate* | Combination medications for treatment of heartburn | Headache, nausea, stomach pain, vomiting |
| **Zelnorm**, *Tegaserod* | Medication for treatment of constipation in irritable bowel syndrome | Nausea |
| **Zestril, Prinivil**, *Lisinopril* | Used to treat high blood pressure and heart failure and for preventing kidney failure due to high blood pressure and diabetes | Altered taste, dizziness, nausea, vomiting; use of epinephrine or levonordefrin in local anesthetic should be minimized; angioedema, hypotension |
| **Zetia**, *Ezetimibe* | Treatment to lower high cholesterol to prevent coronary artery disease | Muscle pain |
| **Zithromax, Z-Pak**, *Azithromycin* | Antibiotic | Nausea, headache |
| **Zocor**, *Simvastatin* | Treatment to lower high cholesterol to prevent coronary artery disease | Muscle pain, tenderness, or weakness with fever or flu symptoms; or nausea, stomach pain, low fever, loss of appetite |
| **Zofran**, *Ondansetron* | Medication for prevention and treatment in nausea from chemotherapy | Xerostomia, drowsiness |
| **Zoloft**, *Sertraline* | Medication for depression | Anxiety, irritability |

*(continued)*

**READY REFERENCE 5-2** COMMONLY PRESCRIBED DRUGSᵃ *(CONTINUED)*

| Drug | Use | Concerns/Oral Manifestations |
|---|---|---|
| *Zolpidem*, **Ambien** | Sleep aid | Xerostomia |
| **Zomig**, *Zolmitriptan* | Medication for migraine headaches and symptoms | Xerostomia, dysphagia |
| *Zonisamide*, **Zonegran** | Medication to prevent seizures | Xerostomia |
| **Zyprexa**, *Olanzapine* | Medication for depression, an antipsychotic for depression with bipolar episodes | Xerostomia, tooth disorder, altered taste |
| **Zyrtec**, *Cetirizine HCl* | Antihistamine: allergic rhinitis | Xerostomia |
| **Zyvox**, *Linezolid* | Antibiotic, oxazolidinone: vancomycin-resistant infections, such as Methicillin-resistant Staphylococcus aureus (MRSA) | Discolored tongue, bad taste |

## REFERENCE

1. Biron Leisica C. Unpublished handout.

# 6 Dental Health History

## MODULE OVERVIEW

The dental health history provides information about the patient's past and present dental experiences. The information gathered from taking the dental health history allows the clinician to determine whether dental treatment alterations are necessary for the patient to undergo dental treatment safely. This module reviews the kinds of information commonly found on dental health history questionnaires.

## MODULE OUTLINE

## OBJECTIVES

- Explain the importance of the dental health history in planning and preparing for patient treatment activities.
- Given a dental health history questionnaire, identify those elements that would be important in modifying the planned treatment.

SECTION 1:

# Adult Dental Health History Questionnaire

A **dental health history** provides a record of a patient's previous dental experiences. Like the medical history, the dental health history is essential in providing safe dental care for the patient. The dental health history is a quick and effective way to obtain important information about the patient's past and present dental experiences. Most dental practices will use a dental health questionnaire to obtain relevant information from the patient.

The information requested in a dental health history varies significantly depending on the type of dental practice. For example, a general dental practitioner may use a dental history questionnaire that covers a broad range of dental conditions, whereas an office specializing in pedodontics, orthodontics, cosmetic dentistry, periodontics, prosthodontics, or oral surgery may use a dental history format that is more narrowly focused to that type of dental specialty practice. An Internet search of the keywords "dental health history" will provide literally hundreds of examples of questionnaires used by various dental practices; all have similarities, but no two are exactly the same.

The dental health questionnaire is a highly effective tool permitting the dental team to identify the patient's potential dental needs and risks. Information gained from the questionnaire can be addressed more carefully and thoroughly at chairside. In addition, the questionnaire can provide opportunities for enriched communication opportunities for the dental team related to addressing potential dental anxiety, oral hygiene/preventive therapy regimens, dietary counseling, esthetic considerations, and treatment alternatives.

It is always assumed that the dental health history provides supplemental information important to the dental practice team *and* is always used in the context of having first taken a complete medical history. The dental health history is never used independent of the medical health history.

## QUESTIONNAIRE FORMAT

There is no standardized format for a dental health questionnaire. Common formats include "fill-in-the-blank" type questions, checkmarks, boxes, and circling the correct response (Fig. 6-1).

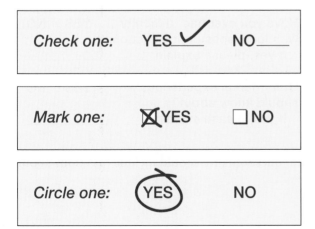

**Figure 6-1. Questionnaire formats.** Common questionnaire formats include the use of check marks, boxes, and circling the correct answer.

## REASON FOR APPOINTMENT

For a new patient, the dental health questionnaire very likely would include some of the elements included in Figure 6-2.

---

### Reason for Today's Visit/Chief Complaint

What is the main reason for your visit today? _____

Have you seen another dentist within the last year? _____

When was your last dental visit?_____
   Reason for the above visit?_____
   Name of previous dentist:_____

Have you had x-rays of your teeth taken recently?
   NO      YES, when: _____

How did you hear of our practice?_____

Referred by: _____

---

**Figure 6-2.   Reason for appointment.** Questions such as these commonly are found on a dental questionnaire regarding the reason for the appointment.

## PREVIOUS DENTAL EXPERIENCES

Many dental questionnaires attempt to identify whether or not the patient has had any previous negative dental experiences that might require special considerations during the current episode of treatment. Examples of special considerations are antianxiety premedication, intravanous (IV) sedation, or nitrous oxide sedation. Some examples of the types of questions that could be used to elicit information about previous dental experiences are listed in Figures 6-3 and 6-4.

---

### Tell Us About Your Previous Dental Experiences

Have your previous dental visits  YES    NO
been favorable/comfortable
emotionally?
   If no, please explain: _____

In general, do you feel positive  YES    NO
about your previous dental
treatment?
   If no, please explain: _____

Have you ever had an adverse  YES    NO
reaction to dental treatment?
   If yes, please explain: _____

Have you ever had any allergic  YES    NO
reactions associated with
dental treatment?
   If yes, please explain: _____

Have you ever had  difficulty  YES    NO
with local anesthetic injections?
   If yes, please explain: _____

Other dental experiences we  YES    NO
should know about?
   If yes, please explain: _____

---

**Figure 6-3.   Previous dental experiences.** A dental questionnaire should include questions about the patient's previous experiences with dental care.

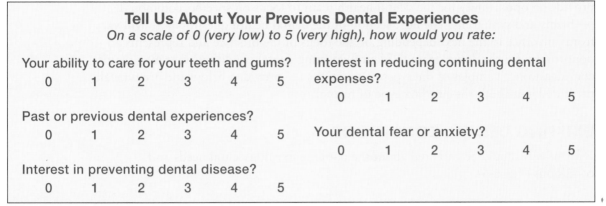

**Figure 6-4. Previous dental experiences.** An alternative way of obtaining information about previous dental experiences is to use a scale assessment, either 0 to 5 or 0 to 10.

## DENTAL CONCERNS

The next section of the dental health questionnaire generally involves identifying specific potential dental concerns that the patient may have regarding possible treatment options. These questions can be used to focus the dental team on issues that the patient feels are important. Examples of typical questions are shown in Figure 6-5.

---

### Tell Us About Any Dental Concerns You May Have

Are you satisfied with your teeth   YES   NO
and their appearance?
 If no, please explain: _____

Are you interested in having   YES   NO
your teeth a lighter color?
 If yes, please explain: _____

Are you interested in any   YES   NO
specific type of dental treatment
at this time?
*Please circle all that apply*:
    implants, cosmetic dentistry,
    replacing missing teeth, dentures,
    replacing old fillings, other dental
    treatments

A lot can be done to prevent dental
diseases (teeth and gum disease).
Would you like to know   YES   NO
more about preventing
dental disease for yourself
or your family?
 If yes, please explain: _____

Do you feel your present   YES   NO
oral hygiene is effective in
cleaning your mouth?
 If no, please explain _____

---

**Figure 6-5. Patient's dental concerns.** The dental questionnaire should include questions about the patient's dental concerns.

The elements in the previous dental health questionnaire not only provide an overview of the patient's past dental experiences, they also help prompt a patient to identify issues that he or she wants addressed by the dental team. These types of questions provide the clinician with a potential "head's up" regarding whether or not this patient has had prior positive or negative dental experiences and alerts the clinician to any potential problems with local anesthesia, the need for anxiety premedication, and other important treatment considerations. The preceding questions, however, do not provide an opportunity for the dental health team to focus on specific, common dental problems and symptoms. The next section of the dental health questionnaire will vary from one office to the next depending on the focus of the practice and represents an opportunity for the dental team to identify existing dental conditions that may require consideration. Examples of the types of questions are provided below and are typically presented in a check-the-line/box type of format.

## EXISTING DENTAL CONDITIONS

Information should be gathered about the patient's existing dental needs and conditions (Fig. 6-6).

---

### Existing Dental Needs and Conditions
*Please indicate with a check if you have had or have any of the following:*

____ Sensitive teeth
   ____ Hot
   ____ Cold
   ____ Sweet
   ____ Pressure
____ Broken teeth or fillings
____ Joint pain or popping or clicking of jaw
____ Gum boils or other infections
____ Swollen/painful or bleeding gums
____ Gum recession
____ Periodontal treatments (gum)
____ Frequent filling replacement
____ Discolored teeth
____ Crooked teeth
____ Orthodontic treatment (braces)
____ Injury to the face, jaws, teeth
____ Root canal therapy

____ Removal of teeth
____ Sores or growths
____ Dry mouth
____ Pain upon swallowing
____ Grinding or clenching teeth
____ Persistent headaches, ear aches, or muscle pain
____ Bad breath, or bad taste in mouth
____ Food catches between teeth when you eat
____ Loose teeth
____ Denture or partial denture
____ Your bite is changing
____ Problems chewing
____ Sore jaws upon awakening. How frequently:
____ Do you prefer to breathe through your
   ____ nose or ____ mouth?
____ Abnormal swallowing habit—tongue thrusting
____ Biting your lip or cheek frequently

---

**Figure 6-6.  Existing dental needs and conditions.**

## DAILY SELF-CARE

Other helpful elements in a dental health questionnaire may relate to identifying the patient's home care/self-care effectiveness. Examples of typical questions are shown in Figure 6-7.

---

### Daily Self-Care Activities

On a daily basis, how many times do you brush your teeth? *(please circle)*

Brush only      0  1  2  3  4+
Floss only       0  1  2+
Brush and floss  0  1  2  3+
____Do not routinely brush or floss on a
   daily basis

What type of toothbrush do you use?
  — Hard      — Medium
  — Soft       — Don't know

Do you use any other dental aids on a regular basis?
  — Bridge cleaners  — Proxabrush
  — Stimudents     — Other
  — Rubber tip

---

**Figure 6-7.  Daily self-care activities.** It is helpful to gather information about the patient's current daily self-care habits.

## DIETARY HABITS

Some dental health questionnaires specifically address dietary activities that might potentially have a significant negative impact on dental health (Fig. 6-8). For example, a history of consuming sugary drinks may increase the risk of dental decay.

---

### Dietary Activities
*Please circle:*

How many caffeinated beverages do you drink daily?
  0   1   2   3   4+   less than 2-3/week

How many alcoholic beverages do you drink daily?
  0   1   2   3   4+   less than 2-3/week

How many sugar-containing carbonated beverages do you drink daily?
  0   1   2   3   4+   less than 2-3/week

How many "diet" sugar substitute carbonated beverages do you drink daily?
  0   1   2   3   4+   less than 2-3/week

How many "sport/energy" beverages do you drink daily?
  0   1   2   3   4+   less than 2-3/week

How many candy bars or energy/power bars do you eat daily?
  0   1   2   3   4+   less than 2-3/week

Do you regularly eat hard candies or breath mints?
  YES   NO   Occasionally

Do you regularly use tobacco products?
  YES   NO   Occasionally

Do you use recreational/street drugs?
  YES   NO   Occasionally

---

**Figure 6-8. Dietary activities.** Information about dietary habits that could be a contributing factor in dental disease can be helpful to the clinician.

**SECTION 2:**

# Child Dental Health History Questionnaire

For offices that treat young children, a special children's dental health questionnaire is required. A typical children's dental health history would include some of the elements illustrated in Figure 6-9.

---

**Children's Dental Heath Questionnaire**

Is this your child's first visit to a dentist?
YES    NO

Do you anticipate that your child will be cooperative?   YES    NO

If this is not your child's first visit, has his/her previous dental experience been:
(circle one)    Positive    Negative

**REASON FOR VISIT**

What is the main purpose of your visit today? _____

Has your child bumped or cracked any front teeth?    NO    YES, when? _____

Has your child ever complained of head-ache, pain, popping, or clicking of the jaws?          YES    NO

**FLUORIDE EXPOSURE**

Is your water supply at home fluoridated?
YES    NO    Don't know

Does your child take any of the following?
(circle all appropriate)    Fluoride tablets
Fluoride drops    Fluoride in vitamins

**PREVENTIVE DENTAL HISTORY**

How often does your child brush?_____

Is the child's brushing supervised? YES NO

Does the child use dental floss?    YES  NO

**CHILD'S HABITS**

Does your child have a night time bottle?
YES    NO

Does your child do any of the following:

Grinding teeth:    How long _____
Still active?    YES    NO

Thumb sucking:    How long _____
Still active?    YES    NO

Finger habit:    How long _____
Still active?    YES    NO

Pacifier:    How long _____
Still active?    YES    NO

Other (lip, cheek, nail biting or biting on foreign objects-pencils, etc.): How long _____
Still active?    YES    NO

---

**Figure 6-9.  Children's dental health questionnaire.**  These questions are examples of questions that would be helpful on a children's health questionnaire.

## SECTION 3:
# Peak Procedure

**PROCEDURE 6-1** REVIEW OF DENTAL HEALTH HISTORY QUESTIONNAIRE

| Action | Rationale |
|---|---|
| 1. Read through every line and check box. Are all the questions answered? | • Complete information is important to protect the patient's health. |
| 2. Can you understand what is written? | • Make a note to ask the patient about anything that is not clear. |
| 3. Did the patient, parent, or guardian sign and date the form? | • The dental history must be signed and dated. |
| 4. Read through the form. Circle concerns in red pencil—such as problems that the patient has experienced in the past with dental treatment. | • Discuss concerns during the patient interview. |
| 5. Read through handwritten responses made by the patient. Circle concerns in red pencil. | • Discuss concerns during the patient interview. |
| 6. Identify any dental treatment alterations that might be necessary for treatment of this patient. | • Examples of treatment alterations include antianxiety medication prior to appointment or use of latex-free gloves for a patient who has experienced an adverse reaction to latex gloves during previous dental treatment. |

**SECTION 4:**

# Module Resources

## Dental Health Questionnaire

Patient_____    Date _____

Student_____

### REASON FOR TODAY'S VISIT - CHIEF COMPLAINT

What is the main reason for your visit today?_____    How did you hear about our practice?_____

_____    _____

_____    Referred by: _____

### PREVIOUS DENTAL TREATMENT

Have you seen another dentist within the last year? ____    Name of previous dentist?_____

When was your last dental visit?_____    Have you had x-rays of your teeth taken ☐ Yes    ☐ No
recently?

Reason for the above visit?_____

### TELL US ABOUT YOUR PREVIOUS DENTAL EXPERIENCES

Have your previous dental visits been    ☐ Yes  ☐ No    Have you ever had any allergic    ☐ Yes  ☐ No
favorable/comfortable emotionally?    reactions associated with dental
    treatment?

  If no, please explain: _____      If yes, please explain:_____

_____    _____

In general, do you feel positive about    ☐ Yes  ☐ No    Have you ever had  difficulty with local    ☐ Yes  ☐ No
your previous dental treatment?    anesthetic injections?

  If no, please explain: _____      If yes, please explain:_____

_____    _____

Have you ever had an adverse    ☐ Yes  ☐ No
reaction to dental treatment?    Other dental experiences we should know about?

  If yes, please explain:_____    _____

_____    _____

### TELL US ABOUT ANY DENTAL CONCERNS YOU MAY HAVE

Are you satisfied with your teeth and    ☐ Yes  ☐ No    Are you interested in any specific type of dental
their appearance?    treatment at this time?
        ☐ Implants
  If no, please explain: _____        ☐ Cosmetic dentistry
        ☐ Replacing missing teeth
_____        ☐ Dentures
Are you interested in having your    ☐ Yes  ☐ No        ☐ Replacing old fillings
teeth a lighter color?        ☐ Other_____

  If yes, please explain:_____    A lot can be done to prevent dental diseases (teeth
    and gum disease). Would you like to know more about
_____    preventing dental disease for yourself
    or your family?    ☐ Yes    ☐ No

      If yes, please explain:_____

    _____

**Figure 6-10A.   Adult dental health questionnaire in English.** Page 1 of an adult dental health questionnaire in English.

# Dental Health Questionnaire (cont)

## EXISTING DENTAL NEEDS/CONDITIONS

*Please indicate with a check if you have had or have any of the following:*

- ☐ Sensitive teeth
  - ☐ Hot
  - ☐ Cold
  - ☐ Sweet
  - ☐ Pressure
- ☐ Broken teeth or fillings
- ☐ Joint pain or popping or clicking of jaw
- ☐ Gum boils or other infections
- ☐ Swollen/painful or bleeding gums
- ☐ Gum recession
- ☐ Periodontal treatments (gum)
- ☐ Frequent filling replacement
- ☐ Discolored teeth
- ☐ Crooked teeth
- ☐ Orthodontic treatment (braces)
- ☐ Injury to the face, jaws, teeth
- ☐ Root canal therapy

- ☐ Removal of teeth
- ☐ Sores or growths
- ☐ Dry mouth
- ☐ Pain upon swallowing
- ☐ Grinding or clenching teeth
- ☐ Persistent headaches, ear aches, or muscle pain
- ☐ Bad breath, or bad taste in mouth
- ☐ Food catches between teeth when you eat
- ☐ Loose teeth
- ☐ Denture or partial denture
- ☐ Your bite is changing
- ☐ Problems chewing
- ☐ Sore jaws upon awakening. How frequently: _____
  - Do you prefer to breathe through your
    - ☐ nose or ☐ mouth?
- ☐ Abnormal swallowing habit - tongue thrusting
- ☐ Biting your lip or cheek frequently

## DAILY SELF-CARE ACTIVITIES

Do you feel your present daily self-care ☐ Yes ☐ No
is effective in cleaning your mouth?

If no, please explain _____

_____

On a daily basis, how many times do you brush your
teeth? (please circle)

| | | | | | |
|---|---|---|---|---|---|
| Brush only | 0 | 1 | 2 | 3 | 4+ |
| Floss only | 0 | 1 | 2+ | | |
| Brush and floss | 0 | 1 | 2 | 3+ | |

☐ Do not routinely brush or floss on a daily basis

What type of toothbrush do you use?
- ☐ Hard
- ☐ Medium
- ☐ Soft
- ☐ Don't know

Do you use any other dental aids on a regular basis?
- ☐ Bridge cleaners
- ☐ Stimudents
- ☐ Rubber tip
- ☐ Proxabrush
- ☐ Other _____

## DIETARY ACTIVITIES

*Please circle:*

How many caffeinated beverages do you drink daily?
  0   1   2   3   4+   less than 2-3/week
How many alcoholic beverages do you drink daily?
  0   1   2   3   4+   less than 2-3/week
How many sugar-containing sodas do you drink daily?
  0   1   2   3   4+   less than 2-3/week
How many "diet" sodas do you drink daily?
  0   1   2   3   4+   less than 2-3/week
How many "sport/energy" beverages do you drink daily?
  0   1   2   3   4+   less than 2-3/week

How many candy bars or energy/power bars do you
eat daily?
  0   1   2   3   4+   less than 2-3/week

Do you regularly eat hard candies or breath mints?
  ☐ Yes   ☐ No   ☐ Occasionally
Do you regularly use tobacco products?
  ☐ Yes   ☐ No   ☐ Occasionally
Do you use recreational/street drugs?
  ☐ Yes   ☐ No   ☐ Occasionally

Signature of Patient _____  Date _____

Reviewed by _____  Date _____

**Figure 6-10B. Adult dental health questionnaire in English.** Page 2 of an adult dental health questionnaire in English.

# Cuestionario de Salud Oral

Paciente _____ Fecha _____

Estudiante _____

## RAZON POR LA VISITA DE HOY - QUEJA PRINCIPAL

¿Cuál es la razón principal de su visita de hoy? _____

_____

_____

¿Cómo se entero usted de nuestra oficina dental? _____

_____

Referido/recomendado por: _____

## TRATAMIENTO DENTAL PREVIO

¿Ha visto a otro dentista durante el último año? _____

¿Cuándo fue su último visita dental? _____

¿Razón por su visita mencionada en previa pregunta?

Nombre de su dentista previo: _____

¿Recientemente, le han tomado radiografias (rayos x) de sus dientes? ☐Sí ☐No

## DIGANOS DE SUS PREVIAS EXPERIENCIAS DENTALES

¿Han sido sus previas visitas dentales favorables/comfortables emocialmente? ☐Sí ☐No

Si su respuesta es No, por favor explique:_____

¿Por lo general, se siente usted positivo sobre su previo tratamiento dental? ☐Sí ☐No

Si su respuesta es No, por favor explique:_____

¿Alguna vez a tenido usted una reacción adversa al tratamiento dental? ☐Sí ☐No

Si su respuesta es Sí, por favor explique: _____

_____

¿Alguna vez ha tenido usted alguna reacción alérgica relacionada con tratamiento dental? ☐Sí ☐No

Si su respuesta es Sí, por favor explique: _____

¿Ha tenido alguna dificultad con inyecciónes de anestesia local? ☐Sí ☐No

Si su respuesta es Sí, por favor explique: _____

_____

¿Otras experiencias dentales que debemos saber de?

_____

_____

## DIGANOS DE CUALQUIER INQUIETUDE/PREOCUPACION DENTAL QUE PUEDA USTED TENER

¿Está satisfecho con sus dientes y la apariencia de sus dientes? ☐Sí ☐No

Si su respuesta es No, por favor explique:_____

_____

¿Está usted interesado en tener sus dientes de un color más claro? ☐Sí ☐No

Si su respuesta es Sí, por favor explique: _____

_____

¿En este momento está usted interesado en algún tipo específico de tratamiento dental?
☐ Implantes
☐ Estética dental
☐ Reemplazar dientes que faltan
☐ Dentadura postiza
☐ Reemplazar un empaste/relleno viejo
☐ Otro _____

Mucho se puede hacer para prevenir enfermedades dentales (de los dientes y las encías). ¿Le gustaría aprender más sobre como prevenir enfermedades dentales para usted o su familia? ☐Sí ☐No

Si su respuesta es Sí, por favor explique:_____

_____

**Figure 6-11A. Adult dental health questionnaire in Spanish.** Page 1 of an adult dental health questionnaire in Spanish.

# Cuestionario de Salud Oral (cont)

## NECESIDADES/CONDICIONES DENTALES EXISTENTES

*Favor de indicar marcando si ha tenido o tiene cualquiera de lo siguiente:*

- ☐ Dientes sensitivos:
  - ☐ Caliente
  - ☐ Frío
  - ☐ Dulce
  - ☐ Presión
- ☐ Dientes quebrados o rellenos/empastados
- ☐ Dolor en la coyuntura o que se le haya salido o ruido o chaquido de la mandíbula
- ☐ Granos en la encía o otras infecciones
- ☐ Encías inflamadas/con dolor o sangrando
- ☐ Encías en recesión
- ☐ Tratamientos periodontal (encías)
- ☐ Frecuente reemplazo de empastado/relleno
- ☐ Dientes descoloridos
- ☐ Dientes chuecos
- ☐ Tratamientos de ortodoncia (frenos)
- ☐ Daños a la cara, quijada/mandíbula, dientes
- ☐ Terapia root canal

- ☐ Sacaron dientes
- ☐ Llagas o bulto/tumor
- ☐ Boca seca
- ☐ Dolor al tragar
- ☐ Rechina o aprieta sus dientes
- ☐ Dolor de cabeza, oido o muscular persistente
- ☐ Mal aliento o mal sabor en la boca
- ☐ Comida se queda entre los dientes cuando come
- ☐ Dientes sueltos
- ☐ Dentadura postiza o dentatura parcial
- ☐ Cambios al morder
- ☐ Problemas para masticar satisfactoriamente
- ☐ Despierta con dolor de mandíbula
  - ¿Si sí, con que frequencia?_____
  - Prefiere usted respirar por ☐ la nariz o ☐ la boca?
- ☐ Tragar anormal - empujar con la lengua
- ☐ Muerde el labio o la mejilla con frecuencia

## ACTIVIDADES DIARIAS DE CUIDADO PERSONAL

¿Piensa usted que su actual cuidado dental ☐ Sí   ☐ No personal es efectivo para limiar su boca?

Si su respuesta es No, por favor explique:_____

_____

¿En un día normal, cuántas veces se cepilla sus dientes? (por favor marque con un círculo)

| | | | | | |
|---|---|---|---|---|---|
| Sólo se cepilla | 0 | 1 | 2 | 3 | 4+ |
| Hilo dental | 0 | 1 | 2+ | | |
| Cepillar e hilo dental | 0 | 1 | 2 | 3+ | |

- ☐ De manera rutinaria no me cepillo o uso el hilo dental todos los días

¿Que tipo de cepillo de dientes usa?
- ☐ Duro
- ☐ Mediano
- ☐ Blando
- ☐ No sé

¿Utiliza diariamente otro tipo de auxiliar dental?
- ☐ Limpiadores de puentes dentales
- ☐ Stimudents
- ☐ Rubber tip
- ☐ Proxabrush
- ☐ Otro_____

## ACTIVIDADES DIETETICAS

*Por favor marque con un circulo:*

¿Cuántas bebidas con cafeína bebe diariamente?
    0   1   2   3   4+   menos de 2-3/a la semana

¿Cuántas bebidas alcohólicas bebe diariamente?
    0   1   2   3   4+   menos de 2-3/a la semana

¿Cuántas bebidas gaseosas/refrescos con azucar bebe diariamente?
    0   1   2   3   4+   menos de 2-3/a la semana

¿Cuántas bebidas gaseosas/refrescos dietético bebe diariamente?
    0   1   2   3   4+   menos de 2-3/a la semana

¿Cuántos bebidas "deportivas/energéticas" bebe diariamente?
    0   1   2   3   4+   menos de 2-3/a la semana

¿Cuántos dulces o barras energéticas come diariamente?
    0   1   2   3   4+   menos de 2-3/a la semana

¿Regularmente usa dulces fuertes o mentas para el aliento?
    ☐ Sí   ☐ No   ☐ Ocasionalmente

¿Regularmente usa productos de tabaco?
    ☐ Sí   ☐ No   ☐ Ocasionalmente

¿Usa usted drogas recreacionales/comunes?
    ☐ Sí   ☐ No   ☐ Ocasionalmente

Firma del paciente_____   Fecha_____

Repasado por_____   Fecha_____

**Figure 6-11B.   Adult dental health questionnaire in Spanish.** Page 2 of an adult dental health questionnaire in Spanish.

# Children's Dental Health Questionnaire

Patient_____ Date _____

Student_____ Child's age _____

---

Is this your child's first visit to a dentist? ☐Yes ☐No

Date of last visit: _____

If this is not your child's first visit, has his/her previous dental experience been: ☐ Positive ☐ Negative

Do you anticipate that your child will be cooperative? ☐Yes ☐No

## REASON FOR VISIT

What is the main purpose of your visit today?

_____

_____

_____

_____

Has your child bumped or cracked any front teeth? ☐Yes ☐No

If yes, when?_____

Has your child ever complained of headache, pain, popping, or clicking of the jaws? ☐Yes ☐No

## FLORIDE EXPOSURE

Is your water supply at home fluoridated?

☐ Yes      ☐ No      ☐ Don't know

Does your child use fluoridated tooth paste?

☐ Yes      ☐ No      ☐ Don't know

Does your child take any of the following?

☐ Fluoride tablets

☐ Fluoride drops

☐ Fluoride in vitamins

## PREVENTIVE DENTAL HISTORY

How often does your child brush?_____

Is the child's brushing supervised? ☐Yes ☐No

Do you feel your child's daily self-care is effective in cleaning the teeth? ☐Yes ☐No

If no, please explain _____

_____

On a daily basis, how many times does your child brush? (please circle)

| | | | | | |
|---|---|---|---|---|---|
| Brush only | 0 | 1 | 2 | 3 | 4+ |
| Floss only | 0 | 1 | 2+ | | |
| Brush and floss | 0 | 1 | 2 | 3+ | |

☐ Does not routinely brush or floss on a daily basis

---

**Figure 6-12A. Children's dental health questionnaire in English.** Page 1 of a children's dental health questionnaire in English.

# Children's Dental Health Questionnaire (cont)

## CHILD'S EXISTING DENTAL NEEDS/CONDITIONS

*Please indicate with a check if your child has had or has any of the following:*

- ☐ Sensitive teeth
    - ☐ Hot
    - ☐ Cold
    - ☐ Sweet
    - ☐ Pressure
- ☐ Broken teeth or fillings
- ☐ Joint pain or popping or clicking of jaw
- ☐ Gum boils or other infections
- ☐ Swollen/painful or bleeding gums
- ☐ Frequent filling replacement
- ☐ Discolored teeth
- ☐ Crooked teeth
- ☐ Orthodontic treatment (braces)
- ☐ Injury to the face, jaws, teeth
- ☐ Root canal therapy

- ☐ Removal of teeth
- ☐ Sores or growths
- ☐ Dry mouth
- ☐ Pain upon swallowing
- ☐ Grinding or clenching their teeth
- ☐ Persistent headaches, ear aches, or muscle pain
- ☐ Bad breath, or bad taste in their mouth
- ☐ Food catches between teeth when you eat
- ☐ Loose teeth
- ☐ Problems with chewing
- ☐ Sore jaws upon awakening. How frequently:_____
    - Do they prefer to breathe through their:
        - ☐ nose or ☐ mouth?
- ☐ Abnormal swallowing habit - tongue thrusting
- ☐ Biting their lip or cheek frequently

## DIETARY ACTIVITIES

*Please circle:*

How many caffeinated beverages does your child drink daily?

0   1   2   3   4+   less than 2-3/week

How many sugar-containing sodas does your child drink daily?

0   1   2   3   4+   less than 2-3/week

How many "diet" sodas does your child drink daily?

0   1   2   3   4+   less than 2-3/week

How many "sport/energy" beverages does your child drink daily?

0   1   2   3   4+   less than 2-3/week

How many candy bars or energy/power bars does your child eat daily?

0   1   2   3   4+   less than 2-3/week

## HABITS

Does your child have a night-time bottle?   ☐ Yes  ☐ No

*Does your child do any of the following:*

☐ Grinding teeth:  Still active?  ☐ Yes  ☐ No

How long _____

☐ Thumb sucking: Still active?  ☐ Yes  ☐ No

How long _____

☐ Finger habit:    Still active?  ☐ Yes  ☐ No

How long _____

☐ Lip biting:      Still active?  ☐ Yes  ☐ No

How long _____

☐ Cheek biting:    Still active?  ☐ Yes  ☐ No

How long _____

☐ Nail biting:     Still active?  ☐ Yes  ☐ No

How long _____

☐ Biting on foreign objects such as pencils:
                   Still active?  ☐ Yes  ☐ No

How long _____

Signature of Parent or Legal Guardian _____ Date _____

Reviewed by _____ Date _____

**Figure 6-12B. Children's dental health questionnaire in English.** Page 2 of a children's dental health questionnaire in English.

# Cuestionario de Salud Oral para Niños/as

Paciente_____   Fecha_____

Estudiante_____   Edad de niño_____

¿Es esta la primera visita al dentista de su niño/a?   ☐Sí  ☐No

Fecha de la última visita dental:_____

Si esta no es la primera visita de su niño/a, ha sido la previa experiencia dental:   ☐ Positiva  ☐ Negativa

¿Anticipa usted que su niño/a cooperará?   ☐Sí  ☐No

## RAZON POR SU VISITA

¿Cuál es la razón principal de su visita de hoy?

_____

_____

_____

_____

¿Ha el/la niño/a golpeado o quebrado cualquier de los dientes frontales?   ☐Sí  ☐No

¿Si sí, cuando?_____

¿Ha el/la niño/a alguna vez quejadóse de dolor de cabeza, dolor, que se le haya salido o chasquido/ruido en la mandíbula?   ☐Sí  ☐No

## CONTACTO CON EL FLUORURO

¿Esta el agua en su casa fluorizada?

☐Sí      ☐No      ☐No sé

¿Usa su niño/a pasta/goma de dientes conteniendo fluoruro?

☐Sí      ☐No      ☐No sé

¿Toma su niño/a algunos de los siguientes?

☐ Tabletas de fluoruro

☐ Gotas de fluoruro

☐ Vitaminas de fluoruro

## HISTORIA DENTAL PREVENTIVO

¿Qué tan frecuente se cepilla los dientes su niño/a?   _____

¿Es supervisado/a su niño/a cuando se cepilla?   ☐Sí  ☐No

¿Piensa usted que su actual cuidado dental de su niño/a es efectivo para limpiar su boca?   ☐Sí  ☐No

Si no, por favor explique:_____

_____

_____

¿En un día normal, cuántas veces se cepilla sus dientes su niño/a? *(por favor marque con un circulo)*

Sólo se cepilla        0   1   2   3   4+

Hilo dental            0   1   2+

Cepillar e hilo dental  0   1   2   3+

☐ De manera rutinaria no me cepillo o uso el hilo dental todos los días

**Figure 6-13A.   Children's dental health questionnaire in Spanish.** Page 1 of a children's dental health questionnaire in Spanish.

# Cuestionario de Salud Oral para Niños/as (cont)

## NECESIDADES/CONDICIONES DENTALES EXISTENTES DE SU NIÑO/A

*Favor de indicar marcando si ha tenido o tiene cualquiera de lo siguiente:*

☐ Dientes sensitivos:
    ☐ Caliente
    ☐ Frío
    ☐ Dulce
    ☐ Presión
☐ Dientes quebrados o rellenos/empastados
☐ Dolor en la coyuntura o que se le haya salido o ruido o chaquido de la mandíbula
☐ Granos en la encía u otras infecciones
☐ Encías inflamadas/con dolor o sangrando
☐ Frecuente reemplazo de empastado/relleno
☐ Dientes descoloridos
☐ Dientes chuecos
☐ Tratamientos de ortodoncia (frenos)
☐ Daños a la cara, quijada/mandíbula, dientes
☐ Terapia root canal

☐ Sacaron dientes
☐ Llagas o bulto/tumor
☐ Boca seca
☐ Dolor al tragar
☐ Rechina o aprieta sus dientes
☐ Dolor de cabeza, oido, o muscular persistente
☐ Mal aliento o mal sabor en la boca
☐ Comida se queda entre los dientes cuando come
☐ Dientes sueltos
☐ Problemas masticar satisfactoriamente
☐ Despierta con dolor de mandíbula
    ¿Si sí, con que frequencia?_____
    Prefiere usted respirar por ☐la nariz o ☐la boca
☐ Tragar anormal - empujar con la lengua
☐ Muerde el labio o la mejilla con frecuencia

## ACTIVIDADES DIETETICAS

*Por favor marque con un círculo:*

¿Cuántas bebidas con cafeína bebe su niño/a diariamente?

0  1  2  3  4+  menos de 2-3/a la semana

¿Cuántas bebidas gaseosas/refrescos conteniendo azúcar bebe su niño/a diariamente?

0  1  2  3  4+  menos de 2-3/a la semana

¿Cuátas bebidas gaseosas/refrescos con substituto de azúcar dietético bebe so niño/a diariamente?

0  1  2  3  4+  menos de 2-3/a la semana

¿Cuántos bebidas "deportivas"/ "energéticas" bebe su ninño/a diariamente?

0  1  2  3  4+  menos de 2-3/a la semana

¿Cuántos dulces o barras energéticas come su niño/a diariamente?

0  1  2  3  4+  menos de 2-3/a la semana

## HABITOS

¿Tiene su niño/a un biberón/mamila nocturna?   ☐Sí  ☐No

*Hace su niño/a cualquiera de lo siguiente:*

☐ Rechinar los dientes:  ¿Aún activo? ☐Sí  ☐No
    ¿Por cuanto tiempo? _____

☐ Chupar el dedo:  ¿Aún activo? ☐Sí  ☐No
    ¿Por cuanto tiempo? _____

☐ Habito del dedo:  ¿Aún activo? ☐Sí  ☐No
    ¿Por cuanto tiempo? _____

☐ Chupón/chupete:  ¿Aún activo? ☐Sí  ☐No
    ¿Por cuanto tiempo? _____

☐ Morder el lavio o:  ¿Aún activo? ☐Sí  ☐No
  la mejilla:
    ¿Por cuanto tiempo? _____

☐ Morder las uñas:  ¿Aún activo? ☐Sí  ☐No
    ¿Por cuanto tiempo? _____

☐ Morder un objeto extraño como un lapiz:
    ¿Aún activo? ☐Sí  ☐No
    ¿Por cuanto tiempo? _____

Firma de los padres o guardian legal _____ Fecha _____

Revisado por _____ Fecha _____

**Figure 6-13B. Children's dental health questionnaire in Spanish.** Page 2 of a children 's dental health questionnaire in English.

## SECTION 5:

# The Human Element

**Table 6-1** ENGLISH-TO-SPANISH PHRASE LIST FOR DENTAL HISTORY

| | |
|---|---|
| Good morning (afternoon), Mr. _____. | Buenos días (tardes), señor _____. |
| Good morning (afternoon), Mrs. _____. | Buenos días (tardes), señora _____. |
| Good morning (afternoon), Miss _____. | Buenos días (tardes), señorita _____. |
| My name is ____. I am your dental hygienist. | Mi nombre es _____. Soy su higienista dental. |
| It is nice to meet you. | Mucho gusto en conocerlo (conocerla). |
| I do not speak Spanish; I will point to Spanish phrases. | No hablo español; voy a indicar las frases en español. |
| Please answer the questions on this form about your dental health. | Por favor responda a las preguntas en este formulario sobre su salud dental. |
| Please answer the questions on this form about your child's dental health. | Por favor responda a las preguntas en este formulario sobre la salud dental de su niño. |
| Has the dentist ever given you anything to help you be less anxious about your dental appointment? | ¿Usted ha tomado algún calmante recetado por el dentista para estar menos ansioso sobre su cita dental? |
| You forgot to answer this question. | Se olvidó responder a esta pregunta. |
| Please sign here. | Por favor firme aquí. |
| Wait here, I will get the dentist or instructor. | Espere aquí; voy a buscar el dentista o el profesor. |
| We are finished for today. | Hemos terminados por hoy. |
| We will schedule your next appointment. | Vamos a hacer una nueva cita. |
| Goodbye, see you next time. | Hasta luego; la (lo) veremos la próxima cita. |

**SECTION 6:**

# Practical Focus—Fictitious Patient Cases

**DIRECTIONS:**

- Section 6 contains completed dental health questionnaires for patients A–E.
- In a clinical setting, you will gather additional information about your patient with each assessment procedure that you perform. When determining treatment considerations and modifications for patients A–E, you should take into account the health history and over-the-counter/prescription drug information that was revealed for each patient in Module 4: Medical History.
- Review the completed dental health questionnaires for patients A–E in Figures 16-14A to 16-18B. For each patient, make a list of any concerns, problems, or treatment modifications that will be necessary based on the information on the dental health history.

# Dental Health Questionnaire

Patient _ALAN A. ASCARI_   Date _1/15/XX_

Student _TYNE BRUCHEIM_

## REASON FOR TODAY'S VISIT - CHIEF COMPLAINT

What is the main reason for your visit today? _CHECK UP - BAD TASTE IN MY MOUTH AND GUMS BLEED_

How did you hear about our practice? _NEIGHBOR, I JUST MOVED INTO AREA_

Referred by: _____

## PREVIOUS DENTAL TREATMENT

Have you seen another dentist within the last year? _NO_

When was your last dental visit? _5 YEARS AGO_

Reason for the above visit? _GUMS BLEED_

Name of previous dentist? _DR. STEWART TRENTON, NEW JERSEY_

Have you had x-rays of your teeth taken ☐Yes ☒No recently?

## TELL US ABOUT YOUR PREVIOUS DENTAL EXPERIENCES

Have your previous dental visits been favorable/comfortable emotionally? ☒Yes ☐No

If no, please explain: _____

In general, do you feel positive about your previous dental treatment? ☒Yes ☐No

If no, please explain: _____

Have you ever had an adverse reaction to dental treatment? ☒Yes ☐No

If yes, please explain: _FAINTED DURING SHOT FOR TEETH_

Have you ever had any allergic reactions associated with dental treatment? ☒Yes ☐No

If yes, please explain: _DR. GLOVES MADE MY LIPS SWELL UP_

Have you ever had difficulty with local anesthetic injections? ☒Yes ☐No

If yes, please explain: _FAINTED_

Other dental experiences we should know about? _____

## TELL US ABOUT ANY DENTAL CONCERNS YOU MAY HAVE

Are you satisfied with your teeth and their appearance? ☒Yes ☐No

If no, please explain: _____

Are you interested in having your teeth a lighter color? ☐Yes ☒No

If yes, please explain: _____

Are you interested in any specific type of dental treatment at this time?

☐ Implants
☐ Cosmetic dentistry
☐ Replacing missing teeth
☐ Dentures
☒ Replacing old fillings
☐ Other _____

A lot can be done to prevent dental diseases (teeth and gum disease). Would you like to know more about preventing dental disease for yourself or your family? ☒Yes ☐No

If yes, please explain: _____

**Figure 6-14A.  Page 1 of the dental health questionnaire for fictitious patient Mr. Ascari.** Page 2 of Mr. Ascari's form is on the following page.

# Dental Health Questionnaire (cont)

## EXISTING DENTAL NEEDS/CONDITIONS

*Please indicate with a check if you have had or have any of the following:*

☐ Sensitive teeth
    ☐ Hot
    ☒ Cold
    ☒ Sweet
    ☐ Pressure
☒ Broken teeth or fillings
☐ Joint pain or popping or clicking of jaw
☐ Gum boils or other infections
☒ Swollen/painful or bleeding gums
☐ Gum recession
☐ Periodontal treatments (gum)
☐ Frequent filling replacement
☐ Discolored teeth
☐ Crooked teeth
☐ Orthodontic treatment (braces)
☐ Injury to the face, jaws, teeth
☐ Root canal therapy

☐ Removal of teeth
☐ Sores or growths
☒ Dry mouth
☐ Pain upon swallowing
☐ Grinding or clenching teeth
☐ Persistent headaches, ear aches, or muscle pain
☒ Bad breath, or bad taste in mouth
☐ Food catches between teeth when you eat
☐ Loose teeth
☐ Denture or partial denture
☐ Your bite is changing
☐ Problems chewing
☐ Sore jaws upon awakening. How frequently: _____
    Do you prefer to breathe through your
        ☐ nose or ☐ mouth?
☐ Abnormal swallowing habit - tongue thrusting
☐ Biting your lip or cheek frequently

## DAILY SELF-CARE ACTIVITIES

Do you feel your present daily self-care is effective in cleaning your mouth? ☒ Yes ☐ No

    If no, please explain _____

_____

On a daily basis, how many times do you brush your teeth? (please circle)

Brush only      0  1  ②  3  4+
Floss only       ⓪  1  2+
Brush and floss  0  1  2  3+

☐ Do not routinely brush or floss on a daily basis

What type of toothbrush do you use?
☒ Hard
☐ Medium
☐ Soft
☐ Don't know

Do you use any other dental aids on a regular basis?
☐ Bridge cleaners
☐ Stimudents
☐ Rubber tip
☐ Proxabrush
☐ Other _____

## DIETARY ACTIVITIES

*Please circle:*

How many caffeinated beverages do you drink daily?
    0  1  2  ③  4+   less than 2-3/week
How many alcoholic beverages do you drink daily?
    ⓪  1  2  3  4+   less than 2-3/week
How many sugar-containing sodas do you drink daily?
    0  1  2  3  ④₊   less than 2-3/week
How many "diet" sodas do you drink daily?
    ⓪  1  2  3  4+   less than 2-3/week
How many "sport/energy" beverages do you drink daily?
    0  1  2  ③  4+   less than 2-3/week

How many candy bars or energy/power bars do you eat daily?
    0  1  ②  3  4+   less than 2-3/week

Do you regularly eat hard candies or breath mints?
    ☐ Yes  ☒ No  ☐ Occasionally
Do you regularly use tobacco products?
    ☒ Yes  ☐ No  ☐ Occasionally
Do you use recreational/street drugs?
    ☐ Yes  ☒ No  ☐ Occasionally

Signature of Patient _____*Alan Ascari*_____    Date _____1/15/XX_____

Reviewed by _____*Tyne Brucheim*_____    Date _____1/15/XX_____

**Figure 6-14B. Page 2 of Mr. Ascari's dental health questionnaire.**

# Children's Dental Health Questionnaire

Patient _BETHANY BIDDLE_          Date _1/10/XX_

Student _EUGENIA MILLER_          Child's age _9_

---

Is this your child's first visit to a dentist?   ☐ Yes ☒ No

Date of last visit: _6/1/XX_

If this is not your child's first visit, has his/her previous dental experience been:   ☒ Positive ☐ Negative

Do you anticipate that your child will be cooperative?   ☒ Yes ☐ No

## REASON FOR VISIT

What is the main purpose of your visit today?

_CHECK UP_

_____

_____

_____

Has your child bumped or cracked any front teeth?   ☐ Yes ☒ No

If yes, when? _____

Has your child ever complained of headache, pain, popping, or clicking of the jaws?   ☐ Yes ☒ No

## FLORIDE EXPOSURE

Is your water supply at home fluoridated?

☒ Yes    ☐ No    ☐ Don't know

Does your child use fluoridated tooth paste?

☒ Yes    ☐ No    ☐ Don't know

Does your child take any of the following?

☐ Fluoride tablets

☐ Fluoride drops

☐ Fluoride in vitamins

## PREVENTIVE DENTAL HISTORY

How often does your child brush? _2_

Is the child's brushing supervised?   ☒ Yes ☐ No

Do you feel your child's daily self-care is effective in cleaning the teeth?   ☒ Yes ☐ No

If no, please explain _____

_____

On a daily basis, how many times does your child brush? (please circle)

| | | | | | |
|---|---|---|---|---|---|
| Brush only | 0 | 1 | ②  | 3 | 4+ |
| Floss only | ⓪ | 1 | 2+ | | |
| Brush and floss | ⓪ | 1 | 2 | 3+ | |

☐ Does not routinely brush or floss on a daily basis

---

**Figure 6-15A.   Page 1 of the dental health questionnaire for fictitious patient Bethany Biddle.** Page 2 of Bethany Biddle's form is on the following page.

# Children's Dental Health Questionnaire (cont)

## CHILD'S EXISTING DENTAL NEEDS/CONDITIONS

*Please indicate with a check if your child has had or has any of the following:*

☐ Sensitive teeth
    ☐ Hot
    ☐ Cold
    ☐ Sweet
    ☐ Pressure
☐ Broken teeth or fillings
☐ Joint pain or popping or clicking of jaw
☒ Gum boils or other infections
☐ Swollen/painful or bleeding gums
☐ Frequent filling replacement
☐ Discolored teeth
☒ Crooked teeth
☐ Orthodontic treatment (braces)
☐ Injury to the face, jaws, teeth
☐ Root canal therapy

☐ Removal of teeth
☐ Sores or growths
☐ Dry mouth
☐ Pain upon swallowing
☐ Grinding or clenching their teeth
☐ Persistent headaches, ear aches, or muscle pain
☐ Bad breath, or bad taste in their mouth
☐ Food catches between teeth when you eat
☐ Loose teeth
☐ Problems with chewing
☒ Sore jaws upon awakening. How frequently: _2X/WEEK_
    Do they prefer to breathe through their:
      ☐ nose or ☐ mouth?
☐ Abnormal swallowing habit - tongue thrusting
☐ Biting their lip or cheek frequently

## DIETARY ACTIVITIES

*Please circle:*

How many caffeinated beverages does your child drink daily?

0   ①    2   3   4+    less than 2-3/week

How many sugar-containing sodas does your child drink daily?

0   1   2   ③   4+    less than 2-3/week

How many "diet" sodas does your child drink daily?

⓪   1   2   3   4+    less than 2-3/week

How many "sport/energy" beverages does your child drink daily?

⓪   1   2   3   4+    less than 2-3/week

How many candy bars or energy/power bars does your child eat daily?

0   1   ②   3   4+    less than 2-3/week

## HABITS

Does your child have a night-time bottle?    ☐ Yes ☒ No

*Does your child do any of the following:*

☐ Grinding teeth:   Still active?   ☐ Yes ☒ No
     How long _____
☐ Thumb sucking: Still active?   ☐ Yes ☒ No
     How long _____
☐ Finger habit:     Still active?   ☐ Yes ☒ No
     How long _____
☐ Lip biting:       Still active?   ☐ Yes ☒ No
     How long _____
☐ Cheek biting:    Still active?   ☐ Yes ☒ No
     How long _____
☐ Nail biting:      Still active?   ☐ Yes ☒ No
     How long _____
☐ Biting on foreign objects such as pencils:
                 Still active?   ☐ Yes ☒ No
     How long _____

Signature of Parent or Legal Guardian __*Brenda Biddle*__   Date __1/10/XX__

Reviewed by __*Eugenia Miller*__   Date __1/10/XX__

**Figure 6-15B.** Page 2 of the dental health questionnaire for fictitious patient Bethany Biddle.

# Dental Health Questionnaire

Patient _CARLOS C. CHAVEZ_    Date _1/05/XX_

Student _JOEL WEINSTEIN_

## REASON FOR TODAY'S VISIT - CHIEF COMPLAINT

What is the main reason for your visit today? ___
_CHECK UP_
_GUMS BLEED_

How did you hear about our practice? ___
_A FRIEND REFERRED ME_
Referred by: _HECTOR GARCIA_

## PREVIOUS DENTAL TREATMENT

Have you seen another dentist within the last year? _NO_

When was your last dental visit? _2 YEARS AGO_

Reason for the above visit? _CLEANING_

Name of previous dentist? _DR. MALDONALDO_
_MERCEDES, TX_

Have you had x-rays of your teeth taken ☐Yes ☒No
recently?

## TELL US ABOUT YOUR PREVIOUS DENTAL EXPERIENCES

Have your previous dental visits been favorable/comfortable emotionally? ☒Yes ☐No

   If no, please explain: ___

In general, do you feel positive about your previous dental treatment? ☒Yes ☐No

   If no, please explain: ___

Have you ever had an adverse reaction to dental treatment? ☐Yes ☒No

   If yes, please explain: ___

Have you ever had any allergic reactions associated with dental treatment? ☐Yes ☒No

   If yes, please explain: ___

Have you ever had difficulty with local anesthetic injections? ☐Yes ☒No

   If yes, please explain: ___

Other dental experiences we should know about? ___

## TELL US ABOUT ANY DENTAL CONCERNS YOU MAY HAVE

Are you satisfied with your teeth and their appearance? ☐Yes ☒No

   If no, please explain: _BROKEN TEETH,_
_DARK COLOR OF TEETH_

Are you interested in having your teeth a lighter color? ☒Yes ☐No

   If yes, please explain: ___

Are you interested in any specific type of dental treatment at this time?
☐ Implants
☐ Cosmetic dentistry
☒ Replacing missing teeth
☐ Dentures
☒ Replacing old fillings
☐ Other ___

A lot can be done to prevent dental diseases (teeth and gum disease). Would you like to know more about preventing dental disease for yourself or your family? ☒Yes ☐No

   If yes, please explain: _SO MY GUMS_
_WON'T BLEED_

**Figure 6-16A. Page 1 of the dental health questionnaire for fictitious patient Mr. Chavez.** Page 2 of Mr. Chavez's form is on the following page.

# Dental Health Questionnaire (cont)

## EXISTING DENTAL NEEDS/CONDITIONS

*Please indicate with a check if you have had or have any of the following:*

- ☐ Sensitive teeth
  - ☐ Hot
  - ☐ Cold
  - ☐ Sweet
  - ☐ Pressure
- ☒ Broken teeth or fillings
- ☐ Joint pain or popping or clicking of jaw
- ☐ Gum boils or other infections
- ☒ Swollen/painful or bleeding gums
- ☒ Gum recession
- ☐ Periodontal treatments (gum)
- ☐ Frequent filling replacement
- ☒ Discolored teeth
- ☐ Crooked teeth
- ☐ Orthodontic treatment (braces)
- ☐ Injury to the face, jaws, teeth
- ☐ Root canal therapy

- ☐ Removal of teeth
- ☐ Sores or growths
- ☐ Dry mouth
- ☐ Pain upon swallowing
- ☐ Grinding or clenching teeth
- ☐ Persistent headaches, ear aches, or muscle pain
- ☒ Bad breath, or bad taste in mouth
- ☐ Food catches between teeth when you eat
- ☐ Loose teeth
- ☐ Denture or partial denture
- ☐ Your bite is changing
- ☐ Problems chewing
- ☐ Sore jaws upon awakening. How frequently: _____
  - Do you prefer to breathe through your
    - ☐ nose or ☐ mouth?
- ☐ Abnormal swallowing habit - tongue thrusting
- ☐ Biting your lip or cheek frequently

## DAILY SELF-CARE ACTIVITIES

Do you feel your present daily self-care is effective in cleaning your mouth? ☐ Yes ☒ No

If no, please explain ___GUMS BLEED___

On a daily basis, how many times do you brush your teeth? (please circle)

Brush only    0   1   ②  3   4+
Floss only    ⓪   1   2+
Brush and floss   0   1   2   3+

☐ Do not routinely brush or floss on a daily basis

What type of toothbrush do you use?
- ☐ Hard
- ☐ Medium
- ☐ Soft
- ☒ Don't know

Do you use any other dental aids on a regular basis?
- ☐ Bridge cleaners
- ☐ Stimudents
- ☐ Rubber tip
- ☐ Proxabrush
- ☐ Other _____

## DIETARY ACTIVITIES

*Please circle:*

How many caffeinated beverages do you drink daily?
  0   1   ②   3   4+   less than 2-3/week

How many alcoholic beverages do you drink daily?
  0   ①   2   3   4+   less than 2-3/week

How many sugar-containing sodas do you drink daily?
  0   ①   2   3   4+   less than 2-3/week

How many "diet" sodas do you drink daily?
  ⓪   1   2   3   4+   less than 2-3/week

How many "sport/energy" beverages do you drink daily?
  ⓪   1   2   3   4+   less than 2-3/week

How many candy bars or energy/power bars do you eat daily?
  0   1   2   3   4+   (less than 2-3/week)

Do you regularly eat hard candies or breath mints?
  ☐ Yes   ☒ No   ☐ Occasionally

Do you regularly use tobacco products?
  ☐ Yes   ☒ No   ☐ Occasionally

Do you use recreational/street drugs?
  ☐ Yes   ☒ No   ☐ Occasionally

Signature of Patient ___Carlos Chavez___    Date ___1/05/XX___

Reviewed by ___Joel Weinstein___    Date ___1/05/XX___

**Figure 6-16B.** Page 2 of Mr. Chavez's dental health questionnaire.

# Dental Health Questionnaire

Patient _DONNA D. DOI_    Date _1/30/XX_

Student _THALIA JONES_

## REASON FOR TODAY'S VISIT - CHIEF COMPLAINT

What is the main reason for your visit today? _____

_CHECK UP_

_BLEEDING GUMS_

How did you hear about our practice? _____

_YELLOW PAGES_

Referred by: _RECENTLY MOVED TO TOWN_

## PREVIOUS DENTAL TREATMENT

Have you seen another dentist within the last year? _YES_

When was your last dental visit? _6 MONTHS AGO_

Reason for the above visit? _CHECK UP_

Name of previous dentist? _DR. GLASSCOE ALPINE, COLORADO_

Have you had x-rays of your teeth taken ☒Yes  ☐No
recently?

## TELL US ABOUT YOUR PREVIOUS DENTAL EXPERIENCES

Have your previous dental visits been
favorable/comfortable emotionally?    ☒Yes  ☐No

If no, please explain: _____

In general, do you feel positive about
your previous dental treatment?    ☒Yes  ☐No

If no, please explain: _____

Have you ever had an adverse
reaction to dental treatment?    ☐Yes  ☒No

If yes, please explain: _____

Have you ever had any allergic
reactions associated with dental
treatment?    ☐Yes  ☒No

If yes, please explain: _____

Have you ever had difficulty with local    ☐Yes  ☒No
anesthetic injections?

If yes, please explain: _____

Other dental experiences we should know about? _____

## TELL US ABOUT ANY DENTAL CONCERNS YOU MAY HAVE

Are you satisfied with your teeth and
their appearance?    ☐Yes  ☒No

If no, please explain: _____

Are you interested in having your
teeth a lighter color?    ☐Yes  ☒No

If yes, please explain: _____

Are you interested in any specific type of dental
treatment at this time?

☐ Implants
☐ Cosmetic dentistry
☐ Replacing missing teeth
☐ Dentures
☐ Replacing old fillings
☐ Other_____

A lot can be done to prevent dental diseases (teeth
and gum disease). Would you like to know more about
preventing dental disease for yourself
or your family?    ☒Yes  ☐No

If yes, please explain: _GUMS BLEED_

**Figure 6-17A.   Page 1 of the dental health questionnaire for fictitious patient Mrs. Doi.**
Page 2 of Mrs. Doi's form is on the following page.

# Dental Health Questionnaire (cont)

## EXISTING DENTAL NEEDS/CONDITIONS

*Please indicate with a check if you have had or have any of the following:*

- ☐ Sensitive teeth
  - ☐ Hot
  - ☐ Cold
  - ☐ Sweet
  - ☐ Pressure
- ☐ Broken teeth or fillings
- ☐ Joint pain or popping or clicking of jaw
- ☐ Gum boils or other infections
- ☒ Swollen/painful or bleeding gums
- ☐ Gum recession
- ☐ Periodontal treatments (gum)
- ☐ Frequent filling replacement
- ☐ Discolored teeth
- ☐ Crooked teeth
- ☐ Orthodontic treatment (braces)
- ☐ Injury to the face, jaws, teeth
- ☐ Root canal therapy

- ☐ Removal of teeth
- ☐ Sores or growths
- ☐ Dry mouth
- ☐ Pain upon swallowing
- ☐ Grinding or clenching teeth
- ☐ Persistent headaches, ear aches, or muscle pain
- ☐ Bad breath, or bad taste in mouth
- ☐ Food catches between teeth when you eat
- ☐ Loose teeth
- ☐ Denture or partial denture
- ☐ Your bite is changing
- ☐ Problems chewing
- ☐ Sore jaws upon awakening. How frequently:_____
  - Do you prefer to breathe through your
    - ☐ nose or ☐ mouth?
- ☐ Abnormal swallowing habit - tongue thrusting
- ☐ Biting your lip or cheek frequently

## DAILY SELF-CARE ACTIVITIES

Do you feel your present daily self-care ☐ Yes ☒ No
is effective in cleaning your mouth?

If no, please explain _MUST NOT BE,_
_GUMS BLEED_

On a daily basis, how many times do you brush your teeth? (please circle)

| | | | | | |
|---|---|---|---|---|---|
| Brush only | 0 | 1 | ②| 3 | 4+ |
| Floss only | 0 | ①| 2+ | | |
| Brush and floss | 0 | 1 | 2 | 3+ | |

☐ Do not routinely brush or floss on a daily basis

What type of toothbrush do you use?
- ☐ Hard
- ☐ Medium
- ☒ Soft
- ☐ Don't know

Do you use any other dental aids on a regular basis?
- ☐ Bridge cleaners
- ☒ Stimudents
- ☐ Rubber tip
- ☐ Proxabrush
- ☐ Other _____

## DIETARY ACTIVITIES

*Please circle:*

How many caffeinated beverages do you drink daily?
   0  1  ②  3  4+   less than 2-3/week
How many alcoholic beverages do you drink daily?
   ⓪  1  2  3  4+   less than 2-3/week
How many sugar-containing sodas do you drink daily?
   ⓪  1  2  3  4+   less than 2-3/week
How many "diet" sodas do you drink daily?
   0  ①  2  3  4+   less than 2-3/week
How many "sport/energy" beverages do you drink daily?
   ⓪  1  2  3  4+   less than 2-3/week

How many candy bars or energy/power bars do you eat daily?
   0  1  2  3  4+   (less than 2-3/week)

Do you regularly eat hard candies or breath mints?
   ☐ Yes  ☒ No  ☐ Occasionally
Do you regularly use tobacco products?
   ☐ Yes  ☒ No  ☐ Occasionally
Do you use recreational/street drugs?
   ☐ Yes  ☒ No  ☐ Occasionally

Signature of Patient _Donna Doi_   Date _1/30/XX_

Reviewed by _Thalia Jones_   Date _1/30/XX_

**Figure 6-17B.** Page 2 of Mrs. Doi's dental health questionnaire.

# Dental Health Questionnaire

Patient _ESTHER E. EADS_   Date _1/24/XX_

Student _PARKER SHEFFIELD_

## REASON FOR TODAY'S VISIT - CHIEF COMPLAINT

What is the main reason for your visit today? _CHECK UP_

How did you hear about our practice? _LONG TIME PATIENT_

Referred by: _____

## PREVIOUS DENTAL TREATMENT

Have you seen another dentist within the last year? _NO_

When was your last dental visit? _2 YEARS AGO_

Reason for the above visit? _CHECK UP_

Name of previous dentist? _____

Have you had x-rays of your teeth taken recently?  ☒ Yes   ☐ No

## TELL US ABOUT YOUR PREVIOUS DENTAL EXPERIENCES

Have your previous dental visits been favorable/comfortable emotionally?   ☒ Yes   ☐ No

  If no, please explain: _____

In general, do you feel positive about your previous dental treatment?   ☒ Yes   ☐ No

  If no, please explain: _____

Have you ever had an adverse reaction to dental treatment?   ☐ Yes   ☒ No

  If yes, please explain: _____

Have you ever had any allergic reactions associated with dental treatment?   ☐ Yes   ☒ No

  If yes, please explain: _____

Have you ever had difficulty with local anesthetic injections?   ☐ Yes   ☒ No

  If yes, please explain: _____

Other dental experiences we should know about?

_____

## TELL US ABOUT ANY DENTAL CONCERNS YOU MAY HAVE

Are you satisfied with your teeth and their appearance?   ☒ Yes   ☐ No

  If no, please explain: _____

Are you interested in having your teeth a lighter color?   ☐ Yes   ☒ No

  If yes, please explain: _____

Are you interested in any specific type of dental treatment at this time?
- ☐ Implants
- ☐ Cosmetic dentistry
- ☐ Replacing missing teeth
- ☐ Dentures
- ☐ Replacing old fillings
- ☐ Other _____

A lot can be done to prevent dental diseases (teeth and gum disease). Would you like to know more about preventing dental disease for yourself or your family?   ☐ Yes   ☒ No

  If yes, please explain: _____

**Figure 6-18A.  Page 1 of the dental health questionnaire for fictitious patient Ms. Eads.** Page 2 of Ms. Eads's form is on the following page.

# Dental Health Questionnaire (cont)

## EXISTING DENTAL NEEDS/CONDITIONS

*Please indicate with a check if you have had or have any of the following:*

☐ Sensitive teeth
    ☐ Hot
    ☐ Cold
    ☐ Sweet
    ☐ Pressure
☐ Broken teeth or fillings
☐ Joint pain or popping or clicking of jaw
☐ Gum boils or other infections
☐ Swollen/painful or bleeding gums
☐ Gum recession
☐ Periodontal treatments (gum)
☐ Frequent filling replacement
☐ Discolored teeth
☐ Crooked teeth
☐ Orthodontic treatment (braces)
☐ Injury to the face, jaws, teeth
☐ Root canal therapy

☐ Removal of teeth
☐ Sores or growths
☐ Dry mouth
☐ Pain upon swallowing
☐ Grinding or clenching teeth
☐ Persistent headaches, ear aches, or muscle pain
☐ Bad breath, or bad taste in mouth
☐ Food catches between teeth when you eat
☐ Loose teeth
☐ Denture or partial denture
☐ Your bite is changing
☐ Problems chewing
☐ Sore jaws upon awakening. How frequently: _____
    Do you prefer to breathe through your
      ☐ nose or ☐ mouth?
☐ Abnormal swallowing habit - tongue thrusting
☐ Biting your lip or cheek frequently

## DAILY SELF-CARE ACTIVITIES

Do you feel your present daily self-care is effective in cleaning your mouth?  ☒ Yes  ☐ No

If no, please explain _____

_____

On a daily basis, how many times do you brush your teeth? (please circle)

Brush only        0  1  **②**  3  4+
Floss only        0  **①**  2+
Brush and floss  0  1  2  3+

☐ Do not routinely brush or floss on a daily basis

What type of toothbrush do you use?
☐ Hard
☐ Medium
☒ Soft
☐ Don't know

Do you use any other dental aids on a regular basis?
☒ Bridge cleaners
☐ Stimudents
☐ Rubber tip
☐ Proxabrush
☐ Other _____

## DIETARY ACTIVITIES

*Please circle:*

How many caffeinated beverages do you drink daily?
  0  1  2  **③**  4+    less than 2-3/week
How many alcoholic beverages do you drink daily?
  **⓪**  1  2  3  4+    less than 2-3/week
How many sugar-containing sodas do you drink daily?
  **⓪**  1  2  3  4+    less than 2-3/week
How many "diet" sodas do you drink daily?
  **⓪**  1  2  3  4+    less than 2-3/week
How many "sport/energy" beverages do you drink daily?
  **⓪**  1  2  3  4+    less than 2-3/week

How many candy bars or energy/power bars do you eat daily?
  0  1  2  3  4+   **(less than 2-3/week)**

Do you regularly eat hard candies or breath mints?
☒ Yes  ☐ No  ☐ Occasionally
Do you regularly use tobacco products?
☐ Yes  ☒ No  ☐ Occasionally
Do you use recreational/street drugs?
☐ Yes  ☒ No  ☐ Occasionally

Signature of Patient *Esther Eads*  Date *1/24/XX*

Reviewed by *Frasier Fairhall*  Date *1/24/XX*

**Figure 6-18B.  Page 2 of Ms. Ead's dental health questionnaire.**

## SECTION 7:
# Skill Check

**TECHNIQUE SKILL CHECKLIST:** DENTAL HEALTH QUESTIONNAIRE

Student:_____    Evaluator:_____

Date:    _____

**DIRECTIONS FOR STUDENT:** Use **Column S**; evaluate your skill level as **S** (satisfactory) or **U** (unsatisfactory).

**DIRECTIONS FOR EVALUATOR:** Use **Column E**. Indicate **S** (satisfactory) or **U** (unsatisfactory). In the optional grade percentage calculation, each **S** equals 1 point, and each **U** equals 0 points.

| CRITERIA | S | E |
|---|---|---|
| **Reads through every line on the completed dental health questionnaire. Identifies any unanswered questions on the form and follows up to obtain complete information.** | | |
| **Makes notes about any information that is not clear or difficult to read. Confirms that the patient has signed and dated the form.** | | |
| **Circles concerns in red pencil. Reads through all handwritten responses and circles concerns in red.** | | |
| **Formulates a list of follow-up questions to review with the patient.** | | |
| **Formulates a preliminary opinion regarding any treatment alterations that may be needed based on the information gathered during the dental health history assessment. Discusses possible treatment alterations with the clinical instructor.** | | |

OPTIONAL GRADE PERCENTAGE CALCULATION

Each **S** equals 1 point, and each **U** equals 0 points. Using the **E** column, the sum of the "**S**"s _____ divided by the total points possible (5) equals the percentage grade _____.

# NOTES

MODULE

# 7

# Vital Signs: Temperature

## MODULE OVERVIEW

This is the first of three modules covering the assessment of vital signs that provide essential information about a patient's health status. The four vital signs are temperature, pulse, respiration, and blood pressure. This module covers the technique for measuring oral temperature. Pulse and respiration are discussed in Module 8. The technique for blood pressure assessment is described in Module 9.

This module covers oral temperature taking, including:

- How to use a glass fever thermometer
- How to prepare the patient for the procedure
- Step-by-step peak procedures for taking an oral temperature

## MODULE OUTLINE

## OBJECTIVES

- Define the term *vital signs* and discuss how vital signs reflect changes in a person's health status.
- Discuss the dental health care provider's responsibilities in assessing temperature.
- Describe factors that can affect a person's body temperature.
- State the variables that can affect accurate temperature assessment.
- Prior to assessing temperature, explain to the patient why an accurate body temperature is needed.
- Describe the equipment to the patient and explain what to expect during the procedure.
- Answer any questions regarding the procedure that the patient might have.
- Accurately assess, interpret, and document body temperature.
- Provide information to the patient about the readings that you obtain.
- Properly use and care for the equipment used for measuring oral temperature.
- Recognize oral temperature findings that have implications in planning dental treatment.
- Provide appropriate referral to a physician when findings indicate the need for further evaluation.
- Compare temperature findings in the fictitious patient cases A–E (in Module 9) to the normal temperature range.
- Demonstrate knowledge of temperature assessment by applying concepts from this module to the fictitious patient cases A–E in Module 9, Vital Signs: Blood Pressure.

**Note to Course Instructor:** Fictitious patient cases A–E for all the vital signs modules are located in Module 9, Vital Signs: Blood Pressure.

## SECTION 1:
# Introduction to Vital Signs Assessment

## VITAL SIGNS OVERVIEW

1. **Origin of terminology.** The word "vital" means "necessary to life." This is why certain key measurements that provide essential information about a person's health are referred to as vital signs.
2. **Definition.** Vital signs are a person's temperature, pulse, respiration, and blood pressure.
3. **Fifth vital sign.** In addition to these standard vital signs, tobacco use has been suggested as the fifth vital sign because tobacco use is a factor in many medical conditions as well as periodontal disease.
4. **Homeostasis.** The body tries to maintain a state of balance (**homeostasis**) by making adjustments as necessary to keep the body's vital signs within the range of normal.
5. **Assessment.** Vital signs can be observed, measured, and monitored to provide critical information about a person's state of health. Temperature is the measurement of the degree of heat in a living body.
   a. **Pulse** is the measurement of the heart rate in beats per minute. The pulse is a throbbing sensation caused by the contraction and expansion of an artery as blood passes through it.
   b. **Respiration** is the breathing rate of an individual, stated in breaths per minute.
   c. **Blood pressure** is the force exerted against the walls of the blood vessels as the blood flows through them.

## WHY ARE VITAL SIGNS IMPORTANT?

* Changes in a vital sign may indicate that something is out of balance in the body and the body is trying to get that balance back.
* Vital signs tell the dental health care provider about changes in a person's body such as illness, stress, or internal body damage.
* For patient safety, vital signs should be measured before any dental treatment.

## BOX 7-1 How Are Vital Signs Measured?

* Oral temperature is measured in the mouth with a thermometer placed under the tongue. A glass, digital, or disposable thermometer may be used.
* Pulse rate is measured by touch. In the dental setting, the pulse rate is felt at the wrist.
* Breathing rate is measured by watching the rise and fall of the chest wall.
* Blood pressure is measured using a stethoscope and a blood pressure cuff. Digital blood pressure cuffs are an alternative to the traditional stethoscope and blood pressure cuff; digital measurement may not be as accurate as the traditional method of assessment.

# UNDERSTANDING TEMPERATURE SCALES – FAHRENHEIT/ CELSIUS/CENTIGRADE

Three terms—Fahrenheit, Celsius, and centigrade—are encountered when reading or discussing the measuring of body temperature. These terms can be confusing to the novice health care provider. All three terms refer to temperature scales used in both medicine and dentistry.

- The terms **Celsius** and **centigrade** can be used interchangeably in a medical or dental setting, but the term Celsius is the one preferred in most countries.
- The Celsius temperature scale is used in most countries except for the United States. Even in the United States, most of the scientific and engineering communities use the Celsius scale.
- In the United States, most Americans remain more accustomed to the **Fahrenheit** temperature scale, which is the scale that U.S. broadcasters use in weather forecasting. In the United States, the Fahrenheit scale is also used for measuring body temperatures in most dental settings.
- In Canada, due to its close relationship with the United States, kitchen devices, literature, and packaging may include both Fahrenheit and Celsius temperatures.
- In this textbook, temperature measurements are reported in both the Fahrenheit and Celsius scales. Ready Reference 7-2 in this textbook explains how to convert temperatures between the Fahrenheit and Celsius temperature scales.

# EQUIPMENT SELECTION

1. **Glass thermometers.** Glass thermometers provide an inexpensive means for obtaining an accurate oral temperature. Modern glass thermometers are mercury free and contain most commonly either galinstan or alcohol.
2. **Automatic temperature equipment.** Automatic temperature equipment—also called digital temperature equipment—ranges from the highly calibrated types used in hospital settings to less advanced equipment designed for home use.
   a. **Battery-powered devices.** The most common types of automatic temperature equipment found in the dental setting are battery-powered devices.
   b. **Precautions for use**
      1. All automatic equipment should be verified using a traditional fluid-filled thermometer.
      2. *An abnormally high or low temperature reading obtained with an automatic device should be verified by retaking the temperature in a few minutes using a traditional fluid-filled thermometer.*

### SECTION 2:

# Peak Procedures

## TEMPERATURE ASSESSMENT WITH A GLASS THERMOMETER

A common method of taking an oral temperature is with a **glass thermometer** (Fig. 7-1). Reading a glass thermometer accurately requires training, so it is helpful to practice the technique before attempting temperature assessment on a patient.

### PROCEDURE 7-1   READING A GLASS THERMOMETER

| Action |
| --- |
| **1.** Hold the stem—the end of the thermometer opposite the bulb—firmly between the thumb and index finger. |
| **2.** Hold the thermometer horizontally at eye level with the degree lines visible.<br><br>Roll the thermometer slowly back and forth between the fingers until the liquid column is visible. |
| **3.** The point where the liquid column ends marks the temperature.<br> • The division between the long lines is 1° Fahrenheit (F) or Celsius (C).<br> • Each small line in between the long lines equals 0.2° F or 0.1° C. |

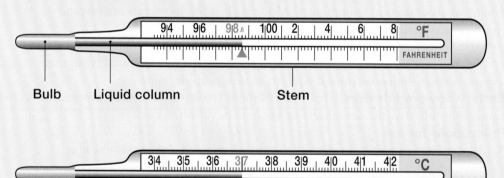

Bulb    Liquid column                    Stem

**Figure 7-1.   Note the location of the liquid column on the scale.** The top thermometer pictured has a Fahrenheit scale. The lower thermometer pictured has a Celsius scale.

## SHAKING DOWN THE LIQUID COLUMN PRIOR TO TAKING A READING

Liquid-in-glass thermometers can be used to measure body temperature because the liquid inside the thermometer expands when exposed to the warmth of the oral cavity. The liquid column should be at a level below 94° F (34.4° C) at the start of the temperature assessment procedure (Fig. 7-2). Shaking down the liquid column requires a rapid snapping motion with the wrist, so practicing this technique is helpful.

### PROCEDURE 7-2    SHAKING DOWN A GLASS THERMOMETER

| Action | Rationale |
|---|---|
| 1. Grasp the stem—the end of the thermometer opposite the bulb—firmly between the thumb and index finger. | • Grasping the bulb may warm the liquid and cause it to rise in the thermometer. |
| 2. Shake the thermometer several times using a quick downward snap of the wrist. Glass thermometers break easily, so shake the thermometer away from counters or objects. | • Moves liquid back into the bulb below 94° F or 34.4° C. |
| 3. Shake the thermometer until the liquid level is below 94° F or 34.4° C. | • If not shaken down, the liquid level could result in an inaccurate temperature reading. For example, the liquid level is at 100° F; however, the patient's temperature is 98°. Forgetting to shake down the liquid level results in an incorrect temperature finding of 100° F. |

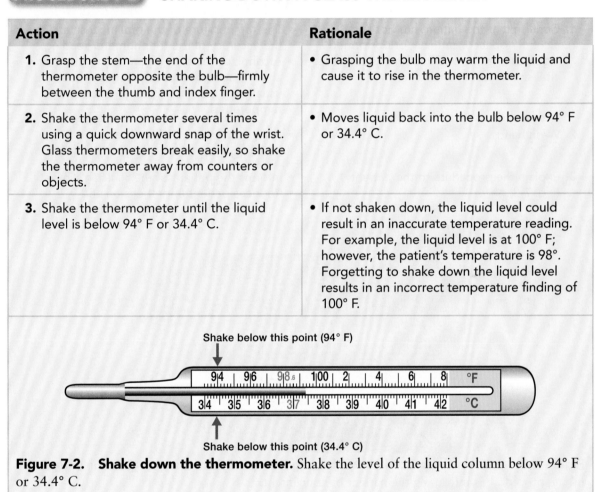

**Figure 7-2.    Shake down the thermometer.** Shake the level of the liquid column below 94° F or 34.4° C.

## PROCEDURE FOR TEMPERATURE TAKING

**PROCEDURE 7-3**    ASSESSING ORAL TEMPERATURE WITH A GLASS THERMOMETER

**Equipment**
Mercury-free glass fever thermometer, stored at room temperature
Tissue
Disposable thermometer sheath
Clock or watch with a second hand
Pen (or computer keyboard)

| Action | Rationale |
|---|---|
| 1. Confirm that the patient has not had alcohol, tobacco, caffeine, or performed vigorous exercise within 30 minutes of the vital signs assessment. | • The temperature of the oral mucosa affects the accuracy of the thermometer reading.<br>• Alcohol, caffeine, or vigorous exercise can alter pulse and respiration; these vital signs usually are assessed in conjunction with temperature. |
| 2. Wash hands. | • Reduces likelihood of transmitting microorganisms. |
| 3. Explain the procedure to the patient (Fig. 7-3). | • Informs the patient of the clinician's intent.<br>• Reduces patient apprehension and encourages patient cooperation. |

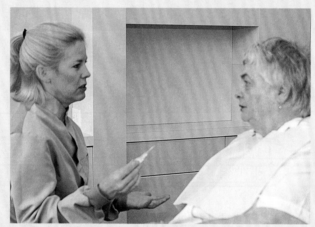

**Figure 7-3.   Explain the procedure to the patient.** An important step in the temperature-taking procedure is informing the patient of your intent.

(continued)

**PROCEDURE 7-3** ASSESSING ORAL TEMPERATURE WITH A GLASS THERMOMETER *(CONTINUED)*

| | |
|---|---|
| **4.** Shake the liquid level below 94° F (34.4° C). | • If not shaken down, the liquid level could result in an inaccurate temperature reading. |
| **5.** Place a disposable sheath on the thermometer (Fig. 7-4). | • Reduces likelihood of cross-contamination. |

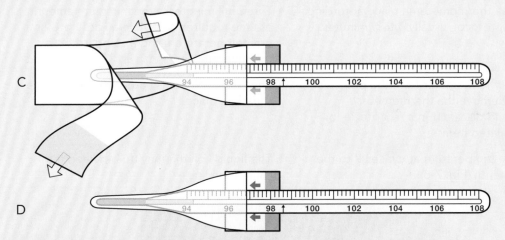

**Figure 7-4A–D. Cover thermometer with a sheath. A.** Gently insert the thermometer into the sheath with the bulb toward the closed end of the sheath. **B.** Tear paper covering at the dotted line. **C.** Hold the small paper section; pull on the larger section to remove it. **D.** The thermometer is now ready to use.

| | |
|---|---|
| **6.** Place the thermometer bulb under the patient's tongue along the gumline—on the right or left side—toward the back of the mouth (Fig. 7-5). <br> • Ask the patient to hold the thermometer in place. <br> • The patient should breathe through the nose, keeping the lips closed. <br> • Caution the patient against biting down on the thermometer. | • The heat from the lingual arteries under the tongue causes the liquid column to rise. Positioning the bulb in this manner places it in close contact with blood vessels lying near to the surface. <br> • Closing the lips helps to keep the bulb in position. <br> • Glass thermometers are easily broken. |

*(continued)*

**PROCEDURE 7-3**    ASSESSING ORAL TEMPERATURE WITH A GLASS
THERMOMETER *(CONTINUED)*

| Action | Rationale |
|---|---|

**Figure 7-5.   Position the bulb under the tongue.** Place the bulb to one side toward the back of the mouth.

| | |
|---|---|
| **7.** Leave the thermometer in place according to clinic protocol, usually 3 to 5 minutes. | • Three full minutes is the minimum amount of time required to obtain an accurate oral temperature using a standard glass thermometer. |
| **8.** Take the thermometer from the patient's mouth. Remove the thermometer sheath and discard it in a receptacle for contaminated items. | • The liquid column is harder to see with the sheath in place. |
| **9.** Read the temperature at eye level to the nearest tenth (Fig. 7-6). | • The liquid column may be between the calibration lines. |

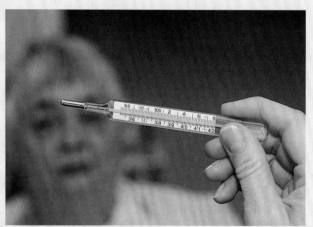

**Figure 7-6.   Read the temperature.** Hold the thermometer in a horizontal orientation and turn it slightly until the liquid column is visible. Note the location of the liquid column on the scale.

*(continued)*

**PROCEDURE 7-3** ASSESSING ORAL TEMPERATURE WITH A GLASS THERMOMETER *(CONTINUED)*

| | |
|---|---|
| **10.** After reading, place the thermometer on a barrier in a safe location. Wash and dry your hands. | • Deters transmission of microorganisms to the paper chart or computer keyboard. |
| Record today's date and time and the temperature reading in the chart or computer record. Discuss findings with the patient. | • Recording the reading promptly facilitates accurate documentation. |
| **11.** Upon completion of the vital signs assessment, report all abnormal findings to a clinical instructor or supervising clinician. | • If the temperature reading is elevated, elective dental treatment should be postponed and the patient is referred to a primary care physician for evaluation. |
| **12.** Wash the thermometer in lukewarm, soapy water. Rinse in cold water and dry.<br><br>Disinfect the thermometer, dry, and place in a storage container. | • Thermometer sheaths can easily tear, allowing oral microorganisms to contaminate the thermometer.<br>• Hot water can cause the liquid column to expand, potentially breaking the thermometer.<br>• Proper containers prevent contamination and protect the delicate thermometer. |

## SECTION 3:
# Ready References

---

**Note:** The Ready References in this book may be removed from the book by tearing along the perforated lines on each page. Laminating or placing these pages in plastic protector sheets will allow them to be disinfected for use in a clinical setting.

---

**READY REFERENCE 7-1**   **BODY TEMPERATURE RANGES**

**Normal Body Temperature**
- The normal adult oral temperature ranges from 96° to 99.6° F (35.5° to 37.5° C).
- The average normal oral temperature is 98.6° F (37° C), however, "normal" varies from person to person.

**Elevation in Body Temperature**
- Fever (pyrexia) is a reading *over* 99.5° F or 37.5° C.

---

**READY REFERENCE 7-2**   **BACK AND FORTH—FROM FAHRENHEIT TO CELSIUS**

| Fahrenheit | Celsius |
|------------|---------|
| 94.0 | 34.4 |
| 95.0 | 35.0 |
| 95.8 | 35.4 |
| 96.0 | 35.5 |
| 98.6 | 37.0 |
| 99.6 | 37.5 |
| 99.8 | 36.6 |
| 100.4 | 38.0 |
| 102.2 | 39.0 |
| 105.8 | 41.0 |

- **To convert Fahrenheit to Celsius:** subtract 32 from the Fahrenheit temperature and divide by 1.8.
- **To convert Celsius to Fahrenheit:** multiply the centigrade temperature by 1.8 and add 32.

**Key:**

Blue shading indicates a below-normal temperature reading.

Green shading indicates a normal temperature reading.

Red shading indicates an elevated temperature reading.

**READY REFERENCE 7-3**  VARIABLES THAT COMMONLY AFFECT TEMPERATURE

- Time of day—temperature varies throughout the day, usually being lowest in the early morning and rising by 0.5° to 1.0° F (0.3° to 0.6° C) in the early evening.
- Exercise—temperature may rise by 1° F (0.6° C) or more after strenuous physical exertion on a hot day.
- Age—the average normal oral temperature for persons over 70 years of age is 96.8° F (36.0° C).
- Environment—a cold or hot environment can alter temperature.
- Stress—a stressful situation can cause body temperature to rise.
- Hormones—a woman's body temperature typically varies by 1° F (0.6° C) or more throughout her menstrual cycle.
- Hot liquids—increase oral temperature for approximately 15 minutes.[1]
- Cold liquids—decrease oral temperature for approximately 15 minutes.[1]
- Smoking—increases oral temperature for approximately 30 minutes.[1]
- Tachypnea (rapid breathing)—decreases oral temperature.[2]
- Infection or inflammation—increases body temperature.

**READY REFERENCE 7-4**  IMPACT OF TEMPERATURE READING ON DENTAL TREATMENT

1. An elevated temperature reading should be reassessed to determine if the initial reading is accurate. Before taking a second temperature reading, reconfirm that the patient has not smoked or consumed a hot beverage for at least 30 minutes. An elevated temperature could also result from spending time in a hot environment, such as driving for an hour in a vehicle with no air-conditioning on a hot day.
2. Temperatures in excess of 101° F (38.3° C) usually indicate the presence of an active disease process.
3. In most cases, dental treatment is contraindicated for a patient with an elevated temperature. The patient should be referred to his or her primary care physician for evaluation.
4. If an elevated temperature is due to a dental infection, immediate dental treatment and antibiotic therapy may be indicated.
5. If the temperature is 104° F (40° C) or higher, a consultation with the patient's primary care physician is indicated.
6. A temperature of 105.8° F (41° C) constitutes a medical emergency. Contact emergency medical services (EMS) to request transport to the hospital.

## READY REFERENCE 7-5  INTERNET RESOURCES FOR INFORMATION GATHERING

**Assessing Body Temperature**

**http:www.webmd.com**
The **WebMD** website has information on body temperature, Fahrenheit and Celsius thermometers, what causes a fever, how to take an oral temperature, how low body temperature can be dangerous, and causes of inaccurate temperature readings.

**http://www.medem.com**
The **American Academy of Pediatrics** website has information for parents on taking a child's temperature.

**Replacing Mercury Thermometers**

**http://www.noharm.org**
The **Healthcare Without Harm** website has online information about mercury thermometers. Click on "Mercury" in the left-hand column.

**http://www.osha.gov/SLTC/etools/hospital/hazards/mercury/mercury.html**
The **U.S. Department of Labor Occupational Safety & Health Administration** website has information about the potential hazards of mercury, health effects of exposure to mercury, and treatment of mercury spills.

**http://www.stanford.edu/dept/EHS**
The **Stanford University** website has information about mercury dangers and replacing mercury thermometers.

## REFERENCES

1. Terndrup TE, Allegra JR, Kealy JA. A comparison of oral, rectal, and tympanic membrane-derived temperature changes after ingestion of liquids and smoking. *Am J Emerg Med.* 1989;7(2):150–154.
2. Tandberg D, Sklar D. Effect of tachypnea on the estimation of body temperature by an oral thermometer. *N Engl J Med.* 1983;308(16):945–946.

## SUGGESTED READINGS

Chester JG, Rudolph JL. Vital signs in older patients: age-related changes. *J Am Med Dir Assoc.* 2011;12(5):337–343.

Wager KA, Schaffner MJ, Foulois B, Swanson Kazley A, Parker C, Walo H. Comparison of the quality and timeliness of vital signs data using three different data-entry devices. *Comput Inform Nurs.* 2010;28(4):205–212.

Wilson LD. Cultural competency: beyond the vital signs. Delivering holistic care to African Americans. *Nurs Clin North Am.* 2011;46(2):219–232, vii.

**SECTION 4:**

# The Human Element

**BOX 7-2**  **Through the Eyes of a Student**

*As a student, I learned an important lesson about people at Mrs. B.'s initial appointment. Mrs. B. was 65 years old, and when she sat down in my chair, she started telling me about her career as a model. She had been a catalog model for a large department store in Toronto for over 40 years. Mrs. B. was dressed meticulously in a three-piece suit. Her shoes were polished and perfectly matched her suit. Her makeup and hair was perfect.*

*Then I began to ask her questions. When was her last dental visit? What was done at that visit? The patient answered my questions, and it became obvious that she had neglected her dental health. I took her vital signs. When she opened her mouth for the thermometer, I saw red swollen gingiva and heavy calculus deposits on her lower anterior teeth.*

*I talked to my instructor in the supply room where the patient would not be able to hear me. I told my instructor how surprised I was that Mrs. B. was neglecting her dental health when "she looked so PERFECT on the outside." My instructor helped me to understand that I should not make assumptions about a patient's values. And even more important, not to expect a patient to have the same health values that I have. My instructor helped me to see that my next task was to talk to my patient without being judgmental. I needed to learn what her values are at the present time. Of course, most important, I learned that I must see each patient as a unique individual with his or her own needs and values.*

*Anonymous graduate*
*George Brown College of Applied Arts and Technology*
*Toronto, Canada*

## ENGLISH-TO-SPANISH PHRASE LIST

**Table 7-1** ENGLISH-TO-SPANISH PHRASE LIST FOR TEMPERATURE ASSESSMENT

| Problem Word | Consider Using |
|---|---|
| I am going to take your temperature. | Voy a tomar su temperatura. |
| Do you have any questions? | ¿Usted tiene alguna pregunta? |
| Open your mouth, please. | Puede abrir la boca. |
| Please keep the thermometer in your mouth, under your tongue. | Por favor mantenga el termómetro bajo de la lengua. |
| Please hold the end of the thermometer with your fingers and keep your lips closed. | Por favor aguante el termómetro con los dedos y mantenga los labios cerrado. |
| Be careful not to bite the thermometer. | Tenga cuidado no morder el termómetro. |
| Please breathe through your nose. | Por favor respire por la nariz y no por la boca. |
| It will take 3 minutes to measure your temperature. | Se demora tres minutos para medir su temperatura. |
| Your temperature is normal. | Su temperatura esta normal. |
| You have a slight fever. | Usted tiene un poco de fiebre. |
| You have a high fever. | Usted tiene una fiebre alta. |
| We cannot treat you today because of your fever. | No podemos hacer ningún tratamiento dental hoy porque de la fiebre que usted tiene. |
| I am concerned about your very high fever; I want to call your doctor. Who is your doctor? | Su fiebre elevada me preocupa, y quiero llamar a su medico. ¿Me puede dar su nombre y numero de teléfono? |
| I recommend that you consult your family doctor about your fever. | Recomendo que usted consulte con su medico sobre la fiebre que tiene. |

## SECTION 5:
# Skill Check

**TECHNIQUE SKILL CHECKLIST:** ORAL TEMPERATURE PROCEDURE

Student: _____ Evaluator: _____

Date: _____

**DIRECTIONS FOR STUDENT CLINICIAN:** Use **Column S**; evaluate your skill level as **S** (satisfactory) or **U** (unsatisfactory).

**DIRECTIONS FOR EVALUATOR:** Use **Column E**. Indicate **S** (satisfactory) or **U** (unsatisfactory). In the optional grade percentage calculation, each **S** equals 1 point, and each **U** equals 0 points.

| CRITERIA | S | E |
|---|---|---|
| Seats the patient in a comfortable upright position. Confirms that the patient has not had a hot or cold beverage or smoked within the previous 30 minutes. | | |
| Washes hands. | | |
| Shakes down the thermometer so that the liquid level is below 94° F or 34.4° C. | | |
| Covers the thermometer with a disposable sheath. | | |
| Asks the patient to open the mouth. Positions the bulb under the tongue on one side toward the back of the mouth. | | |
| Maintains the thermometer in the patient's mouth for 3 to 5 minutes. | | |
| Removes the thermometer from the patient's mouth. Removes and discards the sheath in an appropriate receptacle. | | |
| Holds the thermometer in a horizontal position. Reads the position of the liquid column to the nearest tenth. | | |
| Places the thermometer on a barrier in a safe location. Washes and dries hands. Records today's date, time, and the oral temperature reading in the patient chart or computer record. | | |
| Upon completion of the vital signs assessment, washes the thermometer in lukewarm, soapy water. Rinses it in cold water and dries. Disinfects and dries thermometer; places it in an appropriate container. | | |

OPTIONAL GRADE PERCENTAGE CALCULATION

Each **S** equals 1 point, and each **U** equals 0 points. Using the **E** column, the sum of the "**S**"s _____ divided by the total points possible (10) equals the percentage grade _____.

## COMMUNICATION SKILL CHECKLIST: ROLE-PLAY FOR TEMPERATURE

Student: _____    Evaluator: _____

Date: _____

> **Roles:**
> - Student 1 = Plays the role of the patient.
> - Student 2 = Plays the role of the clinician.
> - Student 3 or instructor = Plays the role of the clinic instructor near the end of the role-play.

**DIRECTIONS FOR STUDENT CLINICIAN:** Use **Column S**; evaluate your skill level as **S** (satisfactory) or **U** (unsatisfactory).

**DIRECTIONS FOR EVALUATOR:** Use **Column E**. Indicate **S** (satisfactory) or **U** (unsatisfactory). In the optional grade percentage calculation, each **S** equals 1 point, and each **U** equals 0 points.

| CRITERIA | S | E |
|---|---|---|
| **Explains what is to be done in terminology that is easily understood by the patient.** | | |
| **Reports the temperature reading to the patient and explains if the reading is normal or outside the normal range and the significance of the finding.** | | |
| **Encourages patient questions before and after the temperature assessment procedure.** | | |
| **Answers the patient's questions fully and accurately.** | | |
| **Communicates with the patient at an appropriate level, avoiding dental/medical terminology or jargon.** | | |
| **Accurately communicates the findings to the clinical instructor. Discusses the implications for dental treatment using correct medical and dental terminology.** | | |

OPTIONAL GRADE PERCENTAGE CALCULATION

Each **S** equals 1 point, and each **U** equals 0 points. Using the **E** column, the sum of the "**S**"s _____ divided by the total points possible (6) equals the percentage grade _____.

MODULE

8

# Vital Signs: Pulse and Respiration

## MODULE OVERVIEW

This is the second of three modules covering the assessment of vital signs. Vital signs are key measurements that provide essential information about a person's state of health. Vital signs include a person's temperature, pulse, respiration, and blood pressure.

This module describes assessment of pulse and respiratory rates, including:

- The anatomy of the brachial and radial arteries
- Palpating the radial pulse point
- Determining the pulse rate
- Measuring respiratory rate

## MODULE OUTLINE

Technique Skill Checklist: Pulse and Respiration
Communication Skill Checklist: Role-Play for Pulse and
   Respiration

## OBJECTIVES

- Define the term *pulse* and describe the factors that may affect a person's pulse.
- Describe the different qualities of the pulse that a clinician should be aware of when taking a pulse.
- Demonstrate the correct technique for locating and assessing the radial pulse.
- Explain why the patient should not be told beforehand that the clinician is assessing his or her respiratory rate.
- Describe the factors that may affect a person's respirations.
- Explain the terms used to describe a person's respirations.
- Demonstrate the correct technique for assessing respiration.
- Provide information to the patient about the pulse and respiration assessment procedure and the readings that you obtain.
- Recognize findings that have implications in planning dental treatment.
- Provide appropriate referral to a physician when findings indicate the need for further evaluation.
- Compare findings in the fictitious patient cases A–E (Module 9) to the normal ranges for pulse and respiration.
- Demonstrate knowledge of the pulse and respiration assessment by applying concepts from this module to the fictitious patient cases A–E in Module 9, Vital Signs: Blood Pressure.

---

**Note to Course Instructor:** Fictitious patient cases A–E for the vital signs modules are located in Module 9, Vital Signs: Blood Pressure.

---

## SECTION 1:
# Peak Procedure For Pulse Assessment

## PULSE RATE

The **pulse rate** is an indication of an individual's heart rate. Pulse rate is measured by counting the number of rhythmic beats that can be felt over an artery in 1 minute. *The normal adult heart rate is between 60 and 100 beats per minute.* Rapid or slow pulse rates are not necessarily abnormal. Athletes tend to have slow pulses at rest. Increased pulse rates may be a normal response to stress, exercise, or pain. Ready Reference 8-1 outlines normal pulse rates at various ages and Ready Reference 8-2 shows some factors that can affect the pulse rate. Ready References 8-3, 8-4, and 8-5 provide details of pulse patterns, pulse amplitude, and pulse pressure.

## PULSE POINTS

As the heart beats and forces blood through the body, a throbbing sensation—the **pulse**—can be felt by putting the fingers over one of the arteries that are close to the surface of the skin. **Pulse points** are the sites on the surface of the body where rhythmic beats of an artery can be easily felt. In the dental setting, the most commonly used pulse point is over the radial artery in the wrist. Before practicing the techniques for assessing the pulse rate and blood pressure, it is helpful to locate and palpate the brachial and radial pulse points on the underside of the arm (Fig. 8-1).

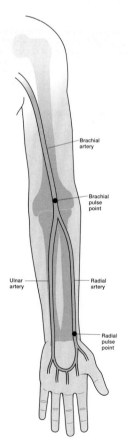

**Figure 8-1.   The anatomy of the brachial and radial arteries of the arm.**
- The **brachial artery** is the main artery of the upper arm; it divides into the radial and ulnar arteries at the elbow. The brachial artery is used when taking blood pressure.
- The **radial artery** is a branch of the brachial artery beginning below the elbow and extending down the forearm on the **thumb side** of the wrist and into the hand.

## ASSESSING PULSE RATE

**PROCEDURE 8-1** PRACTICE LOCATING THE RADIAL ARTERY

| Action | Rationale |
|---|---|
| **1.** Sit or stand facing the patient. Position the patient's arm in a palm-up position with his or her arm resting comfortably on a countertop or chair armrest. | • This position makes it easy to locate the radial pulse point. |
| **2.** Use the finger pads of your index, middle, and ring fingers to locate the radial artery on the wrist at the base of the thumb (Fig. 8-2).<br><br>Feel the throbbing pulse by pressing lightly in the shallow groove at the base of the thumb. | • The sensitive finger pads can feel the pulsation of the artery.<br>• The thumb has a pulse of its own that might be confused with the patient's pulse.<br>• Too much pressure will make it difficult to detect the pulsations under your fingers. |

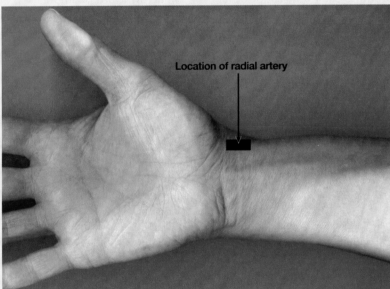

Location of radial artery

**Figure 8-2.** **Location of the radial artery on the thumb side of the wrist.**

## PROCEDURE 8-2   DETERMINING PULSE RATE

**Equipment**
Clock or watch with second hand or digital readout

| Action | Rationale |
|---|---|
| **1.** It takes time to obtain an accurate oral temperature using a glass thermometer. For this reason, pulse, respiration, and blood pressure are assessed during the time needed to determine the oral temperature. | • Assessing the other vital signs while the thermometer registers the patient's temperature makes efficient use of appointment time. |
| **2.** Explain the pulse assessment procedure to the patient. | • Informs the patient of the clinician's intent.<br>• Reduces patient apprehension and encourages cooperation. |
| **3.** The patient's arm should be resting comfortably on the chair armrest or other support, such as a countertop (Fig. 8-3). | • There is no reason for the patient's arm to be in an awkward position. |

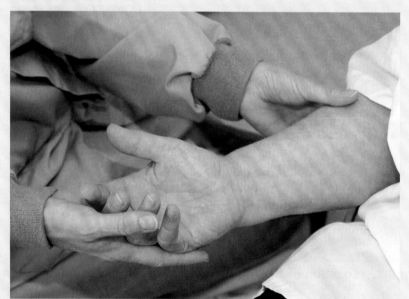

**Figure 8-3.   Arm position.** Position the patient's arm in a comfortable position.

| | |
|---|---|
| **4.** Sit or stand facing the patient. Grasp the patient's wrist with the fingers of your free (non–watch-bearing) hand. | • This position is comfortable for the patient and convenient for the clinician. |

*(continued)*

**PROCEDURE 8-2**   **DETERMINING PULSE RATE** *(CONTINUED)*

| Action | Rationale |
|---|---|
| **5.** Using the finger pads of your first three fingers, locate the radial pulse point on the thumb side of the patient's wrist (Fig. 8-4).<br><br>Apply only enough pressure so that the radial artery can be distinctly felt. | • The thumb is never used to assess the pulse. The thumb has a pulse; this pulse could be confused with the patient's pulse.<br>• Moderate pressure facilitates palpation of the beats. The pulse is imperceptible with too little pressure, whereas too much pressure obscures the pulse. |

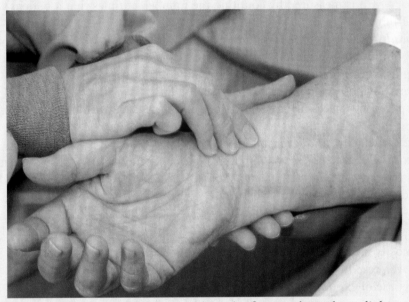

**Figure 8-4. Locate the radial artery.** Place the fingers along the radial artery.

| | |
|---|---|
| **6.** Look at a watch or clock and wait until the second hand gets to the "12" or "6." When the second hand reaches the "12" or "6," begin counting the pulse beats.<br><br>Count for a minimum of 30 seconds. Multiply this number by 2 to calculate the pulse rate for 1 minute.<br>If the pulse is irregular in any way or if your patient has a pacemaker, count the beats for 1 minute. | • Starting with the second hand at the "12" or "6" makes it easy to determine when 30 seconds has passed.<br><br>• Sufficient time is needed to assess the rate and characteristics of the pulse.<br>• With an irregular pulse, the beats counted in a 30-second period may not represent the overall rate. The longer you measure, the more these variations are averaged out. |
| **7.** Make a mental note of the pulse rate and without letting go of the patient's wrist, begin to observe the patient's breathing.<br><br>Assessment of the respiration should begin immediately after taking the patient's pulse. | • The patient may alter the rate of respirations if aware that breathing is being monitored. |

## SECTION 2:
# Peak Procedure For Assessing Respiration

### RESPIRATORY RATE

Respiration is the process that brings oxygen into the body and removes carbon dioxide. With each normal breath, a person inhales 500 ml of air and exhales the same amount. Ready References 8-8 and 8-9 outline terms used when evaluating the respiratory rate and types of respiration.

- The **respiratory rate** is measured by counting the number of times that a patient's chest rises in 1 minute.
- *The normal adult respiratory rate is between 14 and 20 breaths per minute.* Ready Reference 8-6 outlines normal respiration rates at various ages. Young children use their diaphragms when breathing. For this reason, the respiratory rate of a young child is measured by observing the abdomen rise and fall.
- Observing respiration is necessary to detect signs of interference with the breathing process.
- Excitement, exercise, pain, and fever increase respiratory rate.
- Rapid respiration is characteristic of lung diseases such as emphysema. Heart disease also increases the rate of respiration, as do some drugs. Ready Reference 8-7 provides a list of factors that can affect respiration rate.

### CONTROL OF RESPIRATION

Respiration is mostly unconscious; people breathe without thinking about it. Unlike pulse rate, however, respiration is easily brought under voluntary control. Breath-holding, panting, use of expiratory air to speak, singing, or sighing at will are all examples of this **voluntary control**. Just thinking about respiration causes most individuals to alter their breathing rate. Telling someone to "breathe normally" almost certainly will cause that person to begin to breathe more slowly or rapidly. For this reason, the respiratory rate should be measured immediately after taking a pulse. *Counting the respirations while appearing to count the pulse helps to keep the patient from becoming conscious of his or her breathing and possibly altering the usual rate.*

### ASSESSING RESPIRATION

**PROCEDURE 8-3** **COUNT YOUR OWN RESPIRATORY RATE**

| Action | Rationale |
|---|---|
| 1. Place a hand on your own chest and feel your chest rise. One breath in and out is counted as one respiration. | • One inspiration and expiration comprises one respiration. |
| 2. Count the number of times your chest rises for 30 seconds and multiply by 2 to obtain your respiratory rate. | • Sufficient time is needed to observe the breathing rate and characteristics. |
| 3. Note if your breathing is irregular. Listen for unusual breath sounds. Note how much effort is needed for you to breathe. Normal breathing should be quiet and effortless. | • Abnormal respirations may be irregular, rapid, labored, weak, or noisy. |

**PROCEDURE 8-4** **ASSESSING THE RESPIRATORY RATE**

**Equipment:** Clock or watch with second hand or digital readout
Pen (or computer keyboard)

| Action | Rationale |
|---|---|
| **1.** This assessment is best done immediately after taking the patient's pulse. Do not announce that you are measuring the respirations. | • Respiratory rate is under voluntary control. If the patient knows that you are counting the breaths, he or she may change breathing pattern. |
| **2.** After determining the pulse rate, keep your fingers resting on the patient's wrist and begin to assess the patient's respiration (Fig. 8-5).<br><br>Observe respirations inconspicuously; use peripheral vision to observe the chest rise and fall. | • The patient will assume that you are still counting the pulse rate.<br><br>• Breathing rate can be controlled voluntarily. |
| **3.** Look at a watch or clock and wait until the second hand gets to the "12" or "6." When the second hand reaches the "12" or "6," use your peripheral vision to watch the chest and begin counting each rise of the chest as one breath.<br><br>Count the number of breaths for a minimum of 30 seconds. In adults with irregular rates, count for 1 full minute. | • Sufficient time is needed to observe the breathing rate and characteristics. |

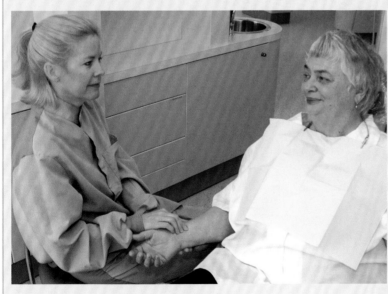

**Figure 8-5. Begin assessment of respiration.** With your fingers still in place after counting the pulse rate, observe the patient's respirations.

*(continued)*

**PROCEDURE 8-4**   **ASSESSING THE RESPIRATORY RATE** *(CONTINUED)*

| Action | Rationale |
|---|---|
| **4.** Pay attention to the depth and rhythm of the patient's respirations by watching the chest rise and fall.<br>• Normal breathing is easy, quiet, and regular.<br>• Abnormal respirations may be irregular, rapid, labored, weak, or noisy.<br>• If breathing is abnormal in any way, count the respirations for at least 1 full minute. | • Increased time allows detection of abnormal characteristics. |
| **5.** Record the pulse and respiratory rates in the patient chart or computer record.<br><br>Discuss the findings with the patient.<br><br>Upon completion of the vital signs assessment, report all abnormal findings to a clinical instructor or supervising clinician. | • Recording findings immediately in the chart facilitates accurate documentation and reporting.<br>• Elective dental treatment may be postponed due to abnormal findings. For example, a patient with labored breathing should be referred to his or her physician for evaluation. |

## SECTION 3:
# Ready References

> **NOTE:** The Ready References in this book may be removed from the book by tearing along the perforated lines on each page. Laminating or placing these pages in plastic protector sheets will allow them to be disinfected for use in a clinical setting.

**READY REFERENCE 8-1** NORMAL PULSE RATES PER MINUTE AT VARIOUS AGES

| Age | Approximate Range | Approximate Average |
|---|---|---|
| 2–6 years | 75–120 | 100 |
| 6–12 years | 75–110 | 95 |
| Adolescent to adult | 60–100 | 80 |

**READY REFERENCE 8-2** FACTORS AFFECTING PULSE RATE

- ✓ Age
- ✓ Medications
- ✓ Stress
- ✓ Exercise

**READY REFERENCE 8-3** PULSE PATTERNS

| |
|---|
| **Regular**—evenly spaced beats; may vary slightly with respiration. |
| **Regularly irregular**—regular pattern overall with "skipped" beats. |
| **Irregularly irregular**—no real pattern, difficult to measure accurately. |
| **Normal amplitude**—full, strong pulse that is easily felt. |
| **Abnormal amplitude**—weak pulse that is not easily felt. |

## READY REFERENCE 8-4    PULSE AMPLITUDE ASSESSMENT

To assess the amplitude of a pulse, use a numerical scale to characterize the strength.

**0**—absent pulse, not palpable

**+1**—weak or thready pulse, hard to feel; the beat is easily eliminated by slight finger pressure

**+2**—normal pulse, easily felt; the beat is eliminated by forceful finger pressure

**+3**—bounding, forceful pulse that is readily felt; the beat is not easily eliminated by pressure from the fingers

## READY REFERENCE 8-5    PULSE PRESSURE

| | |
|---|---|
| **Normal**<br>The pulse pressure is smooth (Fig. 8-6A–C). | A |
| **Weak**<br>The pulse pressure is diminished; the pulse feels weak and small. | B |
| **Bounding**<br>The pulse pressure is increased and the pulse feels strong and bouncing. | C |

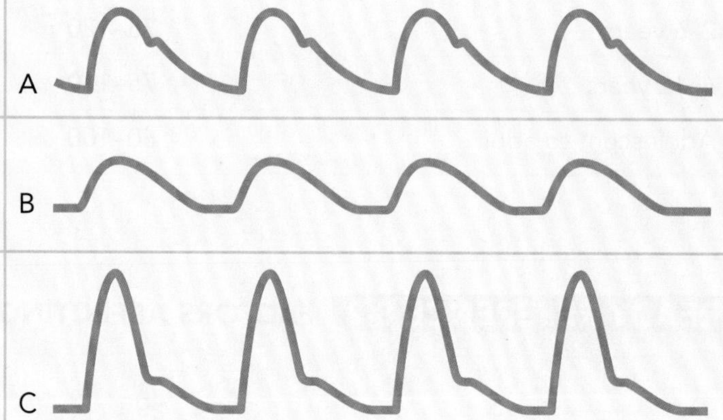

Figure 8-6.    **A.** Normal pulse. **B.** Weak pulse. **C.** Bounding pulse.

## READY REFERENCE 8-6    NORMAL RESPIRATORY RATES PER MINUTE AT VARIOUS AGES

| Age | Approximate Range |
|---|---|
| Preschooler (3–6 years) | 22–34 |
| School age (6–12 years) | 18–30 |
| Adolescent (12–18 years) | 12–16 |
| Adult | 14–20 |

## READY REFERENCE 8-7 FACTORS AFFECTING RESPIRATION RATE

| | |
|---|---|
| ✓ Age | ✓ Altitude |
| ✓ Medications | ✓ Gender |
| ✓ Stress | ✓ Body position |
| ✓ Exercise | ✓ Fever |

## READY REFERENCE 8-8 EVALUATION OF RESPIRATION

**Rhythm**—regularity of respirations

**Ease**—easy, labored, or painful?

**Depth**—deep or shallow?

**Noise**—slight, wheezing, gurgling?

**Abnormal odor**—fruity odor, alcohol on breath?

## READY REFERENCE 8-9 TYPES OF RESPIRATION

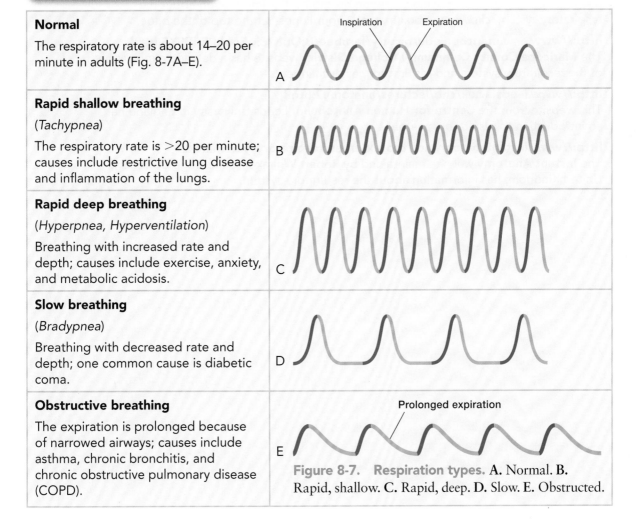

**Normal**

The respiratory rate is about 14–20 per minute in adults (Fig. 8-7A–E).

**Rapid shallow breathing**

(*Tachypnea*)

The respiratory rate is >20 per minute; causes include restrictive lung disease and inflammation of the lungs.

**Rapid deep breathing**

(*Hyperpnea, Hyperventilation*)

Breathing with increased rate and depth; causes include exercise, anxiety, and metabolic acidosis.

**Slow breathing**

(*Bradypnea*)

Breathing with decreased rate and depth; one common cause is diabetic coma.

**Obstructive breathing**

The expiration is prolonged because of narrowed airways; causes include asthma, chronic bronchitis, and chronic obstructive pulmonary disease (COPD).

**Figure 8-7. Respiration types. A.** Normal. **B.** Rapid, shallow. **C.** Rapid, deep. **D.** Slow. **E.** Obstructed.

**READY REFERENCE 8-10**   INTERNET RESOURCES: PULSE AND RESPIRATION

### Pulse

**http://www.bartleby.com/107/**
**Bartleby Great Books Online** website has Gray's Anatomy available for online searches. Enter the anatomical structure that you would like to view in the "Search" box and click on the Go button. Suggested searches: radial artery, brachial artery, and lungs.

**http://www.time-to-run.com/beginners/pulse.htm**
The **Time-To-Run** website has instructions on how to take and record your pulse rate as part of an exercise regimen (running).

**http://my.webmd.com/hw/heart_disease/hw233473.asp**
This **Web MD Health** website has an excellent explanation of pulse measurement.

**http://www.heart.org/HEARTORG/**
The **American Heart Association** website has information such as resting heart rate and how cigarette smoking affects the heart. Enter a topic of interest in the "Search" box.

### Respiration

**http://www.lungusa.org**
The website of the **American Lung Association** has a wealth of information on respiratory diseases and smoking cessation programs. For information about the respiratory system, click on the box marked "Your Lungs" at the top of the page.

**http://www.emc.maricopa.edu/faculty/farabee/BIOBK/BioBookRESPSYS.html**
The **Maricopa County Community College District** website has a detailed explanation of the respiratory system and respiratory gas exchange.

**http://www.leeds.ac.uk/chb/lectures/anatomy7.html**
This website from the **Centre for Human Anatomy** of Leeds University in England has an introduction to respiratory anatomy.

**http://www.instantanatomy.net/thorax/areas/respiratorysystem.html**
The **Instant Anatomy** website maintained by Robert Whitaker, Cambridge University, United Kingdom, has information about the respiratory system.

## SUGGESTED READINGS

Cretikos MA, Bellomo R, Hillman K, Chen J, Finfer S, Flabouris A. Respiratory rate: the neglected vital sign. *Med J Aust.* 2008;188(11):657–659.

Hatlestad D. The anatomy and physiology of respiration. *Emerg Med Serv.* 2002;31(1): 56–65; quiz 80.

Jarvis CM. Vital signs: how to take them more accurately and understand them more fully. *Nursing.* 1976;6(4):31–37.

Krost WS, Mistovich JJ, Limmer DD. Beyond the basics: pediatric assessment and management. *EMS Mag.* 2008;37(10):91–98; quiz 100–101.

Limmer DD, Mistovich JJ, Krost WS. Beyond the basics: putting the vital back in vital signs. *EMS Mag.* 2008;37(9):71–75; quiz 76–77.

Mistovich JJ, Krost WS, Limmer DD. Beyond the basics: interpreting vital signs. *Emerg Med Serv.* 2006;35(12):194–199; quiz 200–201.

Royal College of Nursing. *Standards for Assessing, Measuring and Monitoring Vital Signs in Infants, Children and Young People.* London, United Kingdom: Royal College of Nursing; 2007. www.rcn.org.uk/__data/assets/pdf_file/0004/114484/003196.pdf. Accessed August 15, 2011.

Scharff K. Vital signs revisited. What you may be missing. *Nursing.* 1991;21(6):59.

Streger MR. Taking accurate vital signs. *Emerg Med Serv.* 2000;29(8):63.

## SECTION 4:
# The Human Element

---

## BOX 8-1     Through the Eyes of a Student

*It was my first appointment with Mr. J. As I prepared for his appointment, I noted that he was 70 years of age and had a history of congestive heart failure. When I assessed Mr. J.'s respiration, he seemed breathless and to be having some difficulty in breathing. He seemed to be tired even though this was a morning appointment. I reclined the dental chair so that he could rest while I took his blood pressure. Once he was in a supine position, Mr. J. seemed to have even more difficulty breathing and he asked to sit upright again.*

*I wanted to get on with the appointment because I was worried about completing all my clinic requirements. Something in the back of my mind, however, kept telling me that I should be concerned about Mr. J.'s labored breathing. I decided to report my observations to my clinic instructor.*

*My instructor called an ambulance and the paramedics transported Mr. J. to the hospital. Later I received a telephone call from Mrs. J. telling me that her husband was hospitalized and saying that my actions might have saved his life. I learned that day that even seemly small things like a patient's respiratory rate could be significant. Now, I take the vital signs assessment procedures more seriously and never rush through them.*

*George, student*
*Tallahassee Community College*

**Table 8-1**    ENGLISH-TO-SPANISH PHRASE LIST

| | |
|---|---|
| I am going to take your pulse. | Voy a tomar su pulso. |
| Do you have any questions? | ¿Tiene alguna pregunta? |
| Just relax; this will only take a few minutes. | Cálmese; esto se demora unos minutos. |
| Please breathe through your nose and not through your mouth. | Por favor respire por la nariz, y no por la boca. |
| Your pulse rate is normal. | Su pulso es normal. |
| Your pulse rate is a little fast. | Su pulso es un poco rápido. |
| Do you know what your pulse rate normally is? | ¿Usted sabe cual es su pulso normal? |
| I am concerned about your rapid pulse. I want to call your doctor. Who is your doctor? | Estoy preocupada por su rápido pulso, y quiero llamar a su doctor. ¿Quién es su doctor? |
| Your respiratory rate is normal. | La respiración es normal. |
| Your pulse and respiration are normal. | Su pulso y respiración están normal. |
| It seems to be difficult for you to breathe. Is your breathing normally like this? | Parece que usted tiene un poco de dificultad respirando. ¿Esto es normal para usted? |
| Are you nervous about the dental treatment today? | ¿Esta nervioso/nerviosa sobre su tratamiento dental hoy? |
| I am concerned about your breathing. I want to call your doctor. Who is your doctor? | Estoy preocupado sobre su ritmo de respiración, y quiero llamar a su doctor. ¿Quién es su doctor? |

**NOTE:** The **Practical Focus—Fictitious Patient Cases Section** for all of the vital signs modules is located in Module 9, Vital Signs: Blood Pressure.

## SECTION 5:
# Skill Check

### TECHNIQUE SKILL CHECKLIST: PULSE AND RESPIRATION

Student: _____   Evaluator: _____

Date: _____

**DIRECTIONS FOR STUDENT CLINICIAN:** Using **Column S**, evaluate your skill level as **S** (satisfactory) or **U** (unsatisfactory).

**DIRECTIONS FOR EVALUATOR:** Use **Column E**. Indicate **S** (satisfactory) or **U** (unsatisfactory). In the optional grade percentage calculation, each **S** equals 1 point, and each **U** equals 0 points.

| CRITERIA | S | E |
|---|---|---|
| Positions the patient with the arm resting comfortably on the armrest or other support. | | |
| Faces the patient. Grasps the patient's wrist with the fingers of the free (non–watch-bearing) hand. | | |
| Using the finger pads, locates the radial pulse point on the thumb side of the patient's wrist. Applies only enough pressure so that the radial artery can be distinctly felt. | | |
| Notes whether the pulse is regular or irregular. | | |
| Using a watch with a second hand, counts the beats for a minimum of 30 seconds if the pulse is regular. Counts the pulse for 1 minute if the pulse is irregular. Calculates the pulse rate. | | |
| Makes a mental note of the pulse rate and without letting go of the patient's wrist, begins to observe the patient's breathing. Does not inform the patient that the respirations are being assessed. | | |
| When one complete cycle of inspiration and expiration has been observed, looks at watch in preparation for determining the respiratory rate. Counts the number of breaths for a minimum of 30 seconds. If breathing is abnormal in any way, counts the respirations for 1 minute. Calculates the respiratory rate. | | |
| Records today's date, time, and the pulse and respiratory rates in the patient chart or computer record. | | |
| Reports pulse rate within +/− 2 beats of the evaluator's rate. | | |
| Reports respiratory rate within +/− 2 breaths of the evaluator's rate. | | |

OPTIONAL GRADE PERCENTAGE CALCULATION

Each **S** equals 1 point, and each **U** equals 0 points. Using the **E** column, the sum of the "**S**"s _____ divided by the total points possible (10) equals the percentage grade _____.

## COMMUNICATION SKILL CHECKLIST:  ROLE-PLAY FOR PULSE AND RESPIRATION

Student: _____    Evaluator: _____

Date: _____

---

**Roles:**

- Student 1 = Plays the role of the patient.
- Student 2 = Plays the role of the clinician.
- Student 3 or instructor = Plays the role of the clinic instructor near the end of the role-play.

---

**DIRECTIONS FOR STUDENT CLINICIAN:** Use **Column S**; evaluate your skill level as **S** (satisfactory) or **U** (unsatisfactory).

**DIRECTIONS FOR EVALUATOR:** Use **Column E**. Indicate **S** (satisfactory) or **U** (unsatisfactory). In the optional grade percentage calculation, each **S** equals 1 point and each **U** equals 0 points.

| CRITERIA | S | E |
|---|---|---|
| **Explains what is to be done at the start of the pulse assessment procedure.** | | |
| **At the conclusion of the pulse assessment, does not announce that respiration will be assessed next.** | | |
| **Upon completion of the procedures, reports the pulse and respiration findings to the patient and explains if the readings are normal or outside the normal range and the significance of these findings.** | | |
| **Encourages patient questions before and after the assessment procedure.** | | |
| **Answers the patient's questions fully and accurately.** | | |
| **Communicates with the patient at an appropriate level and avoids dental/medical terminology or jargon.** | | |
| **Accurately communicates the findings to the clinical instructor. Discusses the implications for dental treatment using correct medical and dental terminology.** | | |

OPTIONAL GRADE PERCENTAGE CALCULATION

Each **S** equals 1 point, and each **U** equals 0 points. Using the **E** column, the sum of the "**S**"s _____ divided by the total points possible (7) equals the percentage grade _____.

# MODULE 9

# Vital Signs: Blood Pressure

## MODULE OVERVIEW

This is the third of three modules on vital signs assessment. Vital signs are a person's temperature, pulse, respiration, and blood pressure. In addition to these standard vital signs, tobacco use has been suggested as the fifth vital sign. Tobacco use—smoking cigarettes, cigars, or pipes—is a contributing factor in many medical conditions and, in addition, increases the risk of periodontal disease.

This module describes measurement of blood pressure, including:

- Equipment for blood pressure determination
- Sounds heard during blood pressure measurement
- Critical technique elements
- Peak procedure for blood pressure assessment

## MODULE OUTLINE

## OBJECTIVES

- Define the term *blood pressure* and describe factors that may affect a person's blood pressure.
- Define *systolic* and *diastolic blood pressure* and give their normal values.
- Explain how a sphygmomanometer works and demonstrate how to use this tool to measure blood pressure.
- Diagram the parts of the stethoscope and explain how this tool is used.
- Given a selection of blood pressure cuffs, identify the five basic cuff sizes.
- Identify the bladder width and length of a cuff.
- Check to see if the length, width, and center of the bladder are correctly marked; if not, correctly mark the cuff.
- Explain why the blood pressure cuff is kept at heart level while measuring blood pressure.
- List and describe the Korotkoff sounds that are heard while taking a person's blood pressure.
- Define and discuss the significance of the auscultatory gap.
- Correctly position the patient for blood pressure assessment.
- Locate and palpate the brachial pulse point in the antecubital fossa.
- Demonstrate correct technique for accurately assessing the blood pressure.
- Provide information to the patient about the blood pressure assessment procedure and the readings that you obtain.
- Describe blood pressure findings that have implications in planning dental treatment.
- Provide appropriate referral to a physician when findings indicate the need for further evaluation.
- Compare findings for the fictitious patient cases A–E to the normal range for blood pressure.
- Demonstrate knowledge of blood pressure assessment by applying concepts from this module to the fictitious patient cases A–E found in Section 8.

**SECTION 1:**

# Blood Pressure Assessment in the Dental Setting

The National Heart, Lung, and Blood Institute (NHLBI) estimates that 65 million Americans have high blood pressure (hypertension). Of those 65 million, nearly 20 million are not aware they have the condition. There is a high prevalence of undiagnosed hypertension and prehypertension.[1] As the population ages, the prevalence of hypertension will increase even further unless broad-based measures are implemented for blood pressure screening. Dental health care providers can play an important role in improving the current levels of detection for hypertension by implementing routine blood pressure screening[1] (Boxes 9-1 and 9-2).

---

**BOX 9-1  Standard of Care for Blood Pressure Assessment**

- The American Dental Association (ADA) recommends that blood pressure assessment should be a routine part of the initial appointment for all new dental patients—including children—as a screening tool for undiagnosed high blood pressure.[2]
- In addition, the ADA suggests that a blood pressure assessment should be performed routinely at continuing care appointments (3-, 4-, 6-, or 12-month recall appointments).
- The ADA, Academy of Pediatrics, and American Heart Association (AHA) recommend that blood pressure measurements be taken at all pediatric health care visits—including dental appointments—at 3 to 18 years of age.[3]

---

1. **Blood Pressure Overview.** Arterial **blood pressure** is the pressure exerted against the blood vessel walls as blood flows through them. Every time the heart contracts, it forces 6 qt of blood beyond the torso and out to the head, hands, and feet. With each contraction, the blood not only pushes through the vessels but also presses outward against the vessel walls.
   a. The highest pressure occurs when blood is propelled through the arteries by the contraction of the heart. The pressure created by the blood as it presses through and against the vessel walls is known as the **systolic pressure**.
   b. When the heart relaxes between beats, the pressure exerted on the vessels lessens, but only to a point. That lower pressure is known as the **diastolic pressure**.
   c. Blood pressure is one clue to the health of the heart and blood vessels; therefore, its measurement is an important part of the patient assessment.
   d. Although both pressures are clinically significant, the latest evidence from research indicates the systolic blood pressure to be the more important of the two in the management of high blood pressure.[4–6]
2. **Hypertension and Hypotension**
   a. Blood pressure measurements indicate if a person is **hypertensive** (has abnormally high blood pressure) or **hypotensive** (has abnormally low blood pressure).
   b. High blood pressure—**hypertension**—is blood pressure that stays at or above 140/90 mm Hg.
   c. Blood pressure increases when larger blood vessels begin to lose their elasticity and the smaller vessels start to constrict, causing the heart to try to pump the same volume of blood through vessels with a smaller internal diameter.

3. **Symptoms, Diagnosis, and Treatment of Hypertension**
   a. Hypertension usually has no symptoms (is **asymptomatic**). For this reason, high blood pressure is often called the "**silent killer**."
   b. The only way for an individual to know if he or she has hypertension is to have a blood pressure screening.
   c. Hypertension is easy and painless to detect in a few minutes using a blood pressure cuff and a stethoscope.
4. **Complications of Uncontrolled Hypertension**
   a. Uncontrolled high blood pressure is a serious condition that can lead to stroke, heart attack, heart failure, or kidney failure.
   b. In pregnant women, hypertension can lead to seizures or death as well as premature births or stillbirths.
5. **Treatment of Hypertension and Patient Compliance with Treatment**
   a. Simple treatments including weight loss, lifestyle changes, and medication are effective in lowering blood pressure.
   b. Blood pressure medications are very effective at lowering blood pressure; however, many of the medications have mild side effects such as fatigue and dry cough.
   c. *For the drugs to work, patients must actually take them. Unfortunately, it is estimated that within a year of receiving a prescription, 50% of patients stop taking their blood pressure medication.*

---

## BOX 9-2 High Blood Pressure Facts

**Hypertension in Adults**
According to the AHA, nearly one in three U.S. adults has high blood pressure.

- *Because there are no symptoms from high blood pressure, nearly one-third of the people with this condition do not know they have it.*
- 69% of Americans who have a first heart attack have blood pressure over 140/90 mm Hg.
- 77% of Americans treated for a first stroke have blood pressure over 140/90 mm Hg.
- 74% of Americans with congestive heart failure have blood pressure over 140/90 mm Hg.
- More men than women have high blood pressure.
- Pregnant women are a high-risk group for high blood pressure whether they had hypertension before becoming pregnant or not.

**Hypertension in Children and Adolescents**

- *The newest at-risk populations for high blood pressure are children and adolescents. As many as 50 million Americans aged 6 years and older have high blood pressure.*
- Epidemiologic studies indicate that 2%–4% of the pediatric population and between 15% and 30% of obese children have hypertension,[7-11] which can lead to cardiovascular disease, type 2 diabetes mellitus, and fatty liver disease.[3,12,13,14]
- Blood pressure levels for children and adolescents have risen substantially from 1988 to 2000, in part linked to an increase in prevalence of overweight and obesity.[15]
- The ADA, Academy of Pediatrics, and AHA recommend that children over 3 years of age who are seen in health care settings should have their blood pressure measured at least once during every health care episode.[3,14]

**SECTION 2:**
# Equipment for Blood Pressure Measurement

The gold standard for clinical blood pressure measurement is the **auscultatory method,** where a trained health care provider uses a **sphygmomanometer** and a **stethoscope** to *listen* for arterial sounds in the brachial artery. This is called the "auscultatory method" because the detection of sound is called "auscultation."

## THE SPHYGMOMANOMETER

A **sphygmomanometer** (sss-fig-mo-ma-*nom*-eter) consists of (1) a cuff with an inflatable bladder, (2) a hand bulb with a valve used to inflate and deflate the bladder, and (3) a pressure gauge. A sphygmomanometer is illustrated in Figure 9-1. Figure 9-2 shows different sizes of blood pressure cuffs.

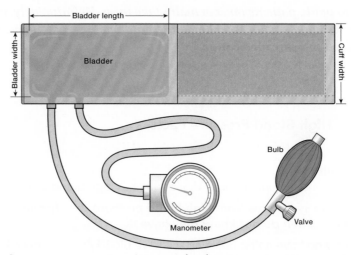

**Figure 9-1.   The sphygmomanometer.** A manual sphygmomanometer consists of a **cuff**—an airtight, flat, inflatable bladder (pouch) covered by a cloth sheath; a **bulb**, which is squeezed to fill the cuff with air; and a **manometer**—a gauge that measures the air pressure in millimeters.

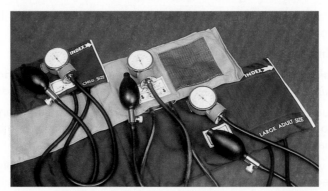

**Figure 9-2.   Blood pressure cuffs in three sizes.** Blood pressure cuffs are available in a wide range of sizes. The correct size is selected in reference to the size of the upper arm midway between the point of the shoulder and the elbow. (Used with permission from Taylor CR, Lillis C, LeMone P, et al. *Fundamentals of Nursing: The Art and Science of Nursing Care.* 7th ed. Philadelphia, PA: Lippincott Williams & Wilkins; 2011.)

## THE MANOMETER PRESSURE GAUGE

A **manometer** is the device that measures the air pressure present in the inflatable pouch. The two traditional types of manometers are aneroid gauges and mercury column gauges (Fig. 9-3).

1. **Aneroid manometers** use a round dial-type gauge to indicate the pressure reading.
   a. The aneroid gauge is the most commonly used type of manometer in a dental office setting.
   b. Aneroid devices are believed to be less accurate than mercury columns because they are so difficult to keep in calibration.[16]
      1. Aneroid manometers require regular checks for common defects such as nonzeroed gauges, cracked faceplates, or defective rubber tubing.[17]
      2. These gauges should be validated for accuracy against a standard mercury manometer at 6-month intervals.[18,19] Refer to Ready Reference 9-8 in the "Ready References" section for information on calibration.
      3. To ensure regular maintenance, the calibration due date should be clearly marked on each gauge.
2. A **mercury manometer** is a device with a column of mercury to indicate the pressure reading.
   a. Mercury manometers are considered the gold standard measuring devices for blood pressure determination. This type may be placed on a table or mounted on the wall.
   b. Mercury manometers pose a health threat if the manometer is broken, causing the mercury to spill.

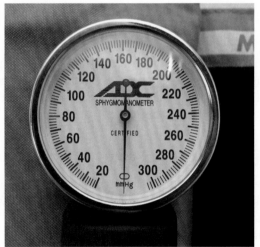
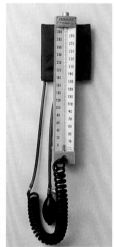

A                                                                              B

**Figure 9-3. Types of manometers. A.** An aneroid manometer is a small, round dial with a needle that indicates the pressure in millimeters (left photo). **B.** A mercury manometer is a device with a column of mercury that indicates the pressure in millimeters (right photo). (Used with permission from Carter, PJ. *Lippincott's Textbook for Nursing Assistants*. 3rd ed. Philadelphia, PA: Lippincott Williams & Wilkins, 2011.)

## THE STETHOSCOPE

A **stethoscope** is a device that makes sound louder and transfers it to the clinician's ears. The parts of a stethoscope are illustrated in Figure 9-4.

1. **Earpieces**, which are placed in the clinician's ears.
2. A **brace and binaurals**, which connect the earpieces to the tubing that conducts the sound.

3. An **amplifying device**, which makes the sound louder; it may be two-sided with a diaphragm and a bell or one-sided with only a diaphragm.
   a. The **diaphragm endpiece** has a large, flat surface that is used to hear loud sounds like the blood rushing through the arteries. The diaphragm endpiece covers a greater area and is easier to hold than a bell endpiece and is recommended for routine measurement of blood pressure in adults.[20]
   b. The **bell endpiece** has a small, rounded surface that is designed to hear faint sounds like heart murmurs. Some authors recommend the bell endpiece for measurement of blood pressure in children because it provides better sound reproduction.[3]

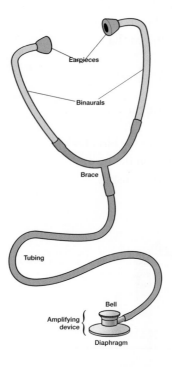

**Figure 9-4.    Parts of a stethoscope.** A stethoscope has the following parts: earpieces, a brace, binaurals, and an amplifying device. The amplifying device may be two-sided, with a diaphragm on one side and a bell on the other.

## AUTOMATIC BLOOD PRESSURE EQUIPMENT

Automatic blood pressure equipment—also called digital or electronic blood pressure equipment—ranges from the highly calibrated types used in hospital settings to less advanced equipment designed for home use.

1. **Electronic Battery-Powered Devices.** The most common types of automatic blood pressure equipment found in the dental setting are electronic battery-powered devices (Fig. 9-5).
   * These devices use a microphone instead of a stethoscope to detect the blood pulsing in the artery.
   * The cuff connects to an electronic monitor that automatically inflates and deflates the cuff when the start button is pressed. There are two types of cuffs, arm and wrist cuffs.
   * A monitor displays the blood pressure reading as a digital display.
2. **Pros and Cons of Electronic Equipment.**
   * Pro: These devices are easiest to use.
   * Con: These devices can be expensive.
   * Con: Many automatic devices do not provide accurate readings.

3. **Types of Automated Devices.** Three categories of automated devices are available: devices that measure blood pressure on the upper arm, the wrist, and the finger.
   - Devices that measure blood pressure at the finger are not recommended.[20]
   - Devices that measure blood pressure at the wrist are more accurate than finger devices but are still not recommended for use in the dental setting.[20]
   - Devices that measure blood pressure in the upper arm have been shown to be the most reliable of the three, both in clinical practice and in the major hypertension trials. The British Hypertension Society (BHS) has established websites to provide updated lists of validated blood pressure measuring devices (http://www.bhsoc.org/blood_pressure_list.stm).
4. **Precautions for Use of Automated Equipment.**
   - The main source of error with automatic devices is that the cuff has not been positioned at the level of the heart when the reading is taken.
   - *Automatic devices are convenient, but they do not provide measurements that are always a close match to the measurements obtained by a standard sphygmomanometer and a stethoscope.*[3, 21, 22] *The preferred method of blood pressure measurement is a traditional sphygmomanometer and a stethoscope (auscultation).*
   - All automatic equipment should be verified using a traditional sphygmomanometer and a stethoscope before its use in a dental setting. An automated device that does not provide readings that are within 1 mm Hg of those obtained with a traditional sphygmomanometer and a stethoscope should not be used in the dental setting. Furthermore, the automatic device must be checked monthly for continued accuracy.
   - *An abnormally high or low reading obtained with an automatic device should be verified by retaking the blood pressure in a few minutes using a traditional sphygmomanometer and a stethoscope.*[3]

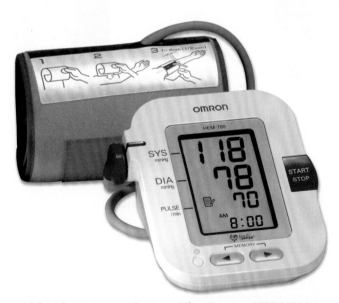

**Figure 9-5. Automatic blood pressure device.** The Omron HEM-780 automatic blood pressure device has been tested for accuracy against two protocols: the Association for the Advancement of Medical Instruments (AAMI) and the International Protocol of the European Society of Hypertension. In March 2001, the *British Medical Journal* published the results of tests on 23 home blood pressure devices. Of the 23 devices tested, only 5 were recommended; all 5 were Omron products. (Courtesy of Omron Healthcare, http://www.omronhealthcare.com.)

**SECTION 3:**

# Measurement and Documentation of Korotkoff Sounds

## BLOOD PRESSURE MEASUREMENTS

1. **Systolic and Diastolic Readings.** Two readings are recorded for blood pressure.
   a. The **systolic reading** is the pressure of the blood flow when the heart beats—the pressure when the first sound is heard. During this stage, the heart is pumping blood through the arteries to the parts of the body.
   b. The **diastolic reading** is the pressure between heartbeats—the pressure when the last sound is heard. During this stage, the heart is relaxed and refills with blood before its next contraction.
2. **Millimeters of Mercury.** Blood pressure readings are recorded in **millimeters of mercury** (mm Hg) because the original mercury manometer devices used a column of mercury.
   a. The pressure is measured by how high a pulsing artery can push a column of mercury in a manometer (Fig. 9-6A).
   b. Measurements made with an aneroid manometer also are recorded in mm Hg despite the fact that these gauges contain no mercury (Fig. 9-6B).
   c. The two blood pressure readings are recorded as a fraction (Box 9-3).

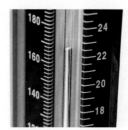

**Figure 9-6A.   Systolic reading on a mercury manometer.** The systolic reading on this gauge is 168 mm Hg.

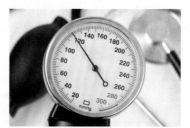

**Figure 9-6B.   Systolic reading on an aneroid manometer.** The systolic reading shown on this gauge is 120 mm Hg.

---

**BOX 9-3    Blood Pressure Measurements**

Blood pressure measurements are recorded as a fraction with the systolic reading as the top number and the diastolic reading as the lower number in the fraction. A typical blood pressure reading for an adult might be 118/78 mm Hg. For example, if an individual's systolic pressure is 118 mm Hg and the diastolic blood pressure is 78 mm Hg, the blood pressure reading is recorded and read as "118 over 78."

$$\frac{\text{Systolic}}{\text{Diastolic}}$$

*To remember that the diastolic number is the lower number, think "diastolic = down."*

**Table 9-1** EFFECTS OF BLOOD PRESSURE CUFF ON BLOOD FLOW

When adequately inflated, the blood pressure cuff stops the blood flow through the brachial artery. A partially inflated cuff allows the blood to push its way, with effort, through the constricted artery. The blood flows easily and freely through the brachial artery when the cuff is not inflated.

| Action | Auscultatory Findings |
|---|---|
| **Cuff pressure stops all blood flow** 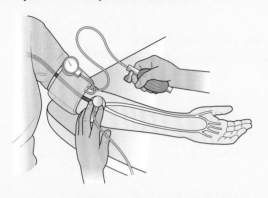 | **Silence** <br> • The cuff is wrapped around the upper arm and inflated. The pressure of the cuff compresses the brachial artery in the arm like a tourniquet, momentarily stopping the blood flow to the lower arm. <br> • With the blood flow to the lower arm temporarily stopped, no sounds can be heard through the stethoscope. |
| **Blood moves through compressed artery** 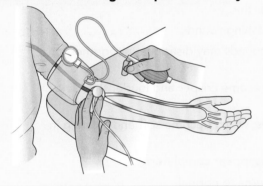 | **Sounds of turbulent flow** <br> Next, air in the cuff is slowly released, and blood begins to push its way through the artery. <br> • The blood flows through in spurts, causing vibrations in the artery walls that can be heard through the stethoscope. <br> • These vibrations are the **Korotkoff sounds**. <br> • Sounds continue to be heard until the pressure in the artery exceeds the pressure of the cuff. |
| **No compression—blood flows freely** 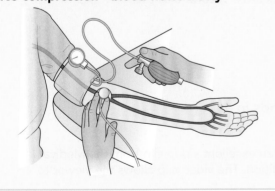 | **Silence** <br> The artery is not compressed; blood flows freely through the artery. No sounds are heard through the stethoscope. |

## THE KOROTKOFF SOUNDS

Blood pressure is most often measured by auscultation using a sphygmomanometer and a stethoscope. Auscultation is the act of listening for sounds within the body to evaluate the condition of the heart, blood vessels, lungs, or other organs. During blood pressure determination, a stethoscope is used to listen to sounds created by the blood as it pushes its way through the constricted brachial artery.

The **Korotkoff** (ko-rot-kov) **sounds** are the series of sounds that are heard as the pressure in the sphygmomanometer cuff is released during the measurement of arterial blood pressure (Boxes 9-4 and 9-5).

- Systolic pressure is defined as "the onset of the tapping Korotkoff sounds."
- The diastolic pressure is defined as "the disappearance of Korotkoff sounds."[3,26,20]

---

**BOX 9-4    Korotkoff Sounds**

| Phase | Sounds and Characteristics |
|-------|----------------------------|
| 1 | The first appearance of repetitive, clear tapping sounds that gradually increase in intensity <br>• The first tapping sound is recorded as the systolic pressure. |
| 2 | A brief period of softer and longer swishing sounds |
| Gap | Auscultatory gap—in some patients, sounds may disappear altogether for a short time |
| 3 | The return of sharper sounds, which become crisper and louder thudding sounds |
| 4 | The distinct, abrupt muffling of sounds, which become soft and blowing in quality |
| 5 | The point at which all sounds finally disappear completely <br>• Silence occurs as the blood flow returns to normal <br>• The point when the last sound is heard is recorded as the diastolic pressure |

---

**BOX 9-5    Hear the Korotkoff Sounds in an Online Video**

"Korotkoff Blood Pressure Sights and Sounds" is an excellent video clip from the Medical Committee of the Virginia Healthy Pathways Coalition. The video clip allows the viewer to hear examples of actual Korotkoff sounds.

Video link: http://vimeo.com/26580985

## AUSCULTATORY PHASES

There are five phases of Korotkoff sounds.

• Each phase is characterized by the volume and quality of sound heard through the stethoscope. Figure 9-7 illustrates these phases.

• These phases were first described by Nicolai Korotkoff and later elaborated by Witold Ettinger.[27-29]

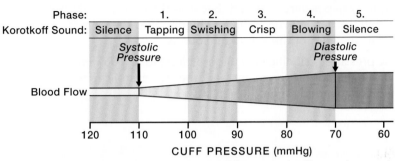

**Figure 9-7. The five phases of Korotkoff sounds.** The Korotkoff sounds are characterized by the volume and quality of sound heard during each phase. In this representation, the systolic pressure is 110 mm Hg and the diastolic pressure is 70 mm Hg.

## THE SILENT AUSCULTATORY GAP

Failure to detect a gap in the Korotkoff sounds is a potential source of error in blood pressure measurement. The **auscultatory gap** is a period of *abnormal silence* that occurs between the Korotkoff phases (Fig. 9-8). Failure to recognize the presence of an auscultatory gap will result in an inaccurate blood pressure reading in which the systolic pressure is underestimated. Box 9-6 provides an example of how failure to recognize the auscultatory gap can result in inaccurate readings.

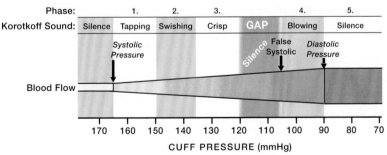

**Figure 9-8. Auscultatory gap—an example.** In this example, the fictitious patient exhibits a gap in sounds between 120 mm Hg and 106 mm Hg; this silent period is known as the auscultatory gap.

## BOX 9-6    The Impact of an Unrecognized Auscultatory Gap

### Technique Error: Gap Mistaken for the Silent Period before Phase 1

1. If the cuff is not inflated high enough, the clinician will mistake the gap in sounds as the silent period before the phase 1 sounds begin.

2. In the example shown below, if the clinician only inflates the cuff to 116 mm Hg:
   - The auscultatory gap is unrecognized. Because the clinician only starts listening at 116 mm Hg (within the gap in sounds), he or she mistakes the sounds he or she hears at 106 mm Hg as the start of the Korotkoff sounds.
   - The systolic pressure is significantly underestimated as 106 mm Hg and interpreted as being within the normal range. Instead, the true systolic reading of 166 mm Hg is above the recommended range.

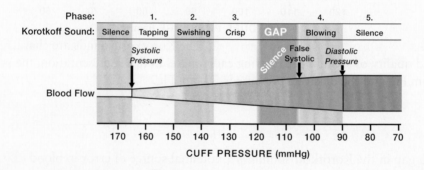

### DETECTION OF AUSCULTATORY GAP

*Palpation of the brachial or radial pulse during cuff inflation ensures that an auscultatory gap is not mistaken for the start of phase I sounds.*[30]

## FLUCTUATIONS IN BLOOD PRESSURE

Blood pressure varies from moment to moment and can be influenced by many factors such as body position, respiration, emotion, anxiety, exercise, meals, tobacco, alcohol, temperature, and pain. Blood pressure also is influenced by age and race and is usually at its lowest during sleep. These influences on blood pressure can be significant, often accounting for rises in systolic blood pressure greater than 20 mm Hg. These factors have to be carefully considered in all circumstances of blood pressure measurement. Insofar as is practical, the patient should be relaxed in a quiet room for a short period of time before measurement.

**White-coat (or office) hypertension** refers to blood pressure that rises above its usual level when it is measured in a health care setting (such as a medical or dental office, where a health care provider may be wearing a white lab coat).[3,31–34] White-coat hypertension is more common in people who have high blood pressure, and in the dental setting, their blood pressure is remarkably higher than normal. This increase in blood pressure tends to subside once the patient becomes more relaxed as the dental appointment progresses. In many cases, continuing with the extraoral examination and then retaking the blood pressure measurement will yield a lower blood pressure reading.

## SECTION 4:
# Critical Technique Elements

The procedure for the measurement of arterial blood pressure using a sphygmomanometer is well established, and consensus recommendations have been produced by the Joint National Committee on Prevention, Detection, Evaluation, and Treatment of High Blood Pressure (USA), the Canadian Hypertension Education Program, the BHS, and the European Society of Hypertension in the interest of standardization.[20,24–25,35–39]

- Every person who performs blood pressure assessments should undergo careful training and be aware of common errors in technique.
- Four of the most critical technique elements for accurate blood pressure determination are the ability to (1) select the proper cuff size, (2) place the cuff, (3) position the patient's arm, and (4) obtain a palpatory estimate of the blood pressure.[16,23,36,37]

### CUFF SIZE

In the case of blood pressure cuffs, one size does *not* fit all. Improper bladder width or length is one of the primary sources of error in accurately assessing blood pressure. Proper technique includes selecting the correct cuff size for the patient's upper arm.[40–42] Each dental office or clinic should have a set of three to four cuffs to properly fit a variety of arm sizes (Fig. 9-2).

- Cuffs are labeled as child, adult small, adult standard, adult large, and adult thigh. Unfortunately, at the current time, there is no universal standardization among manufacturers. For this reason, the bladder dimensions may vary in length and width.
- The AHA guidelines for cuff selection are summarized in Ready Reference 9-1 in the "Ready References" section of this module.
- Ideally, every cuff should be labeled with the dimensions of the enclosed bladder, and a line should mark the center of the bladder. The user should mark unlabeled cuffs by outlining the bladder and indicating its midpoint.
- It is the *length and width of the inflatable bladder*—not its cloth sheath—that affects the accuracy of blood pressure measurement.[43] Figure 9-9 (see Box 9–7) illustrates the bladder length and width.

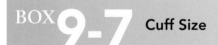

**BOX 9-7**  **Cuff Size**

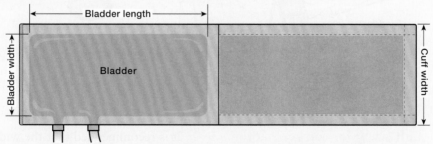

**Figure 9-9.  Bladder size.** The length and width of the bladder are used when selecting the correct cuff size for the patient's arm.

## CORRECT SIZING OF BLADDER

To select the correct cuff size, both the bladder length and width needs to be sized correctly for each individual patient.

- *When placed on the midpoint of the upper arm on an adult patient, the bladder length should encircle at least 80% of the midpoint of the upper arm* (Fig. 9-10).
- *When placed on the midpoint of the arm on an adult patient, the width of the bladder should encircle at least 40% of the arm* (Fig. 9-11).
- A bladder that is too small causes overestimation of the blood pressure—false high readings—because the pressure is not evenly transmitted to the brachial artery. A bladder that is too large may cause underdiagnosing of hypertension—false low readings—because the pressure of the cuff is dispersed over too large a surface of the arm.

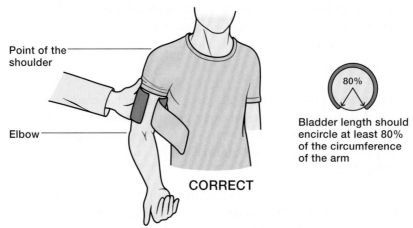

**Figure 9-10.   Cuff sizing for correct bladder length.** The length of the inflatable bladder should encircle at least 80% of the midpoint of the upper arm—almost long enough to encircle the arm.[3,17,23] In children younger than 13 years, the bladder might encircle 100% of the midpoint of the upper arm.

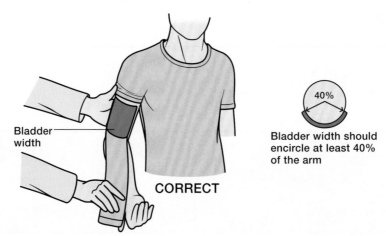

**Figure 9-11.   Cuff sizing for correct bladder width.** It is recommended that the width of the inflatable bladder should encircle at least 40% of the midpoint of the upper arm.[3,17,23]

## ARM POSITION DURING BLOOD PRESSURE ASSESSMENT

1. **Correct Arm Position for Blood Pressure Assessment in the Dental Setting.** Proper positioning of the patient's arm is key to obtaining an accurate blood pressure reading. Blood pressure readings go up or down depending on where the arm is positioned. Recommendations of the AHA, Canadian Hypertension Education Program, and the BHS are all in agreement on the recommendation for arm position (Box 9-8).[20,23,38,44–46]

   a. **Seated Position.** *The patient should be seated comfortably with his or her back supported.*

   b. **Arm Supported By Clinician.**
      1. *The clinician should support the patient's arm by holding it under the elbow.*
      2. The phrase "passively supported arm" indicates that the weight of the patient's arm should be supported by the clinician rather than held in position by the patient.
      3. A rise in blood pressure and heart rate occurs if the patient must tense his or her muscles to support the weight of the arm.

   c. **Antecubital Fossa at Mid-Sternum Level.** *The arm should be horizontal with the antecubital fossa at the level of the patient's heart (about mid-sternum). The patient's arm and hand should be relaxed and the elbow slightly flexed.*
      1. The antecubital fossa is the hollow or depressed area in the underside of the arm at the bend of the elbow (Fig. 9-12).
      2. During blood pressure determination, the antecubital fossa is used as a (1) landmark for locating the brachial pulse point, (2) reference point for cuff placement, and (3) reference point for correct arm position.
         a. The cuff is placed around the upper arm with the lower edge of the cuff about 1 in (2.5 cm) above the antecubital fossa.
         b. The patient's arm is positioned with the antecubital fossa level with the heart. Figure 9-13 in Box 9-8 demonstrates correct arm and cuff position.

   d. **Differences between Arms.** Some studies have demonstrated significant differences between the blood pressure reading obtained from the right arm versus the left arm of an individual.[20] For this reason, the clinician should document the arm used at the initial assessment in the patient record and use the same arm at subsequent visits.

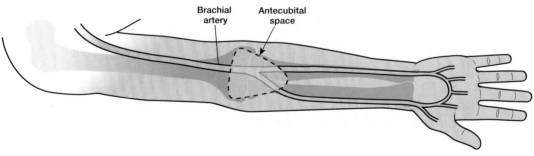

Figure 9-12. Location of the antecubital fossa. The antecubital fossa is the hollow area in the underside of the arm at the bend of the elbow.

**2. Effects of Level of Antecubital Fossa during Blood Pressure Assessment**

**a. Antecubital Fossa Positioned Too Low**

1. Allowing the patient's arm to hang by the patient's side or lie on the dental chair's armrest can result in false high readings.

2. Overestimating the blood pressure in a medical setting might result in overtreatment, for example, prescribing blood pressure medication for a patient who does not really need treatment.

3. Overestimating the blood pressure in a dental setting might needlessly delay dental treatment due to concern that the patient is hypertensive.

**b. Antecubital Fossa Positioned Too High**

1. Positioning the patient's arm so that the antecubital fossa is above mid-sternum level can result in false low readings.

2. Underestimating the blood pressure in a medical setting, in the worst case, could lead to heart attack or stroke.

3. Underestimating the blood pressure in a dental setting is a missed opportunity to identify hypertension and refer the patient to a primary care physician. In addition, it could result in a medical emergency during dental treatment.

---

BOX **9-8** Correct Arm and Cuff Position for Blood Pressure Assessment

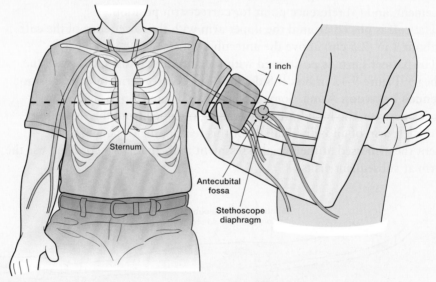

**Figure 9-13. Correct arm position.** For blood pressure determination, the patient's arm should be supported passively with the antecubital fossa at mid-sternum level of the patient.

## PALPATORY ESTIMATION OF BLOOD PRESSURE

To avoid falsely low systolic pressure readings, the systolic pressure should be estimated before the clinician uses the stethoscope by palpating the brachial artery pulse and inflating the cuff until the pulsation disappears. The point at which the pulsation disappears is the **estimated systolic pressure**.

- This palpatory estimation is important, because phase 1 sounds sometimes disappear as pressure is reduced and reappear at a lower level—auscultatory gap—resulting in the systolic pressure being underestimated unless already determined by palpation.[20]
- If the systolic pressure is not first estimated by palpation, insufficient inflation of the cuff may cause the clinician to mistake the lower end of the gap as the systolic pressure.
- Measuring palpable pressure first avoids the risk of seriously underestimating blood pressure because of the auscultatory gap.
- The radial artery is also used for palpatory estimation of the systolic pressure, but by using the brachial artery, the clinician also establishes its location. Later in the procedure, the stethoscope-amplifying device is placed over the brachial artery to listen for the Korotkoff sounds.
- The brachial pulse point is located just above the antecubital fossa toward the inner aspect of the arm (Fig. 9-14).

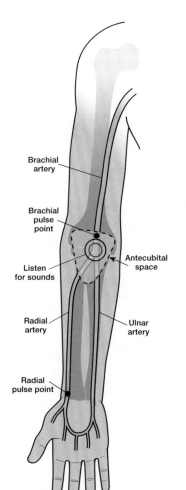

Brachial artery

Brachial pulse point

Listen for sounds

Antecubital space

Radial artery

Ulnar artery

Radial pulse point

**Figure 9-14.   Brachial pulse point and other anatomical landmarks for blood pressure assessment.**

- The brachial artery is palpated just above the antecubital fossa toward the inner aspect (little finger side) of the arm.
- The amplifying endpiece of the stethoscope is placed over the pulse—just above the antecubital fossa toward the inner aspect of the arm—but below the lower edge of the cuff.

## SECTION 5:
# Peak Procedures

---

**PROCEDURE 9-1** **BLOOD PRESSURE DETERMINATION**

**Equipment**
Stethoscope
Sphygmomanometer known to be accurate
Blood pressure cuff of the appropriate size
A watch or a clock displaying seconds
Pen (or computer keyboard)
Patient chart or computer record

**General Considerations**
- The patient should not have had alcohol, tobacco, or caffeine or performed vigorous exercise within 30 minutes of the blood pressure assessment.
- After escorting the patient to the treatment room, allow him or her to relax for at least 5 minutes before beginning the vital signs assessment. If a glass thermometer is used for temperature determination, the pulse, respiration, and blood pressure may be assessed while the thermometer is registering the patient's temperature.
- Delay obtaining the blood pressure if the patient is anxious or in pain.
- *The patient should be sitting in an upright position with his or her back supported and legs uncrossed.[47] The patient should not be moving or speaking during the procedure.*

| Action | Rationale |
|---|---|
| 1. Briefly explain the procedure to the patient. If the patient has never had a blood pressure assessment, explain that some minor discomfort is caused by the inflation of the cuff.[20] | • Reduces patient apprehension and encourages patient cooperation. |
| 2. Select an appropriate arm—no breast cancer surgery involving lymph node removal on that side, cast, injured limb, or other compromising factor. | • Measurement of blood pressure may temporarily impair circulation to the compromised arm. |
| 3. Choose a cuff with an appropriate bladder width and length matched to the size of the patient's upper arm.<br><br>Squeeze the bladder to completely deflate the cuff. | • Using a cuff with the wrong size bladder may result in inaccurate readings.<br><br>• Air remaining in the bladder makes it difficult to wrap the cuff around the arm. |

(continued)

**PROCEDURE 9-1**  BLOOD PRESSURE DETERMINATION *(CONTINUED)*

| Action | Rationale |
|---|---|
| **4.** The patient's upper arm should be bare.<br><br>The sleeve should not be rolled up if doing so creates a tight roll of cloth around the upper arm. | • Clothing over the artery interferes with the ability to hear sounds.<br>• Tight clothing on the arm causes congestion of blood in the arm and probably results in inaccurate readings. Remove arm from sleeve if sleeve cannot be rolled up without creating a tight roll of cloth. |
| **5.** Ask the patient to assume a comfortable position with the palm of the hand upward. | • There is no need for the patient's arm to be in an uncomfortable position. |
| **6.** Position the cuff so that the lower edge is 1–2 in (2–3 cm) above the elbow crease.[20,36]<br><br>Place the cuff so that the midline of the bladder is centered over the brachial artery (Fig. 9-15). Wrap the cuff smoothly and snugly around the arm. Fasten it securely.<br><br>The tubing from the cuff should not cross the auscultatory area. | • Allows sufficient space below the cuff so that the amplifying device of the stethoscope can be placed on the brachial pulse point in the antecubital fossa.<br>• Centering the bladder over the brachial artery assures equal compression of the artery by the bladder pressure.<br>• Loose application of the cuff results in overestimation of the pressure.<br>• Contact of the amplifying device of the stethoscope with the tubing creates noises that make it difficult to hear the Korotkoff sounds. |

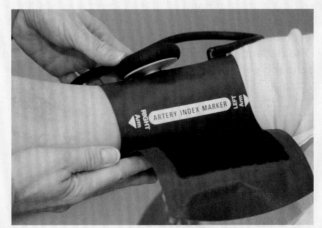

**Figure 9-15.   Position the cuff.** Position the cuff so that the lower edge is 1–2 in (2–3 cm) above the elbow crease and the midline of the bladder is centered over the brachial artery.

*(continued)*

**PROCEDURE 9-1**   **BLOOD PRESSURE DETERMINATION** *(CONTINUED)*

| Action | Rationale |
|---|---|
| **7.** Place the manometer so the mercury column or aneroid dial is easily visible to the clinician and the tubing from the cuff is unobstructed. | • Improper positioning of the gauge can lead to errors in reading the measurements.<br>• Instruct the patient not to talk during the blood pressure procedure. |
| **8.** Place the earpieces of the stethoscope into the ear canals with the *earpieces angled forward* (Fig. 9-16). | • This forward angle directs the earpieces into the canal and not against the ear itself. |

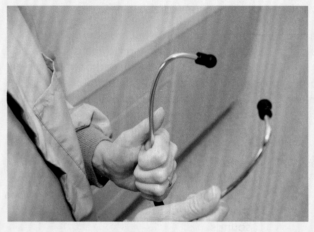

**Figure 9-16.   Position the earpieces.** Direct the stethoscope earpieces forward so that they will be directed into the ear canals and not against the ear itself.

| Action | Rationale |
|---|---|
| **9.** Grasp the patient's elbow with your hand and raise the arm. Support the patient's arm so that the antecubital fossa is at the mid-sternum level. The patient's arm should remain somewhat bent and completely relaxed (Fig. 9-17). | • A lower arm position will result in erroneously high readings.<br>• A higher arm position will result in erroneously low readings.<br>• If the patient does the work of holding up the arm, the readings will be elevated. |

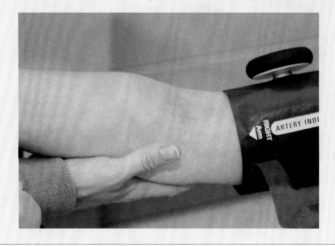

**Figure 9-17.   Establish correct arm position.** Support the patient's arm so that the antecubital fossa is at the mid-sternum level.

*(continued)*

**PROCEDURE 9-1**   BLOOD PRESSURE DETERMINATION *(CONTINUED)*

| Action | Rationale |
|---|---|
| **10.** Palpate the brachial pulse by gently pressing with the fingertips. Use your free hand to tighten the valve on the air pump.<br><br>Inflate the cuff rapidly to 70 mm Hg and then increase by increments of 10 mm Hg. Note the pressure at which the pulse disappears. This is a rough estimate of the systolic pressure. | • Palpation allows for estimation of the systolic pressure.<br>• The bladder will not inflate unless the valve is completely closed.<br>• The palpatory method is used to avoid underinflation of the cuff in patients with an auscultatory gap or overinflation in those with very low blood pressure. |
| **11.** Open the valve, deflate the cuff rapidly, leaving it in place on the arm, and wait 15 seconds. | • Allowing a brief pause before continuing permits the blood to refill and circulate through the arm. |
| **12.** Gently place the amplifying endpiece of the stethoscope over the pulse—just above the antecubital fossa toward the inner aspect of the arm—but below the lower edge of the cuff.<br><br>Hold the amplifying device in place with your fingers, making sure that it makes contact with the skin around its entire circumference (Fig. 9-18). | • Wedging the amplifying device under the edge of the cuff creates extraneous noise that will distract from the sounds made by the blood flowing through the artery.<br>• Heavy pressure on the brachial artery distorts the shape of the artery and the sound.[20]<br>• Moving the amplifying device produces noise that can obscure the Korotkoff sounds. |

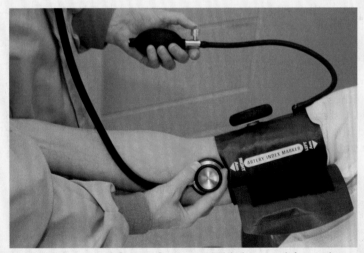

**Figure 9-18.   Position the amplifying device.** Hold the amplifying device firmly in place, making sure that the head contacts the skin around its entire circumference.

*(continued)*

**PROCEDURE 9-1** BLOOD PRESSURE DETERMINATION *(CONTINUED)*

| Action | Rationale |
|---|---|
| **13.** Hold the air pump bulb so that it is easy to reach the valve at the top (Fig. 9-19). Close the valve at the top of the bulb. | • Having the valve within easy reach is important because the other hand is used to hold the amplifying device against the arm. |

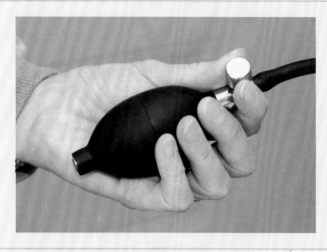

**Figure 9-19.  Grasp the air pump bulb.** Hold the bulb in your hand so the valve is easy to reach.

| Action | Rationale |
|---|---|
| **14.** Using brisk squeezes of the bulb, rapidly inflate the bladder to a pressure 30 mm Hg above the level previously determined by palpation.<br><br>At 30 mm Hg above the systolic estimate, slightly open the valve and release the pressure slowly so that the pressure gauge **drops no faster than 2 mm per second**.[20] | • Rapid inflation of the bladder cuts off the blood flow quickly and intensifies the sounds heard later as the air is slowly released.<br>• Increasing the pressure above that of the palpated pressure ensures a silent period before hearing the first sound.<br>• A slow cuff deflation rate of 2 mm per second is necessary for accurate readings. |
| **15.** Pay careful attention to sounds heard through the stethoscope as the needle on the gauge falls. Listen for the first clear tapping sound (the systolic pressure). Make a mental note of this pressure (Fig. 9-20). | • Systolic pressure is the point at which the blood in the artery is first able to force its way through the vessel. The first clear, tapping sound is the systolic pressure. |

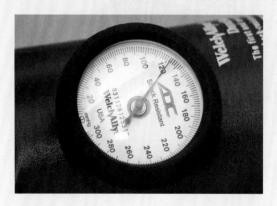

**Figure 9-20.  Note the systolic pressure.** Note the systolic pressure reading when you hear the first clear tapping sound.

*(continued)*

**PROCEDURE 9-1** **BLOOD PRESSURE DETERMINATION** *(CONTINUED)*

| Action | Rationale |
|---|---|
| **16.** Do not reinflate the cuff once the air has been released to recheck the systolic reading.<br><br>If you are uncertain of the systolic reading, continue releasing air and listen carefully for the diastolic pressure. | • Reinflating a partially inflated cuff causes congestion in the lower arm, which lessens the loudness of the Korotkoff sounds.<br>• Obtain the diastolic pressure, wait 30 seconds, and repeat the procedure to obtain the systolic reading. |
| **17.** Continue releasing pressure slowly at a rate of 2 mm per second. The sounds should become louder in intensity, muffle, and then disappear. Listen carefully and note the point at which the sounds disappear (the diastolic pressure). Note the diastolic pressure (Fig. 9-21). | • Diastolic pressure occurs when the blood is able to resume normal flow through the vessel. This smooth flow of blood is silent. |

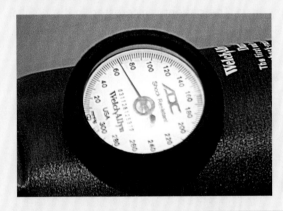

**Figure 9-21. Note the diastolic pressure.** Note the diastolic pressure reading at the point at which the sounds disappear.

| Action | Rationale |
|---|---|
| **18.** After the last Korotkoff sound is heard, the cuff should be deflated slowly for at least another 10 mm Hg. Then, allow the remaining air to escape rapidly.<br><br>If the Korotkoff sounds persist as the pressure level approaches 0 mm Hg, then phase 4 is used to indicate the diastolic pressure. | • Slow deflation for 10 mm Hg ensures that no further sounds are audible.<br>• Once all sounds have disappeared, the cuff is deflated rapidly to prevent venous congestion of the arm.[20]<br>• The AHA recommends using the muffling of sound as the diastolic pressure when recording blood pressure in children. |
| **19.** Immediately record the two numbers as a fraction in whole, even numbers. Also record the arm and the patient's position. An auscultatory gap should always be noted. (112/76 mm Hg, right arm, seated) | • Recording the pressures promptly helps to ensure accuracy.[20]<br>• It is common practice to read blood pressure to the closest 2-mm number. Do not round off the reading to the nearest 5- or 10-mm digit. |

*(continued)*

## PROCEDURE 9-1    BLOOD PRESSURE DETERMINATION *(CONTINUED)*

| Action | Rationale |
|---|---|
| **20.** Blood pressure may be taken in both arms on the patient's initial visit to the dental office or clinic. If there is more than a 10-mm Hg difference between the two arms, the arm with the higher readings should be used at future appointments. | • It is common to have a 5- to 10-mm Hg difference in the systolic reading between the arms. Use the arm with the higher reading for subsequent pressures. |
| **21.** Repeat any reading that is outside the expected range, but wait 30–60 seconds between readings to allow normal circulation to return to the arm.<br><br>Be sure to deflate the bladder completely between attempts to check the blood pressure. | • Repeat reading to confirm the accuracy of the original measurement.<br><br>• False readings are likely to occur if there is congestion of blood in the arm when obtaining repeated readings. |
| **22.** Inform the patient and explain the significance of the blood pressure readings (Fig. 9-22). | • The patient is interested in the results. This is an opportunity to educate the patient about hypertension. |

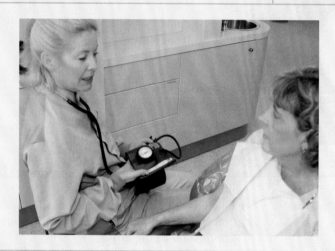

**Figure 9-22.   Inform the patient.** Tell the patient the reading and explain the significance of the reading.

| | |
|---|---|
| **23.** Remove the cuff and clean and store the equipment. | • Equipment should be left in a manner so that it is ready for use. |

## PROCEDURE 9-2    IF KOROTKOFF SOUNDS ARE DIFFICULT TO HEAR

If the Korotkoff sounds are difficult to hear, the following techniques are recommended:

1. Raise the patient's arm—with cuff in place—over his or her head for 15 seconds before rechecking the blood pressure. Raising the arm over the head helps relieve the congestion of blood in the arm, increases pressure differences, and makes the sounds louder and more distinct when blood enters the lower arm.
Reposition any clothing that might be rubbing against the stethoscope tubing (causing extraneous noises).

2. Confirm that the stethoscope earpieces are angled forward and snuggly in ear canals.

3. Hold your hands and tubing as still as possible.

4. Confirm that the amplifying device is over the brachial pulse point and the entire circumference is in contact with the skin.

5. Inflate the cuff rapidly.

6. Inflate the cuff with the antecubital fossa elevated above the heart level, and then gently lower the arm while continuing to support it.

7. Deflate the cuff at a steady rate of 2 mm Hg per second while listening for the Korotkoff sounds.

## SECTION 6:

# Ready References

> **NOTE:** The Ready References in this book may be removed from the book by tearing along the perforated lines on each page. Laminating or placing these pages in plastic protector sheets will allow them to be disinfected for use in a clinical setting.

**READY REFERENCE 9-1**    RECOMMENDED BLADDER DIMENSIONS[a]

| Cuff | Bladder Dimensions in Centimeters (cm) | Maximum Arm Circumference (cm)[b] | Maximum Arm Circumference (in)[b] |
|------|------|------|------|
| **Child** | 9 × 18 | 22 | 8.7 |
| **Adult small** | 10 × 24 | 26 | 10.2 |
| **Adult standard** | 13 × 30 | 34 | 13.4 |
| **Adult large** | 16 × 38 | 44 | 17.3 |
| **Adult thigh** | 20 × 42 | 52 | 20.4 |

[a]**U.S. Department of Health and Human Services, National Institutes of Health, National Heart, Lung, and Blood Institute.** *The Fourth Report on the Diagnosis, Evaluation, and Treatment of High Blood Pressure in Children and Adolescents.* **Bethesda, MD: U.S. Department of Health and Human Services, National Institutes of Health, National Heart, Lung, and Blood Institute; 2005.**
[b]Arm circumference as measured at the midpoint of the upper arm. Midpoint of the arm is defined as half the distance from the highest point of the shoulder to the point of the elbow.

**READY REFERENCE 9-2** CLASSIFICATION OF BLOOD PRESSURE FOR ADULTS AGED 18 YEARS OR OLDER

| Category | Systolic BP in mm Hg | | Diastolic BP in mm Hg |
|---|---|---|---|
| **Normal** | <120 | and | <80 |
| **Prehypertension** | 120–139 | or | 80–89 |
| **Stage 1 hypertension** | 140–159 | or | 90–99 |
| **Stage 2 hypertension** | ≥160 | or | ≥100 |

**KEY:** <, less than; ≥, greater than or equal to.
**NOTE:** The patient's blood pressure is determined by the higher value for either the systolic or diastolic blood pressure.[48]
BP, blood pressure.
Adapted from Chobanian AV, Bakris, GL, Black HR, et al. The seventh report of the Joint National Committee on prevention, detection, evaluation, and treatment of high blood pressure: the JNC 7 report. *JAMA.* 2003;289(19):2560–2572.

**READY REFERENCE 9-3** BLOOD PRESSURE VALUES REQUIRING FURTHER EVALUATION ACCORDING TO AGE AND GENDER FOR CHILDREN AND ADOLESCENTS[a]

| | Blood Pressure in mm Hg | | | | |
|---|---|---|---|---|---|
| | Male | | | Female | |
| Age | Systolic | Diastolic | | Systolic | Diastolic |
| 3 | 100 | 59 | | 100 | 61 |
| 4 | 102 | 62 | | 101 | 64 |
| 5 | 104 | 65 | | 103 | 66 |
| 6 | 105 | 68 | | 104 | 68 |
| 7 | 106 | 70 | | 106 | 69 |
| 8 | 107 | 71 | | 108 | 71 |
| 9 | 109 | 72 | | 110 | 72 |
| 10 | 111 | 73 | | 112 | 73 |
| 11 | 113 | 74 | | 114 | 74 |
| 12 | 115 | 74 | | 116 | 75 |
| 13 | 117 | 75 | | 117 | 76 |
| 14 | 120 | 75 | | 119 | 77 |
| 15 | 120 | 76 | | 120 | 78 |
| 16 | 120 | 78 | | 120 | 78 |
| 17 | 120 | 80 | | 120 | 78 |
| 18 | 120 | 80 | | 120 | 80 |

[a]Any reading equal to or above the readings in Ready Reference 9-3 indicates potentially abnormal blood pressures in one of three ranges—prehypertension, stage 1 hypertension, or stage 2 hypertension—and identifies blood pressures that require additional evaluation.[49]
Used with permission from Kaelber DC, Pickett F. Simple table to identify children and adolescents needing further evaluation of blood pressure. *Pediatrics.* 2009;123(6):e972–e974.

## READY REFERENCE 9-4 · DENTAL MANAGEMENT OF HYPERTENSIVE ADULTS

| Systolic/Diastolic Blood Pressure | Dental Management Recommendations |
| --- | --- |
| <140/90 | 1. Routine dental treatment can be provided; recommend lifestyle modifications (i.e., diet, exercise, quit smoking).<br>2. Retake blood pressure at continuing care appointment as a screening strategy for hypertension. |
| 140–159/90–99 | 1. If the initial reading is in this range, retake blood pressure after 5 minutes and patient has rested. Retaking the blood pressure determines the accuracy of the initial readings.<br>2. Inform patient of blood pressure status; recommend lifestyle modifications.<br>3. Routine treatment can be provided. Employ stress reduction strategies. **Refer to Box 4-4 in Module 4 to review Strategies for Stress Reduction.**<br>4. Measure prior to any appointment. If patient has measurements above normal range on three separate appointments—and is not under the care of a physician for hypertension—refer for medical evaluation. |
| 160–179/100–109 | 1. Retake blood pressure after 5 minutes and patient has rested.<br>2. If still elevated, inform patient of readings.<br>3. Refer for medical evaluation within 1 month; delay treatment if patient is unable to handle stress or if dental procedure is stressful. If local anesthesia is required, use 1:100,000 vasoconstrictor.<br>4. Routine treatment can be provided. Employ stress reduction strategies during dental treatment. |
| ≥180/≥110 | 1. Retake blood pressure after 5 minutes and patient has rested.<br>2. Delay dental treatment until blood pressure is controlled.<br>3. Refer to physician for immediate medical evaluation. Require a medical release form from the patient's physician prior to dental treatment.<br>4. If emergency dental care is needed, it should be done in a setting in which emergency life support equipment is available, such as a hospital dental clinic. |

**KEY:** <, less than; ≥, greater than or equal to. The patient's blood pressure is determined by the higher value for either the systolic or diastolic blood pressure[50]

Modified from Pickett FA, Gurenlian JR. *The Medical History: Clinical Implications and Emergency Prevention in Dental Settings.* Baltimore, MD: Lippincott Williams & Wilkins; 2005, page 9.

**READY REFERENCE 9-5** ASSESSING PEDIATRIC PATIENTS

| Age | Keys to Successful Interaction | Characteristics |
|---|---|---|
| **Preschooler (3–6 years)** | • Explain actions using simple language<br>• Tell child what will happen next<br>• Tell child if something will hurt<br>• Distract child with a story<br>• Praise good behavior | • Normally alert, active<br>• Can sit still on request<br>• Can cooperate with the assessment<br>• Understands speech<br>• Will make up explanations for anything not understood |
| **School-age child (6–12 years)** | • Explain actions using simple language<br>• Explain procedure immediately before performing<br>• Let child make treatment choices when possible<br>• Allow child to participate in exam | • Will cooperate if trust is established<br>• Wants to participate and retain some control |
| **Adolescent (12–17 years)** | • Explain the process as to an adult<br>• Treat the adolescent with respect<br>• Encourage questions | • Able to make decisions about care<br>• Has clear concepts of future |

**READY REFERENCE 9-6** FACTORS AFFECTING THE ACCURACY OF BLOOD PRESSURE MEASUREMENT

- **Time of day**—blood pressure readings are usually lowest in the morning and can increase by as much as 10 mm Hg later in the day.
- **Position**—blood pressure generally is lower when a person is lying down, as compared to when sitting or standing.
- **Arm**—there are pressure differences of more than 10 mm Hg between the arms in 6% of hypertensive patients.
- **Eating**—blood pressure readings usually are slightly higher after a meal, especially if the meal is high in salt content.
- **Exercise**—strenuous activity will temporarily increase the systolic blood pressure.
- **Stress**—anxiety, fear, or pain will temporarily raise a person's blood pressure.

**READY REFERENCE 9-7**    CAUSES OF INACCURACIES IN BLOOD PRESSURE MEASUREMENT

| Problem | Result | Solution |
|---|---|---|
| **Equipment** | | |
| Stethoscope earpieces plugged | Difficulty hearing sounds | Clean earpieces |
| Earpieces fit poorly | Distorted sounds | Angle earpieces forward |
| Aneroid needle not at zero | Inaccurate reading | Recalibrate gauge |
| Bladder too narrow for arm | Inaccurate high reading | Bladder 80% of circumference |
| Bladder too wide for arm | Inaccurate low reading | Use appropriate cuff size |
| Faulty valve | Difficulty inflating cuff | Replace equipment |
| Leaky tubing or bulb | Inaccurate reading | Replace equipment |
| **Patient position** | | |
| Patient arm not at heart level | Inaccurate readings | Position patient with the antecubital fossa at mid-sternum |
| Patient legs dangling | Inaccurate high reading | Legs supported |
| Back unsupported | Inaccurate high reading | Support back |
| **Cuff placement** | | |
| Cuff wrapped too loosely | Reading too high | Rewrap more snugly |
| Applied over clothing | Inaccurate reading | Remove arm from sleeve |
| **Amplifying device** | | |
| Amplifying device not in contact with skin | Extraneous noise | Place amplifying device correctly |
| Amplifying device applied too firmly | Diastolic reading too low | Place amplifying device correctly |
| Amplifying device not over artery | Sounds difficult to hear | Place amplifying device over palpated artery |
| Amplifying device touching tubing or cuff | Extraneous noise | Place below edge of cuff |
| Failure to palpate brachial pulse | Underestimation of systolic pressure | Routinely check systolic pressure by palpation first |
| **Pressure/inflation** | | |
| Inflation level too high | Patient discomfort | Inflate to 30 mm Hg above palpatory blood pressure |
| Inflation level too low | Underestimation of systolic pressure | Inflate to 30 mm Hg above palpatory blood pressure |
| Inflating cuff too slowly | Patient discomfort; over-estimation of diastolic pressure | Inflate the cuff as rapidly as possible |
| Cuff pressure released too fast | Underestimation of systolic pressure; overestimation of diastolic pressure | Release pressure no faster than 2 mm Hg per second |
| Cuff pressure released too slowly | Congestion of blood in forearm; sounds difficult to hear | Remove cuff; ask patient to elevate the arm, then open and close the fist several times |
| **Readings** | | |
| Rounding off readings to 0 or 5 | Inaccurate readings | Record to nearest 2 mm Hg |
| Intra-arm difference | Pressure differences of more than 10 mm Hg between arms | Initially, measure BP in both arms; use arm with higher reading at subsequent appointments |

**READY REFERENCE 9-8**    **EQUIPMENT MAINTENANCE**

**General Maintenance**

- Check the cuff for any breaks in stitching or tears in fabric.
- Check the tubing for cracks or leaks, especially at connections.
- Look to see that the aneroid needle on the gauge is at zero.

**Marking the Cuff**

Unfortunately, not all manufacturers are using the same guidelines to mark blood pressure cuffs. Many cuffs are marked incorrectly; therefore, you will have to correctly mark each cuff.

- The center of the bladder should be positioned over the brachial artery. Locate the center by folding the bladder in half.
- Mark the middle with an "x."
- This is where the cuff should cross the brachial pulse.

**Calibrating an Aneroid Manometer**

The aneroid manometer—because of its design—is prone to mechanical problems that can affect its accuracy. Jolts and bumps that occur during everyday use affect accuracy over time, usually resulting to false low readings.[20] Aneroid gauges require regular calibration and checks for common defects such as nonzeroed gauges, cracked faceplates, or defective rubber tubing.[17] The needle of the aneroid gauge should rest at the zero point before the cuff is inflated and return to zero when the cuff is deflated.

Aneroid manometers should be handled gently to avoid decalibration and require routine maintenance. Every 6 months, the accuracy of the aneroid gauge should be checked at different pressure levels by connecting it with a Y-piece (Fig. 9-23) to the tubing of a standardized mercury column manometer.[18,20]

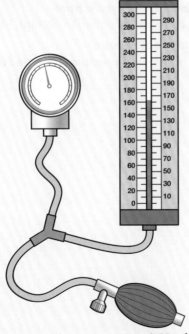

**Figure 9-23. Calibration of an aneroid manometer.** A Y-tube is used to calibrate the aneroid manometer with a mercury manometer.

**READY REFERENCE 9-9**    INTERNET RESOURCES: BLOOD PRESSURE

**http://www.americanheart.org**
The **American Heart Association** website has links to detailed information about hypertension and the treatment of hypertension.

**http://www.nhlbi.nih.gov/guidelines/hypertension/index.htm**
Link to *The Seventh Report of the Joint National Committee on Prevention, Detection, Evaluation, and Treatment of High Blood Pressure (JNC 7)* on the **National Heart, Lung, and Blood Institute's** website.

**http://www.nhlbi.nih.gov/health/prof/heart/hbp/hbp_ped.htm**
*The Fourth Report on the Diagnosis, Evaluation, and Treatment of High Blood Pressure in Children and Adolescents* on the **National Heart, Lung, and Blood Institute's** website.

**http://www.abdn.ac.uk/medical/bhs**
Recommendations on blood pressure measurement on the **British Hypertension Society** website.

**http://www.nlm.nih.gov/medlineplus/highbloodpressure.html**
The **Medline Plus** website has links to a wealth of information on blood pressure, including overviews, diagnosis, treatment, symptoms, prevention, screening, diagrams, health check tools, nutrition, and organizations.

**http://www.bhf.org.uk/heart-health/conditions/high-blood-pressure.aspx**
The **British Heart Foundation** website has information for patients on what blood pressure reading numbers mean, and what causes high blood pressure.

**http://www.diabetes.org**
The **American Diabetes Association** website can be used to access information on topics such as metabolic syndrome and hypertension in diabetics. Type the topic of interest in the "Search" box on the website.

**http://www.fi.edu/learn/heart/healthy/pressure.html**
The **Franklin Institute Online** website has information on high blood pressure.

**http://health.nih.gov/topic/HighBloodPressure**
This link provides information on high blood pressure from the **National Institutes of Health**.

## REFERENCES

1. Al-Zahrani MS. Prehypertension and undiagnosed hypertension in a sample of dental school female patients. *Int J Dent Hyg*. 2011;9(1):74–78.

2. Herman WW, Konzelman JL Jr, Prisant LM. New national guidelines on hypertension: a summary for dentistry. *J Am Dent Assoc*. 2004;135(5):576–584; quiz 653–654.

3. The fourth report on the diagnosis, evaluation, and treatment of high blood pressure in children and adolescents. *Pediatrics*. 2004;114(2 Suppl 4th Report):555–576.

4. Williams B, Poulter NR, Brown MJ, et al. British Hypertension Society guidelines for hypertension management 2004 (BHS-IV): summary. *BMJ*. 2004;328(7440):634–640.

5. Ramsay L, Williams B, Johnston G, et al. Guidelines for management of hypertension: report of the third working party of the British Hypertension Society. *J Hypertens*. 1999;13(9):569–592.

6. Ramsay LE, Williams B, Johnston GD, et al. British Hypertension Society guidelines for hypertension management 1999: summary. *BMJ*. 1999;319(7210):630–635.

7. Angelopoulos PD, Milionis HJ, Moschonis G, et al. Relations between obesity and hypertension: preliminary data from a cross-sectional study in primary schoolchildren: the children study. *Eur J Clin Nutr*. 2006;60(10):1226–1234.

8. Boyd GS, Koenigsberg J, Falkner B, et al. Effect of obesity and high blood pressure on plasma lipid levels in children and adolescents. *Pediatrics*. 2005;116(2):442–446.

9. Falkner B, Gidding SS, Ramirez-Garnica G, et al. The relationship of body mass index and blood pressure in primary care pediatric patients. *J Pediatr*. 2006;148(2):195–200.

10. Manzoli L, Ripari P, Rotolo S, et al. Prevalence of obesity, overweight and hypertension in children and adolescents from Abruzzo, Italy. *Ann Ig*. 2005;17(5):419–431.

11. Sorof JM, Turner J, Martin DS, et al. Cardiovascular risk factors and sequelae in hypertensive children identified by referral versus school-based screening. *Hypertension*. 2004;43(2):214–218.

12. Denney-Wilson E, Hardy LL, Dobbins T, et al. Body mass index, waist circumference, and chronic disease risk factors in Australian adolescents. *Arch Pediatr Adolesc Med*. 2008;162(6):566–573.

13. Urbina EM, Kimball TR, McCoy CE, et al. Youth with obesity and obesity-related type 2 diabetes mellitus demonstrate abnormalities in carotid structure and function. *Circulation*. 2009;119(22):2913–2919.

14. Levey AS, Rocco MV, Anderson S, et al. Kidney Disease Outcomes Quality Initiative (K/DOQI) clinical practice guidelines on hypertension and antihypertensive agents in chronic kidney disease. *Am J Kidney Dis*. 2004;43(5 Suppl 1):S1–S290.

15. Muntner P, He J, Cutler JA, et al. Trends in blood pressure among children and adolescents. *JAMA*. 2004;291(17):2107–2113.

16. Perloff D, Grim C, Flack J, et al. Human blood pressure determination by sphygmomanometry. *Circulation*. 1993;88(5 Pt 1):2460–2470.

17. McAlister FA, Straus SE. Evidence based treatment of hypertension. Measurement of blood pressure: an evidence based review. *BMJ*. 2001;322(7291):908–911.

18. Canzanello VJ, Jensen PL, Schwartz GL. Are aneroid sphygmomanometers accurate in hospital and clinic settings? *Arch Intern Med*. 2001;161(5):729–731.

19. Waugh JJ, Gupta M, Rushbrook J, et al. Hidden errors of aneroid sphygmomanometers. *Blood Press Monit*. 2002;7(6):309–312.

20. O'Brien E, Asmar R, Beilin L, et al. European Society of Hypertension recommendations for conventional, ambulatory and home blood pressure measurement. *J Hypertens*. 2003;21(5):821–848.

21. Gourdeau M, Martin R, Lamarche Y, et al. Oscillometry and direct blood pressure: a comparative clinical study during deliberate hypotension. *Can Anaesth Soc J*. 1986;33(3 Pt 1):300–307.

22. Kaufmann MA, Pargger H, Drop LJ. Oscillometric blood pressure measurements by different devices are not interchangeable. *Anesth Analg*. 1996;82(2):377–381.

23. Chobanian AV, Bakris GL, Black HR, et al. The seventh report of the Joint National Committee on prevention, detection, evaluation, and treatment of high blood pressure: the JNC 7 report. *JAMA*. 2003;289(19):2560–2572.

24. Chobanian AV, Bakris GL, Black HR, et al. Seventh report of the Joint National Committee on prevention, detection, evaluation, and treatment of high blood pressure. *Hypertension*. 2003;42(6):1206–1252.

25. Cuddy ML. Treatment of hypertension: guidelines from JNC 7 (the seventh report of the Joint National Committee on prevention, detection, evaluation, and treatment of high blood pressure 1). *J Pract Nurs*. 2005;55(4):17–21; quiz 2–3.

26. Lewington S, Clarke R, Qizilbash N, et al. Age-specific relevance of usual blood pressure to vascular mortality: a meta-analysis of individual data for one million adults in 61 prospective studies. *Lancet*. 2002;360(9349):1903–1913.

27. O'Brien E, Fitzgerald D. The history of blood pressure measurement. *J Hypertens*. 1994;8(2):73–84.

28. Mancia G, Zanchetti A. One hundred years of auscultatory blood pressure: commemorating N. S. Korotkoff. *J Hypertens*. 2005;23(1):1–2.

29. Multanovsky MP. The Korotkov's method. History of its discovery and clinical and experimental interpretation, and contemporary appraisal of its merits. *Cor Vasa*. 1970;12(1):1–7.

30. Askey JM. The auscultatory gap in sphygmomanometry. *Ann Intern Med*. 1974;80(1):94–97.

31. Gerin W, Ogedegbe G, Schwartz JE, et al. Assessment of the white-coat effect. *J Hypertens*. 2006;24(1):67–74.

32. Pickering TG, Gerin W, Schwartz AR. What is the white-coat effect and how should it be measured? *Blood Press Monit*. 2002;7(6):293–300.

33. Pickering TG, James GD, Boddie C, et al. How common is white coat hypertension? *JAMA*. 1988;259(2):225–228.

34. Verdecchia P, O'Brien E, Pickering T, et al. When can the practicing physician suspect white coat hypertension? Statement from the Working Group on Blood Pressure Monitoring of the European Society of Hypertension. *Am J Hypertens*. 2003;16(1):87–91.

35. National Clinical Guideline Centre. *Hypertension. The Clinical Management of Primary Hypertension in Adults*. London, United Kingdom: The National Clinical Guideline Centre at The Royal College of Physicians; 2011.

36. Beevers G, Lip GY, O'Brien E. ABC of hypertension: blood pressure measurement. Part II-conventional sphygmomanometry: technique of auscultatory blood pressure measurement. *BMJ*. 2001;322(7293):1043–1047.

37. Beevers G, Lip GY, O'Brien E. ABC of hypertension. Blood pressure measurement. Part I-sphygmomanometry: factors common to all techniques. *BMJ*. 2001;322(7292):981–985.

38. Hackam DG, Khan NA, Hemmelgarn BR, et al. The 2010 Canadian Hypertension Education Program recommendations for the management of hypertension: part 2—therapy. *Can J Cardiol*. 2010;26(5):249–258.

39. Hemmelgarn BR, Zarnke KB, Campbell NR, et al. The 2004 Canadian Hypertension Education Program recommendations for the management of hypertension: Part I—blood pressure measurement, diagnosis and assessment of risk. *Can J Cardiol*. 2004;20(1):31–40.

40. Gomez-Marin O, Prineas RJ, Rastam L. Cuff bladder width and blood pressure measurement in children and adolescents. *J Hypertens*. 1992;10(10):1235–1241.

41. Prineas RJ. Measurement of blood pressure in the obese. *Ann Epidemiol*. 1991;1(4):321–336.

42. Sprafka JM, Strickland D, Gomez-Marin O, et al. The effect of cuff size on blood pressure measurement in adults. *Epidemiology*. 1991;2(3):214–217.

43. O'Brien E. Review: a century of confusion; which bladder for accurate blood pressure measurement? *J Hypertens*. 1996;10(9):565–572.

44. Mourad A, Carney S. Arm position and blood pressure: an audit. *Intern Med J*. 2004;34(5):290–291.

45. Netea RT, Lenders JW, Smits P, et al. Both body and arm position significantly influence blood pressure measurement. *J Hypertens*. 2003;17(7):459–462.

46. Netea RT, Lenders JW, Smits P, et al. Influence of body and arm position on blood pressure readings: an overview. *J Hypertens*. 2003;21(2):237–241.

47. Keele-Smith R, Price-Daniel C. Effects of crossing legs on blood pressure measurement. *Clin Nurs Res*. 2001;10(2):202–213.

48. Glick M. The new blood pressure guidelines: a digest. *J Am Dent Assoc*. 2004;135(5):585–586.

49. Kaelber DC, Pickett F. Simple table to identify children and adolescents needing further evaluation of blood pressure. *Pediatrics*. 2009;123(6):e972–e974.

50. Glick M. The new blood pressure guidelines: a digest. *J Am Dent Assoc*. 2004;135(5):585–586.

## SECTION 7:

# The Human Element

---

**BOX 9-9**   **Through the Eyes of a Student:
The Importance of Vital Sign Assessment**

*Just a few weeks ago, I saw Mrs. P., an 81-year-old patient, for her fourth appointment. Mrs. P. is under the care of a physician for blood pressure control and reported taking Toporol 25 mg/day and Prevacid. She had recently been taken off of potassium and had a recent history of low blood pressure. Her blood pressure was 132/92 mm Hg. I double-checked the blood pressure reading to make sure it was accurate. I was a bit concerned about these readings since her blood pressure had ranged from 118/80 mm Hg to 122/78 mm Hg on her other three visits. I asked Mrs. P. how she has been feeling, and she said that she was having a feeling of pressure in her chest. I discussed the blood pressure reading and her symptoms with the dentist. The dentist consulted with her physician who requested that EMS transport her to the hospital.*

*On the way to the hospital, Mrs. P. fainted in the ambulance. Medical tests showed that she had a 96% blockage in one carotid artery and 60% blockage in the other. This experience taught me that it really is important to take vital signs seriously. It is also important to check today's readings with prior readings to look for changes.*

*Charles, student,
Catawba Valley Community College*

---

### PATIENT SCENARIO

Mr. Lester Evans, one of your favorite patients, is scheduled with you at 11:00 for his 4-month recall appointment. Mr. Evans has been a patient in the practice for approximately 10 years. As you seat him in your chair, he tells you that he is leaving his present job and will be starting new employment next week. He wants to make sure that you can complete all of his treatments today because he will not have any time off in the near future.

You take Mr. Evans' vital signs prior to beginning treatment and record his blood pressure as 195/110 mm Hg. His other vital signs are within normal limits. You ask him how he is feeling, and he states that he feels fine. You wait 5 minutes, chatting casually with him, before you repeat his blood pressure assessment. His second reading is 190/110.

1. How should you proceed with Mr. Evans's appointment today?
2. What recommendations can you suggest for Mr. Evans?
3. What treatment modifications can you employ for Mr. Evans' future dental treatment?
4. Because Mr. Evans' schedule is tight, is it appropriate to treat him today and address his blood pressure issue at his next visit? Why or why not?

**Table 9-2** ENGLISH-TO-SPANISH PHRASE LIST FOR BLOOD PRESSURE ASSESSMENT

| | |
|---|---|
| How are you feeling today? | ¿Como se siente hoy? |
| Do you smoke?<br>How many minutes has it been since you smoked a cigarette, cigar, or pipe? | ¿Usted fuma?<br>¿Cuanto tiempo ha pasado desde la última vez que fumó? |
| Did you drink coffee or alcohol before coming here today?<br>About how long ago was that? | ¿Antes de su cita hoy, bebió usted café o alcohol?<br>¿Hace cuanto tiempo? |
| Have you been exercising? | ¿Usted ha estado asiendo ejercicio? |
| I am going to take your blood pressure. | Voy a tomar su presión. |
| Your blood pressure is a clue to the health of your heart and blood vessels. | La presión es una indicación al estado del corazón y de las venas. |
| Have you had your blood pressure taken before? | ¿Le han tomado la presión antes? |
| I am going to pump air into this cuff to take your blood pressure. The cuff will squeeze your arm quite tightly as I pump it up. Then I will begin to release the air from the cuff and you will be more comfortable. | Yo voy ha bombear aire dentro de este cuño de presión, y el cuño apretara su brazo. En un minuto empezaré a dejar que el aire se escape del cuño, y usted estará mas cómodo. |
| Do you have any questions? | ¿Usted tiene alguna pregunta? |
| Would you please roll up your sleeve? | Por favor suba su manga. |
| Please turn your arm over with the palm facing up. | Por favor gire su brazo con la palma arriba. |
| Just relax; this will only take a few minutes. | ¡Tranquilízate! Esto tomará sólo unos minutos. |
| Please remain still and do not talk while I take your blood pressure. | Por favor quédese quieto mientras que tomo su presión. |
| Just relax your arm and hand; let me support your arm for you. | Relajar el brazo y la mano, y déjame soportar el brazo. |
| I will need to take your blood pressure reading again. | Necesito tomar su presión otra vez. |
| Please raise your arm up like this for a few seconds. | Suba su brazo arriba así por unos segundos. |
| Your blood pressure reading is: (Write reading on piece of paper and show to patient.) | Su presión es: |
| This is a normal blood pressure reading. | Su presión está normal. |
| This reading is just a bit higher than recommended. | Su presión está un poco mas alta que se recomenda. |
| This reading is higher than recommended. | Su presión es mas alta que se recomenda. |

*(continued)*

**Table 9-2    ENGLISH-TO-SPANISH PHRASE LIST FOR BLOOD PRESSURE ASSESSMENT** *(CONTINUED)*

| | |
|---|---|
| This reading is higher than it was when you were here before. | Su presión esta mas alta que la ultima vez que usted estaba aquí. |
| Do you know what your blood pressure is usually? | ¿Usted sabe cual es su presión normalmente? |
| Because your blood pressure is a bit higher than ideal, I would recommend that you see your regular doctor and ask him or her to check it. | Porque su presión es un poco mas alta que normal, le recomendo que vaya a ver su medico y le pida que le investigue. |
| I am concerned that your blood pressure is high today. We will not be able to do any dental treatment today. Please make an appointment with your physician as soon as possible. I will need your physician to sign this form before we can schedule your next dental appointment. | Estoy preocupada que su presión esta alta. No vamos hacer ningún tratamiento hoy. Por favor haga una cita con su medico lo mas pronto posible para investigar, y que él llene y firme esta forma. Esta forma es necesaria para hacer una nueva cita para tratamiento dental. |
| Yes, we record everything on a computer now. It is secure, only my clinic instructor and I can see your record. | Su expediente dental está en forma electrónica, pero está protegido. Nadie excepto el instructor(a) clínico y yo puede ver su expediente dental. |
| Are you nervous about the dental treatment today? | ¿Está nervioso sobre su tratamiento dental hoy? |
| I am going to get my clinic instructor. | Voy ha buscar a mi instructor(a) clínico. |

## SECTION 8:
# Practical Focus—Fictitious Patient Cases

---

**DIRECTIONS:**

- The fictitious patient cases in this module involve patients A–E. In a clinical setting, you will gather additional information about your patient with each assessment procedure that you perform. In a similar manner, you will learn additional assessment findings for patients A–E in Modules 10–14.

- In answering the case questions in this module, you should take into account the health history and over-the-counter/prescription drug information that was revealed for each patient in Module 4, Medical History.

---

**FICTITIOUS PATIENT CASE A: Mr. Alan Ascari**

**Synopsis of Information about Mr. Ascari**

Mr. Ascari is a new patient in the dental office. You notice that Mr. Ascari seems to be slightly impatient. As you count his pulse rate, he suddenly removes the thermometer from his mouth and says, "I have had enough of this! First, you ask me all those questions about my health and now, this. I just came in to have my teeth checked, not for a medical exam! Can't you just check my teeth and get it over with?"

---

### Vital Signs

Name _Alan Ascari_         Date _1/15/XX_

Temperature _98.4°F (36.9°C)_     Pulse _____

Respiratory Rate _____     Blood Pressure _____

Tobacco Use:     ☐ Never          ☐ Former

☒ Cigarettes _2_ packs/day     ☐ Pipe     ☒ Smokeless tobacco

---

**Case Questions for Mr. Ascari**

1. How do you think Mr. Ascari is feeling or thinking concerning the health history and vital signs assessment? Why might he feel this way?
2. How would you respond to Mr. Ascari's comments? How would you phrase your response to him?
3. Do you think that it is important to complete the vital signs assessment on Mr. Ascari before proceeding with treatment? Or could you skip this procedure just this once because he is a new patient in the office?

## FICTITIOUS PATIENT CASE B: Bethany Biddle

### Synopsis of Information about Bethany Biddle

Bethany Biddle is a physically active 9-year-old who has been a patient in the dental office since she was 3 years old. Bethany enjoys coming to have her teeth cleaned. She is interested in dental hygiene and always asks a lot of questions about the care that dental hygienists provide.

Bethany hurried into the office 10 minutes late for her appointment. She tells you that her mother was late picking her up at school. Concerned about being late, she ran from the parking lot to the dental office. Remembering that it is 90°F outside, you can understand why she is perspiring and slightly out of breath. Worried about falling behind schedule, you quickly take Bethany's vital signs.

---

### Vital Signs

Name _Bethany Biddle_    Date _1/0/XX_

Temperature _100°F (37.8°C)_    Pulse _112_

Respiratory Rate _36_    Blood Pressure _102/64_

Tobacco Use:    ☒ Never    ☐ Former

☐ Cigarettes ___ packs/day    ☐ Pipe    ☐ Smokeless tobacco

---

### Case Questions for Bethany Biddle

1. At her last four appointments, Bethany's vital signs were all within normal ranges. Identify possible interpretations of Bethany's vital signs at today's appointment. Are you concerned about these findings and what, if any, action would you take?
2. Is there anything about the way in which the vital signs assessment was conducted that could have had an impact on the findings?
3. How would you determine if dental treatment is contraindicated for Bethany? If so, what words would you use to explain the contraindications to Bethany?
4. What will you do next?

FICTITIOUS PATIENT CASE C: Mr. Carlos Chavez

Synopsis of Information about Mr. Chavez

---

## Vital Signs

Name _Carlos Chavez_          Date _1/05/XX_

Temperature _98.6°F (37°C)_          Pulse _100_

Respiratory Rate _20_          Blood Pressure _190/110_

Tobacco Use:    ☒ Never          ☐ Former

☐ Cigarettes ___packs/day    ☐ Pipe    ☐ Smokeless tobacco

---

Case Questions for Mr. Chavez

1. Does Mr. Chavez have any contraindications for dental treatment? If so, what are your concerns?
2. What information would you provide to Mr. Chavez about his vital signs readings? How would you phrase your explanation?
3. After discussing his vital signs, what would you do next?

## FICTITIOUS PATIENT CASE D: Mrs. Donna Doi

### Synopsis of Information about Mrs. Doi

As you seat Mrs. Doi in the dental chair, she tells you that she is grateful for an excuse to get out of the house today. Her 6-year-old daughter, Melanie, has been home sick with a high fever and "strep throat" for the last several days.

---

### Vital Signs

Name _Donna Doi_                    Date _1/30/XX_

Temperature _101.0°F (38.3°C)_      Pulse _80_

Respiratory Rate _15_               Blood Pressure _120/76_

Tobacco Use:   ☒ Never        ☐ Former

   ☐ Cigarettes __packs/day    ☐ Pipe    ☐ Smokeless tobacco

---

### Case Questions for Mrs. Doi

1. Are Mrs. Doi's vital signs within normal ranges?
2. What information would you give Mrs. Doi about her vital signs? How would you phrase your explanation?
3. You note that Mrs. Doi's temperature has been 97.7°F at her last three visits. When you inquire how she is feeling today, she replies, "I was very tired this morning and my throat feels dry and scratchy." Are you concerned about Mrs. Doi's elevated temperature reading? Can you think of any possible causes for her elevated temperature?
4. What will you do next?
5. Does Mrs. Doi have any contraindications for dental treatment? If so, what words would you use to explain these contraindications to Mrs. Doi?

**FICTITIOUS PATIENT CASE E: Ms. Esther Eads**

**Synopsis of Information about Ms. Eads**

Ms. Eads has been a patient in the dental practice for 30 years; she is 79 years of age. Ms. Eads is a retired teacher and is still very active for her age. She enjoys taking day trips with the seniors group at her church. Ms. Eads is here today for a routine checkup.

---

### Vital Signs

Name _Esther Eads_   Date _1/24/XX_

Temperature _95.8°F (37.8°C)_   Pulse _50_

Respiratory Rate _15_   Blood Pressure _118/78_

Tobacco Use:   ☐ Never   ☒ Former

☐ Cigarettes ___packs/day   ☐ Pipe   ☐ Smokeless tobacco

---

**Case Questions for Ms. Eads**

1. Are all of Ms. Eads' vital signs within normal range? What information would you use in determining if her findings today are normal for her?
2. Does Ms. Eads have any contraindications for dental treatment? If so, what words would you use in explaining the contraindications to Ms. Eads?

**SECTION 9:**

# Skill Check

BLOOD PRESSURE ASSESSMENT

Student: _____  Evaluator: _____

Date: _____

**DIRECTIONS FOR STUDENT CLINICIAN:** Use **Column S**; evaluate your skill level as **S** (satisfactory) or **U** (unsatisfactory).

**DIRECTIONS FOR EVALUATOR:** Use **Column E**. Indicate **S** (satisfactory) or **U** (unsatisfactory). In the optional grade percentage calculation, each **S** equals 1 point, and each **U** equals 0 points.

| CRITERIA | S | E |
|---|---|---|
| **Determines that the patient has not had alcohol, tobacco, caffeine, or performed vigorous exercise within 30 minutes of the blood pressure assessment. After seating patient, allows the patient to relax for at least 5 minutes prior to assessment.** | | |
| **Selects an appropriate arm—no breast cancer surgery involving lymph node removal, cast, injured limb, or other compromising factor.** | | |
| **Squeezes the bladder to completely deflate the cuff. Selects a cuff with an appropriate bladder width and length matched to the size of the patient's upper arm.** | | |
| **Asks patient to roll up sleeve. Determines that rolling up the sleeve does not create a tight roll of cloth around the upper arm.** | | |
| **Asks patient to position arm with the palm of the hand upward.** | | |
| **Positions the cuff with the lower edge 1–2 in (2–3 cm) above the elbow with the midline of the bladder centered over the brachial artery. Wraps the cuff smoothly and snugly around the arm and fastens it securely.** | | |
| **Places the manometer so that the mercury column or aneroid dial is easily visible and the tubing from the cuff is unobstructed.** | | |
| **Places the stethoscope earpieces into the ear canals with the earpieces angled forward.** | | |
| **Supports the patient's arm by holding it at the elbow so that the antecubital fossa is level with the patient's mid-sternum. The patient's arm should remain somewhat bent and completely relaxed.** | | |

*(continued)*

## TECHNIQUE SKILL CHECKLIST: BLOOD PRESSURE ASSESSMENT *(CONTINUED)*

| CRITERIA | S | E |
|---|---|---|
| Palpates the brachial pulse with the fingertips. Closes the valve. Inflates the cuff rapidly to 70 mm Hg and then increases the pressure by increments of 10 mm Hg until the pulse disappears. Notes the pressure reading where the pulse disappears. | | |
| Opens the valve, deflates the cuff rapidly, leaving it in place on the arm, and waits 15 seconds. | | |
| Gently places the amplifying device over the pulse—just above the antecubital fossa toward the inner aspect of the arm. Holds the device in place, making sure that it makes contact with the skin around its entire circumference. | | |
| Closes the valve and holds the bulb so that it is easy to reach the valve at the top. Briskly squeezes the bulb to rapidly inflate the bladder to a pressure 30 mm Hg above the palpatory estimate. | | |
| Opens the valve so that the pressure drops no faster than 2 mm per second. | | |
| Pays careful attention to sounds heard through the stethoscope. Notes the point at which the first clear tapping sound occurs. | | |
| Continues releasing the pressure slowly at a rate of 2 mm per second. Notes the point at which the sounds disappear. | | |
| Continues releasing the pressure slowly at a rate of 2 mm per second for at least another 10 mm Hg. Then allows the remaining air to escape rapidly. | | |
| Records the two numbers as a fraction—systolic over diastolic—to the closest 2 mm. Records the arm and the patient's position. Records the auscultatory gap, if present. | | |
| Obtains a systolic reading within +/−2 mm of the evaluator's reading. Obtains a diastolic reading within +/−2 of the evaluator's reading. | | |
| Removes the cuff. Cleans and stores the equipment so that it is ready for use. | | |

**OPTIONAL GRADE PERCENTAGE CALCULATION**

Using the entries in the **E** column, assign a point value of 1 for each **S** and 0 for each **U**. Add the total assigned as 1's _____ and divide by 20 to arrive at the percentage grade. _____

## COMMUNICATION SKILL CHECKLIST: ROLE-PLAY FOR BLOOD PRESSURE

Student: _____   Evaluator: _____

Date: _____

> **Roles:**
> - Student 1 = Plays the role of the patient.
> - Student 2 = Plays the role of the clinician.
> - Student 3 or instructor = Plays the role of the clinic instructor near the end of the role-play.

**DIRECTIONS FOR STUDENT CLINICIAN:** Use **Column S**; evaluate your skill level as **S** (satisfactory) or **U** (unsatisfactory).

**DIRECTIONS FOR EVALUATOR:** Use **Column E**. Indicate **S** (satisfactory) or **U** (unsatisfactory). In the optional grade percentage calculation, each **S** equals 1 point, and each **U** equals 0 points.

| CRITERIA | S | E |
|---|---|---|
| **Explains the blood pressure procedure. If the patient has never had a blood pressure assessment, explains that some minor discomfort is caused by the inflation of the cuff.** | | |
| **Upon completion of the procedure, reports the findings to the patient and explains whether the readings are normal or outside the normal range and the significance of these readings.** | | |
| **Encourages patient questions before and after the blood pressure assessment.** | | |
| **Answers the patient's questions fully and accurately.** | | |
| **Gains the patient's trust and cooperation.** | | |
| **Communicates with the patient at an appropriate level and avoids dental/medical terminology or jargon.** | | |
| **Accurately communicates the findings to the clinical instructor. Discusses the implications for dental treatment. Uses correct medical and dental terminology.** | | |

OPTIONAL GRADE PERCENTAGE CALCULATION

Using the entries in the **E** column, assign a point value of 1 for each **S** and 0 for each **U**. Add the total assigned as 1's _____ and divide by 7 to arrive at the percentage grade. _____

MODULE

# 10

# Tobacco Cessation Counseling

## MODULE OVERVIEW

Consumer survey data collected by the American Dental Association (ADA) shows that half of all smokers visit the dentist annually. A full 75% of these smokers indicate a willingness to hear advice on quitting from dental health care providers. In a 1992 policy statement, the ADA urged dental health care providers to become fully informed about tobacco cessation intervention techniques and educate their patients in methods for overcoming tobacco addiction.

This module is designed to assist dental health care providers in improving their knowledge of tobacco cessation techniques and resources, including:

- Understanding the health risks of tobacco use
- Understanding the health benefits of not using tobacco
- Providing tobacco cessation counseling

## MODULE OUTLINE

## OBJECTIVES

- Explain why tobacco cessation counseling is a valuable part of patient care in the dental setting.
- Value the importance of providing tobacco cessation counseling as a routine part of the dental hygiene appointment.
- Explain a strategy for providing tobacco cessation counseling as a routine part of the dental hygiene appointment.
- Give examples of diseases associated with or linked to tobacco use.
- Give examples of oral diseases and conditions associated with tobacco use.
- Differentiate which components of tobacco/cigarette smoke are (1) addicting and (2) carcinogenic.
- Discuss the hazards of secondhand smoke.
- Identify U.S. Food and Drug Administration (FDA)–approved pharmacotherapies for smoking cessation.
- Explain how to use the American Dental Hygienists Association's "Ask. Advise. Refer." (AAR) program to encourage tobacco cessation.
- Demonstrate knowledge of tobacco cessation counseling by applying information from this module to the fictitious patient case and the communication skills role-play at the end of this module.

## SECTION 1:
# Health Effects of Tobacco Use

### SMOKING: THE FIFTH VITAL SIGN

In addition to the standard vital signs—temperature, pulse, respiration, and blood pressure—tobacco use has been suggested as the fifth vital sign.

- Tobacco use is a contributing factor in many medical conditions and, in addition, increases the risk of periodontal disease. All oral health care professionals should be concerned with their patients' use of tobacco products.
- About 30% of patients in any given dental practice are current smokers.
- The regularly scheduled dental hygiene visit provides a unique opportunity to document tobacco use (Fig. 10-1), relate oral health findings to a patient's use of tobacco, and provide cessation support.

```
                              Vital Signs

        Name_____    Date_____

        Temperature_____    Pulse_____

        Respiratory Rate_____    Blood Pressure_____

        Tobacco Use:    ☐ Never        ☐ Former

                 ☐ Cigarettes ___packs/day   ☐ Pipe   ☐ Smokeless tobacco
```

**Figure 10-1.    Vital signs box.** Tobacco use should be regarded as the fifth vital sign and noted in the patient chart.

### TOBACCO: THE LEADING PREVENTABLE CAUSE OF ILLNESS AND DEATH

Scientific knowledge about the health effects of tobacco use has increased greatly since the first Surgeon General's report published in 1964. Smoking increases the risks of numerous diseases and associated illness and death. In general, smokers have a mortality rate approximately twice that of nonsmokers. Extensive evidence links smoking to cancer, cardiopulmonary disease, and complications of pregnancy.

*Tobacco use has long been identified as the leading preventable cause of illness and death; a fact established by the most substantial body of scientific knowledge ever amassed linking a product to disease.*

- Tobacco claims one life every 8 seconds and kills 1 of 10 adults globally.
- In the United States alone, cigarette use accounts for 1 of every 5 deaths and is responsible for more than 443,000 deaths each year (Fig. 10-2).[1]
- In Canada, more than 37,000 deaths per year are due to smoking (22% of all deaths).
- Smoking causes more deaths alone than AIDS, alcohol, accidents, suicides, homicides, fires, and drugs combined.
- Worldwide, 5 million people die each year from tobacco use. That number has been projected to double by 2020, with more than 70% of those deaths occurring in developing nations.[2]

Average Annual Number of Deaths in the U.S.
Attributable to Cigarette Smoking, 1997-2001

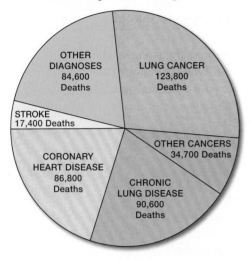

**Figure 10-2. Annual deaths attributable to cigarette smoking.** Source: Centers for Disease Control and Prevention. Annual smoking-attributable mortality, years of potential life lost, and productivity losses—United States, 1997–2001. *MMWR Morb Mortal Wkly Rep.* 2005;54(25):625–628.

## TOBACCO USE AS A RISK FACTOR FOR SYSTEMIC DISEASE

**Risk factors** are conditions that increase a person's chances of getting a disease (such as cancer). There is no doubt that the risk for smoking-related disease increases with the amount a person smokes. However, smoking one to four cigarettes per day is associated with a significantly higher risk of prematurely dying.[3] Cigar use causes cancer of the larynx, mouth, esophagus, and lung; emphysema; and heart disease. The bottom line is that smoking any amount harms nearly every organ of the body, damaging a smoker's overall health even when it does not cause a specific illness (Fig. 10-3A).

### Cancer

Smoking is a known cause of multiple cancers, accounting for 25% to 30% of all cases of cancer and approximately 170,000 cancer deaths every year in the United States.[4]

- The types of cancer associated with tobacco use include those that affect the lung, mouth, nasal passages/nose, larynx, pharynx, breast, esophagus, stomach, pancreas, bladder, kidney, cervix, and possibly the colon and rectum, in addition to acute myelogenous leukemia.
- In particular, smoking has been linked to 90% of cases of lung cancer in males and 78% in females.[5]

### Cardiovascular and Lung Disease

In addition, smoking is a known cause of at least 25% of all heart disease and strokes and no less than 90% of all chronic obstructive pulmonary disease (COPD). Smoking is a major cause of coronary artery disease (CAD), cerebrovascular disease (stroke), peripheral vascular disease (PVD), and abdominal aortic aneurysm.

- **Smoker's cough** is the chronic cough experienced by smokers because smoking impairs the lung's ability to clean out harmful material. Coughing is the body's way of trying to get rid of the harmful material in the lungs.
- **COPD** is a lung disease in which the airways in the lungs produce excess mucus resulting in frequent coughing. Smoking accounts for 80% to 90% of the risk for developing COPD. Only 5% to 10% of patients with COPD have never smoked.
- **CAD**—a thickening of the coronary arteries—is the most common type of heart disease. CAD results in a narrowing of the arteries so that the supply of blood

and oxygen to the heart is restricted or blocked. Smoking is the major risk factor for CAD.

- **PVD** occurs when fat and cholesterol build up on the walls of the arteries, blocking the supply of blood to the arms and legs.
- **Abdominal aortic aneurysm** occurs when part of the aorta—the main artery of the body—becomes weakened. If left untreated, the aorta can burst. Once thought of as an "old man's disease," this disorder has become a major killer in women as well. The disease kills 120,000 Americans per year, is the fourth leading cause of death, and is expected to be the third leading cause of death by 2020.[5]

## Health Risks for Female Smokers

Smoking during pregnancy causes spontaneous miscarriages, low birth weight, placental abruption, fetal heart defects, and sudden infant death syndrome (SIDS). Babies born to women who smoke are more likely to be premature. Women, particularly those older than 35 years of age who smoke and use birth control pills, face an increased risk for heart attack, stroke, and venous thromboembolism.

## Other Conditions

Other conditions that affect smokers include cataracts, macular degeneration, damage to skin, poor dental health, low bone density, early menopause, gastroespohageal reflux, high blood pressure, type 2 diabetes, psoriasis, erectile dysfunction, infertility, and fire-related injury or death.

## Head and Neck Cancer

Smoking also significantly increases the risk for head and neck cancers (more than 500,000 people are diagnosed with these cancers every year). In general, individuals who smoke one pack per day increase their head and neck cancer risk 10-fold, and individuals who smoke two packs per day increase their risk to 25 times that of a nonsmoker.[4]

## MEDICAL HEALTH RISKS OF SECONDHAND SMOKE

**Secondhand smoke** is the term for tobacco smoke that is exhaled by smokers or is produced by a lit cigarette, pipe, or cigar. Secondhand smoke contains the same harmful chemicals that smokers inhale and presents a substantial health risk to nonsmokers (Fig. 10-3B). A 2006 report of the U.S. Surgeon General states that

> "There is no risk-free level of exposure to secondhand smoke. Nonsmokers exposed to secondhand smoke at home or work increase their risk of developing heart disease by 25 to 30 percent and lung cancer by 20 to 30 percent. The finding is of major public health concern due to the fact that nearly half of all nonsmoking Americans are still regularly exposed to secondhand smoke."

## Adult Nonsmokers

- Secondhand smoke exposure is linked to an increase in certain types of cancer among nonsmokers. There are clear associations between secondhand smoke and cancers of the nasal sinus, cervix, breast, and bladder.
- Those exposed to secondhand smoke are at increased risk for cardiopulmonary problems, including decreased lung function, chronic cough, and ischemic heart disease. As many as 60,000 annual heart disease deaths in adult nonsmokers result from secondhand smoke in the United States. Approximately 3,400 lung

cancer deaths per year among adult nonsmokers in the United States are linked to secondhand smoke.[1] In Canada, more than 300 nonsmokers die of lung cancer and at least 700 nonsmokers die of coronary heart disease caused by exposure to secondhand smoke each year.[4]

## Children and Infants

- Exposed children are more likely to have reduced lung capacity, serious lower respiratory tract infections, severe asthma, and middle ear infections.
- The risk for SIDS is higher among babies exposed to smoke, and babies born to women exposed to secondhand smoke are more likely to have low birth weight and to be premature.
- There is a clear link between childhood tooth decay and parental smoking.[6]

## Companion Animals

- Cigarette smoke can cause cancer in dogs, cats, and other pets. Pets don't just inhale smoke; the smoke particles get trapped in their fur and ingested when they groom themselves.
- Dogs living in smoking households have a 60% greater risk of lung cancer, and longer nosed dogs are twice as likely to develop nasal cancer.
- Cats living in smoking households are three times more likely to develop lymphoma, the most common type of feline cancer.
- In addition, secondhand smoke has been associated with lung cancer in pet birds.

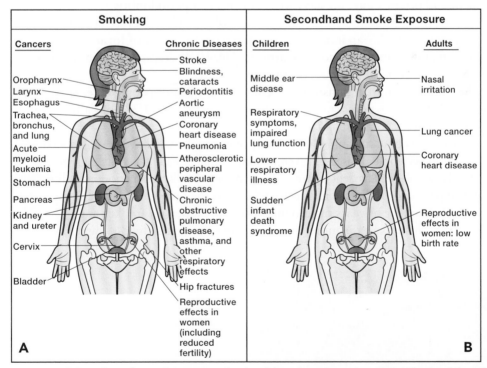

**Figure 10-3.   Health risks of smoking. A.** The health risks of smoking. **B.** The health risks of secondhand smoke exposure. Source: U.S. Dept. of Health & Human Services 2004, 2006. The health consequences of involuntary exposure to tobacco smoke: a report of the Surgeon General. – [Atlanta, Ga.]: U.S. Dept. of Health and Human Services, Centers for Disease Control and Prevention, Coordinating Center for Health Promotion, National Center for Chronic Disease Prevention and Health Promotion, Office on Smoking and Health, [2006]

# HEALTH RISKS TO THE PERIODONTIUM

## The Periodontium

The past effects of smoking on the periodontium, such as bone loss, cannot be reversed; however, smoking cessation is beneficial to the periodontium.

- Several years after quitting, former smokers are no more likely to have periodontal disease than persons who have never smoked. This indicates that quitting seems to gradually erase the harmful effects of tobacco use on periodontal health.
- *Evidence that periodontal health does improve with smoking cessation has led the American Academy of Periodontology to recommend tobacco cessation counseling as an important component of periodontal therapy.*
- Dental hygienists should advise patients of tobacco's negative effects on the periodontium and the benefits of quitting tobacco use. ("As your clinician, I want you to know that quitting smoking is the most important thing you can do to protect your current and future dental health.")

## Smoking and Periodontitis

Smoking appears to be one of the most important risk factors in the development and progression of periodontal disease. Smoking may be responsible for more than half of the cases of periodontal disease among adults in the United States.[4]

- Smokers are 2.6 to 6 times more likely to exhibit periodontal destruction than nonsmokers.[7] Tobacco use is therefore one of the most significant risk factors in the development and progression and successful treatment of periodontitis.
- Smokers are 12 to 14 times more likely than nonsmokers to have severe bone loss.[7]
- Tobacco smoking may play an important role in the development of forms of periodontitis that does not respond to treatment (Fig. 10-4) despite excellent patient compliance and appropriate periodontal therapy.[8]
- Smokers lose more teeth than nonsmokers. Only about 20% of people older than 65 years of age who have never smoked are toothless, whereas 41.3% of daily smokers older than 65 are toothless.
- Current smokers are about four times more likely than people who have never smoked to have advanced periodontal disease.[9] Even in adult smokers with generally high oral hygiene standards and regular dental care habits, smoking accelerates periodontal disease.
- The extent of periodontal disease is directly related to the number of cigarettes smoked and the number of years of smoking. The more a person smokes and the longer a person smokes, the more periodontal disease that individual will have.

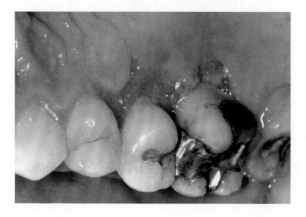

**Figure 10-4. Poor healing after periodontal surgery.** Shown here is a poor healing response to periodontal surgery in a smoker. (Courtesy of Dr. Ralph M. Arnold.)

- Gingival inflammation and gingival bleeding, two of the cardinal signs of periodontal disease, are often reduced or absent in smokers. *For this reason, great care should be taken in performing periodontal screening and examination of smokers. In smokers, the lack of bleeding on probing does not indicate healthy tissue as it does in nonsmokers.*[9]
- Cigarette smoking may be a cofactor in the relationship between periodontal disease and COPD and in the relationship between periodontal disease and coronary heart disease.[9]

## HEALTH RISKS OF SMOKELESS TOBACCO

### Smokeless Tobacco

- **Smokeless tobacco** is tobacco that is not smoked but used in another form. Snuff and chewing tobacco are the two main forms of smokeless tobacco in use in the United States and Canada.
- **Chewing tobacco**—also known as spit tobacco, chew, dip, and chaw—is tobacco cut for chewing.
- **Snuff** is a smokeless tobacco in the form of a powder that is placed between the gingiva and the lip or cheek or inhaled into the nose.
- Smokeless tobacco was formally classified as a "known human carcinogen" by the U.S. Government in 2000. *Smokeless tobacco contains more nicotine than cigarettes.*
- Regular use of smokeless tobacco can cause oral cancers and dental problems, so it should not be used as a substitute for smoking cigarettes. Many people who use smokeless tobacco think it's safer than smoking. However, smokeless tobacco carries many health risks.
  - Gingival recession and decay of exposed root surfaces frequently occurs adjacent to the site of placement of the smokeless tobacco. (Fig. 10-5A)
  - White patches or red sores on the buccal mucosa occur at the site of placement of the smokeless tobacco. (Figs. 10-5B and 10-6)
  - Cancers of the oral cavity (i.e., the mouth, lip, and tongue) have been associated with the use of chewing tobacco as well as snuff. *Studies indicate that the tumors often arise at the site of placement of the tobacco.*
  - Recent research shows the dangers of smokeless tobacco might play a role in cancers of the pancreas, heart disease, and stroke.

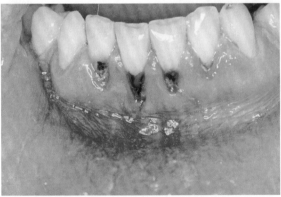 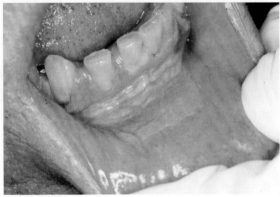

A        B

**Figure 10-5. Oral effects of smokeless tobacco. A.** Gingival recession, red sores, and decayed root surfaces at the site of placement of smokeless tobacco. **B.** A white patch at the site of placement of smokeless tobacco. (Courtesy of Dr. Richard Foster, Guilford Technical Community College, Jamestown, NC.)

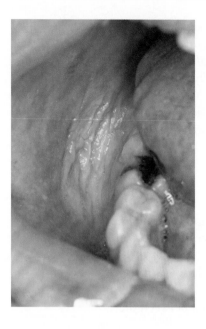

**Figure 10-6.   White patch.** A white patch is evident on the buccal mucosa at the site of placement of smokeless tobacco. (Courtesy of Dr. Richard Foster, Guilford Technical Community College, Jamestown, NC.)

## HEALTH RISKS OF HOOKAH WATER PIPES

A **hookah** is a large water pipe with a hose used to smoke flavored tobacco (Fig. 10-7). A common misconception is that the water in the hookah removes the harmful chemicals from the tobacco smoke. Current research indicates, however, that even after passing through the water, the tobacco smoke still produces high levels of toxins, including carbon monoxide and carcinogens.[10]

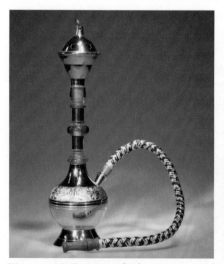
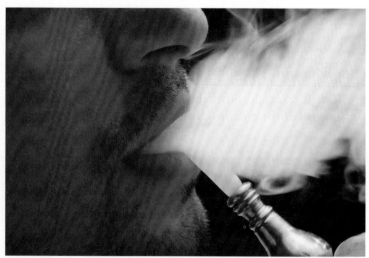

**Figure 10-7.   Hookah.** An example of a hookah water pipe used for smoking flavored tobacco.

**SECTION 2:**
# Harmful Properties of Tobacco

## CHEMICAL COMPONENTS OF TOBACCO PRODUCTS

All tobacco products emit over 7,000 chemicals, 70 of which have been identified as carcinogens (Fig. 10-8).[6] A **carcinogen** is a chemical or other substance that causes cancer.

- The act of burning a cigarette creates the majority of these chemical compounds, many of which are toxic and/or carcinogenic.[10] For example, formaldehyde, benzene, arsenic, ammonia, carbon monoxide, nitrogen oxides, and hydrogen cyanide are all present in cigarette smoke.

- Ironically, low-tar cigarettes often produce higher levels of chemicals like carbon monoxide than regular cigarettes. Also, when smoking a low-tar cigarette, the smoker may inhale more deeply and more often to get the usual amount of nicotine. This is very important because even though nicotine is not a carcinogen, it is the chemical that causes addiction.

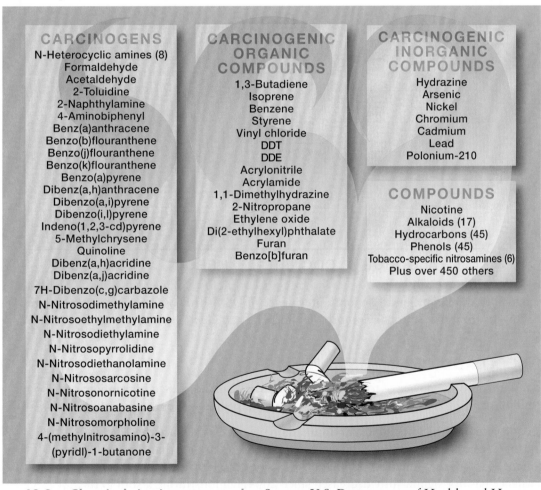

**CARCINOGENS**
N-Heterocyclic amines (8)
Formaldehyde
Acetaldehyde
2-Toluidine
2-Naphthylamine
4-Aminobiphenyl
Benz(a)anthracene
Benzo(b)flouranthene
Benzo(j)flouranthene
Benzo(k)flouranthene
Benzo(a)pyrene
Dibenzo(a,h)anthracene
Dibenzo(a,i)pyrene
Dibenzo(i,l)pyrene
Indeno(1,2,3-cd)pyrene
5-Methylchrysene
Quinoline
Dibenz(a,h)acridine
Dibenz(a,j)acridine
7H-Dibenzo(c,g)carbazole
N-Nitrosodimethylamine
N-Nitrosoethylmethylamine
N-Nitrosodiethylamine
N-Nitrosopyrrolidine
N-Nitrosodiethanolamine
N-Nitrososarcosine
N-Nitrosonornicotine
N-Nitrosoanabasine
N-Nitrosomorpholine
4-(methylnitrosamino)-3-(pyridl)-1-butanone

**CARCINOGENIC ORGANIC COMPOUNDS**
1,3-Butadiene
Isoprene
Benzene
Styrene
Vinyl chloride
DDT
DDE
Acrylonitrile
Acrylamide
1,1-Dimethylhydrazine
2-Nitropropane
Ethylene oxide
Di(2-ethylhexyl)phthalate
Furan
Benzo[b]furan

**CARCINOGENIC INORGANIC COMPOUNDS**
Hydrazine
Arsenic
Nickel
Chromium
Cadmium
Lead
Polonium-210

**COMPOUNDS**
Nicotine
Alkaloids (17)
Hydrocarbons (45)
Phenols (45)
Tobacco-specific nitrosamines (6)
Plus over 450 others

**Figure 10-8. Chemicals in cigarette smoke.** Source: U.S. Department of Health and Human Services. *The Health Consequences of Involuntary Exposure to Tobacco Smoke: A Report of the Surgeon General.* Atlanta, GA: U.S. Department of Health and Human Services, Centers for Disease Control and Prevention, Coordinating Center for Health Promotion, National Center for Chronic Disease Prevention and Health Promotion, Office on Smoking and Health; 2006, pp. 29–45, Table 2.1.

## ADDICTIVE PROPERTIES OF NICOTINE

**Addiction** is a chronic dependence on a substance—such as smoking—despite adverse consequences. The dependence on the substance makes stopping very difficult. All tobacco products contain nicotine. Nicotine is found naturally in tobacco; however, it is classified as an additive because all the tobacco companies increase the amount of nicotine in all tobacco products to ensure continual use.[10]

- Nicotine is powerful, fast acting, and one of the most addictive substances known to humankind (Fig. 10-9).
- Even though nicotine is not a carcinogen, it is the chemical that causes addiction.
- On a milligram-per-milligram basis, it is 10 times more addictive than heroin or cocaine and 6 to 8 times more addictive than alcohol.
- It is therefore imperative that dental hygienists encourage each and every patient who uses tobacco to follow sound advice when making a quit attempt and consider incorporating one of the cessation techniques as part of the quit plan.

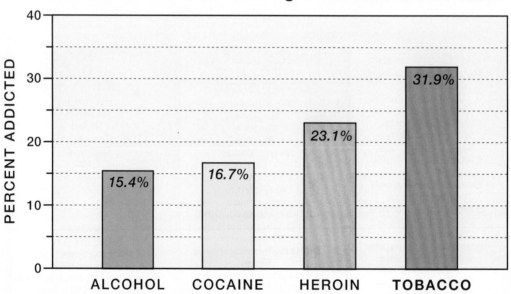

**Figure 10-9. Percent of individuals who become addicted.** Source: Kessler RC, McGonagle KA, Zhao S, et al. Lifetime and 12-month prevalence of DSM-III-R psychiatric disorders in the United States. Results from the National Comorbidity Survey. *Arch Gen Psychiatry.* 1994;51(1):8–19.

## TOBACCO ADDICTION

It is a testament to the power of tobacco addiction that 20.6% of U.S. adults (about 46.6 million) and 21% of Canadians (about 5.3 million people) are current smokers.[2]

- Smoking rates in the United States and Canada have decreased since the 1964 Surgeon General's report linked lung cancer and cigarette use. At that time, an estimated 42% of the American population was smokers. However, the current prevalence has not significantly decreased since 2004, demonstrating a stall in the previous 7-year decline (Fig. 10-10). [11]
- Unfortunately, the incidence is highest in the most vulnerable populations. Those living below poverty line are 31.1% more likely to smoke than those living above the poverty line.[12]

• The most powerless populations—the young, indigent, depressed, uninsured, less educated, blue-collar, and minorities—have the highest percentages of smokers in the United States and in Canada.

• Tragically, tobacco use must be considered a pediatric disease, with more than 2,000 children and adolescents becoming regular users of tobacco each day in the United States alone. Half of all smokers start prior to the age of 14, and 80% begin by age 18. Only 10% of smokers initiate the habit as adults.[12]

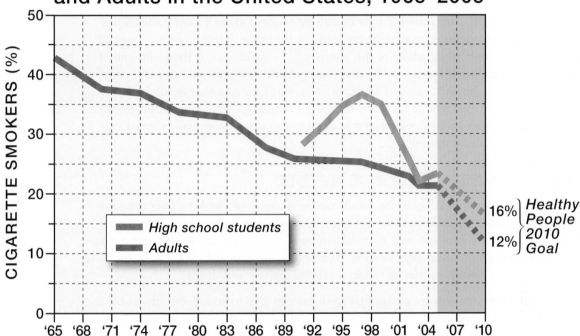

**Figure 10-10.  Current trends in smoking rates.** Source: National Health Interview Surveys: 1965, 1970, 1974, 1978, 1980, 1983, 1985, 1987, 1990, 1993, 1995, 1997, 1999, 2001–2006.

**SECTION 3:**

# Why Should Dental Health Care Providers Intervene?

As one of the most accessible health care professionals, dental hygienists are in an ideal position to provide tobacco cessation services. The more intensive the intervention, the higher the quit rates, but even minimal tobacco interventions—less than 3 minutes— increase the proportion of tobacco users who quit and have a considerable public health impact.

All dental health care professionals should be concerned with their patients' use of tobacco products. Smoking may be responsible for more than half of the cases of periodontal disease among adults in this country.[9,13] Tobacco use is therefore one of the most significant risk factors in the development and progression and successful treatment of periodontitis. Current smokers are about four times more likely than people who have never smoked to have periodontal disease.[9,13] Even in adult smokers with generally high oral hygiene standards and regular dental care habits, smoking accelerates periodontal disease.

## ONE-ON-ONE EDUCATION IS NEEDED

Despite major efforts to educate the public on the dangers of smoking over the past 40 years, the general populace seriously underestimates the magnitude of the harm that tobacco causes. Perhaps even more alarming is that major knowledge gaps exist in what smokers themselves believe to be true about the risks associated with smoking compared to the actual realities of tobacco-related disease and death.

- Although many smokers are aware that smoking can lead to serious health problems including lung cancer, many underestimate the risk of getting the disease from smoking.
- As many as one-third of smokers think that certain activities such as exercise and taking vitamins "undo" most of the detrimental effects of smoking.
- Experts believe these misperceptions may prevent smokers from trying to quit and successfully using proven smoking cessation treatments.
- A century from now, when historians reflect on the account of tobacco in the 20th century, it will surely be looked upon as one of the most intriguing and tragic developments of the period.

## TOBACCO CESSATION COUNSELING WORKS

The effectiveness of even brief tobacco dependence counseling has been well established and is also extremely cost-effective relative to other medical and disease prevention interventions.

- *Smokers cite a health professional's advice to quit as an important motivator for attempting to stop smoking.*
- With effective education, counseling, and support—rather than condemnations and warnings about dangers of smoking—dental health care providers can provide an invaluable service.
- Helping someone overcome a tobacco addiction may be the most broad-reaching health care intervention a dental hygienist can achieve.

## IT'S NEVER TOO LATE TO QUIT

For patients who use tobacco, one of the most important messages is that it is never too late to quit.

- Even for long-term smokers, quitting smoking carries major and immediate health benefits for men and women of all ages (Fig. 10-11). Benefits apply to healthy smokers and to smokers already suffering from smoking-related disease.
- Smoking cessation represents the single most important step that smokers can take to enhance the length and quality of their lives.
- Smokers who quit—even after age 63 years—start repairing their bodies right away. After only 2 weeks, lung function increases by up to 30% in most persons.

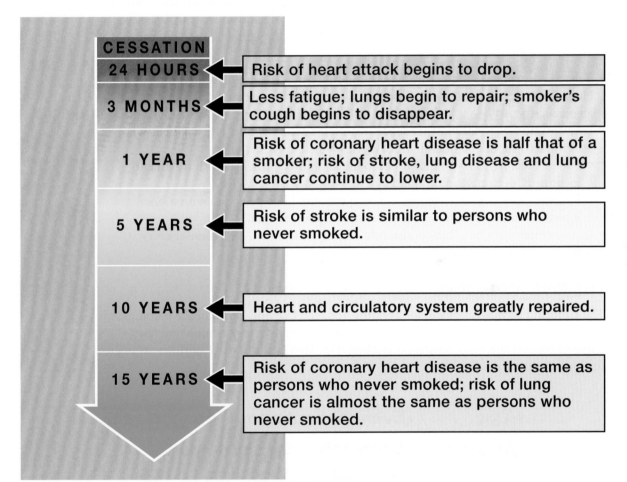

**Figure 10-11. Potential health benefits of quitting.** Source: The health consequences of smoking: a report of the Surgeon General: Dept. of Health and Human Services, Centers for Disease Control and Prevention, National Center for Chronic Disease Prevention and Health Promotion, Office on Smoking and Health; Washington, D.C.[4]

## SECTION 4:
# Guidelines for Tobacco Cessation Counseling

### THE CLINICAL PRACTICE GUIDELINE

The **Clinical Practice Guideline for Treating Tobacco Use and Dependence**, published by the U.S. Department of Health and Human Services, is considered the benchmark for cessation techniques and treatment delivery strategies. The Clinical Practice Guideline may be downloaded at http://www.ahrq.gov/clinic/tobacco/treating_tobacco_use08.pdf. The updated 2008 Guideline reflects the scientific cessation literature published from 1975 to 2007. The guideline contains strategies and recommendations designed to assist clinicians in delivering and supporting effective treatments for tobacco use and dependence. Several key recommendations of the updated guideline are as follows:

- Tobacco dependence is a chronic condition that often requires repeated intervention. However, effective treatments exist that can produce long-term or even permanent abstinence.
- Because effective tobacco dependence treatments are available, every patient who uses tobacco should be offered at least one of these treatments:
  - Patients *willing* to try to quit tobacco use should be provided with treatments identified as effective in this guideline.
  - Patients *unwilling* to try to quit tobacco use should be provided with a brief intervention designed to increase their motivation to quit.
- It is essential that clinicians consistently identify, document, and counsel every tobacco user seen in a health care setting.

### THE FIVE A'S MODEL

The Clinical Practice Guideline for Treating Tobacco Use and Dependence recommends the **Five A's** (Ask, Advise, Assess, Assist, and Arrange) as the key components of comprehensive tobacco cessation counseling (Fig. 10-12). Table 10-1 outlines strategies for implementing the Five A's.

| **ASK** | **Every patient about tobacco use.** |
|---|---|
| **ADVISE** | **Every tobacco user to quit.** |
| **ASSESS** | **Determine willingness to quit.** **Provide information on quitlines.** |
| **ASSIST** | **Refer to quitlines.** |
| **ARRANGE** | **Refer to quitlines.** |

**Figure 10-12.   The Five A's model.** The five steps of the Clinical Practice Guideline's model for tobacco use cessation.

**Table 10-1** STRATEGIES FOR IMPLEMENTING THE FIVE "A's"

| | |
|---|---|
| Ask | • Implement an office-wide system that ensures that for *every* patient at *every* dental appointment, tobacco use status is queried and documented. <br> • Use an identification system that indicates tobacco use status (current, former, never) and level of use (number of cigarettes smoked/chew amount per day) on patient's chart. <br> • Use an open-ended question: *When is the last time you tried a tobacco product?* <br> • **Not asking about tobacco use implies that quitting is not important!** |
| Advise | • Incorporate a consistent, clear, strong, and personalized advice dialogue when urging every tobacco user to quit. <br>   ○ Clear: *It is important for you to quit smoking or using chewing tobacco now, and I can help you.* <br>   ○ Strong: *As your clinician, I know that quitting may be the hardest thing you will ever do, but it is definitely the most important thing you can do for your health.* <br>   ○ Personalized: *Continuing to smoke may worsen these oral findings.* <br> • Express concern for the patient's health and a commitment to aid with quitting. |
| Assess | • Determine the patient's willingness to quit and knowledge of quit resources by asking open-ended questions using a nonjudgmental approach: *How do you feel about quitting at this point in your life? Are you aware that there are tools to make the process a bit easier?* |
| Assist | • Encourage patient to set a quit date—preferably within 1–2 wk of the dental appointment. <br> • Discuss challenges such as withdrawal symptoms, triggers, and vulnerable situations. <br> • Reassure the patient that ambivalence, fear, reluctance, etc. are all normal but should not deter the quit attempt. <br> • Supply information on cessation programs, websites, quitlines, medications, etc. <br> • Provide appropriate cessation referrals for treatment. <br> • Review the options and help the patient determine what would work best for him or her. |
| Arrange | • Follow-up contact should begin soon after the quit date with focus on preventing relapse. <br> • Schedule further follow-up contacts as indicated. <br> • Consider referral for more intensive treatment as indicated. <br> • If tobacco use has occurred, review circumstances and discuss how to avoid another slip in similar circumstances. |

## THE AMERICAN DENTAL HYGIENISTS' ASSOCIATION'S SMOKING CESSATION INITIATIVE

The American Dental Hygienists' Association (ADHA) has developed a condensed, "user-friendly" model for the dental hygienist who does not have the time, inclination, or expertise to provide the more comprehensive tobacco cessation counseling as recommended by the guideline (Fig. 10-13). **Ask. Advise. Refer. (AAR)** is the ADHA's national Smoking Cessation Initiative (SCI) designed to promote cessation intervention by dental hygienists. The AAR approach integrates the "Five A's" into an abbreviated intervention that remains consistent with recommended guidelines.

As part of the AAR campaign, dental hygienists refer their patients who use tobacco to quitlines as well as to Web-based and local cessation programs. Dental hygienists can use a variety of resources to help their patients quit smoking. The AAR program is designed as a program that dental hygienists can easily integrate into their tobacco cessation efforts. See http://www.askadviserefer.org.

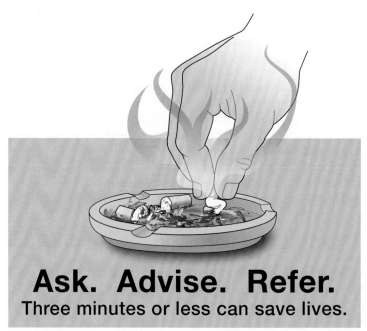

# Ask. Advise. Refer.
## Three minutes or less can save lives.

**Figure 10-13. The "Ask. Advise. Refer." model.** The "Ask. Advise. Refer." program—the American Dental Hygienists' Association's smoking cessation initiative—is an easy-to-use, three-step tobacco use cessation program.

## QUITLINES

**Quitlines** are toll-free telephone centers staffed by trained smoking cessation experts. It takes as little as 30 seconds to refer a patient to a quitline or a website (Fig. 10-14). A list of quitlines is provided in the "Ready Reference" section of this module.

- Evidence suggests quitline use more than triples success in quitting.
- By referring their patients to a quitline, dental hygienists are incorporating all Five A's (Ask, Advise, Assess, Assist, Arrange) of the Smoking Cessation Clinical Practice Guidelines.

- *Quitlines have proven to be one of the more effective methods of promoting smoking cessation.* Canada and the United States have each established publicly financed quitline services.
- Quitline services have the potential to reach large numbers of tobacco users including low income, rural, elderly, uninsured, and racial/ethnic populations who may not otherwise have access to cessation programs.
- Dental hygienists are natural partners for quitlines and can play a major role in increasing their utilization.
- Dental health care providers who ask all patients whether they use tobacco, advise quitting, and refer to quitlines for comprehensive cessation counseling can have a profound impact on patient health. Figure 10-15 outlines a systematic approach to cessation counseling.
- Table 10-2 lists common misconceptions and facts about tobacco cessation counseling.

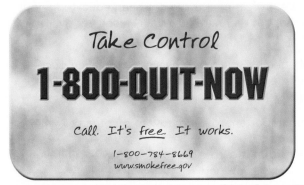
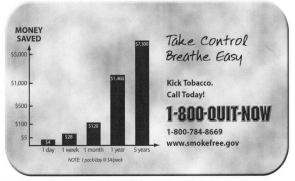

**Figure 10-14.** **U.S. Deparment of Health and Human Services quitline.** The U.S. Department of Health and Human Services has recognized the overwhelming success of quitlines and is dedicated to providing every citizen in every state with this important tool. (Card courtesy of the University of California at San Francisco, Smoking Leadership Center, San Francisco, CA.)

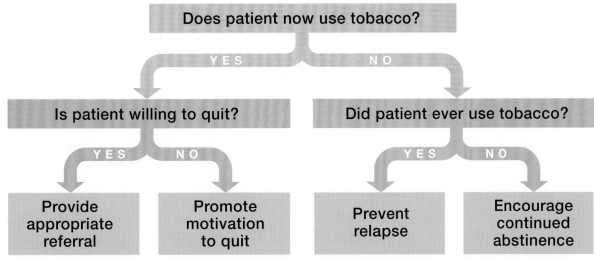

**Figure 10-15.** **Systematic approach to tobacco cessation counseling.** Shown here is a user-friendly decision tree for providing tobacco cessation counseling.

**Table 10-2** COMMON MISCONCEPTIONS: COUNTER MYTH WITH FACTS

| Myth | Fact |
|------|------|
| Tobacco users should not be forced into quitting; professionals should not "nag" them. | • The majority of tobacco users wish to quit but are unable to do so without assistance.<br>• Cessation assistance should be provided at every encounter. |
| Someone already sick as a result from tobacco use should not be made to feel guilty. | • Tobacco addiction is not a moral issue; it is a medical condition similar to any chronic condition such as diabetes. Helping someone maintain blood sugar control decreases risk and enhances quality of life—just as does helping someone quit tobacco use. |
| There is too little time to provide smoking cessation intervention. | • ADHA's "Ask. Advise. Refer." model takes less than 3 min to provide a meaningful intervention. |
| Dental hygienists have not been educated about how to help patients quit smoking. | • Most health care professionals have not been educated about how to intervene, but there are now many resources available to RDHs. |
| Most tobacco users relapse. | • The more quit attempts, the more chance of permanent success.<br>• Educate about the importance of receiving support and follow-up care. |
| Tobacco users have to want to quit in order to quit. | • It is much more important to learn **how** to quit than to **want** to quit.<br>• Educate patients that it is possible to learn how to quit even if the desire to quit is not there.<br>• Quitting is ending a relationship and that is at least a 3-mo process for most.<br>• Using cessation tools and methods increases success rates—the encouragement and tools provided by the dental hygienist are of utmost importance. |

ADHA, American Dental Hygienists' Association; RDH, registered dental hygienist.

## WITHDRAWAL SYMPTOMS

Tobacco use is a complex behavior involving the interplay of physiologic, psychological, and habitual factors that continuously reinforce one another to promote dependence (Fig. 10-16). Two hallmarks of dependency include smoking within 30 minutes of arising from sleep and experiencing withdrawal symptoms if regular pattern of use is disrupted. The cardinal **withdrawal symptoms** include a variety of unpleasant symptoms such as craving for nicotine, irritability, anger, anxiety, fatigue, depressed mood, difficulty concentrating, restlessness, and sleep disturbance.

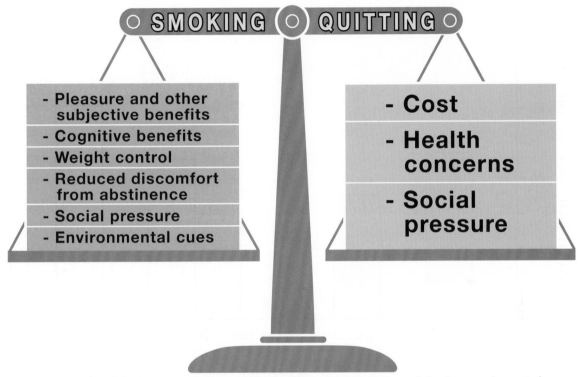

**Figure 10-16.   Addiction versus free will.** Graphic representation of the factors that reinforce continued smoking versus factors that motivate smokers to quit.

## QUIT RATES AND IMPLICATIONS

- The majority of smokers try to quit on their own. For most, relapse occurs quickly. Only half succeed for 2 days and only one-third last for 1 week. Most relapses occur in the first few months. Overall, self-quitters have a success rate of 4% to 6%[15].
- Most smokers make 11 quit attempts before finally succeeding.
- Half of all smokers eventually quit. In the United States, there are now as many former smokers as current smokers.
- *An important implication of the quit rate statistics is that dental health care providers need to understand the importance of helping the tobacco user through not just one quit attempt but rather through several attempts before a final successful one.*
- Another implication is that dental professionals need to prompt and reprompt tobacco users to make efforts to quit. Offering consistent smoking cessation counseling can motivate smokers to *try* to quit.

## SECTION 5:
# Smoking Cessation Products

No matter the level of addiction, all patients attempting to quit should be encouraged to at least try one or more of the effective pharmacotherapies (Fig. 10-17). **Pharmacotherapy** is the treatment of a medical condition using one or more medications. The goal of cessation pharmacotherapy is to alleviate or diminish the symptoms of withdrawal. The more physically comfortable the patient is, the more likely the smoker will make a serious quit attempt and succeed in permanently quitting.

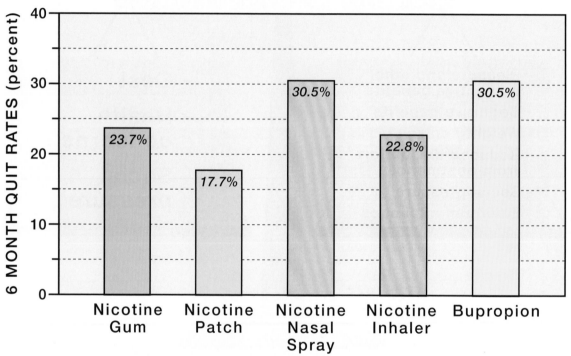

**Figure 10-17.    Six-month quit rates.** Data adapted from *Treating Tobacco Use and Dependence.* Rockville, MD: U.S. Department of Health and Human Services, Public Health Service, June 2000, pp. 72–91.

## NICOTINE REPLACEMENT THERAPY

**Nicotine replacement therapy (NRT)** involves nicotine-containing medications used for smoking cessation.

- Almost all researchers agree that nicotine is not a carcinogen, and there is growing consensus that nicotine derived from medications does not promote cardiovascular disease.
- All of the NRT formulations are associated with slower onset and much lower nicotine levels than cigarettes, and, of course, they do not produce carbon monoxide, toxins, and carcinogens.
- The safety and abuse records of NRT have been excellent. The choice of NRT should be individualized—based on patient preference, past experience, smoking dependence, and habits.

## Label Warning and Contraindications for Nicotine Replacement Therapy Products

The labeling on NRT products still instructs tobacco users to consult their physician if there is a history of heart disease, ulcers, or hypertension, or with pregnancy or breastfeeding.

- The only medical contraindications listed in the guideline are:
  - Immediate myocardial infarction (<2 weeks)
  - Serious arrhythmia
  - Serious or worsening angina pectoris
  - Accelerated hypertension
- There is a documented lack of an association between NRT and acute cardiovascular events.
- The guideline recommends use of NRT in pregnancy if other therapies have failed. Clearly, the fetus is exposed to significantly less nicotine with NRT than with smoking and, most importantly, is not exposed to carbon monoxide, carcinogens, and toxins from cigarettes.

## Nicotine Replacement Therapy Products

- There are five NRT products on the market in both Canada and the United States including the nicotine gum, nicotine lozenge, nicotine patch, nicotine inhaler, and nicotine nasal spray.
  - Nicotine gum first appeared in 1984, and the nicotine patch was made available in 1994. Between 1995 and 1996, both became available without prescription. This resulted in the largest increase in smoking cessation since the 1964 Surgeon General's report on smoking.
  - Two NRT products are still only attainable through prescription. The Nicotrol nasal spray appeared in 1996 and the Nicotrol inhaler in 1998.
  - The final nonprescription NRT product to materialize is the nicotine lozenge, which has been on the market since 2002.
- Light smoking has become more common, perhaps due to smoking restrictions and increases in the price and taxation of tobacco products.
  - Many light smokers have a strong dependence even though they smoke relatively few cigarettes. They are less likely to receive treatment than are heavier smokers, but anecdotal evidence shows an increase in success rates with use of NRT.
  - At the other end of the spectrum, higher-than-recommended doses may be indicated in tobacco users with severe addiction. Failure to respond to NRT products may reflect inadequate dosage, incorrect usage, or both.

## NON-NICOTINE MEDICATIONS

There are two non-nicotine prescription medications specifically developed to help adults quit smoking: bupropion (U.S. trade name Zyban) and varenicline (U.S. trade name Chantix). *It should be noted that the U.S. Food and Drug Administration requires the smoking cessation drugs Chantix and Zyban to carry a strong safety warning.* Both drugs carry "black box" labels warning that people taking the drugs should be closely watched for signs of suicidal thoughts, depression, hostility, or other changes in behavior[18]. This warning should be read and understood by health care providers when considering suggestions for the use of these drugs.

## Bupropion (Zyban)

Bupropion (Zyban)—an atypical antidepressant—is a prescription medication designed to help smokers quit more easily than without the drug.

- It comes in a pill form and has been shown to double quit rates.
- Bupropion works by blocking the reuptake of dopamine and norepinephrine in the central nervous system, which modulates the dopamine reward pathway and reduces cravings for nicotine and symptoms of withdrawal.
- It is effective in those with no current or past depressive symptoms.
- Combining bupropion with NRT often increases success rates over bupropion used alone.

## Varenicline (Chantix)

The most recent non-nicotine medication varenicline (Chantix) was approved in 2006.
- Varenicline contains no nicotine, but it targets the same receptors that nicotine does. Varenicline is believed to block nicotine from these receptors.
- The drug's efficacy is believed to be the result of a sustained, low-level agonist activity at the receptor site, combined with competitive blockade of nicotine binding. The partial agonist activity modestly stimulates receptors, leading to increased dopamine levels that reduce nicotine withdrawal symptoms. By blocking the binding of nicotine to receptors in the central nervous system, varenicline inhibits the surge of dopamine release that occurs immediately (7 to 10 seconds) following each inhalation of tobacco smoke. This effect may help prevent relapse by reducing or even eliminating the pleasure linked with smoking.
- Evidence suggests that using varenicline can increase successful quitting three times more when compared to placebo.

## Table 10-3  PHARMACOTHERAPY TREATMENT OPTIONS

|  | Time Period | Dose | Pros | Cons |
|---|---|---|---|---|
| **Patch** | At least 8 wk, preferably 12 wk | • 21 mg for one pack/day<br>• 14 mg for half a pack/day<br>• 7 mg for five cigarettes per day<br>• Over one pack/day: double up on patches or combine with another product | • Very easy to use<br>• Automatically provides the right dose for a 24-h period<br>• Helps with early morning cravings | • May cause vivid dreams at night<br>• Not orally gratifying<br>• Small possibility of skin reaction to patch |
| **Gum** | Up to 12 wk, then PRN | • 4 mg for one pack/day<br>• 2 mg for less than one pack/day<br>• May chew one piece for every cigarette smoked | • Easy to regulate dose<br>• Can help prevent overeating<br>• Can provide help at difficult moments | • Tricky to use with dentures<br>• Nothing to drink for 20 min prior to use<br>• Must use chew and park technique |
| **Lozenge** | Up to 12 wk, then PRN | • 4 mg for one pack/day<br>• 2 mg for less than one pack/day<br>• May use one lozenge every 1–2 hours | • Easy to adjust dosage<br>• Can help prevent overeating<br>• Can provide help at difficult moments | • Nothing to drink for 20 min prior to use<br>• Must be allowed to dissolve slowly |
| **Nasal spray** | Up to 12 wk, then PRN | • Dose once or twice an hour<br>• Not more than 48 sprays in 24 hours | • Gives fast relief<br>• Easy to adjust dosage | • May cause nasal irritation |
| **Inhaler** | Up to 12 wk, then PRN | • 6–12 cartridges per day | • Keeps hands and mouth busy<br>• Easy to regulate dose<br>• Could help prevent overeating | • Feels like a cigarette<br>• Very conspicuous method that calls attention to quit attempt |

*(continued)*

**Table 10-3** PHARMACOTHERAPY TREATMENT OPTIONS *(CONTINUED)*

| | Time Period | Dose | Pros | Cons |
|---|---|---|---|---|
| Zyban | 12–24 wks; start taking 1–2 wk prior to quitting | • One 150-mg tablet every morning for 3 d; then 150-mg tablet twice a day at least 8 h apart on day 4 and thereafter | • Easy to use<br>• Decreases urge to smoke<br>• May suppress appetite | • Possible sleep disruption<br>• Can cause xerostomia<br>• Contraindicated if with seizure disorder, eating disorder, or taking monoamine oxidase inhibitors (MAOI)<br>• FDA safety warning |
| Chantix | 12–24 wks; start taking 1–2 wk prior to quitting | • One 0.5-mg tablet for 3 d; then one 0.5-mg tablet twice a day for 4 d; then one 1-mg tablet twice a day thereafter | • Easy to use<br>• Decreases urge to smoke<br>• **NO** contraindications<br>• Fewest compliance problems (patients will use it) | • Possible nausea, vomiting, headache, or insomnia<br>• FDA safety warning |

PRN, use as needed.

FDA, U.S. Food and Drug Administration.

## SECTION 6:
# Peak Procedure: Tobacco Cessation

### PROCEDURE 10-1  TOBACCO CESSATION COUNSELING

| | |
|---|---|
| **1. Ask.** Ask if your patient smokes or uses smokeless tobacco products. | • Many smokers want to quit and appreciate the encouragement of health professionals. |
| **2. Advise.** Advise the patient to quit.<br><br>The benefits of quitting include:<br>• Decreased risk of a heart attack; stroke; coronary heart disease; and lung, oral, and pharyngeal cancer<br>• Improved sense of taste and smell<br>• Improved circulation and lung function<br>• Improved health of family members | • Smokers are more likely to quit if advised to do so by health professionals.<br>• The oral examination provides the perfect opportunity to discuss smoking cessation with your patient.<br>• Tobacco use is a major risk factor in oral and pharyngeal cancer as well as periodontal disease.<br>• Tobacco use is a risk factor for coronary heart disease, heart attack, and lung cancer. Secondhand smoke is unhealthy for family members. |
| **3. Refer.** Tell the patient that help is a free phone call away. Provide patient with quitline numbers.<br><br>A list of quitlines for the United States and Canada is located in the "Ready References" section of this module. | • Evidence suggests that quitline use can more than triple success in quitting.<br>• Quitlines provide an easy, fast, and effective way to help smokers quit.<br>• By simply identifying smokers, advising them to quit, and sending them to a free telephone service, clinicians can save thousands of lives. |

## SECTION 7:
# Ready References

### READY REFERENCE 10-1 U.S. NATIONAL QUITLINES

The **U.S. Department of Health and Human Services** has a national quitline number:

**1-800-QUIT-NOW** (1-800-784-8669). This toll-free number is a single access link to the national network of tobacco cessation quitlines. Callers are automatically routed to a state-sponsored quitline.

The **National Cancer Institute quitline** is toll free at **1-877-44U-QUIT** (1-877-448-7848).

Information specialists are available to answer smoking-related questions in English or Spanish, Monday through Friday, 9:00 a.m. to 4:30 p.m. local time.

**American Cancer Society quitline: 1-800-277-2345**

**American Lung Association quitline: 1-800-586-4872**

### READY REFERENCE 10-2 CANADIAN QUITLINES BY PROVINCE

| | |
|---|---|
| New Brunswick<br>Nova Scotia<br>Ontario<br>Manitoba<br>Saskatchewan | 1-877-513-5333 |
| Alberta | 1-866-332-2322 |
| British Columbia | 1-877-455-2233 |
| Newfoundland and Labrador | 1-800-363-5864 |
| Northwest Territories | Call your public health unit |
| Nunavut | 1-866-877-3845 |
| Prince Edward Island | 1-888-818-6300 |
| Quebec | 1-866-527-7383 |
| Yukon | 1-800-661-0408 (ext. 8393) |

**READY REFERENCE 10-3**  PROFESSIONAL INTERNET RESOURCES

**http://www.askadviserefer.org**
Website for the **American Dental Hygienists' Association's** smoking cessation initiative. The site has resources including links to fact sheets, presentations, and quitline resource lists.

**http://www.ada.org/prof/resources/topics/cancer.asp**
The **American Dental Association's** website provides oral cancer information for dental health care providers.

**http://www.cdc.gov/tobacco**
Website of the **Centers for Disease Control and Prevention** that features an online guide for clinicians and helpful links.

**http://smokingcessationleadership.ucsf.edu**
The **Smoking Cessations Leadership Center (SCLC)** is a national program office of the Robert Wood Johnson Foundation that aims to increase smoking cessation rates and increase the number of health professionals who help smokers quit. Click on *Health Profession Resources* for a downloadable tool kit including print-and-post flyers for the dental office and downloadable PowerPoint slide presentations.

**http://www.smokefree.gov/usmap.html#**
On this website, click on a state to find smoking cessation resources in that state.

**http://www.cancer.org/docroot/PED/PED_10_6.asp?sitearea=PED**
**American Cancer Society** website with resources for health professionals. Smoking cessations resources include free brochures to keep smokers motivated, patient education materials, and a link to find a quitline in your area.

**http://www.ahrq.gov/path/tobacco.htm#Clinic**
**Agency for Health Care Research & Quality**

**http://www.chestnet.org/education/online/pccu/vol15/lessons13_14/lesson13.php**
**American College of Chest Physicians**

**http://www.attud.org/**
**Association for the Treatment of Tobacco Use and Dependence**

**http://www.oralcancerfoundation.org/tobacco/index.htm**
**Oral Cancer Foundation**

**http://www.athc.wisc.edu**
**Addressing Tobacco in Healthcare**

**http://tobaccofreenurses.org**
**Tobacco Free Nurses**

**http://www.surgeongeneral.gov/tobacco/default.htm**
**United States Department of Health and Human Services**

# Smoking History

Patient _____ Date _____

1. At what age did you begin to smoke? _____

2. How many cigarettes do you smoke per day now? _____
   Per day at your heaviest? _____

3. How many times have you tried to stop smoking? _____
   ☐ Never tried to stop

4. What is the longest period of time you have gone without smoking? _____

5. What forms of tobacco are you currently using? *(Please check all that apply.)*
   ☐ Cigarettes            ☐ Chewing tobacco
   ☐ Pipes                 ☐ Snuff
   ☐ Cigars                ☐ Other

6. Do your ☐ family members, ☐ friends, ☐ co-workers smoke? *(Please check all that apply. Circle if you live with any of these smokers.)*

7. What smoking cessation methods have you tried? *(Please check all that apply.)*
   ☐ None                  ☐ Self-help programs
   ☐ Cold turkey           ☐ Gradual reduction
   ☐ Hypnosis              ☐ Laser
   ☐ Acupuncture           ☐ Other

8. Are you being ☐ encouraged, or ☐ discouraged to stop smoking by any of the following? *(Please check all that apply.)*
   ☐ Spouse or significant other     ☐ Friend
   ☐ Child                           ☐ Co-worker
   ☐ Other family member

9. Who do you turn to for support? *(Please check all that apply.)*
   ☐ Spouse or significant other     ☐ Counselor
   ☐ Parent                          ☐ Healthcare provider
   ☐ Sibling                         ☐ Friend
   ☐ Other family member             ☐ Co-worker
   ☐ Clergy/rabbi/priest

Please rank the following on a scale of 1 (strongly disagree) to 5 (strongly agree):
   I am ready to stop smoking at this time:         1  2  3  4  5
   I am concerned about weight gain:                1  2  3  4  5
   I am concerned about dealing with stress:        1  2  3  4  5

_____          _____
Patient Signature                        Reviewed by

Figure 10-18.   Smoking history in English.

# Historia de Uso de Tabaco

Nombre _____ Fecha _____

1. ¿Ha que edad usted empezo ha fumar? _____

2. ¿Cuantos cigarillos usted fuma cada dia ahora?_____
   ¿Cual ha sido el máximo por dia? _____

3. ¿Cuantas veces ha tratado de parar ha fumar?_____
   ☐ Nunca trató de parar

4. ¿Cual ha sido el período mas largo que ha dejado de fumar? _____

5. ¿Qué formas de tabaco utiliza usted? *(Por favor indice cuales aplican.)*
   ☐ Cigarillos             ☐ Tabaco de masticar
   ☐ Pipas                  ☐ Snuff
   ☐ Cigarros               ☐ Otro

6. ¿Su ☐familia, ☐amigos, ☐compañeros de trabajo fuman? *(Indice cuales aplican. Si vive con algun fumador, ponga un círculo alrededor de cual aplica.)*

7. ¿Qué método de cesar de fumar ha tratado? *(Por favor indice cuales aplican.)*
   ☐ Ninguno                ☐ Programa de ayuda personal
   ☐ Abrupto                ☐ Rebajo gradual
   ☐ Hipnosis               ☐ Láser
   ☐ Acupuntura             ☐ Otro _____

8. ¿Quien le ☐ayuda o ☐disuade parar de fumar?
   *(Por favor indice cual aplica, y cuales los afecta.)*
   ☐ Esposa/esposo          ☐ Amigos
   ☐ Niños                  ☐ Compañeros de trabajo
   ☐ Otros de su familia

9. ¿Ha quien usted va para ayuda de dejar de fumar? *(Indice cuales aplican.)*
   ☐ Esposa/esposo          ☐ Consejero
   ☐ Mis padres             ☐ Agencia médica
   ☐ Hermanos               ☐ Amigos
   ☐ Otros de su familia    ☐ Compañeros de trabajo
   ☐ Ministro religioso

Indice rango en escala de 1 *(no esta de acuerdo)* ha 5 *(esta de acuerdo)*:
   Estoy listo para parar de fumar ahora:          1  2  3  4  5
   Estoy preocupado sobre aumentar de peso:     1  2  3  4  5
   Estoy preocupado sobre estar estresado:         1  2  3  4  5

Firma del paciente _____   Revisado por _____

Figure 10-19. Smoking history in Spanish.

# REFERENCES

1. Annual smoking-attributable mortality, years of potential life lost, and productivity losses—United States, 1997–2009. *MMWR Morb Mortal Wkly Rep.* 2010;59(35):1135–1140.

2. World Health Organization. Tobacco atlas. 2002. Available from: http://www.who.int/tobacco/publications/surveillance/tobacco_atlas/en. Accessed August 24, 2012.

3. Doll R, Peto R, Boreham J, et al. Mortality in relation to smoking: 50 years' observations on male British doctors. *BMJ.* 2004;328(7455):1519.

4. The 2004 United States Surgeon General's Report: The health consequences of smoking. *N S W Public Health Bull.* 2004;15(5–6):107.

5. U.S. Department of Health and Human Services. *The Health Consequences of Smoking: A Report of the Surgeon General.* Atlanta, GA: U.S. Department of Health and Human Services, Centers for Disease Control and Prevention, National Center for Chronic Disease Prevention and Health Promotion, Office on Smoking and Health, 2004.

6. National Institutes of Health State-of-the-Science conference statement: tobacco use: prevention, cessation, and control. *Ann Intern Med.* 2006;145(11):839–844.

7. Stoltenberg JL, Osborn JB, Pihlstrom BL, et al. Association between cigarette smoking, bacterial pathogens, and periodontal status. *J Periodontol.* 1993;64(12):1225–1230.

8. MacFarlane GD, Herzberg MC, Wolff LF, et al. Refractory periodontitis associated with abnormal polymorphonuclear leukocyte phagocytosis and cigarette smoking. *J Periodontol.* 1992;63(11):908–913.

9. Haber J, Wattles J, Crowley M, et al. Evidence for cigarette smoking as a major risk factor for periodontitis. *J Periodontol.* 1993 Jan;64(1):16–23.

10. Jacob P III, Abu Raddaha AH, Dempsey D, et al. Nicotine, carbon monoxide, and carcinogen exposure after a single use of a water pipe. *Cancer Epidemiol Biomarkers Prev.* 2011;20(11):2345–2353.

11. U.S Department of Health and Human Services. *The Health Consequences of Involuntary Exposure to Tobacco Smoke: A Report of the Surgeon General.* Atlanta, GA: U.S. Department of Health and Human Services, Centers for Disease Control and Prevention, Coordinating Center for Health Promotion, National Center for Chronic Disease Prevention and Health Promotion, Office on Smoking and Health; 2006.

12. National Institute on Drug Abuse. Research report series on nicotine addiction. http://www.nida.nih.gov/researchreports/nicotine/nicotine.html. Accessed August 14, 2012.

13. Centers for Disease Control and Prevention. Cigarette smoking among adults—United States 2004. *MMWR Morb Mortal Wkly Rep.* 2005;54:509–513.

14. U.S. Department of Health and Human Services. *Healthy People 2010 (Conference Edition, in Two Volumes).* Washington, DC: U.S. Department of Health and Human Services; 2000.

15. Tomar SL, Asma S. Smoking-attributable periodontitis in the United States: findings from NHANES III. National Health and Nutrition Examination Survey. *J Periodontol.* 2000;71(5):743–751.

16. Hughes JR. New treatments for smoking cessation. *CA Cancer J Clin.* 2000;50(3):143–151; quiz 152–155.

17. Centers for Disease Control and Prevention. Vital signs: current cigarette smoking among adults aged > or = 18 years—United States, 2009. *MMWR Morb Mortal Wkly Rep.* 2010;59(35):1135–1140.

18. Kuehn BM. Varenicline gets stronger warnings about psychiatric problems, vehicle crashes. *JAMA.* 2009;302(8):834.

**SECTION 8:**

# Patient Education Resources

## AMERICAN DENTAL HYGIENISTS' ASSOCIATION'S SMOKING CESSATION RESOURCES

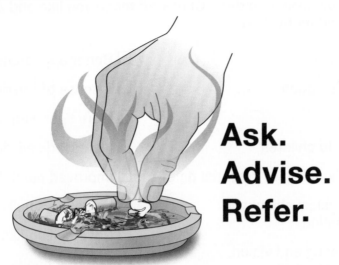

Ask.
Advise.
Refer.

**Figure 10-20. Ask. Advise. Refer.** The ADHA's Smoking Cessation Initiative offers many free resources online at *http://www.askadviserefer.org/about.asp*.

Download the following resources from the website:

### Quit Smoking Products for Clinicians—Order Form

The Quick Reference Guide for Clinicians and the English and Spanish versions of the You Can Quit Smoking Quit Plan are available from the Agency for Healthcare Research and Quality.

### You Can Quit Smoking Consumer Guide

The *You Can Quit Smoking Consumer Guide* is a booklet that will assist smokers in developing a quit plan offering five key steps that embody the key recommendations from the Clinical Practice Guideline: Treating Tobacco Use and Dependence.

### Personalized Quit Plans

The *You Can Quit Smoking* quit plans were developed by the U.S. Department of Health and Human Services and can be used to help prepare smokers for their first call to a quitline and to set a quit date. Quit plans are available for download in the following versions:

- English and English prenatal
- Spanish and Spanish prenatal
- Chinese
- Hmong
- Korean
- Laotian
- Vietnamese

**PATIENT FORMS, HANDOUTS, AND WORKSHEETS**

## Personalized Benefits of Quitting Smoking

The following is a list of benefits one can receive after quitting that was developed by successful quitters. Check off those you like and add your own for increased motivation.

☐ Improved health

☐ Personal satisfaction

☐ Less tension

☐ Better image to children

☐ Improved scheduling of personal time

☐ Increased physical ability and improved stamina

☐ Improved hearing and vision, especially night vision

☐ Fewer dental problems—fresher breath

☐ Clothes, drapes, house, car smell better

☐ Reduced rates for car, health, and life insurance

☐ Reduced litter from filters, ashes, and paper

☐ Removal of film on windows and furniture

☐ Better appearance

☐ A sense of freedom

☐ More spending money

☐ Increased self-discipline

☐ Improved mental abilities

☐ Improved smell and taste

☐ Not smelling like smoke

☐ Two free hands

☐ Fewer colds

☐ Fewer burn holes in clothes

☐ Better social acceptance

☐ Better circulation

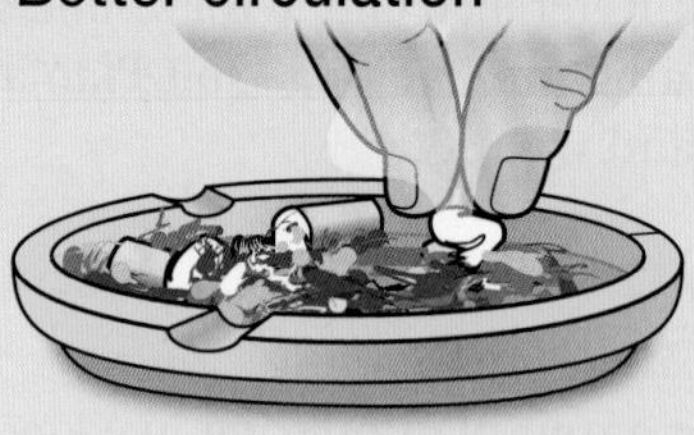

_____

_____

_____

_____

_____

_____

**Figure 10-21.   Personalized Benefits of Quitting Smoking worksheet.**

## Plan of Action

| | |
|---|---|
| Coffee break | 1. Drink juice or dairy product instead<br>2. Skip coffee break |
| Watching television | 1. Do something with your hands, such as knit or play cards<br>2. Sit in another room, go for a walk outside, exercise |
| Getting up in the morning | 1. Get in the shower immediately or do calisthenics<br>2. Roll over and try to sleep an extra 10 minutes |
| Alcohol-related activities | 1.<br><br>2. |
| Special occasions | 1.<br><br>2. |
| Argument with someone | 1.<br><br>2. |
| Waiting for a bus | 1.<br><br>2. |
| Talking on the telephone | 1.<br><br>2. |
| Your own situations: | 1.<br><br>2. |
| | 1.<br><br>2. |

Figure 10-22.   Plan of Action worksheet.

# When the Craving Comes

☐ Take a few deep breaths and remember your determination to be free of the addiction.

☐ Think of your most important reason for wanting to stop and say it aloud in front of the mirror.

☐ Drink lots of water and juices.

☐ Do not start feeling sorry for yourself—feel for those who are still smoking. You were smart enough to join a smoking cessation program and stop smoking.

☐ Seek the company of nonsmokers. Immediately turn you attention to something else. Remember that even the most intense craving lasts only a few minutes —5 at the most. The urge passes whether or not you smoke a cigarette.

☐ Take a break. Get up and walk around.

☐ Do something with your hands. Knit. Doodle. Play with a coin. Write a letter.

☐ Frequent places where you do not smoke rather than places where you used to smoke.

☐ Whistle, sing, brush your teeth, take a shower.

☐ Curb use of alcoholic and caffeinated beverages.

☐ Pop something low calorie into your mouth—gum or crisp vegetables such as carrots or celery.

☐ Concern yourself only with today—get through *today* without smoking.

☐ Be good to yourself in every possible way. Indulge and enjoy a special treat with the money you have saved by not buying cigarettes.

☐ Talk to yourself: *"Take it easy. . . Calm down."*

☐ Practice relaxation techniques. Stretch, yawn, do deep knee bends, touch your toes, shrug your shoulders.

☐ Pretend you are smoking a cigarette. It is a very helpful breathing exercise. Breathe in and out slowly and deeply—sigh!

☐ Think of quitting as an act of love and a gift of love—*to yourself.*

Figure 10-23.   When the Craving Comes handout.

QUITTING TAKES HARD WORK AND A LOT OF EFFORT, BUT—

# You Can Quit Smoking
SUPPORT AND ADVICE
FROM YOUR CLINICIAN

## A PERSONALIZED QUIT PLAN FOR: _____

### WANT TO QUIT?
- ▶ Nicotine is a powerful addiction.
- ▶ Quitting is hard, but don't give up.
- ▶ Many people try 2 or 3 times before they quit for good.
- ▶ Each time you try to quit, the more likely you will be to succeed.

### GOOD REASONS FOR QUITTING:
- ▶ You will live longer and live healthier.
- ▶ The people you live with, especially your children, will be healthier.
- ▶ You will have more energy and breathe easier.
- ▶ You will lower your risk of heart attack, stroke, or cancer.

### TIPS TO HELP YOU QUIT:
- ▶ Get rid of ALL cigarettes and ashtrays in your home, car, or workplace.
- ▶ Ask your family, friends, and coworkers for support.
- ▶ Stay in nonsmoking areas.
- ▶ Breathe in deeply when you feel the urge to smoke.
- ▶ Keep yourself busy.
- ▶ Reward yourself often.

### QUIT AND SAVE YOURSELF MONEY:
- ▶ At $3.00 per pack, if you smoke 1 pack per day, you will save $1,100 each year and $11,000 in 10 years.
- ▶ What else could you do with this money?

**U.S. Department of Health and Human Services**
Public Health Service

ISSN 1530-6402

(over)

Figure 10-24A. Page 1 of the quit plan in English.

# FIVE KEYS FOR QUITTING | YOUR QUIT PLAN

## 1. GET READY.

- ▶ Set a quit date and stick to it—not even a single puff!
- ▶ Think about past quit attempts. What worked and what did not?

## 1. YOUR QUIT DATE:

## 2. GET SUPPORT AND ENCOURAGEMENT.

- ▶ Tell your family, friends, and coworkers you are quitting.
- ▶ Talk to your doctor or other health care provider.
- ▶ Get group, individual, or telephone counseling.

## 2. WHO CAN HELP YOU:

## 3. LEARN NEW SKILLS AND BEHAVIORS.

- ▶ When you first try to quit, change your routine.
- ▶ Reduce stress.
- ▶ Distract yourself from urges to smoke.
- ▶ Plan something enjoyable to do every day.
- ▶ Drink a lot of water and other fluids.

## 3. SKILLS AND BEHAVIORS YOU CAN USE:

## 4. GET MEDICATION AND USE IT CORRECTLY.

- ▶ Talk with your health care provider about which medication will work best for you:
- ▶ Bupropion SR—available by prescription.
- ▶ Nicotine gum—available over-the-counter.
- ▶ Nicotine inhaler—available by prescription.
- ▶ Nicotine nasal spray—available by prescription.
- ▶ Nictone patch—available over-the-counter.

## 4. YOUR MEDICATION PLAN:

Medications:

Instructions:

## 5. BE PREPARED FOR RELAPSE OR DIFFICULT SITUATIONS.

- ▶ Avoid alcohol.
- ▶ Be careful around other smokers.
- ▶ Improve your mood in ways other than smoking.
- ▶ Eat a healthy diet and stay active.

## 5. HOW WILL YOU PREPARE?

**Quitting smoking is hard. Be prepared for challenges, especially in the first few weeks.**

Followup plan: _____

Other information: _____

Referral: _____

Clinician          Date

**Figure 10-24B. Page 2 of the quit plan in English.**

VENCER EL TABACO ES DURO Y REQUIERE UN GRAN ESFUERZO, PERO —

# Usted puede dejar de fumar

**APOYO Y CONSEJOS DE SU PROFESIONAL DE SALUD**

**UN PLAN PERSONALIZADO PARA VENCER EL TABACO:**

## ¿QUIERE DEJAR DE FUMAR?

▶ Nicotina es un vicio poderoso.
▶ Dejar el tabaco es duro, pero no se rinda.
▶ Muchas personas lo intentan 2 o 3 veces antes de vencerlo para siempre.
▶ Cada vez que usted intenta vencer el tabaco, es más probable que usted triunfe.

## RAZONES BUENAS PARA DEJAR DE FUMAR:

▶ Usted vivirá más y vivirá más saludable.
▶ Las personas con que usted vive, especialmente sus hijos, serán más saludables.
▶ Usted tendrá más energía y respirará más fácil.
▶ Usted bajará su riesgo de ataque al corazón, de derrame cerebral, o de cáncer.

## DATOS PARA AYUDARLE DEJAR DE FUMAR:

▶ Retire TODOS los cigarrillos y ceniceros de su casa, su auto, o de su trabajo.
▶ Pídale apoyo a su familia, amigos, y compañeros de trabajo.
▶ Permanezca en áreas de no fumar.
▶ Respire profundo cuando sienta la necesidad de fumar.
▶ Manténgase ocupado.
▶ Recompénsese a menudo .

## DEJE DE FUMAR Y AHORRE DINERO:

▶ A $3.00 por cajetilla, si usted fuma una cajetilla por día, usted ahorraría $1,100 cada año y $11,000 en 10 años.
▶ ¿Qué más podría hacer usted con este dinero?

**U.S. Department of Health and Human Services**
Public Health Service

ISSN 1530-6402

(próxima página)

**Figure 10-25A.    Page 1 of the quit plan in Spanish.**

| CINCO CLAVES PARA DEJAR DE FUMAR | SU PLAN PARA VENCER EL TABACO |
|---|---|
| **1. PREPARESE.**<br>▶ Establezca una fecha y no la cambie - ni un solo soplo!<br>▶ Piense en sus previos intentos . ¿Qué trabajó y qué no? | **1. SU FECHA DE VENCER EL HABITO:** |
| **2. OBTENGA APOYO Y ALIENTO.**<br>▶ Dígale a su familia, amigos y compañeros de trabajo que usted va dejar de fumar.<br>▶ Hable con su doctor u otro profesional de salud.<br>▶ Obtenga apoyo por medio de grupos, individuos o el teléfono. | **2. QUIEN LO PUEDE AYUDAR:** |
| **3. APRENDA NUEVA HABILIDADES Y CONDUCTAS.**<br>▶ Cuándo comience a dejar de fumar, cambie su rutina.<br>▶ Reduzca el stress.<br>▶ Distráigase de los impulsos de fumar.<br>▶ Planee hacer algo agradable todos los días.<br>▶ Beba mucha agua y otros líquidos. | **3. HABILIDADES Y CONDUCTAS QUE USTED PUEDE UTILIZAR:** |
| **4. OBTENGA MEDICAMENTOS Y USELOS CORRECTAMENTE.**<br>▶ Hable con su profesional de salud acerca de cuál medicamento sería mejor para usted:<br>▶ Bupropion SR—disponible por receta médica.<br>▶ Chicle de nicotina—disponible sin receta médica.<br>▶ Inhalador de nicotina—disponible por receta médica.<br>▶ Rocío nasal de nicotina—disponible por receta médica.<br>▶ Parche de nicotina—disponible sin receta médica. | **4. SU PLAN DE MEDICAMENTOS:**<br>Medicamentos :<br><br>Instrucciones : |
| **5. ESTE PREPARADO PARA RECAER O PARA SITUACIONES DIFICILES.**<br>▶ Evite el alcohol.<br>▶ Tenga cuidado alrededor de otros fumadores.<br>▶ Mejore su estado de ánimo en maneras que no incluya fumar.<br>▶ Coma una dieta saludable y permanezca activo. | **5. ¿COMO SE VA PREPARAR?:** |

**Dejar de fumar es difícil. Prepárese al desafío, especialmente en las primeras semanas.**

Plan a seguir: _____

Otra información: _____

Referencia: _____

_____          _____
Clínico                                          Fecha

**Figure 10-25B.    Page 2 of the quit plan in Spanish.**

BOX **10-1**    Websites To Help You Quit

**http://www.cdc.gov/tobacco/how2quit.htm**
Website of the **Centers for Disease Control and Prevention** that focuses on how to quit smoking. Features an online consumer guide, quit tips, guide for clinicians, and helpful links.

**http://www.nlm.nih.gov/medlineplus/smoking.html**
The **MedlinePlus** website provides accurate information regarding all aspects of the effects of tobacco on health, ways to avoid tobacco, and smoking cessation.

**http://smokingcessationleadership.ucsf.edu/**
The **Smoking Cessation Leadership Center** (SCLC) is a national program office of the Robert Wood Johnson Foundation. SCLC aims to increase smoking cessation rates and increase the number of health professionals who help smokers quit.

**http://www.drugfree.org/join-together**
The **Join Together** website sponsored by the **Boston University School of Publish Health** provides resources for smokers to quit smoking. Site includes interactive tools, e-mail reminders, chat rooms, nicotine news, and other resources to help people quit smoking.

**http://www.cancer.org/Healthy/StayAwayfromTobacco/GuidetoQuittingSmoking/index**
**American Cancer Society**

**http://www.lungusa.org/stop-smoking/**
**American Lung Association**

**www.quitnet.com**
**Quit Net**

**http://www.cdc.gov/tobacco/**
**Centers for Disease Control and Prevention**

**http://www.ahrq.gov/consumer/tobacco/**
**U.S. Department of Health and Human Services** link to an easy-to-read brochure: "Help for Smokers and Other Tobacco Users" (PDF file).

**http://www.niddk.nih.gov/health/nutrit/pubs/quitsmok/index.htm**
The Weight-Control Information Network, an informational service of the **National Institute of Diabetes, Digestive, and Kidney Disease (NIDDK)** provides helpful information for people who are worried about gaining weight when they stop smoking. This site will alleviate fears about gaining weight.

**http://www.becomeanex.org**
BecomeAnEX.org is a project of the **National Alliance for Tobacco Cessation** to help people quit smoking.

## Section 9:
# The Human Element

---

BOX **10-2**    **Through the Eyes of the Clinician**

*Mr. R. is a 60-year-old male who started smoking at age 14. By 17, he was smoking daily—as much as one to three packs a day. Mr. R's current daily consumption was two packs a day. Typically, Mr. R. smoked immediately upon waking and if he woke in the middle of the night. This information indicated to me that Mr. R. had a strong physical addiction.*

*Mr. R. told me that a year ago, he met a wonderful woman, Helen, and that they were going to be married in 7 months. He was very defensive about his smoking and said that Helen really wanted him to quit before their wedding. Mr. R. confided that he found the pressure from his fiancée about quitting decidedly unhelpful! He felt that he did not have the "willpower" to quit. He also expressed concern that since he had been smoking for so long, it was probably pointless to quit at his age.*

*I encouraged Mr. R. to just listen to the cessation options available to him. I assured him that it wasn't nearly as necessary* **to want to quit** *as it was* **to decide to quit***, and I could help by offering him tools to assist in the quitting process. I spoke to Mr. R. about nicotine addiction and explained that through no fault of his own, he most likely had a genetic predisposition to nicotine addiction. I told him that even though taking control of a nicotine addiction was more difficult than heroin, cocaine, or alcohol, it was very possible. Although quitting may be the most difficult thing he would ever do, it would also be the most worthwhile.*

*In speaking with Mr. R., I stressed the* **health benefits of quitting** *rather than talking about health risks from smoking. I explained that the goal of quitting was not to stop wanting to smoke but to stop the behavior of smoking. He may want a cigarette for the rest of his life—not to the degree upon first quitting—but that doesn't mean he has to smoke the rest of his life. Quitting isn't about willpower—it is about taking control over an addiction that now controls his life.*

*I also spoke to Mr. R. about cessation medications. He decided he would try Chantix. Mr. R. decided to set a quit date 3 weeks after our meeting. I asked him to follow up with me by phone, and he did. Mr. R. reported that he pushed his quit date back by 1 week. He decided to cut down a bit first. He was on Chantix for 4 full weeks before noticing any effect, but after that, he felt it was very beneficial in the quitting process.*

*Six months after our meeting, Mr. R. e-mailed me from Paris. He and Helen were enjoying a very happy honeymoon; Mr. R. was still not smoking and very confident that he would remain tobacco free. Mr. R. stayed on Chantix for 4 months and knows he can use it again should the need arise. He did gain a bit of weight but felt that with exercise, he would soon lose those extra pounds. He felt "tremendous" and was so glad that Helen had encouraged him to quit.*

*Carol Southard, RN, MSN, Project Consultant*
*ADHA Smoking Cessation Initiative*

## PATIENT SCENARIO

As you enter the waiting room to call your next patient, Jeremy M., the scent of smoke surrounds you. Jeremy, who is 13 years old, attends the local middle school. His mother has dropped him off for his prophylaxis appointment. You review Jeremy's medical history and are anxious to hear his response to your questions about smoking. At first, he denies the use of tobacco, but upon further pressing, he states, "Yeah I smoke ... what's the big deal? Both my parents smoke too." You are disturbed by his response, but grateful for his honesty.

1. What do you do to educate Jeremy about the dangers of tobacco use?
2. Is it ethical to share this information with his parents?
3. How can you intervene to make Jeremy aware of the necessity of tobacco cessation?
4. How can you help Jeremy quit smoking?

### Section 10:

# Practical Focus—Fictitious Patient Case for Tobacco Cessation

---

**DIRECTIONS:**

**FICTITIOUS PATIENT CASE A: Mr. Alan Ascari**

- The fictitious patient case in this module involves Patient A, Mr. Alan Ascari.

- While completing the Practical Focus section in this module, you should take into account the health history and over-the-counter/prescription drug information that was revealed for Mr. Ascari in Module 4, Medical History and Module 9, Vital Signs: Blood Pressure.

- Review Mr. Ascari's smoking history form on the next page of this module.

- Using Peak Procedure 10-1 for guidance, role-play tobacco cessation counseling with a classmate portraying Mr. Ascari. Remember to use the patient resource handouts from section during the role-play.

---

# Smoking History

Patient ___ALAN ASCARI___ Date ___1/15/XX___

1. At what age did you begin to smoke? ___15___

2. How many cigarettes do you smoke per day now? ___2 PACKS___
   Per day at your heaviest? ___2 PACKS___

3. How many times have you tried to stop smoking? ___2___
   ☐ Never tried to stop

4. What is the longest period of time you have gone without smoking? ___2 DAYS___

5. What forms of tobacco are you currently using? *(Please check all that apply.)*
   ☒ Cigarettes          ☒ Chewing tobacco ___AT WORK___
   ☐ Pipes               ☐ Snuff
   ☐ Cigars              ☐ Other

6. Do your ☐ family members, ☐ friends, ☒ co-workers smoke? *(Please check all that apply. Circle if you live with any of these smokers.)*

7. What smoking cessation methods have you tried? *(Please check all that apply.)*
   ☐ None                ☐ Self-help programs
   ☒ Cold turkey         ☐ Gradual reduction
   ☒ Hypnosis            ☐ Laser
   ☐ Acupuncture         ☐ Other ___

8. Are you being ☒ encouraged, or ☐ discouraged to stop smoking by any of the following? *(Please check all that apply.)*
   ☒ Spouse or significant other    ☐ Friend
   ☒ Child                          ☐ Co-worker
   ☐ Other family member

9. Who do you turn to for support? *(Please check all that apply.)*
   ☒ Spouse or significant other    ☐ Counselor
   ☐ Parent                         ☐ Healthcare provider
   ☐ Sibling                        ☐ Friend
   ☐ Other family member            ☐ Co-worker
   ☐ Clergy/rabbi/priest

Please rank the following on a scale of 1 (strongly disagree) to 5 (strongly agree):
I am ready to stop smoking at this time:        1  2  ③  4  5
I am concerned about weight gain:               ①  2  3  4  5
I am concerned about dealing with stress:       1  2  3  4  ⑤

*Alan Ascari*                              *John Schiff*, DH1
Patient Signature                          Reviewed by

Figure 10-26.   Mr. Ascari's completed smoking history form.

Section 11:
# Skill Check

---

**SKILL CHECKLIST:** ROLE-PLAY TOBACCO CESSATION COUNSELING

---

Student: _____ Evaluator: _____

Date: _____

> **Roles:**
> * Student 1 = Plays the role of the patient.
> * Student 2 = Plays the role of the clinician.

**DIRECTIONS FOR STUDENT CLINICIAN:** Use **Column S**; evaluate your skill level as **S** (satisfactory) or **U** (unsatisfactory).

**DIRECTIONS FOR EVALUATOR:** Use **Column E**. Indicate **S** (satisfactory) or **U** (unsatisfactory). In the optional grade percentage calculation, each **S** equals 1 point, and each **U** equals 0 points.

| CRITERIA | S | E |
|---|---|---|
| **Asks the patient if he or she uses tobacco.** | | |
| **Advises the patient that quitting is important for wellness and longevity. Asks the patient if he or she is interested in learning about tobacco cessation.** | | |
| **Encourages patient questions about the health risks of tobacco use and the tools for tobacco cessation.** | | |
| **Answers the patient's questions fully and accurately.** | | |
| **Communicates with the patient at an appropriate level and avoids dental/medical terminology or jargon.** | | |
| **Provides the patient with quitline telephone numbers or websites and patient education materials on tobacco cessation.** | | |

OPTIONAL GRADE PERCENTAGE CALCULATION

Using the entries in the **E** column, assign a point value of 1 for each **S** and 0 for each **U**. Add the total assigned as 1's _____ and divide by 6 to arrive at the percentage grade. _____

# NOTES

# 11 Soft Tissue Lesions

## MODULE OVERVIEW

This module discusses recognition of soft tissue lesions of the skin and oral mucosa. It presents a systematic approach to describing pertinent characteristics of soft tissue lesions. The ability to formulate a concise, accurate verbal and written description of any lesion is a necessary skill when communicating and documenting findings from the extraoral and intraoral examination.

This module covers:

- Recognizing the primary types of soft tissue lesions
- Formulating a written description of a soft tissue lesion
- Prevention of skin and oral cancers

## MODULE OUTLINE

- Explain the importance of inspecting the head, neck, and oral cavity for the presence of oral lesions.
- Define the following key terms used in this module:

| | |
|---|---|
| Discrete | Nodule |
| Grouped | Wheal |
| Confluent | Vesicle |
| Linear | Bulla |
| Macule | Pustule |
| Patch | Ulcer |
| Papule | Fissure |
| Plaque | |

- Given an image of a lesion, use the Lesion Descriptor Worksheet (Fig. 11-31A,B) to identify the location and characteristics of the lesion and to develop a written description of the lesion.
- Describe findings that have implications in planning dental treatment.
- Provide appropriate referral to a physician or dental specialist when findings indicate the need for further evaluation.
- Demonstrate knowledge of soft tissue lesions by applying information from this module to the fictitious patient cases A–E found in Modules 12 and 13.

---

**Note to Course Instructor:** Skill checklists and fictitious patient cases A–E for this topic are located in Modules 12 (Head and Neck Examination) and 13 (Oral Examination).

## SECTION 1:
# Learning to Look at Lesions

Inspection of the skin and oral mucosa for soft tissue lesions is an important part of every head and neck examination and intraoral examination. By performing routine screenings, dental health care providers can reduce deaths from skin, oral, and pharyngeal cancers.

## WHY LOOK FOR LESIONS?

The most effective approach to decreasing the number of deaths associated with soft tissue cancers is through early detection and appropriate treatment and referral. In June 2003, the American Dental Association (ADA) launched a campaign urging dental professionals to examine patients for signs of early soft tissue lesions. Most Americans visit a dental office or clinic at least once a year. For this reason, dental health care providers have a unique opportunity to help decrease skin and oral cancer rates by routinely performing head, neck, and intraoral examinations. Early detection of skin and oral cancers is critical in the prevention of cancer deaths. When detected at its earliest stage, skin and oral cancers are more easily treated and cured.

## CANCER FACTS AND STATISTICS

1. **Skin Cancer**
   a. Skin cancer is the most common of all cancer types.
   b. More than 1 million skin cancers are diagnosed each year in the United States. The number of skin cancers has been on the rise steadily for the past 30 years.
   c. There are two main types of skin cancers—melanomas and nonmelanomas.
   d. Melanomas are much more likely to spread to other parts of the body and account for over 60% of skin cancer deaths. *Melanoma is almost always curable in its early stages.*
   e. Nonmelanomas—such as basal cell and squamous cell cancers—are the most common cancers of the skin. Nonmelanomas rarely spread elsewhere in the body and are less likely than melanomas to be fatal.
2. **Oral and Pharyngeal Cancer**
   a. Approximately 30,000 new cases of oral and pharyngeal cancer are diagnosed each year in the United States.
   b. More than one in four people affected with oral cancer will die—about one person each hour. According to the American Cancer Society, oral cancer claims almost as many lives as melanoma cancer.

## WHAT IS A SOFT TISSUE LESION?

A soft tissue lesion is an area of abnormal-appearing skin or mucosa that does not resemble the soft tissue surrounding it. Lesions are variations in color, texture, or form of an area of skin or mucosa. A soft tissue lesion may be:

• Present at birth—such as a mole or birthmark
• Associated with an infection—such as warts or acne
• Associated with an allergic reaction—such as hives
• Associated with an injury—such as a blister from a burn or scar from a cut

# CHARACTERISTICS OF SOFT TISSUE LESIONS

## Lesion Border Traits

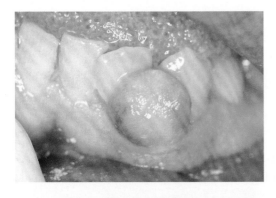

**Figure 11-1. Regular border.** The border of a lesion is regular if it resembles a symmetrical circle or an oval shape.

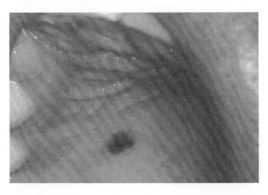

**Figure 11-2. Irregular border.** The border of a lesion is irregular if it is not uniform or has deviations from a circular or oval shape.

## Lesion Margin Traits

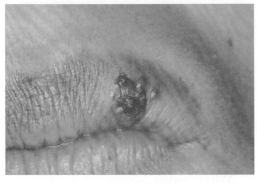

**Figure 11-3. Smooth margin.** The margin of a lesion is smooth if it is level with the surface of the lesion.

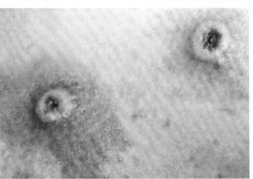

**Figure 11-4. Raised margin.** The margin of a lesion is raised if it is above the level of the surface of the lesion.

## Lesion Color

Lesions can be red, white, red and white, blue, yellow, brown, or black. Some examples are shown here.

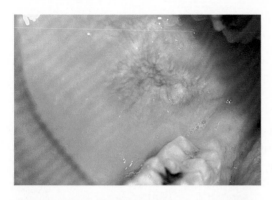

**Figure 11-5. Red and white lesion.** Shown here is an example of a red and white lesion on the buccal mucosa.

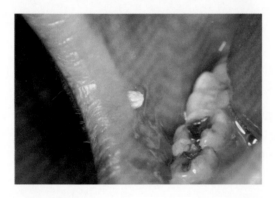

**Figure 11-6. White lesion.** Shown here is an example of a raised white lesion on the buccal mucosa.

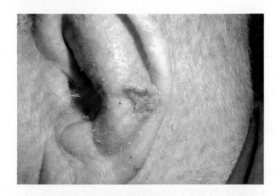

**Figure 11-7. Yellow lesion.** Shown here is a yellow, crusty lesion on the ear.

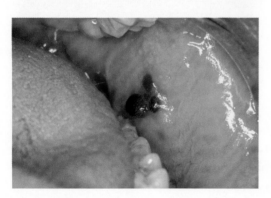

**Figure 11-8. Blue lesion.** Shown here is a group of blue lesions on the buccal mucosa.

## Common Lesion Configurations

Configuration refers to the way that multiple lesions are arranged.

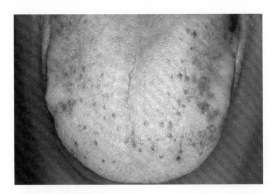

**Figure 11-9. Discrete configuration.** Discrete lesions are individual lesions that are separate and distinct from one another. The individual tiny areas (spots) of brown pigmentation on this tongue are examples of discrete lesions.

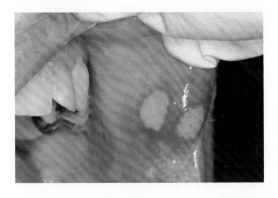

**Figure 11-10. Grouped configuration.** Lesions that are clustered together are described as grouped.

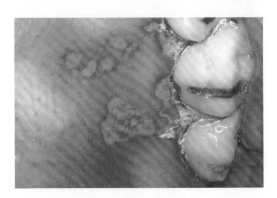

**Figure 11-11. Confluent configuration.** Lesions that have merged together so that individual lesions are not distinguishable are termed confluent.

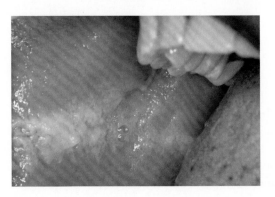

**Figure 11-12. Linear configuration.** Lesions that form a line have a linear configuration.

# BASIC TYPES OF SOFT TISSUE LESIONS

## Flat Lesions

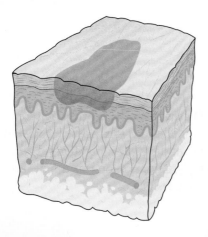

**Figure 11-13. Flat lesion.** A flat lesion is one in which the *surface of the lesion is the same as the normal level* of the skin or oral mucosa. The only way that flat lesions can be detected is through a change in color from the surrounding skin or oral mucosa.

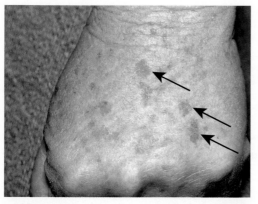

**Figure 11-14. Macule.** A macule is a small flat, discolored spot on the skin or mucosa that does not include a change in skin texture or thickness.
- A macule is less than 1 cm in size; the discoloration can be brown, black, red, or lighter than the surrounding skin.
- Examples: freckles, petechia, amalgam tattoo

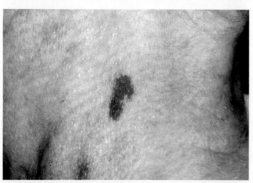

**Figure 11-15. Macule.** This flat red lesion is an example of a macule on a patient's neck.

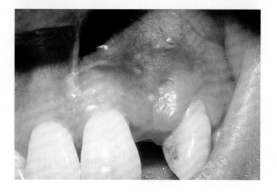

**Figure 11-16. Patch.** A patch is a flat, discolored spot on the skin or mucosa.
- A patch is larger than 1 cm in size.
- Examples: lichen planus, snuff dipper's patch, port-wine stain, amalgam tattoo

## Elevated Lesions

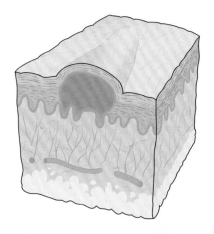

**Figure 11-17. Elevated lesion.** An elevated lesion is one in which the *surface of the lesion is raised above* the normal level of the skin or oral mucosa.

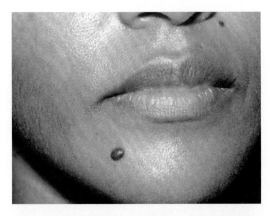

**Figure 11-18. Papule.** A papule is a solid raised lesion that is usually less than 1 cm in diameter.
- A papule may be any color.
- Example: an elevated mole

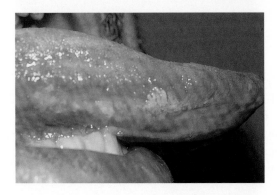

**Figure 11-19. Plaque.** A plaque is a superficial raised lesion often formed by the coalescence (joining) of closely grouped papules.
- A plaque is more than 1 cm in diameter; a plaque differs from a nodule in its height—a plaque is flattened, and a nodule is a bump.
- Examples: leukoplakia, psoriasis

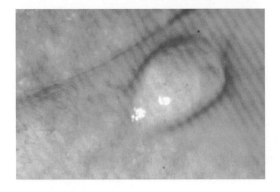

**Figure 11-20. Nodule.** A nodule is a raised marble-like lesion detectable by touch, usually 1 cm or more in diameter.
- It can be felt as a hard mass distinct from the tissue surrounding it
- Examples: wart, basal cell carcinoma, melanoma, enlarged lymph node

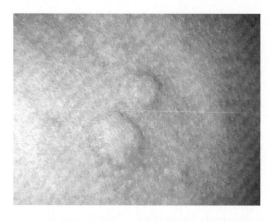

**Figure 11-21.   Wheal.** A wheal is a raised, somewhat irregular area of localized edema.
* Wheals are often itchy, lasting 24 hours or less; they are usually due to an allergic reaction, such as to a drug or insect bite
* Examples: Mosquito bite, hives

## Fluid-Filled Lesions

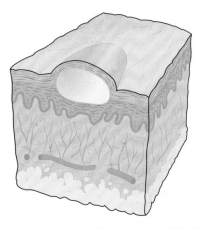

**Figure 11-22.   Fluid-filled lesion.** A fluid-filled lesion is an elevated lesion filled with clear fluid or pus.

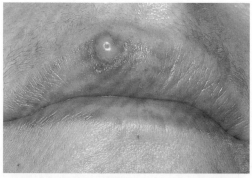

**Figure 11-23.   Vesicle.** A vesicle is a small blister filled with fluid.
* A vesicle usually is 1 cm or less in diameter.
* Example: herpes simplex, herpes zoster, chicken pox and smallpox lesions

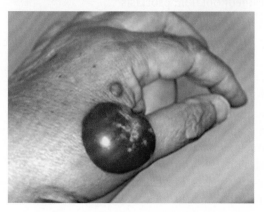

**Figure 11-24.   Bulla.** A bulla is a large blister filled with fluid.
* A bulla is usually over 1 cm in diameter
* Example: blister as seen in burns or from trauma

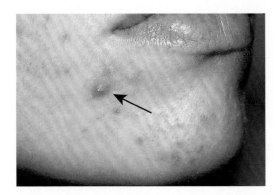

**Figure 11-25. Pustule.** A pustule is a small raised lesion filled with pus.
• Example: acne, boil, abscess

## Depressed Lesions

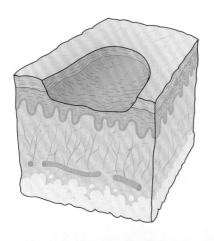

**Figure 11-26. Depressed lesion.** A depressed lesion is one in which the surface of the lesion is below the normal level of the skin or oral mucosa. Erosion is the loss of the top layer of skin. Most depressed lesions are ulcers. The depth of a depressed lesion is the distance from the base to the top of the lesion's margin. The depth of a lesion may be superficial or deep.

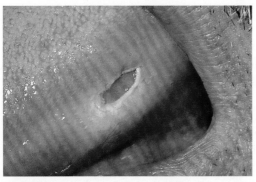

**Figure 11-27. Ulcer.** An ulcer is a craterlike lesion of the skin or mucosa where the top two layers of the skin are lost.
• The depth is superficial if it is less than 3 mm.
• Example: Aphthous ulcer, chicken pox lesions

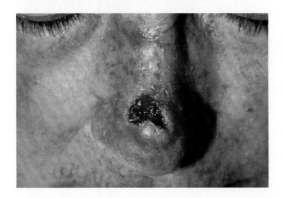

**Figure 11-28. Deep ulcer.** An example of a deep ulcer with a depth that is more than 3 mm.

## Linear Cracks

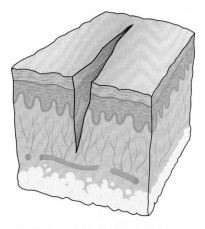

**Figure 11-29. Crack.** A crack is a linear break in the surface of the skin or mucosa.

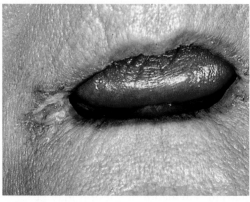

**Figure 11-30. Fissure.** A fissure is a linear crack in the top two layers of the skin or mucosa.
- Examples: fissured tongue, angular cheilitis

## THE ABCD-T APPROACH TO FORMULATING LESION DESCRIPTIONS

The description of a soft tissue lesion has two components: (1) *characteristics of the lesion* and (2) *type of lesion*. A lesion's characteristics include its anatomic location, border traits, color, configuration, and diameter or dimensions. Primary types of lesions are flat, elevated, fluid-filled, and depressed lesions.

Because each lesion has so many characteristics, it is common for clinicians to feel overwhelmed when trying to create a verbal description of a lesion. To assist clinicians in remembering the characteristics to document, it is helpful to remember the letters **A, B, C, D,** and **T** (Box 11-1).

---

BOX **11-1** Remembering What to Look For

*Use the letters A, B, C, D, and T to help you remember the characteristics to look for on a lesion.*
- **A**—*Anatomic location*
- **B**—*Border*
- **C**—*Color and configuration*
- **D**—*Diameter or dimensions*
- **T**—*Type*

**SECTION 2:**

# Peak Procedure: Describing Lesions

**PROCEDURE 11-1** DETERMINING AND DESCRIBING LESION CHARACTERISTICS

| Action | Rationale |
|---|---|
| **1. Determine lesion characteristics.** Use the **Lesion Descriptor Worksheet** (Fig. 11-31A,B) from the Ready References section of this module. Circle or highlight the words that describe the lesion. | • The Lesion Descriptor Worksheet makes it easy to identify the characteristics of a particular lesion. |
| **A—Anatomic location.** Describe the anatomic location of the lesion. | • This allows other clinicians to locate the lesion from your written description. |
| **B—Border.** Examine the lesion to see if the border is symmetrical (having balanced proportions, equal halves from the center dividing line) or asymmetrical (unequal halves). Examine the border to see if it is well demarcated, regular, or irregular. | • An asymmetrical lesion with an irregular border may indicate a malignant lesion. |
| **C—Color and configuration.** Note the color of the lesion. Record the configuration of the lesion(s). Is this a single lesion? Are the lesions separate, clustered together, grouped, confluent, or linear? | • Lesions can change color over time. A color change may indicate a malignant lesion.<br>• Many skin diseases have lesions in a typical configuration. |
| **D—Diameter or dimensions.** Measure the size of the lesion using a plastic millimeter ruler if the lesion is on the skin. Use a periodontal probe for intraoral lesions. | • Over time, a change in size may indicate a malignant lesion. |
| **T—Type.** Identify the type of lesion, such as macule, vesicle, etc. | • The type of lesion is an important component of the description of a lesion. |

*(continued)*

**PROCEDURE 11-1** DETERMINING AND DESCRIBING LESION CHARACTERISTICS (*CONTINUED*)

| | |
|---|---|
| 2. **Document lesion location.** Indicate the location of lesion on the appropriate illustration on the Lesion Descriptor Worksheet. | • The rationale for drawing the lesion is **NOT** to create an artistic likeness of it.<br>• Drawing the lesion on an anatomical illustration assists other clinicians in quickly locating the lesion now and at future appointments, if applicable. |

3. **Develop a written description.** After circling or highlighting the words on the **Lesion Descriptor Worksheet** that pertain to the lesion, you are ready to formulate a description for the lesion.

For example:
**A**—Anatomic location: left buccal mucosa near tooth #14
**B**—Border: well demarcated
**C**—Color and configuration: blue; single lesion
**D**—Diameter or dimensions: 4 mm × 2mm
**T**—Type: macule

4. **Finalize the description.** Next, use the outline to create a description and enter it at the bottom of page 2 of the **Lesion Descriptor Worksheet**.
For example, using the words outlined above, the description might be: *On the left buccal mucosa near tooth #14, a single, well-demarcated, blue, 4 mm × 2 mm macule.*

5. **Document the lesion.** Enter the lesion description and date in the patient's chart or computerized record.

**SECTION 3:**

# Detection and Prevention

## TOOLS FOR CANCER DETECTION OF SKIN AND ORAL CANCERS

In the dental setting, the three primary tools for the detection of soft tissue lesions are the head and neck examination, oral examination, and patient history. Medical history questionnaires should include questions that elicit information about tobacco and alcohol use as well as interest in smoking cessation programs. Box 11-2 outlines the role of a dental professional in cancer detection.

---

**BOX 11-2**   **Dental Professional's Role in Cancer Detection**

*A thorough examination of the head, neck, and oral cavity should be a routine part of each dental visit. Clinicians should be particularly vigilant with patients who use tobacco and alcohol.*

- **EXAMINE** the patient at each visit using a systematic visual inspection of the head, neck, and oral cavity.
- **ENSURE** the health history questionnaire elicits information about tobacco and alcohol use.
- **EDUCATE** the patient that tobacco and alcohol use dramatically increases the risk of oral cancer.
- **IDENTIFY** and document any suspicious soft tissue lesions.
- **REFER** to a dermatologist—for skin lesions—or an oral maxillofacial surgeon—for oral lesions—to obtain a definitive diagnosis of the suspicious lesion.
- **FOLLOW UP** to make sure that a definitive diagnosis was obtained.

---

## IMPORTANCE OF SMOKING CESSATION COUNSELING

*The oral examination provides the perfect opportunity to discuss smoking cessation with your patient.* By advising patients to quit smoking, dental professionals can assist patients in reducing their risk of oral cancer and other life-threatening diseases, such as coronary heart disease. Dental health care providers can promote health wellness by counseling patients about the *three primary controllable risk factors for skin and oral cancers: (1) sun exposure, (2) smoking, and (3) alcohol consumption.* Smoking cessation counseling is covered in Module 10.

**SECTION 4:**
# Ready References

## Lesion Descriptor Worksheet

*Directions: Highlight or circle the applicable descriptors*

| | |
|---|---|
| **(A)** **Anatomic Location** | *Head:* Scalp, eye, ear, nose, cheek, chin, neck; right or left side <br> *Neck:* Midline, right, left; near certain anatomic structure <br> *Lip:* Upper, lower, commissure, vermillion border; labial mucosa <br> *Buccal mucosa:* Parotid papilla; mucobuccal fold; near tooth # <br> *Gingiva:* Free, attached; near tooth # <br> *Tongue:* Anterior-third, middle-third, posterior-third; dorsal, ventral, right lateral, left lateral <br> *Floor of mouth:* Lingual frenum, sublingual folds, sublingual caruncle; near tooth # <br> *Palate:* Hard, soft; midline, incisive papilla; right side, left side <br> *Oropharynx:* Pillars, midline, uvula |
| **(B)** **Border** | *Well-demarcated:* Easy to see where lesion begins and ends <br> *Poorly demarcated:* Difficult to see where lesion begins and ends <br> *Regularly shaped:* Uniform border <br> *Irregularly shaped:* Border not uniform |
| **(C)** **Color Change Configuration** | *Color:* Red, white, red and white, blue, yellow, brown, black <br> *Lesion pattern:* Single lesion or multiple lesions (discrete, grouped, confluent, linear) |
| **(D)** **Diameter/ Dimension** | *If oblong or irregular in shape:* Length and width <br> *If circular or round in shape:* Diameter (measurement of a line running from one side of a circle through the center to the other side) |
| **(T)** **T y p e** | **Nonpalpable Flat Lesions** — *Macule* - Flat discolored spot, less than 1 cm in size <br> *Patch* - Flat discolored spot, larger than 1 cm in size <br><br> **Palpable, Elevated, Solid Masses** — *Papule* - Solid raised lesion, less than 1 cm in diameter <br> *Plaque* - Superficial raised lesion, larger than 1 cm in diameter <br> *Nodule* - Marble-like lesion, larger than 1 cm in diameter <br> *Wheal* - Localized area of skin edema <br><br> **Fluid-Filled Lesions** — *Vesicle* - Small blister filled with clear fluid, less than 1 cm in diameter <br> *Bulla* - Larger fluid-filled lesion, larger than 1 cm in diameter <br> *Pustule* - Small raised lesion filled with pus <br><br> **Loss of Skin or Mucosal Surface** — *Erosion* - Loss of top layer of skin or mucosa <br> *Ulcer* - Craterlike lesion where top two layers of skin or mucosa are lost <br> *Fissure* - A linear crack |

**Figure 11-31A. Page 1 of the Lesion Descriptor Worksheet.**

# Lesion Descriptor Worksheet

*Directions:* Draw the lesion(s) on the appropriate illustration, showing the anatomic location, relative shape, and size.

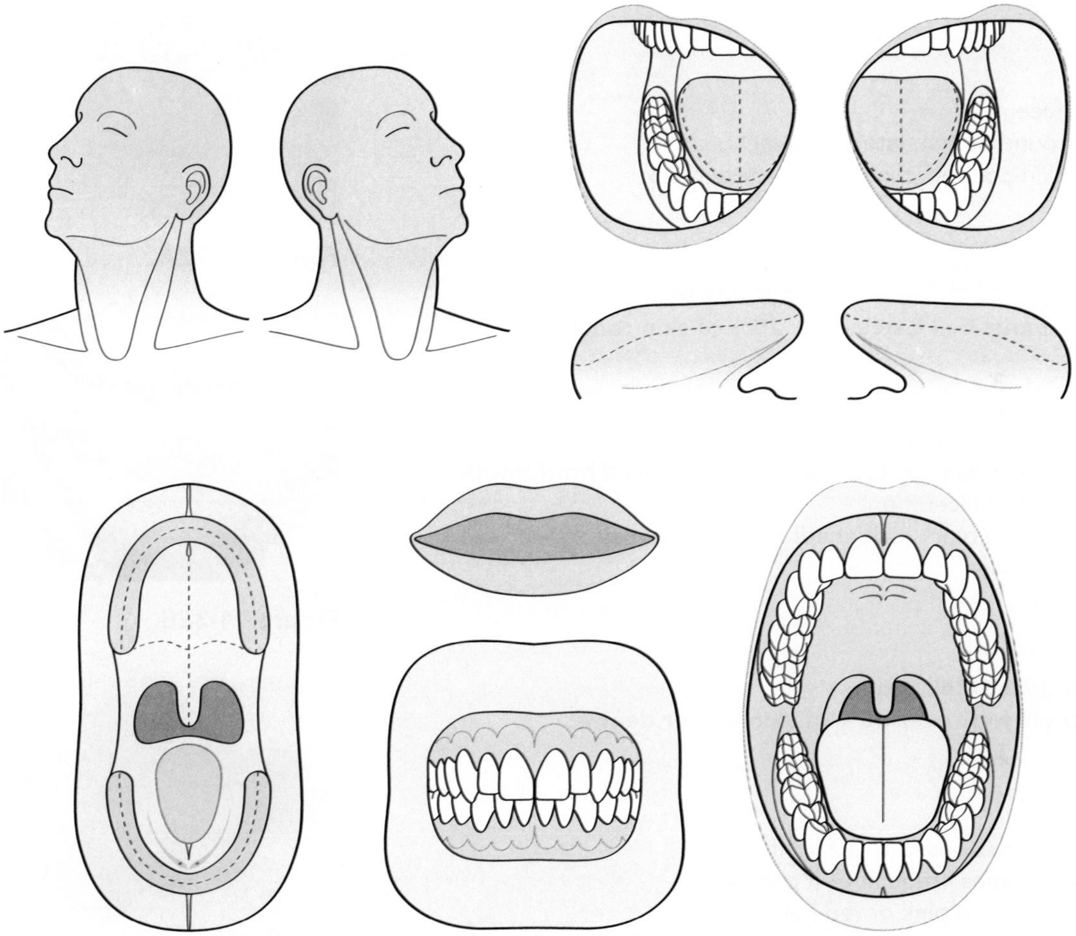

*Develop a Chart Entry:* Using each descriptor circled and the location indicated on this worksheet, develop a written description of the lesion(s). After you have perfected the written description, enter it in the paper or computerized patient chart. Remember the A, B, C, D, T plan for formulating a description.

_____

_____

_____

_____

**Figure 11-31B. Page 2 of the Lesion Descriptor Worksheet.**

## READY REFERENCE 11-1  CHARACTERISTICS OF COMMON CANCEROUS LESIONS

| Type | Appearance |
|---|---|
| **Basal Cell Carcinoma, 60% of skin cancers.**<br><br>**A**—face<br>**B**—round at first, later irregular<br>**C**—skin-colored, pink, dark brown, black | 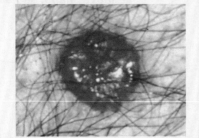<br>Figure 11-32A. |
| **Squamous Cell Carcinoma, 20% of skin cancers.**<br><br>**A**—areas exposed to sunlight; lip<br>**B**—poorly demarcated raised border; raised border with central ulceration<br>**C**—skin-colored, reddened; new lesions may appear near old ones | 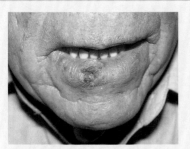<br>Figure 11-32B. |
| **Malignant Melanoma,** **accounts for over 60% of skin cancer deaths.**<br><br>**A**—areas exposed to sunlight<br>**B**—becomes irregular as it grows<br>**C**—may have pink or red halo | 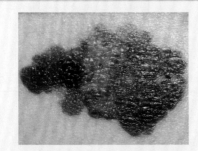<br>Figure 11-32C. |
| **Kaposi Sarcoma**<br><br>**A**—skin; mucous membranes<br>**B**—raised border; well demarcated<br>**C**—intense red, blue, or brown: color does not blanch | 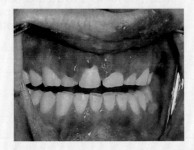<br>Figure 11-32D. |

**READY REFERENCE 11-2** INTERNET RESOURCES: LESIONS

**http://www.dermnetnz.org**
**Derm Net Nz** is the website of the New Zealand Dermatological Society. This website has a list of skin disorders and conditions that includes descriptions and often images.

**http://www.dentistry.vcu.edu/about/departments/opath/labcasex/textfiles/descriptions/softissdescintro.html**
**Basic Diagnostic Skills: Describing Soft Tissue Lesions** on the website of Virginia Commonwealth University School of Dentistry, Oral and Maxillofacial Pathology Diagnostic Service. This module discusses the site, morphology, and color of soft tissue lesions.

**http://www.pediatrics.wisc.edu/education/derm**
**Primary Care Dermatology Module Nomenclature of Skin Lesions** on the website of the University of Wisconsin, Madison. Click on the "Tutorials" box for descriptions and images of common skin lesions. An excellent site with three tutorials: (1) primary lesions, (2) secondary lesions, and (3) patterns and distributions.

**http://www.library.vcu.edu/tml/oralpathology**
**Oral Pathology Review Images** on the Virginia Commonwealth University School of Dentistry, Department of Oral Pathology website is an excellent collection of images of the most common abnormalities of the oral cavity.

**http://www.uiowa.edu/~oprm/AtlasHome.html**
The **Oral Pathology Database** on the website of the University of Iowa College of Dentistry. This atlas shows multiple examples of important lesions of the oral cavity.

**http://www.dent.ohio-state.edu/oralpath2/**
Common oral lesions on the website of **Ohio University College of Dentistry**.

**http://www.aafp.org/afp/980915ap/rose.html**
The website of the American Family Physician Journal includes the online article, **Recognizing Neoplastic Skin Lesions: A Photo Guide**. This article contains excellent information and images of cancerous skin lesions.

**http://www.cancer.org/docroot/PED/ped_0.asp**
Information on cancer prevention and detection on the website of the **American Cancer Society**.

**http://www.nci.nih.gov**
The **National Cancer Institute** (U.S. National Institutes of Health) website is an outstanding source of information on cancer prevention, detection, treatment, and cancer statistics.

## SECTION 5:
# The Human Element

---

### BOX 11-3  Through the Eyes of a Student

*Our school had just switched to a new medical history form and the new form has two columns of information. Even after using this new form for some time, I think that it is easy to miss some of the questions when reviewing the patient's answers.*

*Today, I was seeing a new patient, Mr. U. I had forgotten to look at the tobacco use question. So, I did not read that my patient had been chewing tobacco for over 10 years. If I had read this information, I would not have made my next mistake.*

*I did a quick oral exam and accidentally overlooked some suspicious tissue changes on the lower anterior mucolabial fold. I did not notice until my instructor came to assist me. She showed me where Mr. U. held his tobacco in his mouth and how the tissue looked different. He had what would be considered precancerous tissue changes. I explained to Mr. U. the risk of developing cancer and he seemed ready to change this habit. I may have helped to save my patient's life or at least decreased his risk of developing oral cancer. You can bet that I will never take the oral exam lightly ever again.*

*Kimberly, student*
*Tallahassee Community College*

**PATIENT SCENARIO**

As a first-year dental hygiene student in your second semester, you have just started treating patients. Today, a group of patients from a local adolescent correctional facility will be the patients in the clinic. You will be treating Grace, a 16-year-old female who has an uneventful medical history assessment, which you have reviewed with the social worker accompanying the group.

You begin treatment and perform an extraoral examination on Grace. Because everything is within normal limits, you proceed to the intraoral examination. You retract the right cheek of the buccal mucosa and find a large red and white lesion in the mucobuccal fold that extends the entire length of the cheek. Because this is the first soft tissue lesion that you have ever found on a patient, you are not sure what to do next.

1. Is it ethical to share this information with your instructor/social worker?
2. How do you inform/educate Grace about the lesion?
3. How do you document the lesion in Grace's chart or computerized record?
4. What to you teach Grace about her own oral health?

## SOURCES OF CLINICAL PHOTOGRAPHS

The authors gratefully acknowledge the sources of the following clinical photographs in this module.

- Figure 11-1. Dr. John S. Dozier, Tallahassee, Florida.
- Figure 11-2. Dr. Michaell A. Huber, University of Texas Health Science Center at San Antonio.
- Figure 11-3. Dr. Michaell A. Huber, University of Texas Health Science Center at San Antonio.
- Figure 11-4. Centers for Disease Control and Prevention Public Health Image Library.
- Figure 11-5. From Langlais RP, Miller CS, Nield-Gehrig JS. *Color Atlas of Common Oral Diseases.* 4th ed. Philadelphia, PA: Lippincott Williams & Wilkins; 2009.
- Figure 11-6. Dr. Richard Foster, Guilford Technical Community College, Jamestown, NC.
- Figure 11-7. Dr. Charles Goldberg, University of California San Diego School of Medicine.
- Figure 11-8. Dr. Richard Foster, Guilford Technical Community College, Jamestown, NC.
- Figure 11-9. Dr. Richard Foster, Guilford Technical Community College, Jamestown, NC.
- Figure 11-10. Dr. Richard Foster, Guilford Technical Community College, Jamestown, NC.
- Figure 11-11. Courtesy of Dr. Michaell A. Huber, University of Texas Health Science Center at San Antonio.
- Figure 11-12. Dr. Richard Foster, Guilford Technical Community College, Jamestown, NC.
- Figure 11-14. From Goodheart HP. *Goodheart's Photoguide of Common Skin Disorders.* 2nd ed. Philadelphia, PA: Lippincott Williams & Wilkins; 2003.
- Figure 11-16. From Langlais RP, Miller CS, Nield-Gehrig JS. *Color Atlas of Common Oral Diseases.* 4th ed. Philadelphia, PA: Lippincott Williams & Wilkins; 2009.
- Figure 11-18. From Goodheart HP. *Goodheart's Photoguide of Common Skin Disorders.* 2nd ed. Philadelphia, PA: Lippincott Williams & Wilkins; 2003.
- Figure 11-19. From Goodheart HP. *Goodheart's Photoguide of Common Skin Disorders.* 2nd ed. Philadelphia, PA: Lippincott Williams & Wilkins; 2003.
- Figure 11-20. Dr. Michaell A. Huber, University of Texas Health Science Center at San Antonio.

## SOURCES OF CLINICAL PHOTOGRAPHS *(CONTINUED)*

The authors gratefully acknowledge the sources of the following clinical photographs in this module.

- Figure 11-21. From Goodheart HP. *Goodheart's Photoguide of Common Skin Disorders*. 2nd ed. Philadelphia, PA: Lippincott Williams & Wilkins; 2003.
- Figure 11-23. From Langlais RP, Miller CS, Nield-Gehrig JS. *Color Atlas of Common Oral Diseases*. 4th ed. Philadelphia, PA: Lippincott Williams & Wilkins; 2009.
- Figure 11-24. From Langlais RP, Miller CS, Nield-Gehrig JS. *Color Atlas of Common Oral Diseases*. 4th ed. Philadelphia, PA: Lippincott Williams & Wilkins; 2009.
- Figure 11-25. From Goodheart HP. *Goodheart's Photoguide of Common Skin Disorders*. 2nd ed. Philadelphia, PA: Lippincott Williams & Wilkins; 2003.
- Figure 11-27. From Langlais RP, Miller CS, Nield-Gehrig JS. *Color Atlas of Common Oral Diseases*. 4th ed. Philadelphia, PA: Lippincott Williams & Wilkins; 2009.
- Figure 11-28. From the National Cancer Institute, Bethesda, Maryland.
- Figure 11-30. From Neville B, Damm DD, White DK. *Color Atlas of Clinical Oral Pathology*. Philadelphia, PA: Lea & Febiger; 1991.
- Figure 11-32A. From the National Cancer Institute, Bethesda, Maryland.
- Figure 11-32B. From Goodheart HP. *Goodheart's Photoguide of Common Skin Disorders*. 2nd ed. Philadelphia, PA: Lippincott Williams & Wilkins; 2003.
- Figure 11-32C. From the National Cancer Institute, Bethesda, Maryland.
- Figure 11-32D. From Weber J, Kelley J. *Health Assessment in Nursing*. 2nd ed. Philadelphia, PA: Lippincott Williams & Wilkins; 2003.
- Figure 11-33. From Goodheart HP. *Goodheart's Photoguide of Common Skin Disorders*. 2nd ed. Philadelphia, PA: Lippincott Williams & Wilkins; 2003.
- Figure 11-35. Dr. Richard Foster, Guilford Technical Community College, Jamestown, NC.
- Figure 11-37. Dr. Richard Foster, Guilford Technical Community College, Jamestown, NC.
- Figure 11-39. Dr. Richard Foster, Guilford Technical Community College, Jamestown, NC.
- Figure 11-41. Dr. Richard Foster, Guilford Technical Community College, Jamestown, NC.
- Figure 11-43. Dr. Richard Foster, Guilford Technical Community College, Jamestown, NC.

**SECTION 6:**

# Practical Focus—Describing and Documenting Lesions

---

**DIRECTIONS:**

- Use the steps outlined in **Procedures 11-1** and the **Lesion Descriptor Worksheet** to develop descriptions for the four lesions in this section.

- An example is provided as a guide for completing this section of the module.

- The pages in this section may be removed from the book for easier use by tearing along the perforated lines on each page.

**EXAMPLE:**

**Location:** Mucosa of left cheek

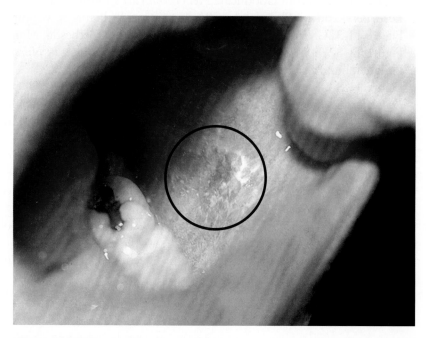

**Figure 11-33. Lesion example.**

**EXAMPLE: Worksheet page 1**

# Lesion Descriptor Worksheet

*Directions: Highlight or circle the applicable descriptors*

| | |
|---|---|
| **Ⓐ Anatomic Location** | *Head:* Scalp, eye, ear, nose, cheek, chin, neck; right or left side<br>*Neck:* Midline, right, left; near certain anatomic structure<br>*Lip:* Upper, lower, commissure, vermillion border; labial mucosa<br>*Buccal mucosa:* Parotid papilla; mucobuccal fold; near tooth #<br>*Gingiva:* Free, attached; near tooth #<br>*Tongue:* Anterior-third, middle-third, posterior-third; dorsal, ventral,<br>    right lateral, left lateral<br>*Floor of mouth:* Lingual frenum, sublingual folds, sublingual caruncle;<br>    near tooth #<br>*Palate:* Hard, soft; midline, incisive papilla; right side, left side<br>*Oropharynx:* Pillars, midline, uvula |
| **Ⓑ Border** | *Well-demarcated:* Easy to see where lesion begins and ends<br>*Poorly demarcated:* Difficult to see where lesion begins and ends<br>*Regularly shaped:* Uniform border<br>*Irregularly shaped:* Border not uniform |
| **Ⓒ Color Change Configuration** | *Color:* Red, white, red and white, blue, yellow, brown, black<br>*Lesion pattern:* Single lesion or<br>    multiple lesions (discrete, grouped, confluent, linear) |
| **Ⓓ Diameter/ Dimension** | *If oblong or irregular in shape:* Length and width<br>*If circular or round in shape:* Diameter (measurement of a line running<br>    from one side of a circle through the center to the other side) |
| **Ⓣ Type** — Nonpalpable Flat Lesions | *Macule* - Flat discolored spot, less than 1 cm in size<br>*Patch* - Flat discolored spot, larger than 1 cm in size |
| Palpable, Elevated, Solid Masses | *Papule* - Solid raised lesion, less than 1 cm in diameter<br>*Plaque* - Superficial raised lesion, larger than 1 cm in diameter<br>*Nodule* - Marble-like lesion, larger than 1 cm in diameter<br>*Wheal* - Localized area of skin edema |
| Fluid-Filled Lesions | *Vesicle* - Small blister filled with clear fluid, less than 1 cm in diameter<br>*Bulla* - Larger fluid-filled lesion, larger than 1 cm in diameter<br>*Pustule* - Small raised lesion filled with pus |
| Loss of Skin or Mucosal Surface | *Erosion* - Loss of top layer of skin or mucosa<br>*Ulcer* - Craterlike lesion where top two layers of skin or mucosa are lost<br>*Fissure* - A linear crack |

**Figure 11-34A.   Page 1 of Lesion Descriptor Worksheet for example of lesion.**

**EXAMPLE: Worksheet page 2**

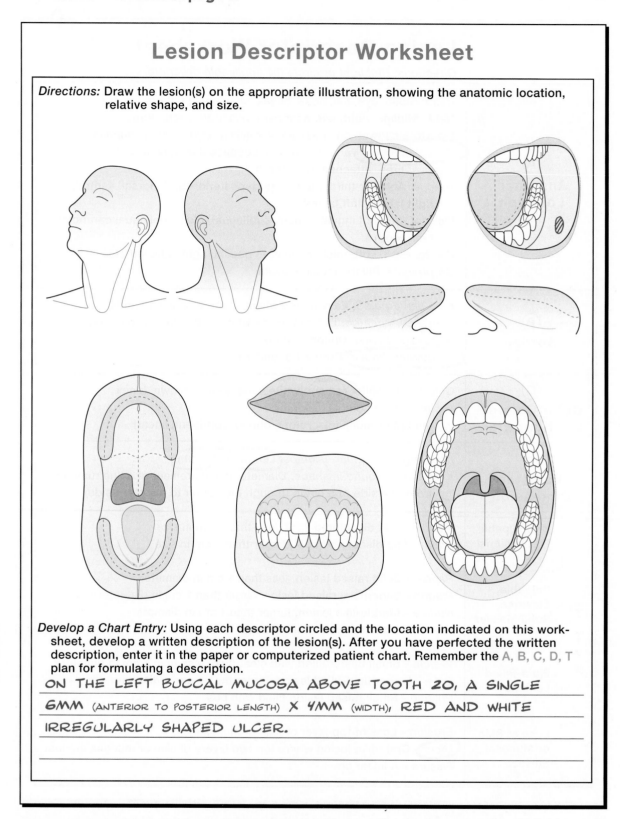

# Lesion Descriptor Worksheet

*Directions:* Draw the lesion(s) on the appropriate illustration, showing the anatomic location, relative shape, and size.

*Develop a Chart Entry:* Using each descriptor circled and the location indicated on this worksheet, develop a written description of the lesion(s). After you have perfected the written description, enter it in the paper or computerized patient chart. Remember the A, B, C, D, T plan for formulating a description.

ON THE LEFT BUCCAL MUCOSA ABOVE TOOTH 20, A SINGLE 6MM (ANTERIOR TO POSTERIOR LENGTH) X 4MM (WIDTH), RED AND WHITE IRREGULARLY SHAPED ULCER.

**Figure 11-34B. Page 2 of Lesion Descriptor Worksheet for example of lesion.**

## Lesion 1:

**Location:** Palate, right side of midline

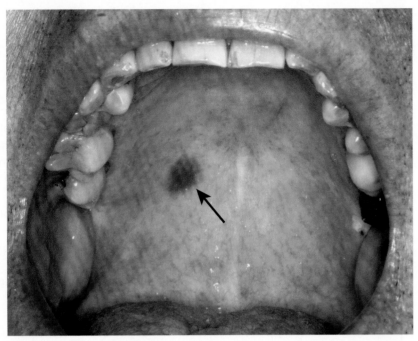

**Figure 11-35.    Lesion 1.**

**Lesion 1**

# Lesion Descriptor Worksheet

*Directions: Highlight or circle the applicable descriptors*

| | |
|---|---|
| **Ⓐ Anatomic Location** | *Head:* Scalp, eye, ear, nose, cheek, chin, neck; right or left side<br>*Neck:* Midline, right, left; near certain anatomic structure<br>*Lip:* Upper, lower, commissure, vermillion border; labial mucosa<br>*Buccal mucosa:* Parotid papilla; mucobuccal fold; near tooth #<br>*Gingiva:* Free, attached; near tooth #<br>*Tongue:* Anterior-third, middle-third, posterior-third; dorsal, ventral, right lateral, left lateral<br>*Floor of mouth:* Lingual frenum, sublingual folds, sublingual caruncle; near tooth #<br>*Palate:* Hard, soft; midline, incisive papilla; right side, left side<br>*Oropharynx:* Pillars, midline, uvula |
| **Ⓑ Border** | *Well-demarcated:* Easy to see where lesion begins and ends<br>*Poorly demarcated:* Difficult to see where lesion begins and ends<br>*Regularly shaped:* Uniform border<br>*Irregularly shaped:* Border not uniform |
| **Ⓒ Color Change Configuration** | *Color:* Red, white, red and white, blue, yellow, brown, black<br>*Lesion pattern:* Single lesion or<br>multiple lesions (discrete, grouped, confluent, linear) |
| **Ⓓ Diameter/ Dimension** | *If oblong or irregular in shape:* Length and width<br>*If circular or round in shape:* Diameter (measurement of a line running from one side of a circle through the center to the other side) |
| **Ⓣ T y p e** / **Nonpalpable Flat Lesions** | *Macule* - Flat discolored spot, less than 1 cm in size<br>*Patch* - Flat discolored spot, larger than 1 cm in size |
| **Palpable, Elevated, Solid Masses** | *Papule* - Solid raised lesion, less than 1 cm in diameter<br>*Plaque* - Superficial raised lesion, larger than 1 cm in diameter<br>*Nodule* - Marble-like lesion, larger than 1 cm in diameter<br>*Wheal* - Localized area of skin edema |
| **Fluid-Filled Lesions** | *Vesicle* - Small blister filled with clear fluid, less than 1 cm in diameter<br>*Bulla* - Larger fluid-filled lesion, larger than 1 cm in diameter<br>*Pustule* - Small raised lesion filled with pus |
| **Loss of Skin or Mucosal Surface** | *Erosion* - Loss of top layer of skin or mucosa<br>*Ulcer* - Craterlike lesion where top two layers of skin or mucosa are lost<br>*Fissure* - A linear crack |

**Figure 11-36A.   Page 1 of Lesion Descriptor Worksheet for use with lesion 1.**

**Lesion 1**

# Lesion Descriptor Worksheet

*Directions:* Draw the lesion(s) on the appropriate illustration, showing the anatomic location, relative shape, and size.

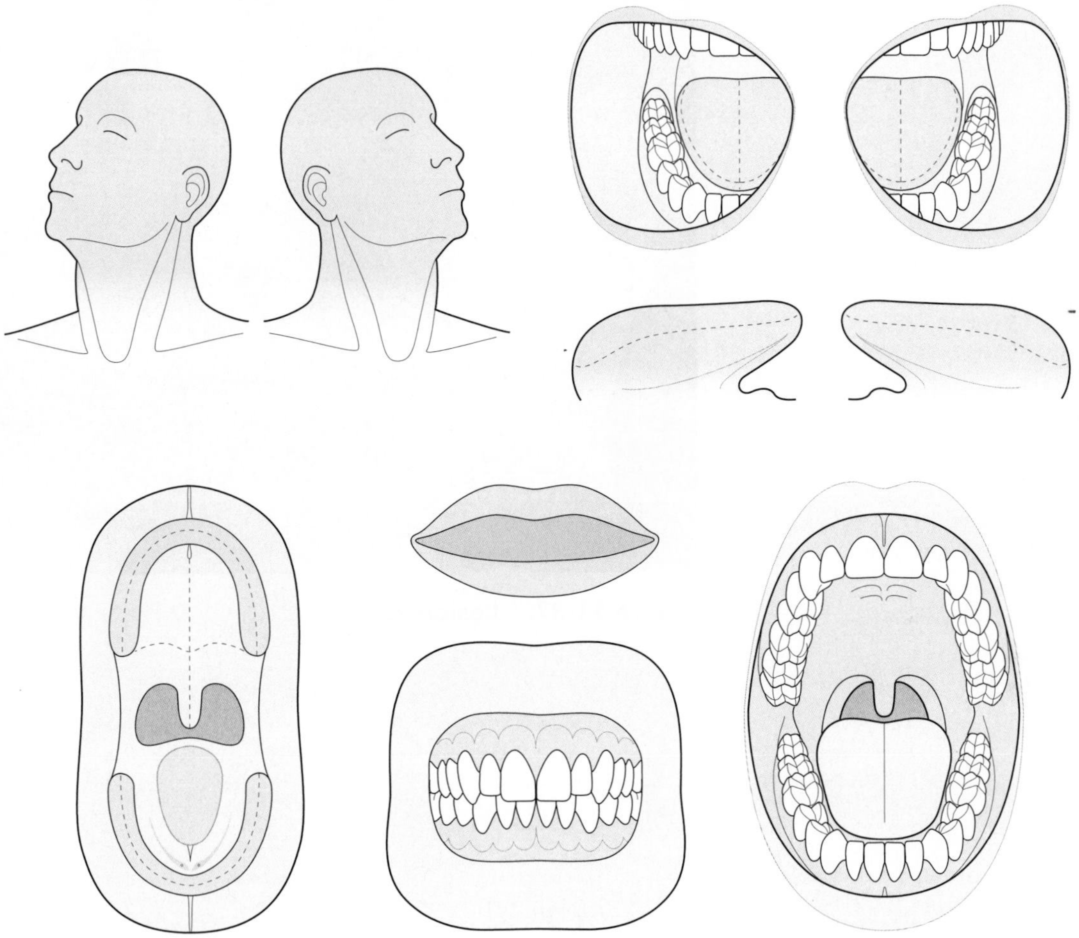

*Develop a Chart Entry:* Using each descriptor circled and the location indicated on this worksheet, develop a written description of the lesion(s). After you have perfected the written description, enter it in the paper or computerized patient chart. Remember the A, B, C, D, T plan for formulating a description.

_____

_____

_____

_____

**Figure 11-36B. Page 2 of Lesion Descriptor Worksheet for use with lesion 1.**

## Lesion 2:

**Location:** Mucosa of right cheek

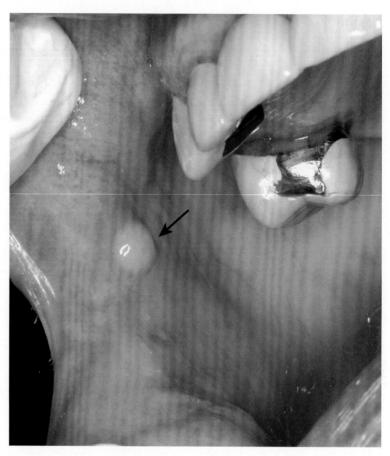

**Figure 11-37.** Lesion 2.

Lesion 2

# Lesion Descriptor Worksheet

*Directions: Highlight or circle the applicable descriptors*

| | |
|---|---|
| **Ⓐ** <br> **Anatomic Location** | *Head:* **Scalp, eye, ear, nose, cheek, chin, neck; right or left side** <br> *Neck:* **Midline, right, left; near certain anatomic structure** <br> *Lip:* **Upper, lower, commissure, vermillion border; labial mucosa** <br> *Buccal mucosa:* **Parotid papilla; mucobuccal fold; near tooth #** <br> *Gingiva:* **Free, attached; near tooth #** <br> *Tongue:* **Anterior-third, middle-third, posterior-third; dorsal, ventral, right lateral, left lateral** <br> *Floor of mouth:* **Lingual frenum, sublingual folds, sublingual caruncle; near tooth #** <br> *Palate:* **Hard, soft; midline, incisive papilla; right side, left side** <br> *Oropharynx:* **Pillars, midline, uvula** |
| **Ⓑ** <br> **Border** | *Well-demarcated:* **Easy to see where lesion begins and ends** <br> *Poorly demarcated:* **Difficult to see where lesion begins and ends** <br> *Regularly shaped:* **Uniform border** <br> *Irregularly shaped:* **Border not uniform** |
| **Ⓒ** <br> **Color Change Configuration** | *Color:* **Red, white, red and white, blue, yellow, brown, black** <br> *Lesion pattern:* **Single lesion or** <br>    **multiple lesions (discrete, grouped, confluent, linear)** |
| **Ⓓ** <br> **Diameter/ Dimension** | *If oblong or irregular in shape:* **Length and width** <br> *If circular or round in shape:* **Diameter (measurement of a line running from one side of a circle through the center to the other side)** |
| **Ⓣ** <br> **T y p e** | **Nonpalpable Flat Lesions** — *Macule* - **Flat discolored spot, less than 1 cm in size** <br> *Patch* - **Flat discolored spot, larger than 1 cm in size** <br><br> **Palpable, Elevated, Solid Masses** — *Papule* - **Solid raised lesion, less than 1 cm in diameter** <br> *Plaque* - **Superficial raised lesion, larger than 1 cm in diameter** <br> *Nodule* - **Marble-like lesion, larger than 1 cm in diameter** <br> *Wheal* - **Localized area of skin edema** <br><br> **Fluid-Filled Lesions** — *Vesicle* - **Small blister filled with clear fluid, less than 1 cm in diameter** <br> *Bulla* - **Larger fluid-filled lesion, larger than 1 cm in diameter** <br> *Pustule* - **Small raised lesion filled with pus** <br><br> **Loss of Skin or Mucosal Surface** — *Erosion* - **Loss of top layer of skin or mucosa** <br> *Ulcer* - **Craterlike lesion where top two layers of skin or mucosa are lost** <br> *Fissure* - **A linear crack** |

**Figure 11-38A.   Page 1 of Lesion Descriptor Worksheet for use with lesion 2.**

**Lesion 2**

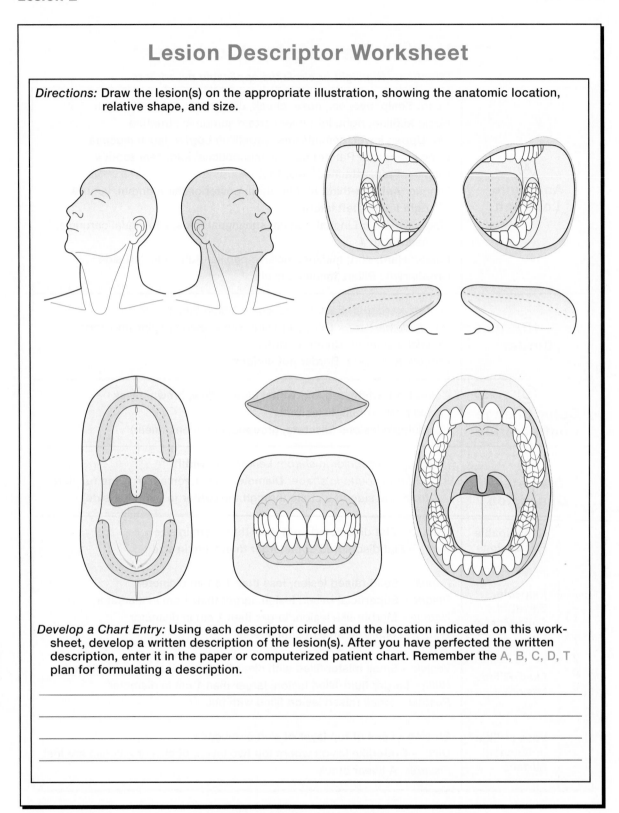

# Lesion Descriptor Worksheet

*Directions:* Draw the lesion(s) on the appropriate illustration, showing the anatomic location, relative shape, and size.

*Develop a Chart Entry:* Using each descriptor circled and the location indicated on this worksheet, develop a written description of the lesion(s). After you have perfected the written description, enter it in the paper or computerized patient chart. Remember the A, B, C, D, T plan for formulating a description.

**Figure 11-38B.   Page 2 of Lesion Descriptor Worksheet for use with lesion 2.**

**Lesion 3:**

**Location:** Palate

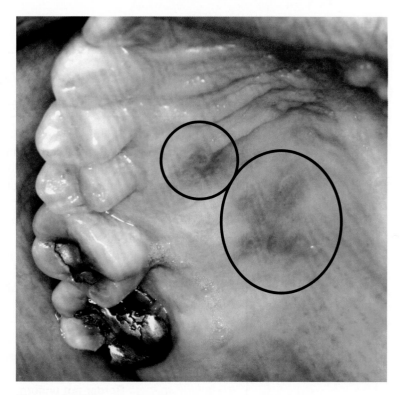

**Figure 11-39. Lesion 3.**

## Lesion 3

# Lesion Descriptor Worksheet

*Directions: Highlight or circle the applicable descriptors*

| | |
|---|---|
| **Ⓐ Anatomic Location** | *Head:* Scalp, eye, ear, nose, cheek, chin, neck; right or left side<br>*Neck:* Midline, right, left; near certain anatomic structure<br>*Lip:* Upper, lower, commissure, vermillion border; labial mucosa<br>*Buccal mucosa:* Parotid papilla; mucobuccal fold; near tooth #<br>*Gingiva:* Free, attached; near tooth #<br>*Tongue:* Anterior-third, middle-third, posterior-third; dorsal, ventral, right lateral, left lateral<br>*Floor of mouth:* Lingual frenum, sublingual folds, sublingual caruncle; near tooth #<br>*Palate:* Hard, soft; midline, incisive papilla; right side, left side<br>*Oropharynx:* Pillars, midline, uvula |
| **Ⓑ Border** | *Well-demarcated:* Easy to see where lesion begins and ends<br>*Poorly demarcated:* Difficult to see where lesion begins and ends<br>*Regularly shaped:* Uniform border<br>*Irregularly shaped:* Border not uniform |
| **Ⓒ Color Change Configuration** | *Color:* Red, white, red and white, blue, yellow, brown, black<br>*Lesion pattern:* Single lesion or multiple lesions (discrete, grouped, confluent, linear) |
| **Ⓓ Diameter/ Dimension** | *If oblong or irregular in shape:* Length and width<br>*If circular or round in shape:* Diameter (measurement of a line running from one side of a circle through the center to the other side) |
| **Ⓣ T y p e** | **Nonpalpable Flat Lesions** | *Macule* - Flat discolored spot, less than 1 cm in size<br>*Patch* - Flat discolored spot, larger than 1 cm in size |
| | **Palpable, Elevated, Solid Masses** | *Papule* - Solid raised lesion, less than 1 cm in diameter<br>*Plaque* - Superficial raised lesion, larger than 1 cm in diameter<br>*Nodule* - Marble-like lesion, larger than 1 cm in diameter<br>*Wheal* - Localized area of skin edema |
| | **Fluid-Filled Lesions** | *Vesicle* - Small blister filled with clear fluid, less than 1 cm in diameter<br>*Bulla* - Larger fluid-filled lesion, larger than 1 cm in diameter<br>*Pustule* - Small raised lesion filled with pus |
| | **Loss of Skin or Mucosal Surface** | *Erosion* - Loss of top layer of skin or mucosa<br>*Ulcer* - Craterlike lesion where top two layers of skin or mucosa are lost<br>*Fissure* - A linear crack |

**Figure 11-40A.   Page 1 of Lesion Descriptor Worksheet for use with lesion 3.**

**Lesion 3**

# Lesion Descriptor Worksheet

*Directions:* Draw the lesion(s) on the appropriate illustration, showing the anatomic location, relative shape, and size.

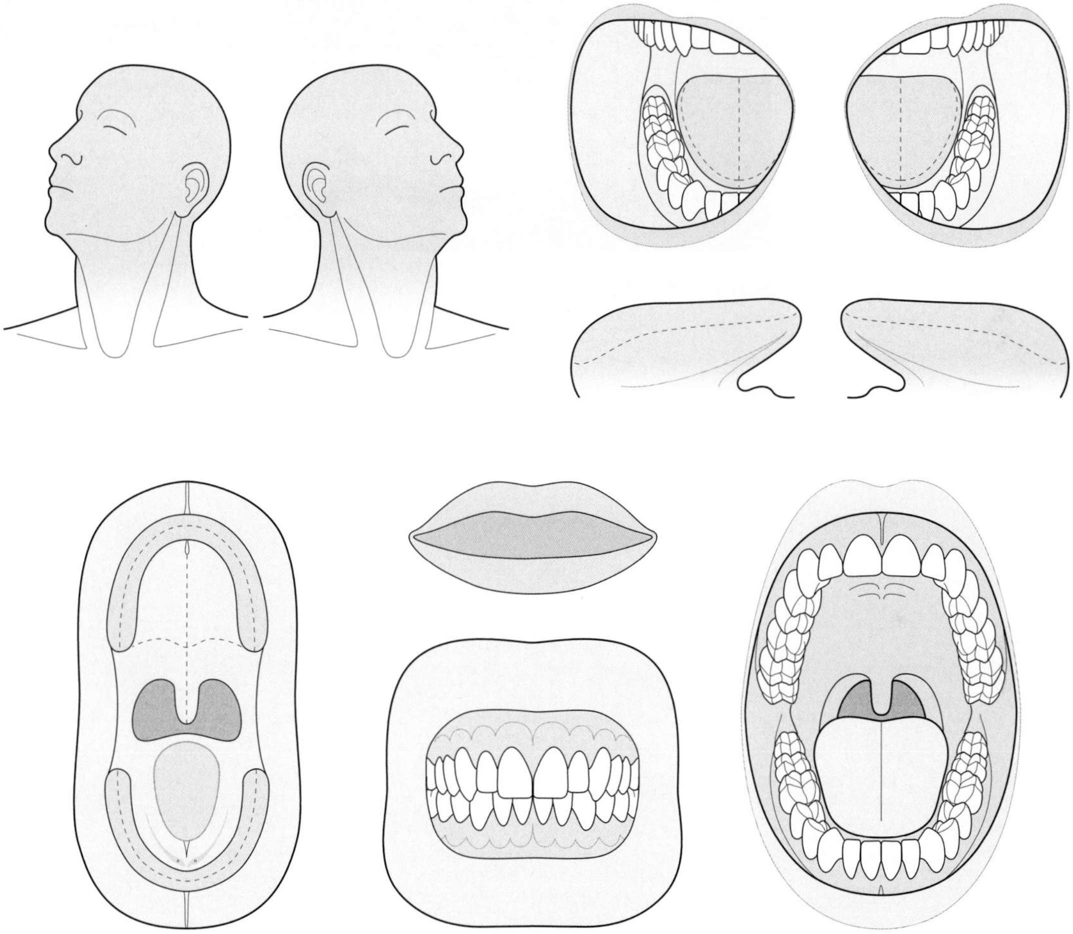

*Develop a Chart Entry:* Using each descriptor circled and the location indicated on this worksheet, develop a written description of the lesion(s). After you have perfected the written description, enter it in the paper or computerized patient chart. Remember the A, B, C, D, T plan for formulating a description.

**Figure 11-40B.   Page 2 of Lesion Descriptor Worksheet for use with lesion 3.**

## Lesion 4:

**Location:** Gingiva and alveolar mucosa, right side of oral cavity

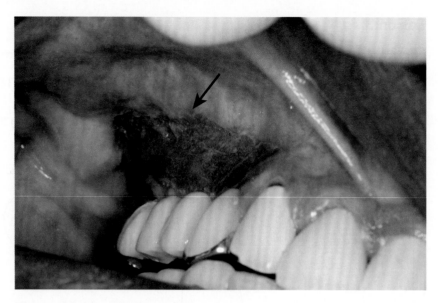

**Figure 11-41.    Lesion 4.**

**Lesion 4**

# Lesion Descriptor Worksheet

*Directions: Highlight or circle the applicable descriptors*

| | |
|---|---|
| **Ⓐ Anatomic Location** | *Head:* Scalp, eye, ear, nose, cheek, chin, neck; right or left side<br>*Neck:* Midline, right, left; near certain anatomic structure<br>*Lip:* Upper, lower, commissure, vermillion border; labial mucosa<br>*Buccal mucosa:* Parotid papilla; mucobuccal fold; near tooth #<br>*Gingiva:* Free, attached; near tooth #<br>*Tongue:* Anterior-third, middle-third, posterior-third; dorsal, ventral, right lateral, left lateral<br>*Floor of mouth:* Lingual frenum, sublingual folds, sublingual caruncle; near tooth #<br>*Palate:* Hard, soft; midline, incisive papilla; right side, left side<br>*Oropharynx:* Pillars, midline, uvula |
| **Ⓑ Border** | *Well-demarcated:* Easy to see where lesion begins and ends<br>*Poorly demarcated:* Difficult to see where lesion begins and ends<br>*Regularly shaped:* Uniform border<br>*Irregularly shaped:* Border not uniform |
| **Ⓒ Color Change Configuration** | *Color:* Red, white, red and white, blue, yellow, brown, black<br>*Lesion pattern:* Single lesion or multiple lesions (discrete, grouped, confluent, linear) |
| **Ⓓ Diameter/ Dimension** | *If oblong or irregular in shape:* Length and width<br>*If circular or round in shape:* Diameter (measurement of a line running from one side of a circle through the center to the other side) |
| **Ⓣ Type** — Nonpalpable Flat Lesions | *Macule* - Flat discolored spot, less than 1 cm in size<br>*Patch* - Flat discolored spot, larger than 1 cm in size |
| Palpable, Elevated, Solid Masses | *Papule* - Solid raised lesion, less than 1 cm in diameter<br>*Plaque* - Superficial raised lesion, larger than 1 cm in diameter<br>*Nodule* - Marble-like lesion, larger than 1 cm in diameter<br>*Wheal* - Localized area of skin edema |
| Fluid-Filled Lesions | *Vesicle* - Small blister filled with clear fluid, less than 1 cm in diameter<br>*Bulla* - Larger fluid-filled lesion, larger than 1 cm in diameter<br>*Pustule* - Small raised lesion filled with pus |
| Loss of Skin or Mucosal Surface | *Erosion* - Loss of top layer of skin or mucosa<br>*Ulcer* - Craterlike lesion where top two layers of skin or mucosa are lost<br>*Fissure* - A linear crack |

**Figure 11-42A. Page 1 of Lesion Descriptor Worksheet for use with lesion 4.**

**Lesion 4**

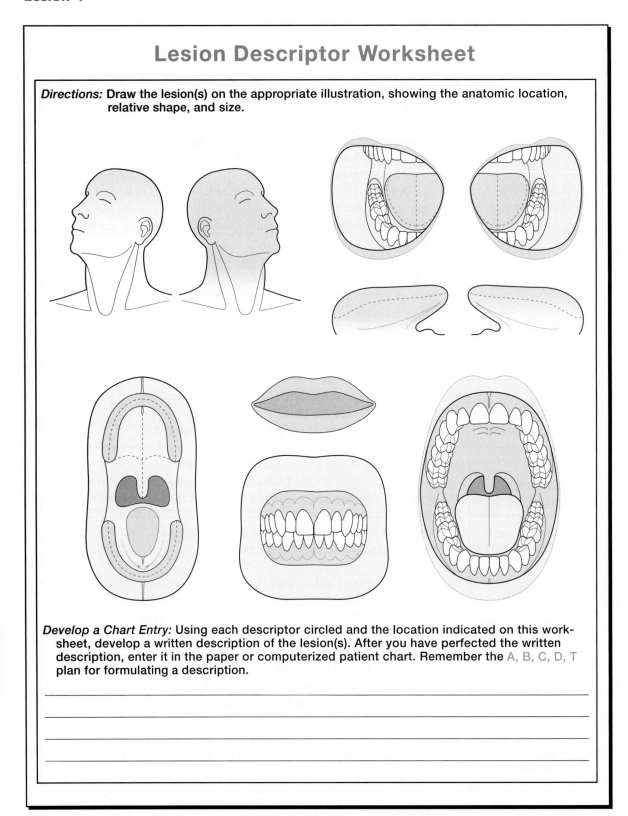

## Lesion Descriptor Worksheet

*Directions:* **Draw the lesion(s) on the appropriate illustration, showing the anatomic location, relative shape, and size.**

*Develop a Chart Entry:* **Using each descriptor circled and the location indicated on this worksheet, develop a written description of the lesion(s). After you have perfected the written description, enter it in the paper or computerized patient chart. Remember the A, B, C, D, T plan for formulating a description.**

**Figure 11-42B.   Page 2 of Lesion Descriptor Worksheet for use with lesion 4.**

## Lesion 5:

**Location:** Gingiva, maxillary left posterior sextant, facial aspect

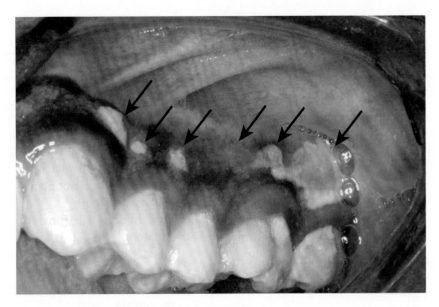

**Figure 11-43.** Lesion 5.

**Lesion 5**

## Lesion Descriptor Worksheet

*Directions: Highlight or circle the applicable descriptors*

| Ⓐ Anatomic Location | *Head*: Scalp, eye, ear, nose, cheek, chin, neck; right or left side<br>*Neck:* Midline, right, left; near certain anatomic structure<br>*Lip:* Upper, lower, commissure, vermillion border; labial mucosa<br>*Buccal mucosa:* Parotid papilla; mucobuccal fold; near tooth #<br>*Gingiva:* Free, attached; near tooth #<br>*Tongue:* Anterior-third, middle-third, posterior-third; dorsal, ventral, right lateral, left lateral<br>*Floor of mouth:* Lingual frenum, sublingual folds, sublingual caruncle; near tooth #<br>*Palate:* Hard, soft; midline, incisive papilla; right side, left side<br>*Oropharynx:* Pillars, midline, uvula |
|---|---|
| Ⓑ Border | *Well-demarcated:* Easy to see where lesion begins and ends<br>*Poorly demarcated:* Difficult to see where lesion begins and ends<br>*Regularly shaped:* Uniform border<br>*Irregularly shaped:* Border not uniform |
| Ⓒ Color Change Configuration | *Color:* Red, white, red and white, blue, yellow, brown, black<br>*Lesion pattern:* Single lesion or multiple lesions (discrete, grouped, confluent, linear) |
| Ⓓ Diameter/ Dimension | *If oblong or irregular in shape:* Length and width<br>*If circular or round in shape:* Diameter (measurement of a line running from one side of a circle through the center to the other side) |

| Ⓣ<br>T<br>y<br>p<br>e | Nonpalpable Flat Lesions | *Macule* - Flat discolored spot, less than 1 cm in size<br>*Patch* - Flat discolored spot, larger than 1 cm in size |
|---|---|---|
| | Palpable, Elevated, Solid Masses | *Papule* - Solid raised lesion, less than 1 cm in diameter<br>*Plaque* - Superficial raised lesion, larger than 1 cm in diameter<br>*Nodule* - Marble-like lesion, larger than 1 cm in diameter<br>*Wheal* - Localized area of skin edema |
| | Fluid-Filled Lesions | *Vesicle* - Small blister filled with clear fluid, less than 1 cm in diameter<br>*Bulla* - Larger fluid-filled lesion, larger than 1 cm in diameter<br>*Pustule* - Small raised lesion filled with pus |
| | Loss of Skin or Mucosal Surface | *Erosion* - Loss of top layer of skin or mucosa<br>*Ulcer* - Craterlike lesion where top two layers of skin or mucosa are lost<br>*Fissure* - A linear crack |

**Figure 11-44A.   Page 1 of Lesion Descriptor Worksheet for use with lesion 5.**

**Lesion 5**

# Lesion Descriptor Worksheet

*Directions:* Draw the lesion(s) on the appropriate illustration, showing the anatomic location, relative shape, and size.

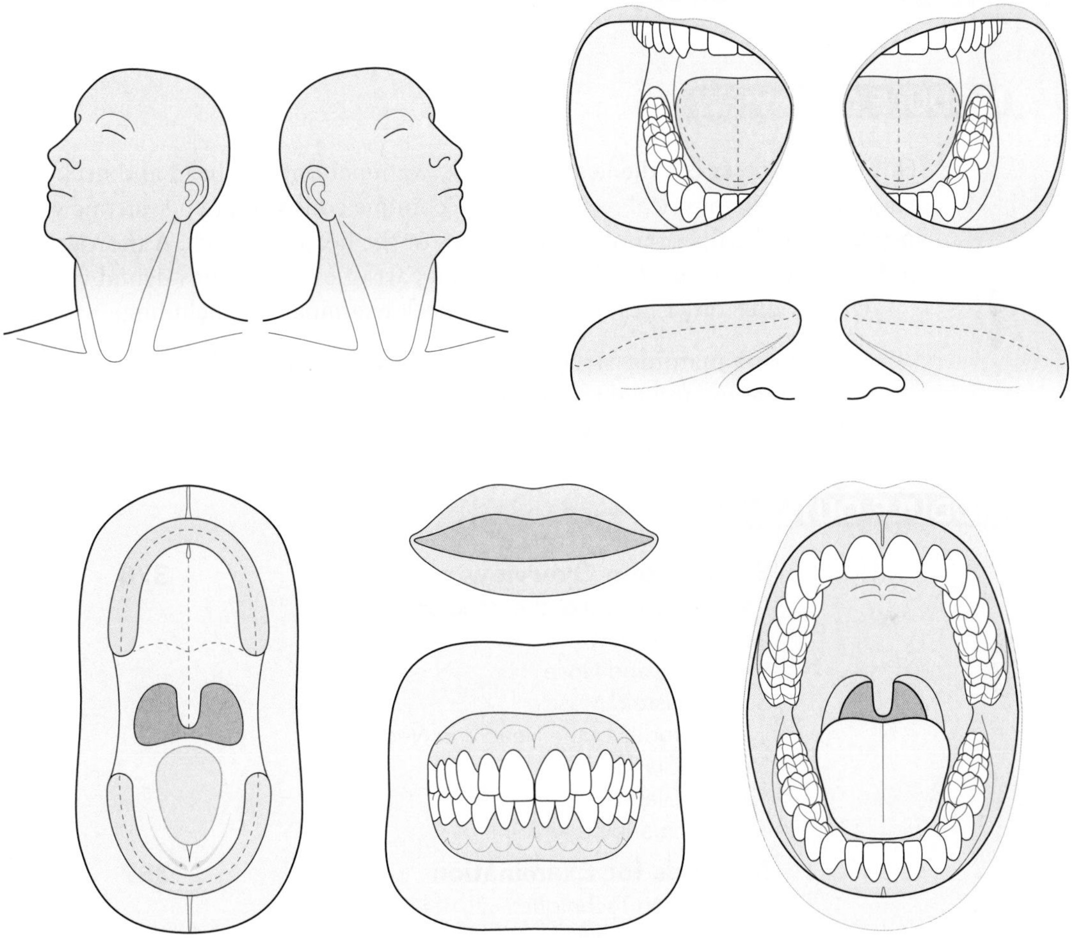

*Develop a Chart Entry:* Using each descriptor circled and the location indicated on this work-sheet, develop a written description of the lesion(s). After you have perfected the written description, enter it in the paper or computerized patient chart. Remember the A, B, C, D, T plan for formulating a description.

Figure 11-44B.  Page 2 of Lesion Descriptor Worksheet for use with lesion 5.

MODULE OVERVIEW

This module describes the head and neck examination. The head and neck examination is a physical examination technique consisting of a systemic visual inspection and palpation of the structures of the head and neck. A thorough head and neck examination should be a routine part of each patient's dental visit.

This module describes the head and neck examination, including:

- Review of anatomic structures of the head and neck
- Examination and palpation techniques
- Peak procedure for a systematic head and neck examination

MODULE OUTLINE

## OBJECTIVES

- Locate the (1) lymph nodes of the head and neck, (2) salivary and thyroid glands, and (3) temporomandibular joint (TMJ).
- Describe the normal anatomy of the structures of the head and neck.
- Identify deviations from normal of the skin, lymph nodes, and salivary and thyroid glands.
- Position the patient correctly for the head and neck examination.
- Provide information to the patient about the head and neck examination and any notable findings.
- Demonstrate the head and neck examination using correct technique and a systematic sequence of examination.
- Document notable findings in the patient chart or computerized record.
- Explain findings that have implications in planning dental treatment.
- Provide referral to an appropriate specialist when findings indicate the need for further evaluation.
- Demonstrate knowledge of the head and neck exam by applying concepts from this module to the fictitious patient cases A–E found in Section 6.

## SECTION 1:
# Examination Overview

The head and neck examination is a physical examination technique consisting of a systematic visual inspection of the skin of the head and neck combined with palpation of the lymph nodes, salivary glands, thyroid gland, and temporomandibular joint. This procedure takes only minutes and allows the clinician to gather general information on the health of a patient, note early indications of some diseases, and detect abnormalities and potentially life-threatening malignancies at an early stage. *The head and neck and oral examinations are the two most important clinical procedures that a clinician will ever master because these examinations can literally save a patient's life.* The oral examination is presented in Module 13.

There are many structures to be assessed during the head and neck examination. To assist the clinician in performing a systematic examination, the structures are organized into four subgroups: (1) the overall appraisal of the head, neck, face, ears, and skin; (2) lymph nodes of the head and neck; (3) salivary and thyroid glands; and (4) temporomandibular joint (TMJ).

## OVERALL APPRAISAL OF THE HEAD AND NECK

The head and neck examination begins while greeting and seating the patient. While chatting with the patient, unobtrusively examine the head and neck area including assessment of facial form and symmetry and inspection of the skin (Fig. 12-1).

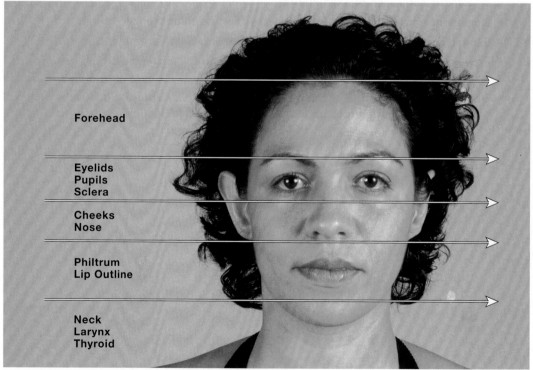

Forehead

Eyelids
Pupils
Sclera

Cheeks
Nose

Philtrum
Lip Outline

Neck
Larynx
Thyroid

**Figure 12-1. Overall appraisal.** Divide the face and neck into imaginary zones. Scanning from right to left, inspect each zone carefully but unobtrusively. Note signs of asymmetry, hair loss, dilated or unequal pupils, involuntary facial movements, and variations such as changes in color, scars, lesions, or fissuring of the skin.

## ANATOMY REVIEW

To perform an accurate head and neck examination, the clinician needs to know the anatomy of the eyes, ears, nose, and neck and recognize the clinical appearance of normal structures.

## EYES, EARS, AND NOSE

Knowledge of the landmarks of the eyes, ears, and nose is useful when recording the location of a soft tissue lesion or other notable findings (Figs. 12-2 and 12-3).

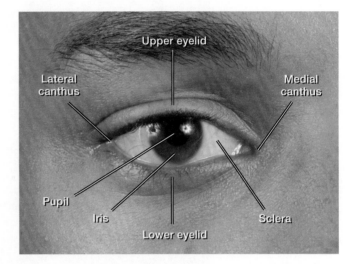

**Figure 12-2. Landmarks of the eye.** The sclera (white of the eye), pupil, and eyelids are anatomical landmarks of the eye.

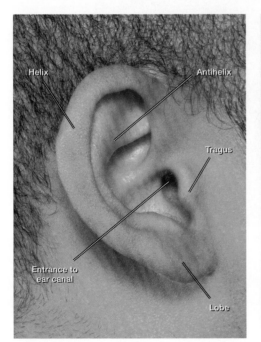

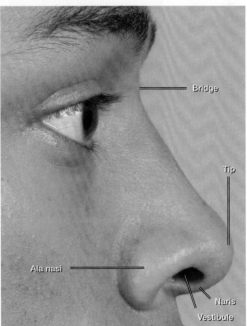

**Figure 12-3. Landmarks of the ear and nose.** External ear landmarks include the earlobe, tragus, helix, antihelix, and entrance to the ear canal. Landmarks of the nose include the bridge, tip, anterior naris, and ala nasi.

## STERNOMASTOID MUSCLE

The **sternomastoid muscle**—also known as the **sternocleidomastoid muscle**—is a long, thick superficial muscle on each side of the head with its origin on the mastoid process and insertion on the sternum and clavicle (Fig. 12-4).

- This muscle acts to bend, rotate, and flex head.
- The ability to locate the sternomastoid muscle is significant because *the cervical lymph nodes lie above, beneath, and posterior to this muscle.*

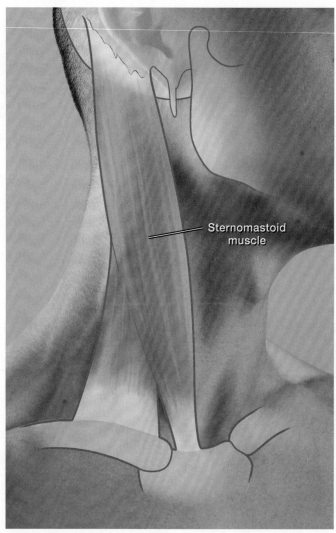

Sternomastoid muscle

**Figure 12-4.   The sternomastoid muscle of the neck.**

## LYMPH NODES OF THE HEAD AND NECK

The lymphatic system is a network of lymph nodes connected by lymphatic vessels that plays an important part in the body's defense against infection. This system transports lymph—a clear fluid that carries nutrients and waste materials between the body tissues and the bloodstream. Lymph nodes (pronounced "limf") are small, bean-shaped structures that filter out and trap bacteria, fungi, viruses, and other unwanted substances to safely eliminate them from the body (Fig. 12-5). All substances transported by the lymphatic system pass through at least one lymph node, where foreign substances can be filtered out and destroyed before fluids are returned to the bloodstream.

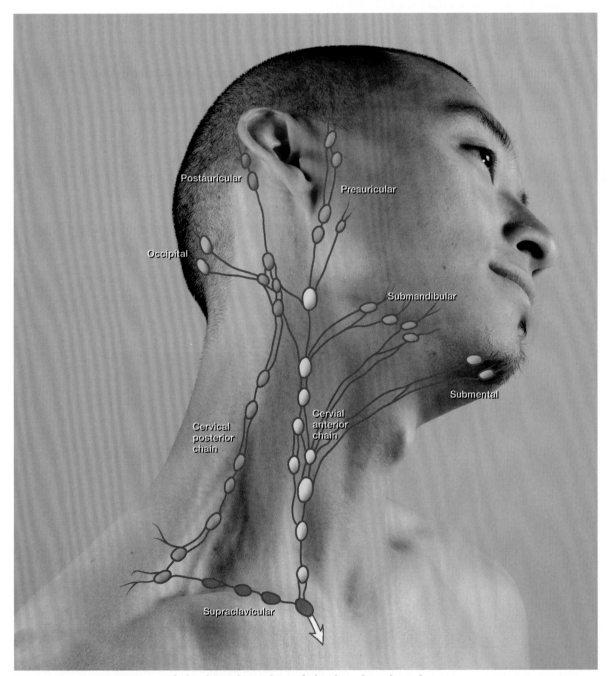

**Figure 12-5.** Location of the lymph nodes of the head and neck.

There are 400 to 700 lymph nodes in the body, *170 to 200 of which are located in the neck*. The major lymph node groups are located along the anterior and posterior aspects of the neck and on the underside of the jaw (Fig. 12-5).

1. Normal lymph nodes can be as small as the head of a pin or the size of a pea or baked bean.
2. Lymph nodes can become enlarged due to infection, inflammatory conditions, an abscess, or cancer.
   a. Lymphadenopathy (lymph·ad·e·nop·a·thy) is the term for enlarged lymph nodes.
   b. If the nodes are quite big, they may be visible bulging under the skin (Fig. 12-6), particularly if the enlargement is asymmetric (i.e., it will be more obvious if one side of the neck is larger than the other).
3. By far, the most common cause of lymph node enlargement is infection. In general, when swelling appears suddenly and is tender to the touch, it is usually caused by injury or infection.
   a. When a part of the body is infected, the nearby lymph nodes become swollen as they collect and destroy the infecting organisms. For example, if a person has a throat infection, the lymph nodes in the neck may swell and become tender to the touch.
   b. Nodes with a viral infection are usually 1/2 to 1 in across.
   c. Nodes with a bacterial infection usually are larger than 1 in across, about the size of a quarter.
4. Node enlargement that comes on gradually and painlessly may result from cancer.
   a. An enlarged lymph node might be a sign that the cancer has spread to a lymph node.
   b. Metastasis is the spread of cancer from the original tumor site to other parts of the body by tiny clumps of cells transported by the blood or lymphatic system.
   c. When oral cancer metastasizes, it most commonly spreads through the lymphatic system to the cervical chain of lymph nodes in the neck.
   d. Lymph nodes can play a role in the spread of cancer because the lymphatic system can transport cancer cells throughout the body.

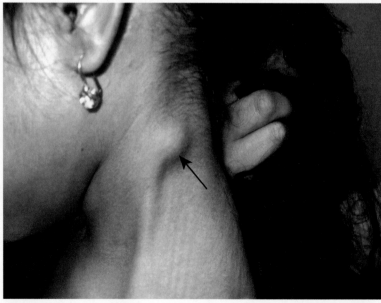

**Figure 12-6.   Lymphadenopathy.** An enlarged cervical lymph node. (Image provided by Stedman's Medical Dictionary.)

## SALIVARY GLANDS

Salivary glands produce saliva and have ducts that release saliva into the mouth (Fig. 12-7). Problems of the salivary glands include obstruction of the flow of saliva, inflammation, infection, and salivary gland tumors.

There are three main pairs of salivary glands:
- The parotid glands are the largest of the salivary glands. Each gland is located on the surface of the masseter muscle between the ear and the jaw.
- The submandibular glands sit below the jaw toward the back of the mouth.
- The sublingual glands are located under the tongue, beneath the mucous membrane of the floor of the mouth.

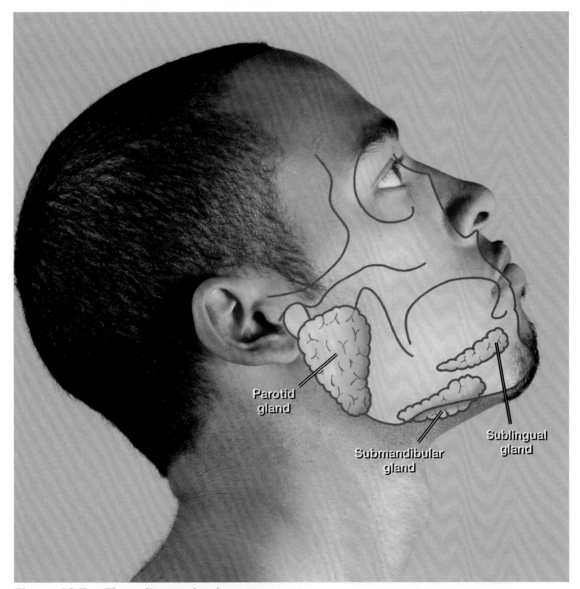

Figure 12-7.   The salivary glands.

## THYROID GLAND

The **thyroid gland** (THIGH-royd), one of the endocrine glands, secretes thyroid hormone, which controls the body's metabolic rate. The thyroid gland is located in the middle of the lower neck and is covered by layers of skin and muscles (Fig. 12-8). It is situated below the larynx (voice box), over the trachea, and just above the clavicles (collarbones). The small 2-in gland has a right and left lobe joined by a narrow isthmus, giving the gland the shape of a bow tie.

Disorders of the thyroid gland are very common, affecting millions of Americans. The most common disorders of the thyroid are an overactive or underactive gland. Examination of the thyroid is done to look at the size of the gland, as well as for **nodules** (lumps or masses). Normally, the thyroid gland cannot be seen and can barely be felt, but if it becomes enlarged, it can be felt and it may appear as a bulge below or to the side of the Adam's apple (Figs. 12-9 and 12-10).

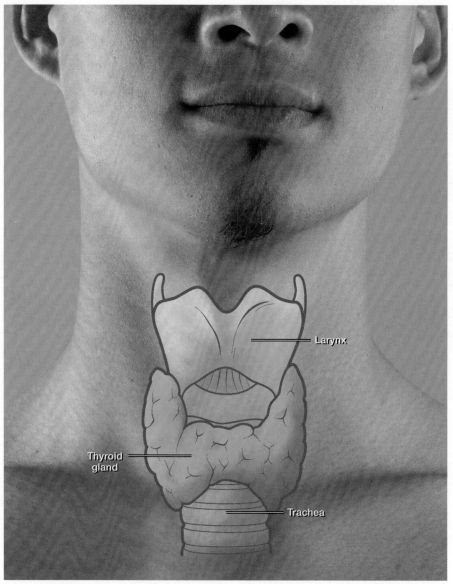

**Figure 12-8. The thyroid and larynx.** The thyroid gland is made up of two lobes that are connected by an isthmus and thus has a bow tie–shaped appearance. A portion of each lobe lies behind the sternomastoid muscle.

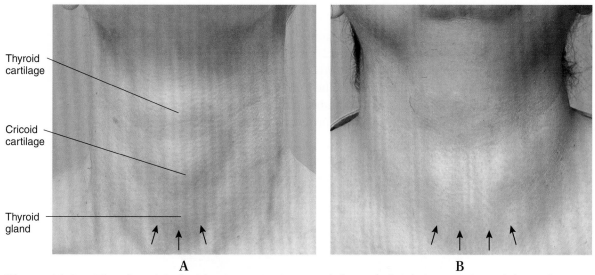

Thyroid cartilage

Cricoid cartilage

Thyroid gland

A

B

**Figure 12-9.   The thyroid gland at rest. A.** A normal thyroid gland. **B.** An enlarged thyroid gland. Goiter is the term for an enlarged thyroid gland. (From Bickley LS, Szilagyi P. *Bates' Guide to Physical Examination and History Taking.* 8th ed. Philadelphia, PA: Lippincott Williams & Wilkins; 2003.)

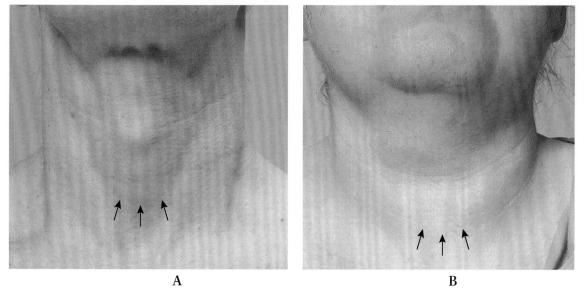

A

B

**Figure 12-10.   The thyroid gland during swallowing. A.** A normal thyroid gland during swallowing. **B.** An enlarged thyroid—the enlarged gland is more evident as it rises during the act of swallowing. (From Bickley LS, Szilagyi P. *Bates' Guide to Physical Examination and History Taking.* 8th ed. Philadelphia, PA: Lippincott Williams & Wilkins; 2003.)

## TEMPOROMANDIBULAR JOINT

The **temporomandibular joint (TMJ)** is the joint that connects the mandible to the temporal bone at the side of the head (Figs. 12-11 and 12-12). It is one of the most complicated joints in the body, allowing the jaw to open and close, move forward and backward, and move from side to side. The joint contains a piece of cartilage called a disk that keeps the skull and the mandible from rubbing against each other. Temporomandibular disorders include problems with the joints, the muscles surrounding them, or both.

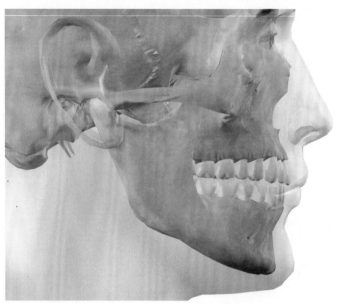

**Figure 12-11.    Lateral view of the temporomandibular joint.** (Courtesy of LifeART. Copyright 2006 Lippincott Williams & Wilkins. All rights reserved.)

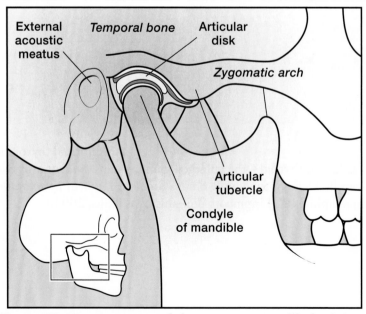

**Figure 12-12.    Anatomy of the temporomandibular joint.**

SECTION 2:
# Methods for Examination

## EXAMINATION TECHNIQUES

1. **Examination Techniques.** The two primary examination techniques are inspection and palpation.
   A. Inspection is a systematic visual examination of a patient's general appearance, skin, or a part of the body to observe its condition.
   B. Palpation is the examination of a part of the body by using the fingertips to move or compress a structure against the underlying tissue. The most sensitive part of the hand—the fingertips—should be used for palpation.
2. **Keys to Effective Examination Technique**
   A. **Consistent sequence.** The sequence for examination of the head and neck must be followed consistently with every patient so as not to accidentally skip an area or structure. The specific order can vary from clinician to clinician. It is most important, however, that once a clinician chooses a particular sequence, he or she must keep the same sequence of examination every time to ensure thoroughness.
   B. **Good palpation technique.** Correct palpation technique is critical to the success of a head and neck examination. Suggestions for effective palpation technique are listed in Box 12-1.
   C. **Careful documentation.** All findings should be documented on the patient chart or computerized record. Documentation of unusual or abnormal findings with a camera is extremely helpful.

---

BOX **12-1** Technique for Effective Palpation

1. To detect abnormalities such as swelling, tumors, or enlarged lymph nodes, the structure being examined must be compressed against a firm, underlying structure or between the examiner's fingers.
2. To compress a structure against an underlying structure, use the fingertips to depress the structure being examined about 1/2 in against the underlying tissue.
3. Depress the structure, applying consistent light pressure and a circular motion.
4. When ready to palpate another area, lift the fingers, move to the next area, and repeat the process, applying light, consistent pressure against the underlying tissue.
5. Incorrect palpation technique involves lightly "walking" or "dancing" the fingertips over a structure. This light dancing technique usually is unsuccessful in detecting nodules, tumors, swelling, or enlarged lymph nodes.
6. Rather than dancing your fingertips over a structure, use the fingertips to compress the structure against the underlying tissues using a circular motion.

## COMPRESSION TECHNIQUES

To detect abnormalities such as swelling, tumors, or enlarged lymph nodes, the structure being examined must be compressed against a firm structure or between the examiner's fingers (Table 12-1). The fingertips are used during palpation by placing the sensitive palmar surfaces of the fingertips against the tissues (Fig. 12-17).

Two basic compression techniques are employed during palpation:
1. Compressing the soft tissue between the examiner's fingertips; and
2. Compressing the soft tissue against underlying structures or tissues of the head or neck.

### Table 12-1  METHODS FOR DETECTING ABNORMALITIES
**Compression Techniques**

| | |
|---|---|
| 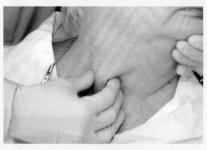 **Figure 12-13.** | **Compression between the fingers of one hand**—the technique of compressing the tissue between the fingers and thumb of the same hand.<br><br>Example: Compressing the sternomastoid muscle of the neck between the fingers and thumb |
| 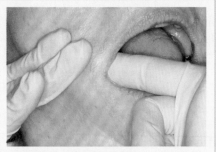 **Figure 12-14.** | **Compression between the fingers of both hands**—the technique of compressing the tissues between the fingers of both hands in coordination to assess a structure.<br><br>Example: Using an index finger intraorally to compress the tissue of the buccal mucosa against the fingers of the extraoral hand |
| 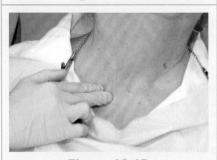 **Figure 12-15.** | **Compression against an underlying structure**—this technique uses one or two fingers to move or depress a structure against the underlying tissues.<br><br>Example: Using the fingers to compress the supraclavicular lymph nodes of the neck against the underlying tissues |
| 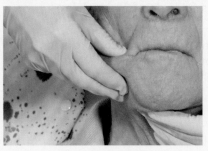 **Figure 12-16.** | **Compression against and over an underlying structure**—this palpation technique uses the fingertips to move or compress a structure against the underlying the tissue.<br><br>Example: Using the fingers of the right hand to roll the tissue from under the chin up and over the inferior border of the mandible |

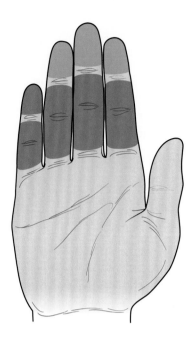

**Figure 12-17. Fingertips.** The sensitive palmar surfaces of the fingertips (shown in green) are used to palpate structures of the head, neck, and oral cavity.

## PALPATION EXPECTATIONS

In health, the lymph nodes, salivary glands, and thyroid are rarely detectible by palpation. For this reason, many beginning clinicians express their concern saying, "But I don't feel anything." Table 12-2 outlines findings that can be detected by palpation.

- Palpating the structures of the head and neck can be likened to our observations in everyday life.
- Think about the skin of the arm. When touched, the skin on an arm is smooth, even, soft, and intact. This is the normal finding.
- If the arm is stung by a bee, however, there will be a red, raised welt on the skin. The area of the sting is swollen, tender, and warm to the touch. The welt is an example of an abnormal finding.
- Thus, an infected, injured, or diseased structure—like a lymph node—may be palpable when normally it is not detectible.

**Table 12-2** FINDINGS DETECTED BY PALPATION

| Quality | Characteristics |
|---|---|
| **Surface** | Smooth or rough<br>Flat or a raised knob, lump, or swelling |
| **Shape** | Irregular, round, or oval |
| **Consistency** | Firm, hard, or spongy |
| **Mobility** | Mobile (moves independently of the underlying structure)<br>Fixed (not freely mobile; stuck to underlying structures) |
| **Tenderness** | Amount of tenderness, if any, experienced by the patient when the structure is palpated |

**SECTION 3:**

# Peak Procedure

The head and neck examination involves the inspection and palpation of the structures of the head and neck. It is helpful to organize the structures to be examined into four subgroups:

**1.** Overall appraisal, head, neck, face, and skin
**2.** Lymph nodes of the head and neck
**3.** Salivary and thyroid glands
**4.** The temporomandibular joint (TMJ)

## PROCEDURE 12-1. HEAD AND NECK EXAMINATION
## SUBGROUP 1: OVERALL APPRAISAL OF HEAD, NECK, FACE, AND SKIN

**Table 12-3** OVERALL APPRAISAL: WHAT CAN I EXPECT TO FEEL?

| | |
|---|---|
| **Normal Findings** | • The face and neck appear symmetrical.<br>• The skin is intact and of uniform color.<br>• There is an even distribution of hair on the scalp. |
| **Notable Findings** | • Lesions or color changes of the skin<br>• Uneven pattern of hair loss<br>• Masses in the neck<br>• Wounds, bruises, scars<br>• Swelling of the face or neck<br>• Asymmetry of the face or neck<br><br>Remember to request information from the patient. The patient will have valuable information about the duration and possibly know the cause of any notable findings, such as a scar due to injury or surgery. |

## PROCEDURE 12-1   HEAD AND NECK EXAMINATION

**Equipment:**
Gloves and optional overgloves
Small cup of water for patient use during thyroid exam

### Subgroup 1: Overall Appraisal of Head, Neck, Face, and Skin

| Action | Rationale |
|---|---|
| **1. General appraisal.** While seating and chatting with the patient, unobtrusively inspect the skin and facial symmetry of the face and neck.<br><br>If problems are detected, question the patient about the onset, duration, and possible causes of any surface variations of the skin, such as lesions or scars. | 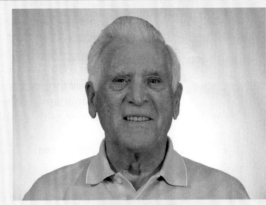<br>**Figure 12-18.** |
| **2. Preparation and positioning.** Position the patient in an upright seated position. The patient should support his or her head in an upright position rather than resting it against the headrest.<br><br>Ask the patient to remove eyeglasses and loosen clothing that limits examination of the neck. Wash and dry hands, don gloves.<br><br>Donning overgloves at this time is optional. | • An upright head position makes the structures of the neck stand out for easier examination.<br>• The height of the patient chair should be positioned so that the clinician can easily reach all the structures to be examined.<br>• Gloves prevent direct contact with open wounds, cuts, sores, or contagious skin conditions.<br>• Donning overgloves at this time facilitates moving directly from the head and neck examination to the intraoral examination. The overgloves are removed before proceeding to the intraoral examination. |
| **3. Provide information.** Briefly explain the examination procedure to the patient. | • Reduces patient apprehension and encourages patient cooperation |
| **4. Head, scalp, and ears.** Change your position so that you are standing directly behind the patient. Visually inspect the head and scalp for any abnormalities. Inspect the ears. | • Lesions and head lice are common conditions that may be detected on the skin and scalp of the head.<br>• The ears are common sites for lesions, such as basal cell carcinoma. |

*(continued)*

## SUBGROUP 2: LYMPH NODES OF THE HEAD AND NECK

**Table 12-4** LYMPH NODES: WHAT CAN I EXPECT TO FEEL?

| Normal Findings | • Lymph nodes are usually not detectible.<br>• No tenderness. |
|---|---|
| Notable Findings | **Infected lymph nodes:**<br>• Firm<br>• Tender<br>• Enlarged and warm<br>• Bilateral (on both sides of the head)<br>• Freely movable from underlying structures<br>• Feel a bit like a swollen grape<br>• Following an infection, lymph nodes occasionally remain permanently enlarged; these will be small (less than 1 cm), non-tender, with a rubbery consistency<br><br>**Malignancies:**<br>• Firm<br>• Nontender<br>• Matted (stuck to each other)<br>• Fixed (stuck to underlying tissue)<br>• Unilateral (only enlarged on one side) |

**PROCEDURE 12-1** **HEAD AND NECK EXAMINATION** *(CONTINUED)*

### Subgroup 2: Lymph Nodes of the Head and Neck

**1. Occipital lymph nodes.** The occipital nodes are located at the base of the skull.

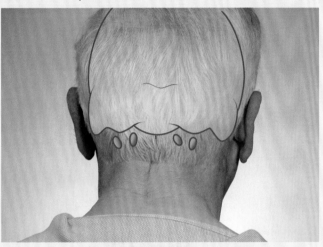

**Figure 12-19.**

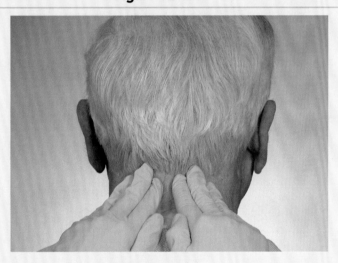

**Figure 12-20.**

1. **Your position.** Stand behind the patient.
2. **Patient's position.** Ask the patient to tip the head forward slightly. If applicable, the patient can assist by holding up long hair so that the neck is fully visible to the examiner.
3. **Palpation technique.**
   - Position your fingertips at the base of the skull.
   - Begin at the midline of the neck, working outward along the hairline until the sternomastoid muscle is reached.
   - Use circular motions with your fingertips to compress the tissues against the base of the underlying bone.
   - Cover the area slightly above and below the hairline because the location of lymph nodes varies among patients.

*(continued)*

**PROCEDURE 12-1**    **HEAD AND NECK EXAMINATION** *(CONTINUED)*

### Subgroup 2: Lymph Nodes of the Head and Neck

**2. Posterior auricular lymph nodes.** The posterior auricular nodes are located behind each ear.

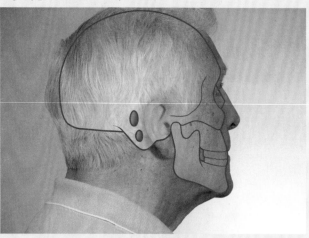

**Figure 12-21.**

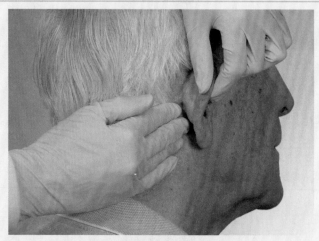

**Figure 12-22.**

1. **Your position.** Stand behind the patient.
2. **Patient's position.** Head in an upright position. If applicable, the patient can assist by holding up long hair so that the neck is fully visible to the examiner.
3. **Palpation technique.**
   - *Inspect each ear separately, beginning with the right ear.*
   - Displace the right ear forward to visually inspect the back of the ear and the skin behind the ear. The ears are common sites for lesions, such as basal cell carcinoma.
   - Palpate the posterior auricular nodes using steady, gentle circular motions with your fingertips to compress the tissues against the bone of the patient's skull.
   - Repeat this procedure to examine the back of the left ear and the skin behind it.

*(continued)*

**PROCEDURE 12-1**  **HEAD AND NECK EXAMINATION** *(CONTINUED)*

## Subgroup 2: Lymph Nodes of the Head and Neck

**3. Preauricular lymph nodes.** The preauricular nodes are located in front of the ears.

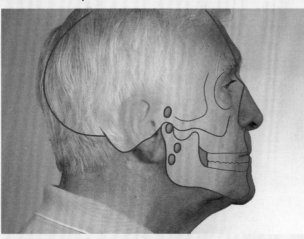

**Figure 12-23.**

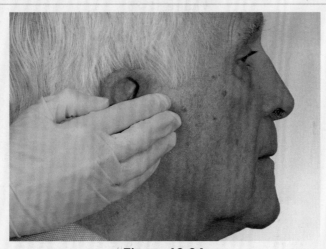

**Figure 12-24.**

1. **Your position.** Stand behind the patient.
2. **Patient's position.** Head in an upright position.
3. **Palpation technique.**
   - Palpate the preauricular nodes using steady, gentle circular motions with your fingertips against the underlying bone.
   - Note tender or enlarged lymph nodes.

*(continued)*

**PROCEDURE 12-1**    **HEAD AND NECK EXAMINATION** *(CONTINUED)*

### Subgroup 2: Lymph Nodes of the Head and Neck

4. **Submental lymph nodes.** The submental nodes are located under the jaw on either side of the midline of the mandible.

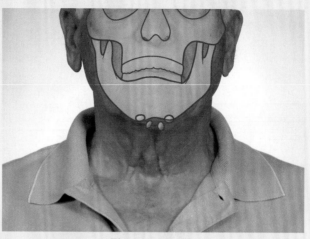

**Figure 12-25.**

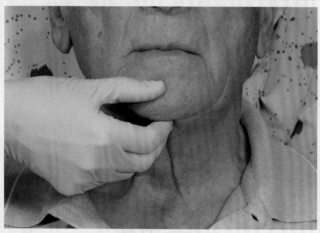

**Figure 12-26.**

1. **Your position.** Stand behind or to the side of the patient.
2. **Patient's position.** Head in an upright position.
3. **Palpation technique.**
   - Use your thumb and index finger to compress the area behind and beneath the symphysis (midline area) of the mandible.
   - Note tender or enlarged nodes.

*(continued)*

## Subgroup 2: Lymph Nodes of the Head and Neck

5. **Submandibular lymph nodes.** The submandibular nodes are under the jaw, along the side of the mandible.

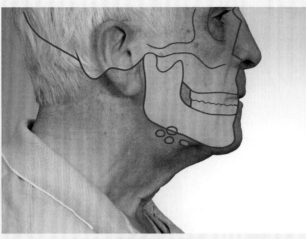

**Figure 12-27.**

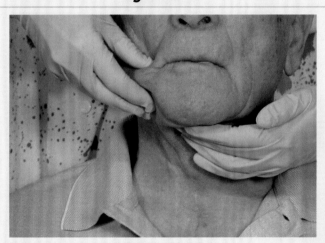

**Figure 12-28.**

1. **Your position.** Stand behind the patient.
2. **Patient's position.** Head in an upright position.
3. **Palpation technique.**
   - Begin with the submandibular nodes on the right side of the head.
   - To facilitate palpation, ***use your left hand as a stabilizing hand*** to move the tissue under the chin toward the right side of the neck. Moving the tissue toward the right side assists the examiner in rolling the tissue over the right side of the mandible.
   - ***Your right hand is used for palpation.*** Cup your fingers under the chin; roll the tissue up and over the inferior border of the mandible. Keeping the fingertips in place, allow the tissue to slowly slide down over the mandible, back into normal position. As the tissue moves over the mandible, you can detect enlarged nodes.
   - Examine the submandibular nodes on the left side of the jaw using a similar procedure.

*(continued)*

**PROCEDURE 12-1**    HEAD AND NECK EXAMINATION *(CONTINUED)*

### Subgroup 2: Lymph Nodes of the Head and Neck

6. **Cervical lymph nodes to muscle.** The anterior chain of cervical lymph nodes lies above the sternomastoid muscle.

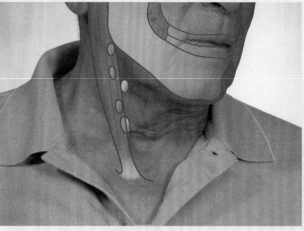

**Figure 12-29.**

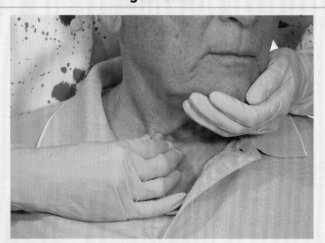

**Figure 12-30.**

1. **Your position.** Stand behind the patient.
2. **Patient's position.** Ask the patient to tip the chin down slightly and turn the head to the left. This position makes the sternomastoid muscle stand out. ***Support the patient's chin with your left hand.***
3. **Palpation technique.**
   - Palpate the cervical nodes medial to the sternomastoid muscle, beginning with those on the right side of the neck.
   - With your *right hand*, grasp the body of the muscle between your fingertips and thumb.
   - Rotate your fingertips back and forth over of the muscle, covering its entire length from behind the ear to the clavicle.

*(continued)*

**PROCEDURE 12-1** HEAD AND NECK EXAMINATION *(CONTINUED)*

### Subgroup 2: Lymph Nodes of the Head and Neck

7. **Cervical lymph nodes posterior to muscle.** The posterior chain of cervical lymph nodes lies beneath and posterior to the sternomastoid muscle.

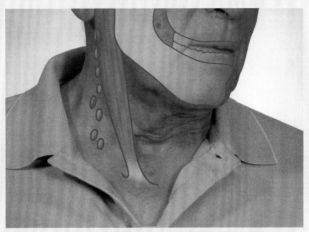

**Figure 12-31.**

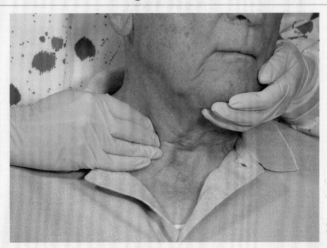

**Figure 12-32.**

1. **Your position.** Stand behind the patient.
2. **Patient's position.** Ask the patient to maintain the same head position as when palpating the lymph nodes medial to the muscle.
3. **Palpation technique.**
   - Begin by palpating the nodes on the right side of the neck.
   - Palpate the nodes by positioning the fingertips of your index and middle fingers under (behind) the muscle and applying gentle compression against the underlying tissues along the entire length of the muscle from behind the ear to the clavicle.
   - Repeat this procedure to examine the cervical nodes medial and posterior to the sternomastoid muscle on the left side of the neck.

*(continued)*

**PROCEDURE 12-1**    **HEAD AND NECK EXAMINATION** *(CONTINUED)*

## Subgroup 2: Lymph Nodes of the Head and Neck

**8. Supraclavicular lymph nodes.** The supraclavicular nodes are located in the angle formed between the sternomastoid muscle and the clavicle.

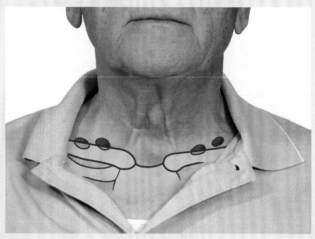

**Figure 12-33.**

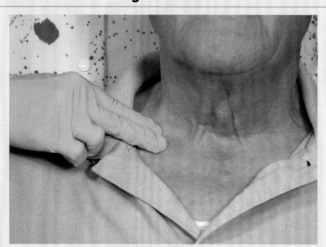

**Figure 12-34.**

**1. Your position.** Stand to the side of or behind the patient.

**2. Patient's position.** Ask the patient to face forward with the chin tipped slightly downward. This position facilitates palpation by relaxing the muscles in the neck.

**3. Palpation technique.**

- Place your index and middle fingers above the clavicle on the right side of the neck and apply circular compression.
- Palpate the supraclavicular nodes on the left side using the same technique.

*(continued)*

## SUBGROUP 3: SALIVARY AND THYROID GLANDS

**Table 12-5** SALIVARY AND THYROID GLANDS: WHAT CAN I EXPECT TO FEEL?

| Normal Findings | Usually not detectible; no tenderness |
|---|---|
| Notable Findings | **Salivary glands:**<br>• Swollen or enlarged<br>• Firm, hard consistency<br>• Tender to palpation<br><br>**Thyroid gland:**<br>• Palpable gland<br>• Deviates from the midline of the neck<br>• Asymmetrical lobes<br>• Enlarged lobes, diffuse enlargement; irregular borders<br>• Nodules present<br>• Hard, firm consistency<br>• Fixed to underlying structures |

**PROCEDURE 12-1**    **HEAD AND NECK EXAMINATION** *(CONTINUED)*

### Subgroup 3: Salivary and Thyroid Glands

**1. Parotid glands.** The parotid gland is located between the ear and the jaw.

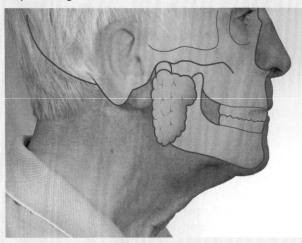

**Figure 12-35.**

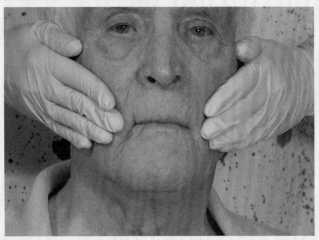

**Figure 12-36.**

1. **Your position.** Stand behind or slightly to the side of the patient.
2. **Patient's position.** Head in an upright position.
3. **Palpation technique.**
   - Place the palms of your hands in front of the ears with your fingers extending the full length of the cheek so that you can palpate the entire gland.
   - Use circular compression to compress the tissue against the cheekbones.
   - A normal parotid gland is difficult to detect by palpation; however, an enlarged gland or nodules in the gland are palpable.
   - Pain or tenderness may be related to salivary stones, inflammation, or cancer.

*(continued)*

## PROCEDURE 12-1   HEAD AND NECK EXAMINATION *(CONTINUED)*

### Subgroup 3: Salivary and Thyroid Glands

2. **Submandibular glands—Locate.** The submandibular gland sits below the jaw toward the back of the mouth.

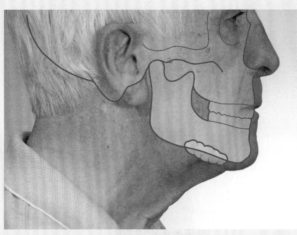

**Figure 12-37.**

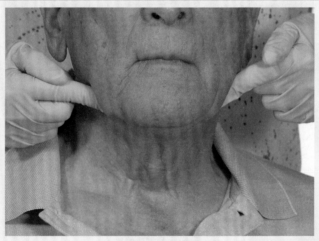

**Figure 12-38.**

1. **Your position.** Stand behind the patient.
2. **Patient's position.** Head in an upright position.
3. **Locate the submandibular gland.**
   - Locate the submandibular salivary glands by placing your index fingers near the angle of the mandible and then moving forward along the mandible to locate the slight depression in the inferior border of the mandible—the **antegonial notch**.
   - *Continue to the next page for the palpation technique for the submandibular glands.*

*(continued)*

**PROCEDURE 12-1** HEAD AND NECK EXAMINATION *(CONTINUED)*

## Subgroup 3: Salivary and Thyroid Glands

### 3. Submandibular glands—Palpate.

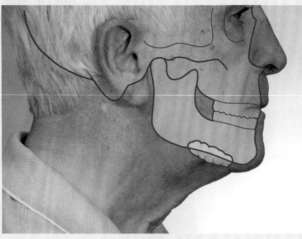

**Figure 12-39.**

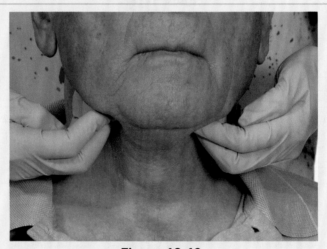

**Figure 12-40.**

1. **Your position.** Stand behind the patient.
2. **Patient's position.** Head in an upright position.
3. **Palpation technique.**
   - Move your fingers under the chin to locate the gland on both sides of the head.
   - Ask the patient to press the tip of his or her tongue against the roof of his or her mouth. This causes the mylohyoid and tongue muscles to tense, making it easier to palpate the submandibular gland.
   - Bilaterally compress the glands upward against the tensed muscles.

*(continued)*

**PROCEDURE 12-1** HEAD AND NECK EXAMINATION *(CONTINUED)*

### Subgroup 3: Salivary and Thyroid Glands

4. **Thyroid gland—Locate.** The thyroid gland is located in the middle of the lower neck. It is situated below the larynx, over the trachea, and just above the clavicles.

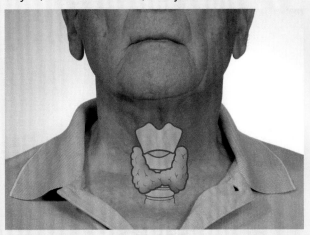

**Figure 12-41.**

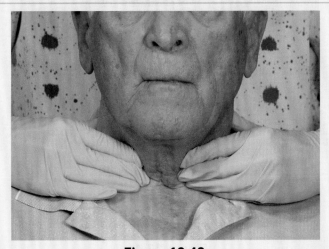

**Figure 12-42.**

1. **Your position.** Stand behind the patient.
2. **Patient's position.** Head in an upright position.
3. **Locate the thyroid gland.**
   - Find the thyroid cartilage (the Adam's apple) at the midline of the neck. The thyroid gland lies approximately 2 to 3 cm below the thyroid cartilage.
   - Give the patient a cup of water and ask him or her to swallow as you watch this region. The thyroid gland, along with the adjacent structures, will move up and down with swallowing.
   - The normal thyroid is not visible, so observing the neck during swallowing is helpful in locating the gland. Once you have located the gland, you are ready to palpate it.
   - ***Continue to the next page for the palpation technique for the thyroid gland.***

*(continued)*

**PROCEDURE 12-1**    HEAD AND NECK EXAMINATION *(CONTINUED)*

## Subgroup 3: Salivary and Thyroid Glands

**5. Thyroid gland—Palpate right lobe.**

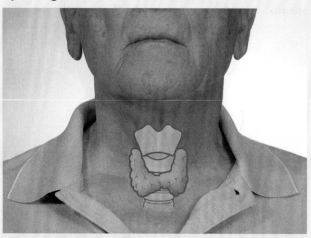

**Figure 12-43.**

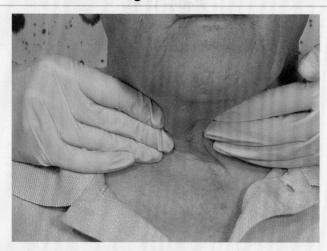

**Figure 12-44.**

1. **Your position.** Stand behind the patient and position your hands with thumbs on the nape of the neck.
2. **Patient's position.** Ask the patient to flex the neck forward and tilt the head slightly to the right. This relaxes the neck muscles for easier palpation.
3. **Palpation technique.** Begin with the right lobe of the gland.
   - *Use your left hand as a stabilizing hand* to displace the trachea slightly to the right.
   - *Use your right hand for palpation*. Position your fingers between the Adam's apple and the sternomastoid muscle. *Rest your fingers lightly in a stationary position.*
   - Ask the patient to take a sip of water and swallow as the fingers of your right hand rest lightly on the neck. The gland slides beneath your fingers as it moves up and down during swallowing. Repeat this process several times.
   - A normal gland is undetectable or barely detectable. Do not be disappointed if you do not identify the gland. If the gland is detectable, this is a notable finding.
   - Repeat a similar maneuver to examine the left lobe of the thyroid gland.

*(continued)*

## SUBGROUP 4: TEMPOROMANDIBULAR JOINT (TMJ)

**Table 12-6** TMJ: WHAT CAN I EXPECT TO FEEL?

| Normal Findings | • Smooth motions as the jaw is moved<br>• Symmetrical movement |
|---|---|
| Notable Findings | • Abnormal sounds (popping, clicking)<br>• Grating sensations as the jaw opens and closes<br>• Asymmetrical movements<br>• Limited range of movement<br>• Tenderness or pain reported by the patient |

**PROCEDURE 12-1** **HEAD AND NECK EXAMINATION** *(CONTINUED)*

### Subgroup 4: Temporomandibular Joint (TMJ)

**1. TMJ—Locate.**

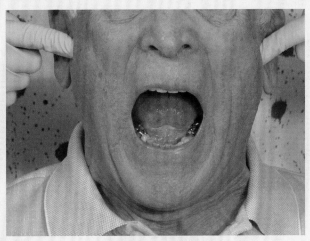

Figure 12-45.

1. **Your position.** Stand behind the patient.
2. **Patient's position.** Head in an upright position.
3. **Locate the TMJ.**
   * Locate the joints by placing your index fingers just in front of the tragus of each ear.
   * Ask the patient to open and close the mouth. As the mouth is opened and closed, your fingertips should drop into the joint spaces.
   * ***Continue to the next page for directions on palpating the TMJ.***

*(continued)*

**PROCEDURE 12-1**    HEAD AND NECK EXAMINATION *(CONTINUED)*

### Subgroup 4: Temporomandibular Joint (TMJ)

**2. TMJ—Palpate.**

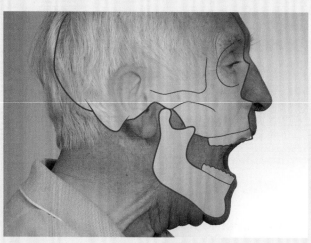

**Figure 12-46.**

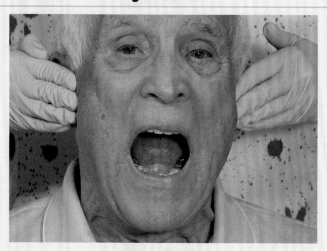

**Figure 12-47.**

1. **Your position.** Stand behind the patient.
2. **Patient's position.** Head in an upright position.
3. **Palpation technique.**
   - Place your fingertips over the joints. Palpate the joints as the patient slowly opens and closes the mouth several times.
   - Note any deviations during opening.
   - ***Continue to the next page for directions on palpation during lateral excursions.***

*(continued)*

**PROCEDURE 12-1**    HEAD AND NECK EXAMINATION *(CONTINUED)*

### Subgroup 4: Temporomandibular Joint (TMJ)

**4. TMJ—Lateral excursions (side to side movements of the jaw).**

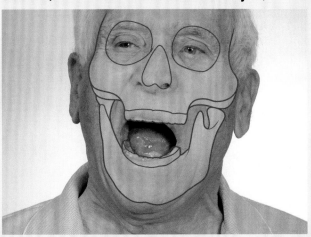

**Figure 12-48.**

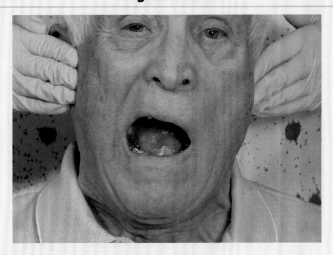

**Figure 12-49.**

1. **Your position.** Stand behind the patient.
2. **Patient's position.** Head in an upright position.
3. **Palpation technique.**
   - Maintaining your hands in the same position, ask the patient to open the mouth slightly and move the lower jaw laterally to the right.
   - Repeat this maneuver, with the patient moving the lower jaw to the left.
   - Finally, ask the patient to protrude the lower jaw forward.
   - Listen for abnormal sounds such as popping or clicking.

*(continued)*

**PROCEDURE 12-1**    HEAD AND NECK EXAMINATION *(CONTINUED)*

### Subgroup 4: Temporomandibular Joint (TMJ)

**5. Optional examination: TMJ—Range of motion.**

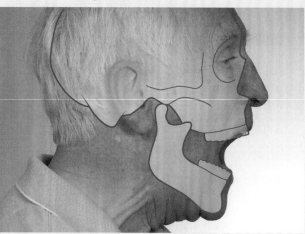

**Figure 12-50.**

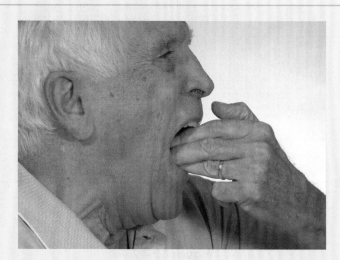

**Figure 12-51.**

**Assessment of the range of motion is optional, based on notable findings from the TMJ assessment.**

- Assess normal range of motion by asking the patient to place the index, middle, and ring fingers between the incisal edges of the upper and lower incisors. The patient's own fingers are proportional to his or her jaw and are a good indication of adequate range of motion.

**6. Document.** Document all notable findings in the patient chart or computerized record.

## SECTION 4:
## Ready References

**READY REFERENCE 12-1** **INTERNET RESOURCES FOR INFORMATION GATHERING**

**http://www.cancer.gov/cancertopics/types/head-and-neck**
The website of the **National Cancer Institute** has a wealth of information on head and neck cancer.

**http://www.cancer.gov/dictionary**
The National Cancer Institute's **Dictionary of Cancer Terms**, which contains more than 3,500 terms related to cancer and medicine.

**http://www.slideshare.net/rdhms/oral-cancer-exam**
An online slide program on detecting oral cancer: A Guide for Health Care Professionals.

**http://oralcancerfoundation.org/dental/slide_show.htm**
Oral Cancer Foundation's oral cancer gallery. This collection of photos contain both cancers and noncancerous diseases of the oral environment that may be mistaken for malignancies. Click on each slide to obtain a brief patient history and the actual diagnosis of the lesion.

**oralcancerfoundation.org/dental/additional_dental.htm**
A wealth of information on oral cancer assembled by the Oral Cancer Foundation that can be downloaded in PDF format.

**oralcancerfoundation.org/dental/pdf/screening.pdf**
Instructional booklet on oral cancer screening by the British Dental Association.

**http://www.health.gov/nhic/**
The **National Health Information Center (NHIC)** is a health information referral service. NHIC puts health professionals and consumers who have health questions in touch with those organizations that are best able to provide answers.

**http://www.mdanderson.org/diseases/head_neck/**
Website of **MD Anderson Cancer Center**, a leading head and neck cancer facility, has information on head and neck cancer and tobacco and cancer.

**http://www/mskcc.org/mskcc/html/338.cfm**
The website of **Memorial Sloan-Kettering Cancer Center**, a leading head and neck cancer facility, has information on the risk factors, prevention, symptoms, and early detection of head and neck cancer.

**http://www.mskcc.org/mskcc/html/420.cfm**
The website of **Memorial Sloan-Kettering Cancer Center** has information on skin cancer and melanoma, basal cell carcinoma, and squamous cell carcinoma.

*(continued)*

**READY REFERENCE 12-1** INTERNET RESOURCES FOR INFORMATION GATHERING
*(CONTINUED)*

**http://www.oralcancerfoundation.org/dental/slide_show.htm**
**Oral pathology images on the Oral Cancer Foundation website.** This collection of photos contains both cancers and noncancerous diseases of the oral environment that may be mistaken for malignancies. Some contain a brief patient history that may add insight to the actual diagnosis of the disease. As you review these images and their descriptions, you will be presented with what the referring doctor originally diagnosed and treated the patient for. Clicking on the "Diagnosis" button will reveal the actual results of biopsy.

**http://www.oralcancerfoundation.org/tobacco/index.htm**
The website of the **Oral Cancer Foundation** has information on the connection of tobacco and cancer.

**http://www.nlm.nih.gov/medlineplus/oralcancer.html**
The **MedlinePlus** website has a wealth of information on head and neck cancer.

## SUGGESTED READINGS

Bagan J, Scully C. Oral cancer: comprehending the condition, causes, controversies, control and consequences. 5. Clinical features and diagnosis of cancer. *Dent Update*. 2011;38(3): 209–211.

Balevi B. Assessing the usefulness of three adjunctive diagnostic devices for oral cancer screening: a probabilistic approach. *Community Dent Oral Epidemiol*. 2011;39(2): 171–176.

Barasch A, Litaker M. Nutrition and the risk of oral and pharyngeal cancer: the evidence for any association remains weak and clinical significance remains limited. *J Evid Based Dent Pract*. 2011;11(2):120–121.

Chainani-Wu N, Epstein J, Touger-Decker R. Diet and prevention of oral cancer: strategies for clinical practice. *J Am Dent Assoc*. 2011;142(2):166–169.

Dedhia RC, Smith KJ, Johnson JT, et al. The cost-effectiveness of community-based screening for oral cancer in high-risk males in the United States: a Markov decision analysis approach. *Laryngoscope*. 2011;121(5):952–960.

Deng H, Sambrook P, Logan R. The treatment of oral cancer: an overview for dental professionals. *Aust Dent J*. 2011;56(3):244–252.

Dios PD, Scully C. Oral cancer: comprehending the condition, causes, controversies, control and consequences. 7. Staging and diagnostic clinical aids. *Dent Update*. 2011;38(5): 354–356.

Elango KJ, Anandkrishnan N, Suresh A, et al. Mouth self-examination to improve oral cancer awareness and early detection in a high-risk population. *Oral Oncol*. 2011;47(7): 620–624.

Hapner ER, Bauer KL, Wise JC. The impact of a community-based oral, head, and neck cancer screening for reducing tobacco consumption. *Otolaryngol Head Neck Surg*. 2011;145(5):778–782

Hertrampf K, Wenz HJ, Koller M, et al. Public awareness about prevention and early detection of oral cancer: a population-based study in Northern Germany. *J Craniomaxillofac Surg*. 2012;40(3):e82–86.

Irwin JY, Thyvalikakath T, Spallek H, et al. English and Spanish oral cancer information on the Internet: a pilot surface quality and content evaluation of oral cancer web sites. *J Public Health Dent*. 2011;71(2):106–116.

Kallergis G. Informing cancer patient in relation to his type of personality: the dependent (oral) patient. *J BUON*. 2011;16(2):366–371.

Kruse AL, Bredell M, Gratz KW. Oral cancer in men and women: are there differences? *Oral Maxillofac Surg*. 2011;15(1):51–55.

MacCarthy D, Flint SR, Healy C, et al. Oral and neck examination for early detection of oral cancer—a practical guide. *J Ir Dent Assoc*. 2011;57(4):195–199.

Margolis F. Oral pathology of tots and teens. The identification, etiology, and treatment of common oral lesions in infants, children, and adolescents. *Dimens Dent Hyg*. 2010;8(2): 58–61.

McGurk M. Summary of: Patient awareness of oral cancer health advice in a dental access centre: a mixed methods study. *Br Dent J*. 2011;210(6):262–263.

Meurman JH, Scully C. Oral cancer: comprehending the condition, causes, controversies, control and consequences. 3. Other risk factors. *Dent Update*. 2011;38(1):66–68.

Natarajan E, Eisenberg E. Contemporary concepts in the diagnosis of oral cancer and precancer. *Dent Clin North Am.* 2011;55(1):63–88.

Newton T, Scully C. Oral cancer: comprehending the condition, causes, controversies, control and consequences. 8. Communicating about cancer. *Dent Update.* 2011;38(6):426–428.

Palmer O, Grannum R. Oral cancer detection. *Dent Clin North Am.* 2011;55(3):537–548, viii–ix.

Scott SE, Weinman J, Grunfeld EA. Developing ways to encourage early detection and presentation of oral cancer: What do high-risk individuals think? *Psychol Health.* 2011;26(10):1392–1405.

Seoane J, Corral-Lizana C, Gonzalez-Mosquera A, Esparza G, Sanz-Cuesta T, Varela-Centelles P. The use of clinical guidelines for referral of patients with lesions suspicious for oral cancer may ease early diagnosis and improve education of healthcare professionals. *Med Oral Patol Oral Cir Bucal.* 2011;16(7):e864–e869.

Steele TO, Meyers A. Early detection of premalignant lesions and oral cancer. *Otolaryngol Clin North Am.* 2011;44(1):221–229, vii.

van der Waal I, Scully C. Oral cancer: comprehending the condition, causes, controversies, control and consequences. 6. Co-morbidities. *Dent Update.* 2011;38(4):283–284.

van der Waal I, Scully C. Oral cancer: comprehending the condition, causes, controversies, control and consequences. 4. Potentially malignant disorders of the oral and oropharyngeal mucosa. *Dent Update.* 2011;38(2):138–140.

Warnakulasuriya S. Waterpipe smoking, oral cancer and other oral health effects. *Evid Based Dent.* 2011;12(2):44–45.

Williams M, Bethea J. Patient awareness of oral cancer health advice in a dental access centre: a mixed methods study. *Br Dent J.* 2011;210(6):E9.

Zygogianni AG, Kyrgias G, Karakitsos P, et al. Oral squamous cell cancer: early detection and the role of alcohol and smoking. *Head Neck Oncol.* 2011;3:2.

**SECTION 5:**
# The Human Element

| BOX **12-2** | **Through the Eyes of a Patient** |
|---|---|

*About 10 years ago, while I was pregnant with my first child, my mother urged me to go and have the small brown spot above my upper lip checked by a doctor. At the time, I was excited and busy getting ready for my first child, and I decided that the brown spot was just like a beauty mark. I knew that it had only appeared about a year ago, but I did not want to worry about it. After all, I saw my obstetrician each month and I had just had a dental exam last month. Surely, my doctor or my dentist would have noticed the brown spot above my lip and told me if it was a problem. Wouldn't they?*

*Well, finally, because my mother just insisted, I went to see my regular doctor to ask about the brown "beauty" mark. I was shocked when he wanted to remove the spot and send it off to the lab. The test results showed that the brown spot was cancer and I had to have additional surgery to make sure that all the cancer cells had been removed.*

*Six years ago, I went back to school and became a dental hygienist. Today, as a dental hygienist, I stress the importance of a yearly head, neck, and oral cancer examination to all my patients. My experience made me so aware that many health professionals have tunnel vision. My obstetrician concentrated on my pregnancy. My dentist looked at my teeth but did not look up an inch to notice the brown spot above my upper lip. As future dental health care providers, I strongly urge you to remember that doing a cancer exam and following up on any changes could save a patient's life.*

*Cathy, R.D.H*
*Cancer Survivor*

**PATIENT SCENARIO**

Utsava is in her last semester of dental hygiene school, and her patient for the day just cancelled. Desperate, she calls any relative or friend that she can think of who may be available for this last-minute appointment. Her brother-in-law, Paresh, a 32-year-old engineer who owns his own company, agrees to be her patient for the day.

Paresh's medical history assessment indicates that although he appears to be in good health, he has not seen a physician or dentist for over 10 years. Utsava performs a head and neck examination and asks her instructor, Professor Miller, to check it so she can progress with the appointment.

Utsava reports to her instructor that all areas of the head and neck examination were all "within normal limits." Professor Miller asks Paresh to tip his head forward so she can both observe and palpate his occipital lymph nodes. As soon as she does, Professor Miller both notices and palpates an enlargement in Paresh's occipital area, which extends from the nape of his neck all the way under his hairline. Professor Miller points out the enlargement to Utsava, who states that she just thought that it was part of Paresh's normal anatomy. Utsava states that as long as she has known Paresh, his occipital area has looked like this. Utsava does admit that looking closely at it now, the area appears to have enlarged over the last few years. Professor Miller is very concerned about the finding because she feels that it is outside the limits of normal.

1. What ethical principles are involved in this scenario?
2. How should Utsava address Paresh's treatment?
3. What should Utsava do when treating future patients?

| Table 12-4 | ENGLISH-TO-SPANISH PHRASE LIST FOR HEAD AND NECK EXAMINATION |

| | |
|---|---|
| Next, I will do a head and neck exam. | Ahora voy a hacer una examinación de la cabeza y el cuello. |
| Just relax. This examination is not painful and only takes a few minutes. | No tenga miedo. La examinación no duele, y solamente toma unos minutos. |
| At any time during the examination, please tell me if any area is tender. | A cualquier tiempo durante la examinación, por favor digame si tiene algun area que está sensible. |
| Please tilt your head forward (back). | Por favor incline la cabeza hacia delante. Por favor incline la cabeza hacia atrás. |
| Please **turn** your head to the right (left). | Por favor vuelta la cabeza a la derecha. Por favor vuelta la cabeza a la izquierda. |
| Please **tilt** your head to the right (left). | Por favor incline la cabeza a la derecha. Por favor incline la cabeza a la izquierda. |
| Please look straight ahead. | Por favor mire al frente. |
| I will check the lymph nodes in your head and neck. | Voy a examinar las glandulas tiroides en la cabeza y el cuello. |
| The lymph nodes are part of the body's defenses; they act as a filtering system to remove bacteria and viruses from your system. | Las glandulas tiroides son parte de las defensas naturales del cuerpo; estas filtran fluidos en el cuerpo y protegen contra bacterias y virus. |
| Please press your tongue against the roof of your mouth. | Por favor aprete la lengua contra el techo de la boca. |
| Now, I will check your saliva glands. | Ahora voy a examinar la glandula de saliva. |
| Next, I will check your thyroid gland. | Ahora voy a examiner la glandula. |
| Please take a sip of water and hold it in your mouth. Please swallow. | Tome un poco de agua y aguántela en la boca. Por favor trage. |
| Now, I will check the joint in your jaw. | Ahora examinaré la articulación de la mandibula. |
| Please slowly open and close your mouth. | Por favor abra y cierre la boca, pero despacio. |
| Please move your lower jaw to the right (left). | Por favor vuelta la mandibula a la derecha. Por favor vuelta la mandibula a la izquierda. |
| Several of your lymph nodes are swollen. Have you been ill or had an infection? | Varios de las glandulas tiroides están hinchadas. ¿Ha estado enfermo o ha tenido alguna infección? |

*(continued)*

**Table 12-4    ENGLISH-TO-SPANISH PHRASE LIST FOR HEAD AND NECK EXAMINATION (*CONTINUED*)**

| | |
|---|---|
| Everything looks (feels) fine. | Todo parece (se siente) bien. |
| Your _____ is swollen. | El/la _____ esta hinchado. |
| I am concerned about this area on your skin. | Estoy preocupado por esta area de la piel. |
| Do you spend much time outside in the sun? | ¿Usted pasa mucho tiempo afuera en el sol? |
| How long have you had this spot on your skin? | ¿Hace mucho tiempo que tiene esta mancha en la piel? |
| How did you get this scar? | ¿Como recibió esta cicatriz? |
| Does anyone in your family have thyroid problems? | ¿Algun miembro de su familia ha tenido problemas con tiroides? |
| Does your jaw ever bother you? | ¿Le ha molestado la mandibula alguna vez? |
| Do you have frequent headaches? | ¿Usted tiene dolor de la cabeza con frecuencia? |
| Does your mouth ever lock in the open position? | ¿Se le ha atascado la boca en posición abierta? |
| I am concerned about this area and would like to have it examined by a physician/specialist. | Estoy preocupado sobre esta zona, y quiero que sea examinada por un médico/especialista. |
| Do you have a physician that you see regularly? | ¿Usted tiene un médico personal? |
| Here are the names of several physicians/ specialists in our area. | Aqui tiene los nombres de varios médicos/ especialistas en esta area. |
| I can set up an appointment with the specialist of your choice. | Yo le puedo hacer una cita con el especialista de su preferencia. |
| I will write a note to the specialist explaining my concerns. | Le voy a escribir una nota al especialista para explicarle la preocupación. |
| I am going to get my clinic instructor. | Voy a buscar mi instructor. |

## SECTION 6:

# Practical Focus—Fictitious Patient Cases

---

**DIRECTIONS:**

- The photographs in this section show the findings from the head and neck examination of five fictitious patients, patients A–E. Refer to previous modules to refresh your memory regarding each patient's health history and vital signs because there may be a connection between the patient's systemic health status or habits and the findings from the head and neck examination.

- Use the Lesion Descriptor Worksheet to develop descriptions for the notable findings of fictitious patients A–E.

- The pages in this section may be removed from the book for easier use by tearing along the perforated lines on each page.

---

## SOURCES OF CLINICAL PHOTOGRAPHS

The authors gratefully acknowledge the sources of the following clinical photographs in the Practical Focus section of this module.

- Figure 12-52. From Goodheart HP. *Goodheart's Photoguide of Common Skin Disorders*. 2nd ed. Philadelphia, PA: Lippincott Williams & Wilkins; 2003.
- Figure 12-54. From Langlais RP, Miller CS, Nield-Gehrig JS. *Color Atlas of Common Oral Diseases*. 4th ed. Philadelphia, PA: Lippincott Williams & Wilkins; 2009.
- Figure 12-58. Dr. Richard Foster, Guildford Technical Community College, Jamestown, NC.
- Figure 12-60. Image provided by Stedman's Medical Dictionary.

## FICTITIOUS PATIENT CASE A: MR. ALAN ASCARI

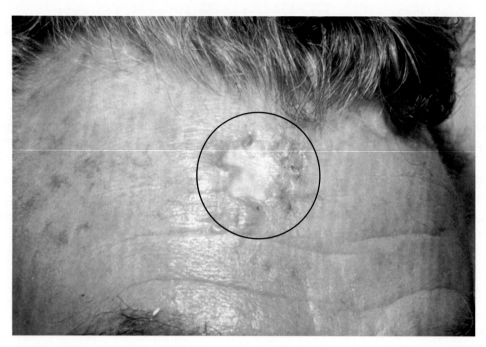

Figure 12-52.   Mr. Ascari: Finding on forehead.

# Lesion Descriptor Worksheet

*Directions: Highlight or circle the applicable descriptors*

| | |
|---|---|
| **Ⓐ**<br>**Anatomic Location** | *Head*: Scalp, eye, ear, nose, cheek, chin, neck; right or left side<br>*Neck*: Midline, right, left; near certain anatomic structure<br>*Lip*: Upper, lower, commissure, vermillion border; labial mucosa<br>*Buccal mucosa*: Parotid papilla; mucobuccal fold; near tooth #<br>*Gingiva*: Free, attached; near tooth #<br>*Tongue*: Anterior-third, middle-third, posterior-third; dorsal, ventral, right lateral, left lateral<br>*Floor of mouth*: Lingual frenum, sublingual folds, sublingual caruncle; near tooth #<br>*Palate*: Hard, soft; midline, incisive papilla; right side, left side<br>*Oropharynx*: Pillars, midline, uvula |
| **Ⓑ**<br>**Border** | *Well-demarcated:* Easy to see where lesion begins and ends<br>*Poorly demarcated:* Difficult to see where lesion begins and ends<br>*Regularly shaped:* Uniform border<br>*Irregularly shaped:* Border not uniform |
| **Ⓒ**<br>**Color Change Configuration** | *Color:* Red, white, red and white, blue, yellow, brown, black<br>*Lesion pattern:* Single lesion or<br>multiple lesions (discrete, grouped, confluent, linear) |
| **Ⓓ**<br>**Diameter/ Dimension** | *If oblong or irregular in shape:* Length and width<br>*If circular or round in shape:* Diameter (measurement of a line running from one side of a circle through the center to the other side) |
| **Ⓣ**<br>**T y p e** | **Nonpalpable Flat Lesions**<br><br>*Macule* - Flat discolored spot, less than 1 cm in size<br>*Patch* - Flat discolored spot, larger than 1 cm in size<br><br>**Palpable, Elevated, Solid Masses**<br><br>*Papule* - Solid raised lesion, less than 1 cm in diameter<br>*Plaque* - Superficial raised lesion, larger than 1 cm in diameter<br>*Nodule* - Marble-like lesion, larger than 1 cm in diameter<br>*Wheal* - Localized area of skin edema<br><br>**Fluid-Filled Lesions**<br><br>*Vesicle* - Small blister filled with clear fluid, less than 1 cm in diameter<br>*Bulla* - Larger fluid-filled lesion, larger than 1 cm in diameter<br>*Pustule* - Small raised lesion filled with pus<br><br>**Loss of Skin or Mucosal Surface**<br><br>*Erosion* - Loss of top layer of skin or mucosa<br>*Ulcer* - Craterlike lesion where top two layers of skin or mucosa are lost<br>*Fissure* - A linear crack |

**Figure 12-53A.** Page 1 of Lesion Descriptor Worksheet for Mr. Ascari.

# Lesion Descriptor Worksheet

*Directions:* Draw the lesion(s) on the appropriate illustration, showing the anatomic location, relative shape, and size.

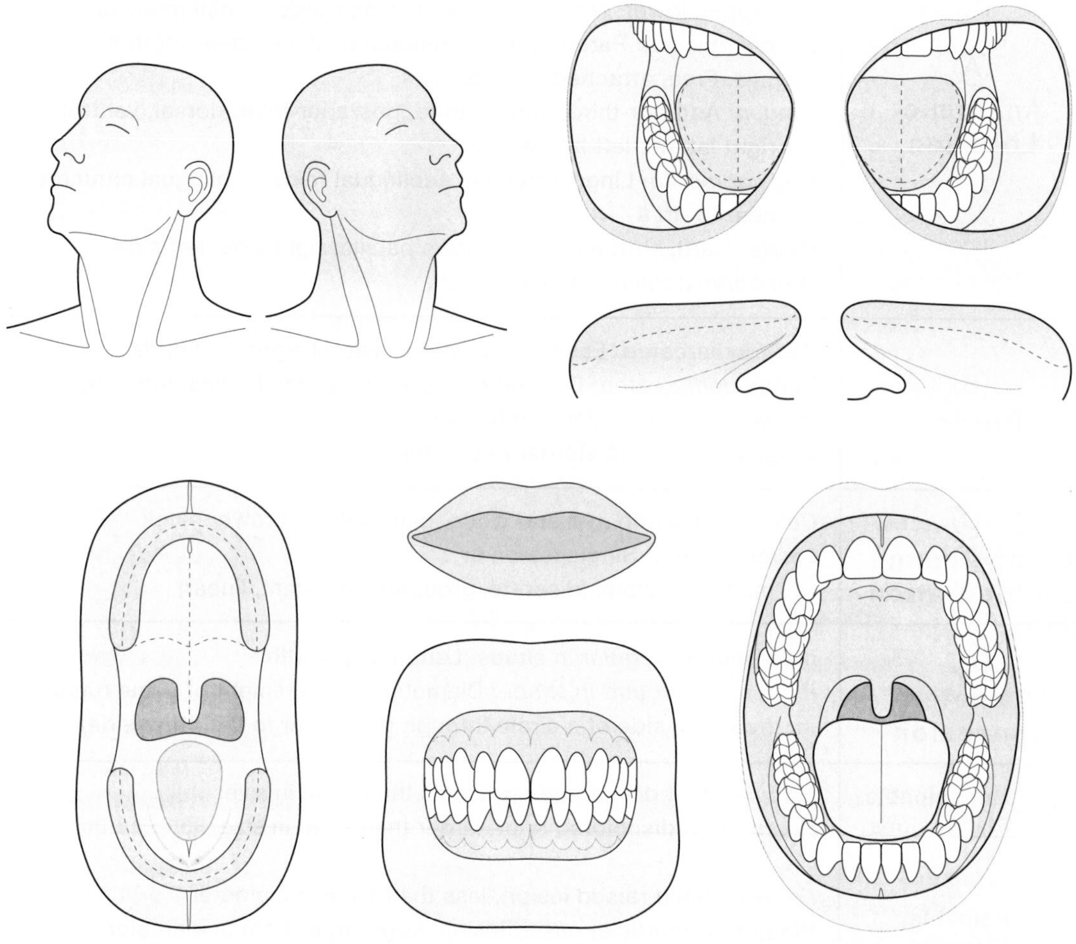

*Develop a Chart Entry:* Using each descriptor circled and the location indicated on this worksheet, develop a written description of the lesion(s). After you have perfected the written description, enter it in the paper or computerized patient chart. Remember the A, B, C, D, T plan for formulating a description.

Figure 12-53B.    Page 2 of Lesion Descriptor Worksheet for Mr. Ascari.

# FICTITIOUS PATIENT CASE B: BETHANY BIDDLE

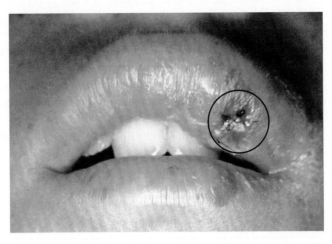

Figure 12-54.    Bethany Biddle: Finding on upper lip.

# Lesion Descriptor Worksheet

*Directions: Highlight or circle the applicable descriptors*

| | |
|---|---|
| **(A)** **Anatomic Location** | *Head:* Scalp, eye, ear, nose, cheek, chin, neck; right or left side<br>*Neck:* Midline, right, left; near certain anatomic structure<br>*Lip:* Upper, lower, commissure, vermillion border; labial mucosa<br>*Buccal mucosa:* Parotid papilla; mucobuccal fold; near tooth #<br>*Gingiva:* Free, attached; near tooth #<br>*Tongue:* Anterior-third, middle-third, posterior-third; dorsal, ventral, right lateral, left lateral<br>*Floor of mouth:* Lingual frenum, sublingual folds, sublingual caruncle; near tooth #<br>*Palate:* Hard, soft; midline, incisive papilla; right side, left side<br>*Oropharynx:* Pillars, midline, uvula |
| **(B)** **Border** | *Well-demarcated:* Easy to see where lesion begins and ends<br>*Poorly demarcated:* Difficult to see where lesion begins and ends<br>*Regularly shaped:* Uniform border<br>*Irregularly shaped:* Border not uniform |
| **(C)** **Color Change Configuration** | *Color:* Red, white, red and white, blue, yellow, brown, black<br>*Lesion pattern:* Single lesion or<br>multiple lesions (discrete, grouped, confluent, linear) |
| **(D)** **Diameter/ Dimension** | *If oblong or irregular in shape:* Length and width<br>*If circular or round in shape:* Diameter (measurement of a line running from one side of a circle through the center to the other side) |
| **(T)** **Type** | **Nonpalpable Flat Lesions**<br>*Macule* - Flat discolored spot, less than 1 cm in size<br>*Patch* - Flat discolored spot, larger than 1 cm in size<br><br>**Palpable, Elevated, Solid Masses**<br>*Papule* - Solid raised lesion, less than 1 cm in diameter<br>*Plaque* - Superficial raised lesion, larger than 1 cm in diameter<br>*Nodule* - Marble-like lesion, larger than 1 cm in diameter<br>*Wheal* - Localized area of skin edema<br><br>**Fluid-Filled Lesions**<br>*Vesicle* - Small blister filled with clear fluid, less than 1 cm in diameter<br>*Bulla* - Larger fluid-filled lesion, larger than 1 cm in diameter<br>*Pustule* - Small raised lesion filled with pus<br><br>**Loss of Skin or Mucosal Surface**<br>*Erosion* - Loss of top layer of skin or mucosa<br>*Ulcer* - Craterlike lesion where top two layers of skin or mucosa are lost<br>*Fissure* - A linear crack |

**Figure 12-55A. Page 1 of Lesion Descriptor Worksheet for Bethany Biddle.**

# Lesion Descriptor Worksheet

*Directions:* Draw the lesion(s) on the appropriate illustration, showing the anatomic location, relative shape, and size.

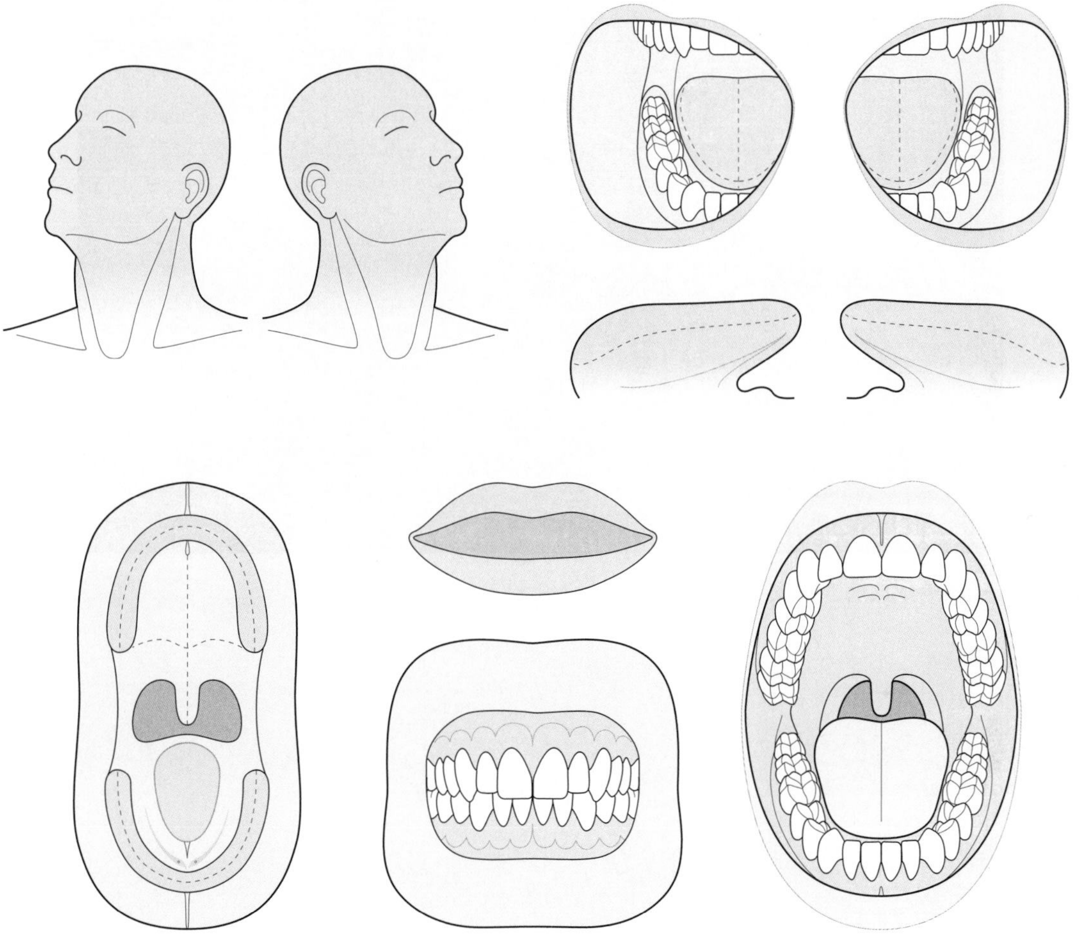

*Develop a Chart Entry:* Using each descriptor circled and the location indicated on this worksheet, develop a written description of the lesion(s). After you have perfected the written description, enter it in the paper or computerized patient chart. Remember the A, B, C, D, T plan for formulating a description.

Figure 12-55B.    Page 2 of Lesion Descriptor Worksheet for Bethany Biddle.

# FICTITIOUS PATIENT CASE C: MR. CARLOS CHAVEZ

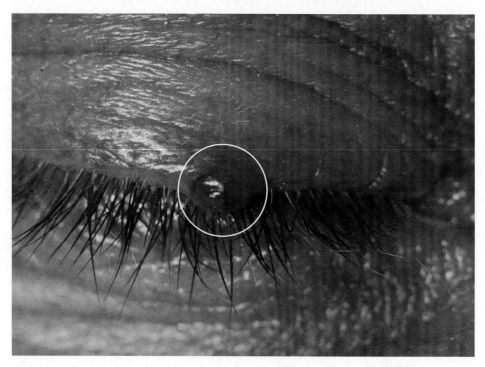

Figure 12-56.   Mr. Chavez: Finding on upper eyelid.

# Lesion Descriptor Worksheet

*Directions: Highlight or circle the applicable descriptors*

| | |
|---|---|
| **Ⓐ**<br>**Anatomic**<br>**Location** | *Head:* Scalp, eye, ear, nose, cheek, chin, neck; right or left side<br>*Neck:* Midline, right, left; near certain anatomic structure<br>*Lip:* Upper, lower, commissure, vermillion border; labial mucosa<br>*Buccal mucosa:* Parotid papilla; mucobuccal fold; near tooth #<br>*Gingiva:* Free, attached; near tooth #<br>*Tongue:* Anterior-third, middle-third, posterior-third; dorsal, ventral,<br>     right lateral, left lateral<br>*Floor of mouth:* Lingual frenum, sublingual folds, sublingual caruncle;<br>     near tooth #<br>*Palate:* Hard, soft; midline, incisive papilla; right side, left side<br>*Oropharynx:* Pillars, midline, uvula |
| **Ⓑ**<br>**Border** | *Well-demarcated:* Easy to see where lesion begins and ends<br>*Poorly demarcated:* Difficult to see where lesion begins and ends<br>*Regularly shaped:* Uniform border<br>*Irregularly shaped:* Border not uniform |
| **Ⓒ**<br>**Color Change**<br>**Configuration** | *Color:* Red, white, red and white, blue, yellow, brown, black<br>*Lesion pattern:* Single lesion or<br>     multiple lesions (discrete, grouped, confluent, linear) |
| **Ⓓ**<br>**Diameter/**<br>**Dimension** | *If oblong or irregular in shape:* Length and width<br>*If circular or round in shape:* Diameter (measurement of a line running<br>     from one side of a circle through the center to the other side) |

| **Ⓣ**<br>**T**<br>**y**<br>**p**<br>**e** | **Nonpalpable**<br>**Flat Lesions** | *Macule* - Flat discolored spot, less than 1 cm in size<br>*Patch* - Flat discolored spot, larger than 1 cm in size |
|---|---|---|
| | **Palpable,**<br>**Elevated,**<br>**Solid Masses** | *Papule* - Solid raised lesion, less than 1 cm in diameter<br>*Plaque* - Superficial raised lesion, larger than 1 cm in diameter<br>*Nodule* - Marble-like lesion, larger than 1 cm in diameter<br>*Wheal* - Localized area of skin edema |
| | **Fluid-Filled**<br>**Lesions** | *Vesicle* - Small blister filled with clear fluid, less than 1 cm in diameter<br>*Bulla* - Larger fluid-filled lesion, larger than 1 cm in diameter<br>*Pustule* - Small raised lesion filled with pus |
| | **Loss of Skin**<br>**or Mucosal**<br>**Surface** | *Erosion* - Loss of top layer of skin or mucosa<br>*Ulcer* - Craterlike lesion where top two layers of skin or mucosa are lost<br>*Fissure* - A linear crack |

**Figure 12-57A.   Page 1 of Lesion Descriptor Worksheet for Mr. Chavez.**

# Lesion Descriptor Worksheet

*Directions:* Draw the lesion(s) on the appropriate illustration, showing the anatomic location, relative shape, and size.

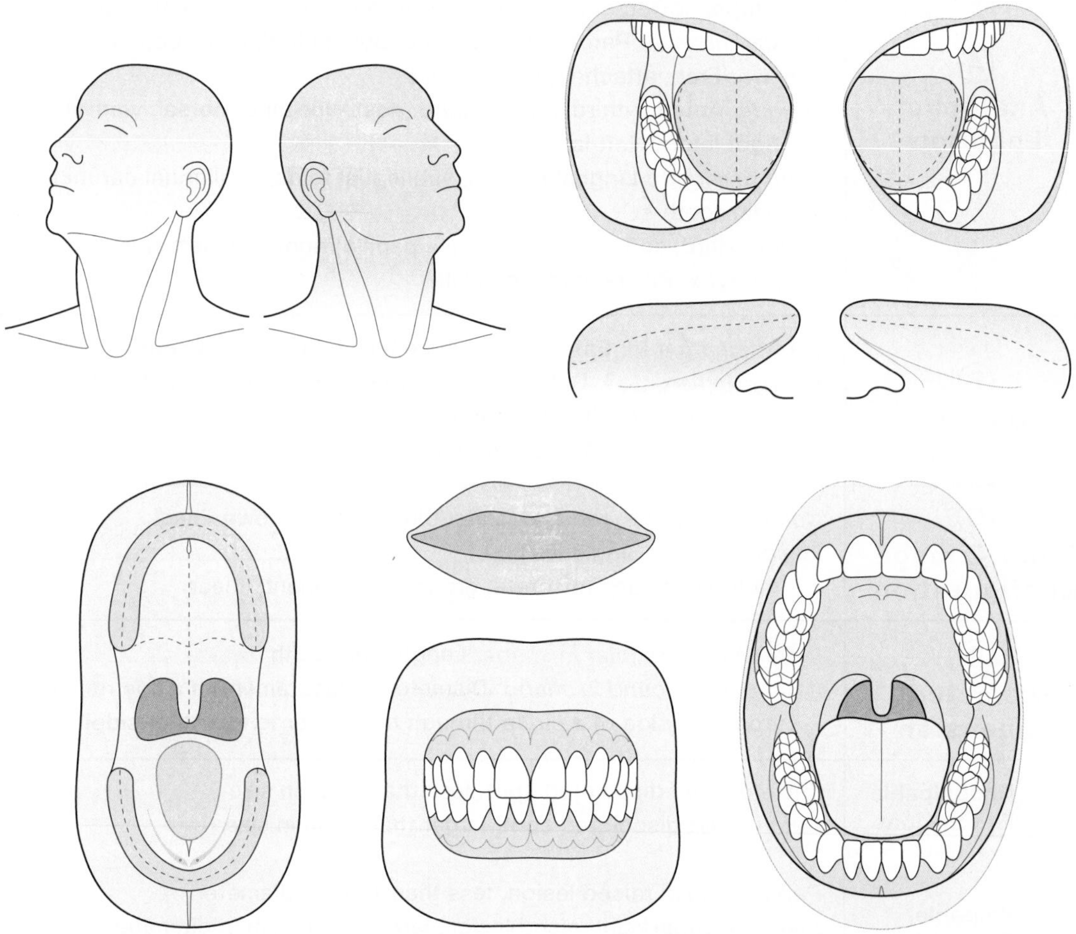

*Develop a Chart Entry:* Using each descriptor circled and the location indicated on this worksheet, develop a written description of the lesion(s). After you have perfected the written description, enter it in the paper or computerized patient chart. Remember the A, B, C, D, T plan for formulating a description.

_____

_____

_____

_____

**Figure 12-57B.   Page 2 of Lesion Descriptor Worksheet for Mr. Chavez.**

# FICTITIOUS PATIENT CASE D: MRS. DONNA DOI

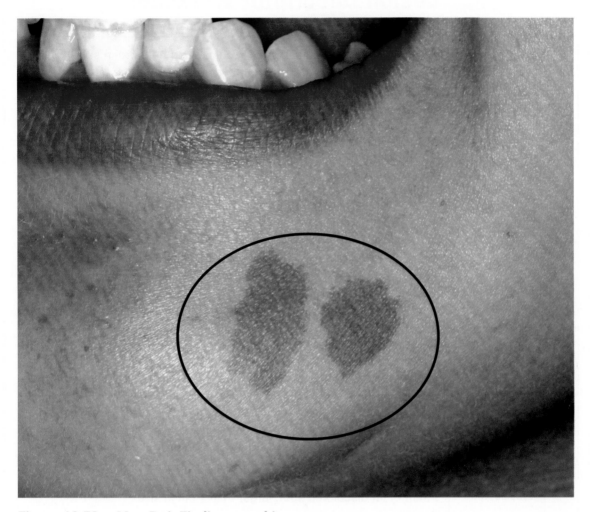

Figure 12-58. Mrs. Doi: Findings on chin.

# Lesion Descriptor Worksheet

*Directions: Highlight or circle the applicable descriptors*

| | |
|---|---|
| **Ⓐ** <br> **Anatomic Location** | *Head*: Scalp, eye, ear, nose, cheek, chin, neck; right or left side <br> *Neck:* Midline, right, left; near certain anatomic structure <br> *Lip:* Upper, lower, commissure, vermillion border; labial mucosa <br> *Buccal mucosa:* Parotid papilla; mucobuccal fold; near tooth # <br> *Gingiva:* Free, attached; near tooth # <br> *Tongue:* Anterior-third, middle-third, posterior-third; dorsal, ventral, right lateral, left lateral <br> *Floor of mouth:* Lingual frenum, sublingual folds, sublingual caruncle; near tooth # <br> *Palate:* Hard, soft; midline, incisive papilla; right side, left side <br> *Oropharynx:* Pillars, midline, uvula |
| **Ⓑ** <br> **Border** | *Well-demarcated:* Easy to see where lesion begins and ends <br> *Poorly demarcated:* Difficult to see where lesion begins and ends <br> *Regularly shaped:* Uniform border <br> *Irregularly shaped:* Border not uniform |
| **Ⓒ** <br> **Color Change Configuration** | *Color:* Red, white, red and white, blue, yellow, brown, black <br> *Lesion pattern:* Single lesion or <br> multiple lesions (discrete, grouped, confluent, linear) |
| **Ⓓ** <br> **Diameter/ Dimension** | *If oblong or irregular in shape:* Length and width <br> *If circular or round in shape:* Diameter (measurement of a line running from one side of a circle through the center to the other side) |

| **Ⓣ** <br> **T y p e** | **Nonpalpable Flat Lesions** | *Macule* - Flat discolored spot, less than 1 cm in size <br> *Patch* - Flat discolored spot, larger than 1 cm in size |
|---|---|---|
| | **Palpable, Elevated, Solid Masses** | *Papule* - Solid raised lesion, less than 1 cm in diameter <br> *Plaque* - Superficial raised lesion, larger than 1 cm in diameter <br> *Nodule* - Marble-like lesion, larger than 1 cm in diameter <br> *Wheal* - Localized area of skin edema |
| | **Fluid-Filled Lesions** | *Vesicle* - Small blister filled with clear fluid, less than 1 cm in diameter <br> *Bulla* - Larger fluid-filled lesion, larger than 1 cm in diameter <br> *Pustule* - Small raised lesion filled with pus |
| | **Loss of Skin or Mucosal Surface** | *Erosion* - Loss of top layer of skin or mucosa <br> *Ulcer* - Craterlike lesion where top two layers of skin or mucosa are lost <br> *Fissure* - A linear crack |

**Figure 12-59A.   Page 1 of Lesion Descriptor Worksheet for Mrs. Doi.**

# Lesion Descriptor Worksheet

*Directions:* Draw the lesion(s) on the appropriate illustration, showing the anatomic location, relative shape, and size.

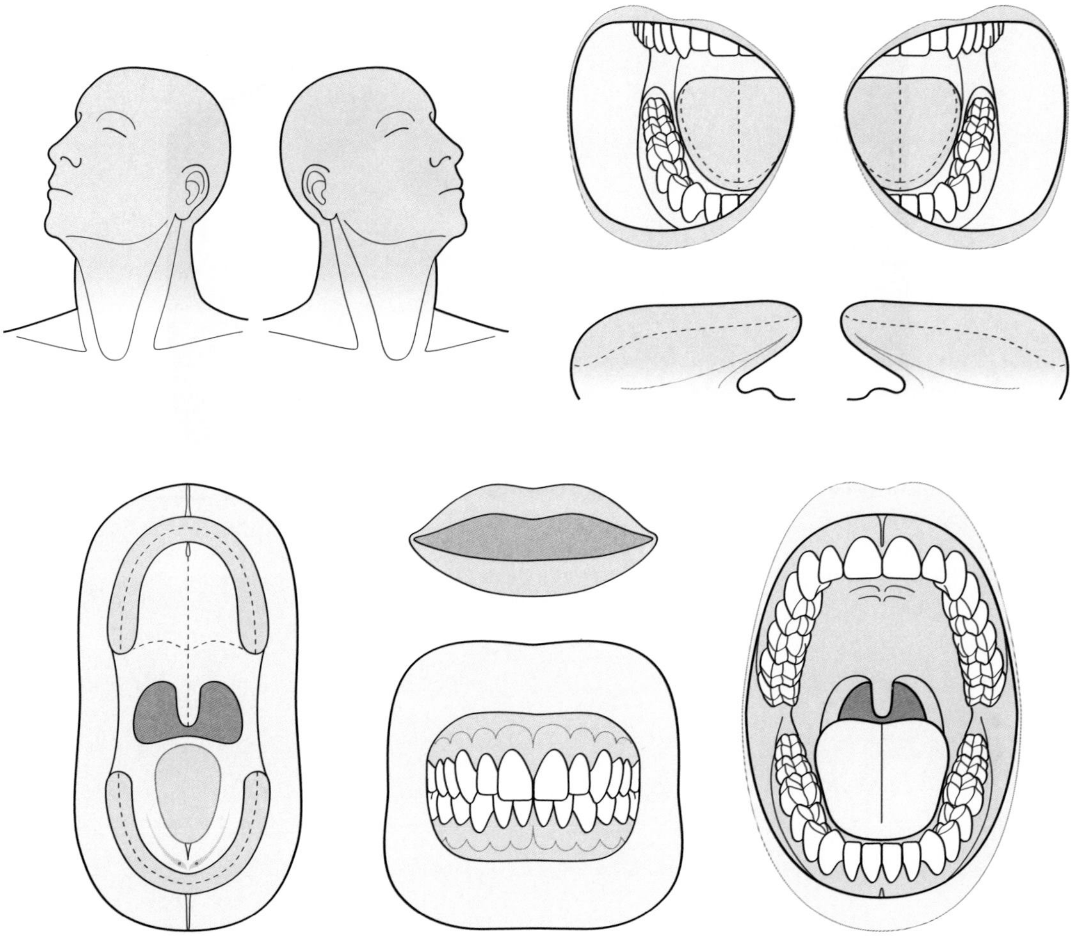

*Develop a Chart Entry:* Using each descriptor circled and the location indicated on this work-sheet, develop a written description of the lesion(s). After you have perfected the written description, enter it in the paper or computerized patient chart. Remember the A, B, C, D, T plan for formulating a description.

_____

_____

_____

_____

**Figure 12-59B.** Page 2 of Lesion Descriptor Worksheet for Mrs. Doi.

# FICTITIOUS PATIENT CASE E: MS. ESTHER EADS

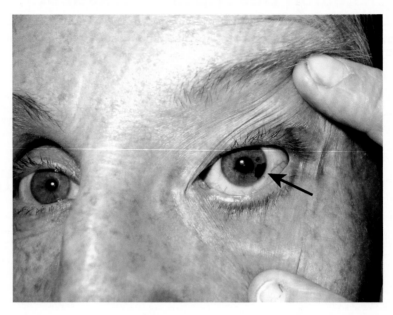

Figure 12-60. Ms. Eads: Finding on iris of left eye.

# Lesion Descriptor Worksheet

*Directions: Highlight or circle the applicable descriptors*

| | |
|---|---|
| **Ⓐ** <br> **Anatomic Location** | *Head*: Scalp, eye, ear, nose, cheek, chin, neck; right or left side <br> *Neck:* Midline, right, left; near certain anatomic structure <br> *Lip:* Upper, lower, commissure, vermillion border; labial mucosa <br> *Buccal mucosa:* Parotid papilla; mucobuccal fold; near tooth # <br> *Gingiva:* Free, attached; near tooth # <br> *Tongue:* Anterior-third, middle-third, posterior-third; dorsal, ventral, right lateral, left lateral <br> *Floor of mouth:* Lingual frenum, sublingual folds, sublingual caruncle; near tooth # <br> *Palate:* Hard, soft; midline, incisive papilla; right side, left side <br> *Oropharynx:* Pillars, midline, uvula |
| **Ⓑ** <br> **Border** | *Well-demarcated:* Easy to see where lesion begins and ends <br> *Poorly demarcated:* Difficult to see where lesion begins and ends <br> *Regularly shaped:* Uniform border <br> *Irregularly shaped:* Border not uniform |
| **Ⓒ** <br> **Color Change Configuration** | *Color:* Red, white, red and white, blue, yellow, brown, black <br> *Lesion pattern:* Single lesion or <br>     multiple lesions (discrete, grouped, confluent, linear) |
| **Ⓓ** <br> **Diameter/ Dimension** | *If oblong or irregular in shape:* Length and width <br> *If circular or round in shape:* Diameter (measurement of a line running <br>     from one side of a circle through the center to the other side) |

| Ⓣ T y p e | **Nonpalpable Flat Lesions** | *Macule* - Flat discolored spot, less than 1 cm in size <br> *Patch* - Flat discolored spot, larger than 1 cm in size |
|---|---|---|
| | **Palpable, Elevated, Solid Masses** | *Papule* - Solid raised lesion, less than 1 cm in diameter <br> *Plaque* - Superficial raised lesion, larger than 1 cm in diameter <br> *Nodule* - Marble-like lesion, larger than 1 cm in diameter <br> *Wheal* - Localized area of skin edema |
| | **Fluid-Filled Lesions** | *Vesicle* - Small blister filled with clear fluid, less than 1 cm in diameter <br> *Bulla* - Larger fluid-filled lesion, larger than 1 cm in diameter <br> *Pustule* - Small raised lesion filled with pus |
| | **Loss of Skin or Mucosal Surface** | *Erosion* - Loss of top layer of skin or mucosa <br> *Ulcer* - Craterlike lesion where top two layers of skin or mucosa are lost <br> *Fissure* - A linear crack |

**Figure 12-61A. Page 1 of Lesion Descriptor Worksheet for Ms. Eads.**

# Lesion Descriptor Worksheet

*Directions:* Draw the lesion(s) on the appropriate illustration, showing the anatomic location, relative shape, and size.

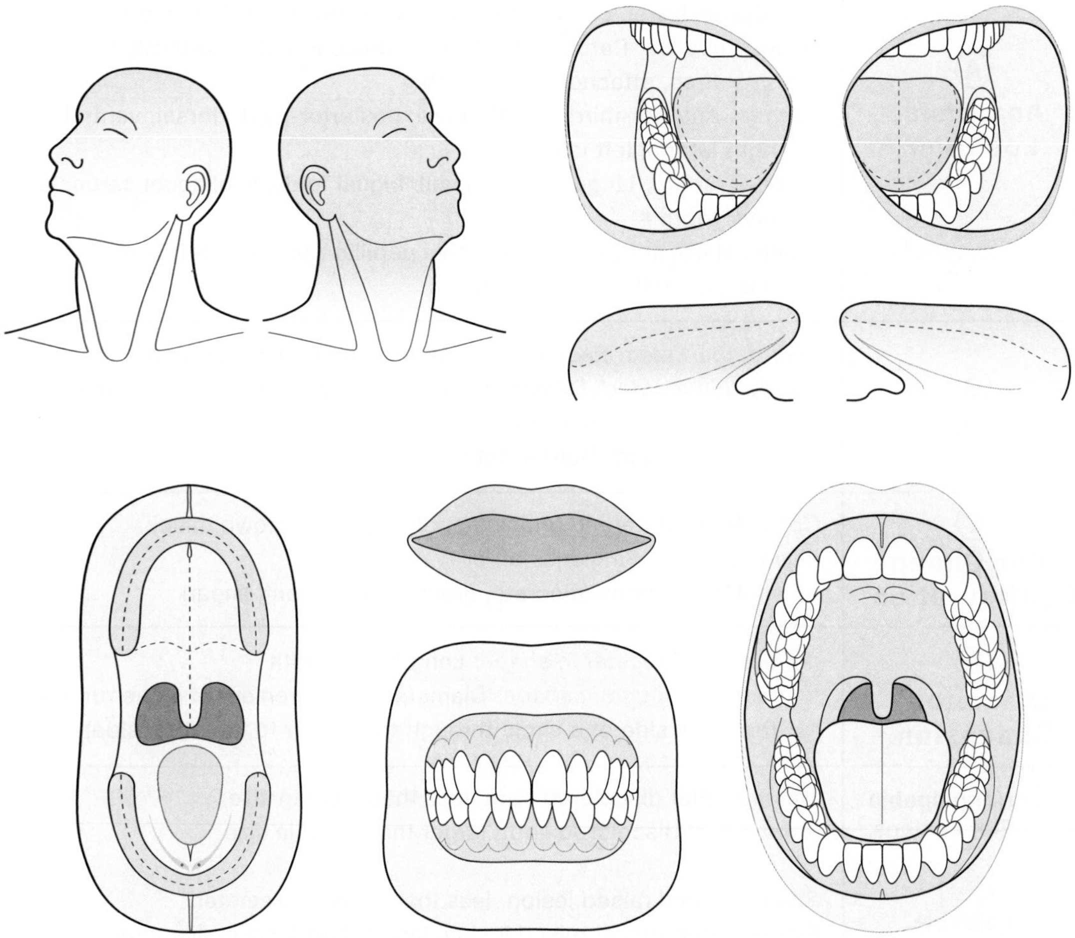

*Develop a Chart Entry:* Using each descriptor circled and the location indicated on this worksheet, develop a written description of the lesion(s). After you have perfected the written description, enter it in the paper or computerized patient chart. Remember the A, B, C, D, T plan for formulating a description.

_____

_____

_____

_____

Figure 12-61B.    Page 2 of Lesion Descriptor Worksheet for Ms. Eads.

## SECTION 7:

# Skill Check

**TECHNIQUE SKILL CHECKLIST:** HEAD AND NECK EXAMINATION

Student: _____ Evaluator: _____

Date: _____

**DIRECTIONS FOR STUDENT:** Use **Column S**; evaluate your skill level as **S** (satisfactory) or **U** (unsatisfactory).

**DIRECTIONS FOR EVALUATOR:** Use **Column E**. Indicate **S** (satisfactory) or **U** (unsatisfactory). In the optional grade percentage calculation, each **S** equals 1 point, and each **U** equals 0 points.

| CRITERIA | S | E |
|---|---|---|
| **Subgroup 1: Overall Appraisal of the Head, Neck, Face, and Skin** | | |
| Unobtrusively inspects the skin and facial symmetry of the face and neck. | | |
| Positions the patient in an upright seated position. Asks patient to remove eyeglasses and loosen clothing that limits examination of the neck. Requests that the patient not lean the head against the headrest. | | |
| Visually inspects the head, scalp, and ears. | | |
| Washes and dries hands. Follows clinic protocol regarding gloves. | | |
| **Subgroup 2: Lymph Nodes of the Head and Neck** | | |
| Palpates the occipital nodes. | | |
| Palpates the posterior auricular lymph nodes by applying circular compression with the fingertips. | | |
| Palpates the preauricular lymph nodes by applying circular compression with the fingertips. | | |
| Palpates the submental nodes using digital compression with the thumb and index finger. | | |
| Palpates the submandibular nodes by rolling the tissue over the mandible. | | |
| Palpates the cervical nodes medial to the muscle by grasping the muscle and rotating the fingertips back and forth over the muscle. Covers the entire length of the muscle from the ear to the clavicle. | | |
| Palpates the cervical lymph nodes posterior to the muscle by applying gentle compression under the muscle against the underlying tissues along the entire length of the muscle. | | |
| Palpates the supraclavicular lymph nodes using circular compression. | | |
| **Subgroup 3: Salivary and Thyroid Glands** | | |
| Palpates the parotid glands using circular compression. | | |

*(continued)*

**SKILL CHECKLIST:**  HEAD AND NECK EXAMINATION *(CONTINUED)*

| CRITERIA | S | E |
|---|---|---|
| **Locates submandibular glands by finding the antegonial notch. Asks the patient to press the tip of the tongue against the roof of the mouth while compressing the glands upward against the tensed muscles.** | | |
| **Locates the thyroid gland below the thyroid cartilage. Asks patient to swallow a sip of water, if necessary, to facilitate locating the gland. Keeping the hand in a stationary position, palpates the gland as the patient swallows sips of water.** | | |
| Subgroup 4: Temporomandibular Joint<br>**Locates the joints near the tragus of each ear and palpates as the patient slowly opens and closes the mouth.** | | |
| **Palpates the TMJ as the patient makes lateral excursions to the right and then to the left.** | | |
| OPTIONAL: **Assesses the range of motion by asking the patient to place the index, middle, and ring fingers between the incisal edges of the upper and lower incisors.** | | |
| **Documents notable findings in the patient chart or computerized record.** | | |

OPTIONAL GRADE PERCENTAGE CALCULATION

Each **S** equals 1 point, and each **U** equals 0 points. Using the **E** column, total the sum of the "**S**"s _____ divided by the total points possible (18 or 19 if optional step is included) to calculate the percentage grade.

**COMMUNICATION SKILL CHECKLIST:** HEAD AND NECK EXAMINATION

Student: _____     Evaluator: _____

Date:     _____

---

**Roles:**

- Student 1 = Plays the role of a fictitious patient.
- Student 2 = Plays the role of the clinician.
- Student 3 or instructor = Plays the role of the clinic instructor near the end of the role-play.

---

**DIRECTIONS FOR STUDENT CLINICIAN:** Use **Column S**; evaluate your skill level as **S** (satisfactory) or **U** (unsatisfactory).

**DIRECTIONS FOR EVALUATOR:** Use **Column E** to record your evaluation of the student clinician's communication skills during the role-play. Indicate **S** (satisfactory) or **U** (unsatisfactory). In the optional grade percentage calculation, each **S** equals 1 point, and each **U** equals 0 points.

| CRITERIA | S | E |
|---|---|---|
| **Explains what is to be done.** | | |
| **Reports notable findings to the patient. As needed, makes referrals to a physician or dental specialist.** | | |
| **Encourages patient questions before and during the head and neck examination.** | | |
| **Answers the patient's questions fully and accurately.** | | |
| **Communicates with the patient at an appropriate level and avoids dental/medical terminology or jargon.** | | |
| **Accurately communicates the findings to the clinical instructor. Discusses the implications for dental treatment using correct medical and dental terminology.** | | |

OPTIONAL GRADE PERCENTAGE CALCULATION

Each **S** equals 1 point, and each **U** equals 0 points. Using the **E** column, total the sum of the "**S**"s _____ divided by the total points possible (6) to calculate the percentage grade.

# NOTES

# 13 Oral Examination

## MODULE OVERVIEW

This module describes the oral examination. The oral examination is a physical examination technique that consists of a systemic visual inspection and/or palpation of the structures of the oral cavity and oropharynx. This examination should be a routine part of each patient's dental visit.

This module describes the oral examination, including:

- An anatomy review of oral structures
- Peak procedure for a systematic oral examination

## MODULE OUTLINE

## OBJECTIVES

- Recognize the normal anatomy of the oral cavity.
- Locate the following oral structures: parotid ducts, sublingual fold, sublingual caruncles, papillae, anterior and posterior pillars, and the tonsils.
- Recognize and describe deviations from normal in the oral cavity.
- Position the patient correctly for the oral examination.
- Provide information to the patient about the oral examination and any notable findings.
- Demonstrate the oral examination using correct technique and a systematic sequence of examination.
- Document notable findings in the patient chart or computerized record.
- Explain findings that have implications in planning dental treatment.
- Provide referral to a physician or dental specialist when findings indicate the need for further evaluation.
- Demonstrate knowledge of the soft tissue findings by applying concepts from this module to the fictitious patient cases A–E found in Section 5.

**SECTION 1:**

# Examination Overview

A comprehensive oral examination is a physical examination technique consisting of a systemic inspection of the oral structures. Like the head and neck examination, this procedure takes only minutes. The oral examination allows the clinician to gather general information on the health of a patient, note early indications of some diseases, and detect abnormalities and potentially life-threatening malignancies at an early stage. Tissue changes in the mouth that signal the beginnings of cancer often can be seen and felt easily.

With early detection and timely treatment, deaths from oral cancer could be dramatically reduced. When detected at the earliest stages, oral cancer has an 80% survival rate. At present, only one-third of oral cancers are diagnosed in the early stage. Only 13% of Americans recall having an oral examination performed in the past year.[1] Healthy People 2020 targets the goal of increasing this statistic to 20% so that more individuals receive an annual comprehensive oral examination.[2] The American Dental Association (ADA) recommends that a thorough oral examination should be a routine part of each patient's dental visit. Teaching patients about oral cancer screenings and performing oral cancer examinations at every appointment is part of the dental hygiene process of care and policy of the American Dental Hygienists' Association.[3,4]

## INCIDENCE

In the United States, it is estimated that 36,540 men and women (25,420 men and 11,120 women) will be diagnosed with cancer of the oral cavity and pharynx in 2010.[5,6] Oral cancer will cause over 8,000 deaths, killing roughly 1 person per hour, 24 hours per day.[6] Worldwide, the problem is much greater, with over 640,000 new cases being found each year.[6] Of the oral structures, the tongue is the site with the highest incidence rate (Fig. 13-1).

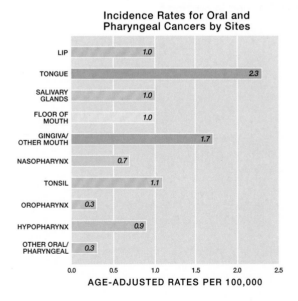

**Figure 13-1.   Incidence rates for oral and pharyngeal cancers by sites.** The rates are per 100,000 and are age adjusted to the 1970 U.S. standard population. (Source: National Institute of Dental and Craniofacial Research, National Institutes of Health and the Division of Oral Health. Centers for Disease Control and Prevention.)

## RISK FACTORS, SIGNS, AND SYMPTOMS

The public domain publications of the U.S. Department of Health and Human Services, National Institutes of Health, and National Institutes of Dental and Craniofacial Research contain information about risk factors, prevention, signs, and symptoms of oral cancer. A summary of this information is found below.

### Risk Factors for Oral Cancer

1. **Age.**
   * The incidence of oral cancer rises steadily with age, usually because older persons have had a longer exposure to risk factors, such as exposure to sunlight.
   * Incidence peaks in persons aged 55 to 74 years.
2. **Gender.** Men are two times more likely to develop oral cancer than women.
3. **Sunlight.** Exposure to sunlight is a risk factor for lip cancer.
4. **Tobacco and Alcohol Use.**
   * Tobacco and excessive alcohol use increases the risk of oral cancer.
   * Using tobacco and alcohol in combination poses a much higher risk than using either substance alone. Those who both smoke and drink alcohol have a 15 times greater risk of developing oral cancer than others.[2]

---

**BOX 13-1**    **Signs and Symptoms of Oral Cancer**

**LESIONS THAT MIGHT SIGNAL ORAL CANCER**

* Leukoplakia (white lesions): possible precursor to cancer
* Erythroplakia (red lesions): less common than leukoplakia but with greater potential for becoming cancerous

**SYMPTOMS THAT YOUR PATIENT MIGHT REPORT**

* Soreness
* A lump or thickening
* Numbness in the tongue or other areas of the mouth
* Feeling that something is caught in the throat, hoarseness
* Difficulty chewing or swallowing
* Ear pain
* Difficulty moving the jaw or tongue
* Swelling of the jaw that causes dentures to fit poorly

**MANAGEMENT OF SUSPICIOUS LESIONS**

* White or red lesions should be reevaluated in 2 weeks
* Any white or red lesion that does not resolve itself in 2 weeks should be biopsied to obtain a definitive diagnosis
* Any symptom listed previously that persists for more than 2 weeks indicates the need for referral to an appropriate specialist for definitive diagnosis

## ANATOMY REVIEW

### Landmarks of the Lips

Two important landmarks of the lips are the vermillion border and the commissure (Fig. 13-2). Both of these landmarks are useful when recording the location of a soft tissue lesion or other notable finding. Figures 13-3 and 13-4 illustrate some conditions that can cause an alteration in the normal appearance of the lip.

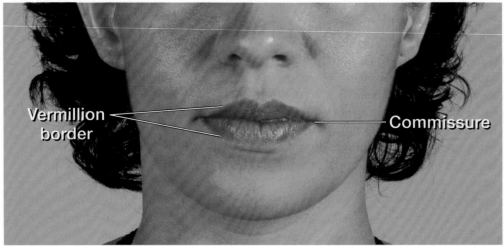

**Figure 13-2.   The lips.** The **vermillion border** and **commissures** of the lips are useful landmarks when recording the location of a soft tissue lesion or other notable finding.

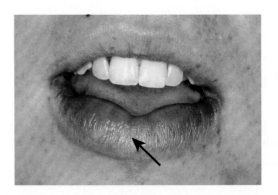

**Figure 13-3.   Angioedema of the lower lip.** This swollen lower lip was caused by an allergic reaction to the latex gloves. Questions that screen for a history and symptoms of latex sensitivity should be included on the health history form. (Courtesy of Dr. Richard Foster, Guilford Technical Community College.)

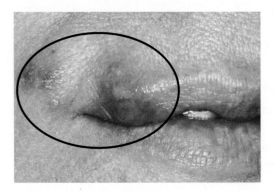

**Figure 13-4.   Recurrent herpes simplex.** These recurrent herpes labialis vesicles contain the herpes simplex virus (HSV). Contact with the fluid can result in the spread of this viral infection to other epidermal sites. (Courtesy of Dr. Richard Foster, Guilford Technical Community College.)

## Salivary Glands

The major salivary glands are three pairs of glands that produce saliva (Fig. 13-5).

1.  The parotid glands are the largest of the salivary glands. Each gland is located on the surface of the masseter muscle between the ear and the jaw.
    *   Each parotid gland has a duct that opens into the oral cavity opposite the maxillary first molar (Fig. 13-6).

2.  The submandibular glands sit below the jaw toward the back of the mouth.
    *   Each submandibular gland has a duct that extends forward in the floor of the mouth to open into the sublingual caruncles.
    *   Refer to Figure 13-7 for the anatomy of the anterior floor of the mouth.

3.  The sublingual glands are located in the anterior floor of the mouth next to the mandibular canines.
    *   Each has one major duct that opens—along with the submandibular glands— into the sublingual caruncles.
    *   In addition, the sublingual gland has several minor ducts, which open in a line along the fold of tissue beneath the tongue known as the sublingual fold.

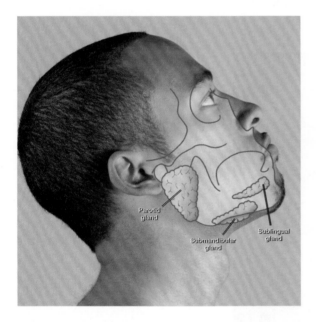

Figure 13-5.   The major salivary glands.

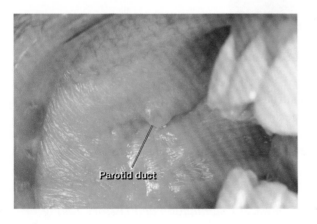

Figure 13-6.   Parotid duct. The parotid duct starts at the anterior part of the gland and opens on the inside of the cheek opposite the second molar. (Courtesy of Dr. Richard Foster, Guilford Technical Community College.)

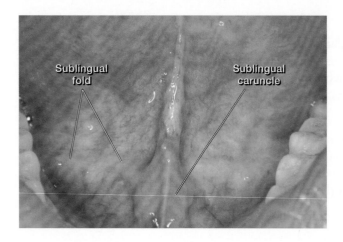

**Figure 13-7.  Salivary ducts.** The submandibular and sublingual glands have ducts that open into the sublingual caruncles on the floor of the mouth. The sublingual gland also has several minor ducts that open along the sublingual fold. (Courtesy of Dr. Richard Foster, Guilford Technical Community College.)

## Ventral Surface of the Tongue and Anterior Floor of Mouth

Landmarks of the ventral surface of the tongue and anterior floor of the mouth include the sublingual caruncles, the lingual frenum, the sublingual fold, and the sublingual veins. Some of these landmarks are shown in Figure 13-8.

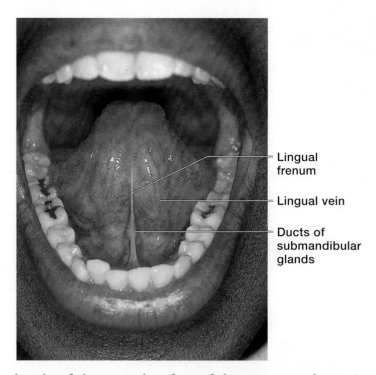

**Figure 13-8.   Landmarks of the ventral surface of the tongue and anterior floor of the mouth.** The anterior view of the mouth and ventral surface of the tongue, showing the:

- **Sublingual caruncles**—located on either side of the **lingual frenum** (the tissue that attaches the tongue to the floor of the mouth)
- Minor ducts of the submandibular gland that open in the fold of tissue beneath the tongue known as the **sublingual fold**
- **Sublingual veins** of the tongue

(Adapted from Bickley LS, Szilagyi P. *Bates' Guide to Physical Examination and History Taking.* 8th ed. Philadelphia, PA: Lippincott Williams & Wilkins; 2003.)

## Dorsal Surface of the Tongue

The dorsal surface of the tongue has a complex arrangement of papillae that serve as taste sensitive structures. Figure 13-9 illustrates this arrangement of papillae. Figures 13-11 and 13-12 show variations in the appearance (pigmentation) and anatomy (ankyloglossia) of the tongue.

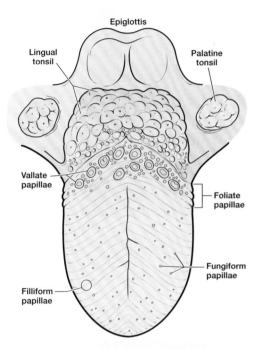

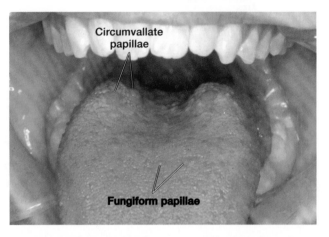

(Courtesy of Dr. Richard Foster, Guilford Technical Community College)

**Figure 13-9.   Dorsum of the tongue and its papillae.** The papillae are the taste-sensitive structures of the tongue.

- The largest and most posterior papillae are the circumvallate papillae.
- The long, thin, grey, hair-like filiform papillae cover the anterior two-thirds of the dorsal surface of the tongue.
- The fungiform papillae are broad, round, red, mushroom-shaped papillae.
- The foliate papillae are three to five large, red, leaf-like projections on the lateral border of the posterior third of the tongue (Fig. 13-10).
- The circumvallate papillae are 8 to 12 large papillae that form a V-shaped row.

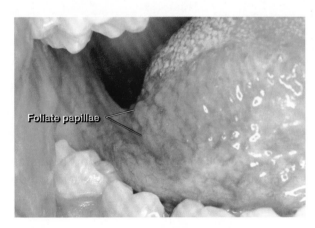

**Figure 13-10.   Foliate papillae.** The foliate papillae are large, leaf-like projections on the lateral border of the posterior third of the tongue. (Courtesy of Dr. Richard Foster, Guilford Technical Community College.)

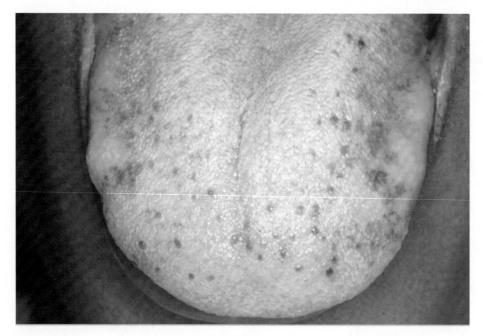

**Figure 13-11.   Pigmented tongue.** Pigmentation of the tongue is a normal finding most commonly seen in dark-skinned individuals. (Courtesy of Dr. Richard Foster, Guilford Technical Community College.)

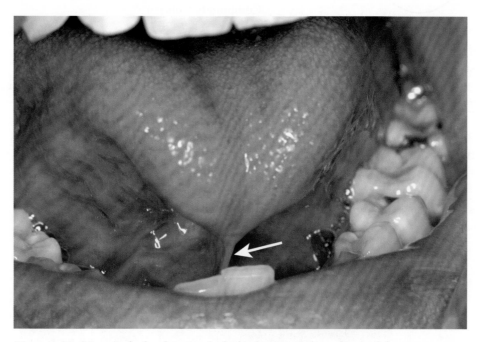

**Figure 13-12.   Ankyloglossia.** Ankyloglossia, a short lingual frenum, limits tongue movement. (Courtesy of Dr. Richard Foster, Guilford Technical Community College.)

## Palate, Tonsils, and Oropharynx

Figure 13-13 illustrates the normal anatomy of the palate, tonsils, and oropharynx. Figures 13-14 and 13-15 show conditions that can alter the appearance of the anatomy of the palate, tonsils, and oropharynx.

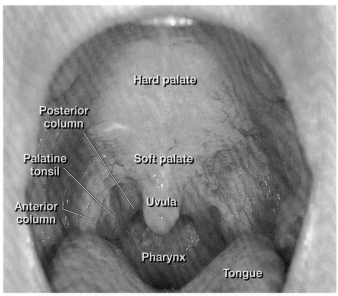

**Figure 13-13.  Landmarks of the hard and soft palate, tonsils, and oropharynx.** (From Bickley LS, Szilagyi P. Bates' *Guide to Physical Examination and History Taking.* 8th ed. Philadelphia, PA: Lippincott Williams & Wilkins; 2003.)

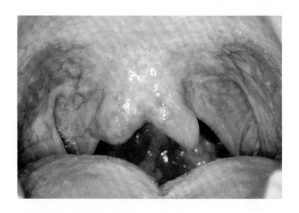

**Figure 13-14.  Bifid uvula.** A bifid uvula is a minor cleft of the posterior soft palate. (Courtesy of Dr. Richard Foster, Guilford Technical Community College.)

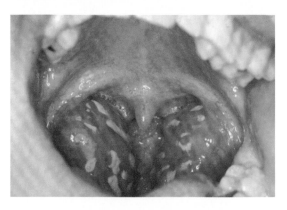

**Figure 13-15.  Tonsillitis.** Tonsillitis is an infection or inflammation of the tonsils characterized by severe sore throat, fever, headache, enlarged tender lymph nodes in the neck, and enlarged red tonsils. (Courtesy of Dr. Richard Foster, Guilford Technical Community College.)

## SECTION 2:

# Peak Procedure

Evidence-based clinical recommendations developed by a panel convened by the ADA Council on Scientific Affairs advocates the comprehensive oral examination as the "gold standard" for early oral cancer detection.[7]

   The oral examination involves the inspection and/or palpation of the structures of the oral cavity and oropharynx. To assist the examiner, it is helpful to organize the structures to be examined into seven subgroups:

- Subgroup 1: Lips and Vermillion Border
- Subgroup 2: Oral Cavity and the Mucosal Surfaces
- Subgroup 3: Underlying Structures of the Lips and Cheeks
- Subgroup 4: Floor of the Mouth
- Subgroup 5: Salivary Gland Function
- Subgroup 6: The Tongue
- Subgroup 7: Palate, Tonsils, and Oropharynx

## SUBGROUP 1: VISUAL INSPECTION OF LIPS AND VERMILLION BORDER

**Table 13-1**  LIPS AND VERMILLION BORDER: WHAT CAN I EXPECT?

| Normal findings | • At rest, the lips normally touch<br>• The surface of the lips is smooth and intact with a normal color and texture<br>• The vermillion border is even and not raised |
|---|---|
| Notable findings | • Changes in shape or texture (fissuring, desquamation, crusts)<br>• Chapped, or cracked lips<br>• Pigment changes or variations in color<br>• Lip pits<br>• Irregular vermillion border<br>• Lips that do not meet at rest<br>• Cheilosis at the commissures<br>• Herpetic lesions<br>• Soft tissue lesions<br>• Swelling of the lips; trauma or lip biting<br>• Asymmetrical mouth; may indicate a neurological condition, tumors, or infections |

**PROCEDURE 13-1**   **ORAL EXAMINATION**

**Equipment:**
Gloves and protective gear for the clinician
Safety glasses for the patient
2″ × 2″ gauze squares, cotton-tipped applicators, and a dental mirror

### Subgroup 1: Visual Inspection of the Lips and Vermillion Border

**1.** Preparation for the examination.

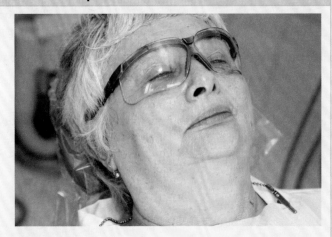

**Figure 13-16.**

- After briefly explaining the procedure to the patient, ask him or her to remove partial or complete dentures, if applicable. Give female patients a tissue to remove lipstick.
- Provide the patient with safety glasses.
- Wash your hands and don gloves.
- *Place the patient in a supine position.*
- *Position yourself in a seated position.*

**2.** Lips and vermillion border—visual inspection.

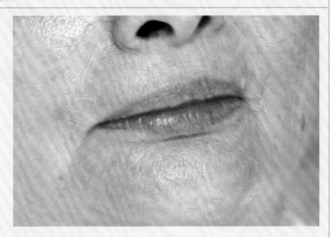

**Figure 13-17.**

- Visually inspect the lips and the vermillion border.

*(continued)*

## SUBGROUP 2: INSPECTION OF THE ORAL CAVITY AND MUCOSAL SURFACES

**Table 13-2**  MUCOSAL SURFACES: WHAT CAN I EXPECT?

| **Normal findings** | • Smooth, intact, and coral pink to bluish brown in color<br>• No lesions<br>• Minor salivary glands in the lips feel like small beads when palpated<br>• Intact frenum on maxillary and mandibular arches<br>• Normal variations: Fordyce granules (ectopic sebaceous glands) |
|---|---|
| **Notable findings** | • Note changes in color or texture<br>• Swelling<br>• Trauma<br>• Lesions<br>• Pale or reddened mucosa; dry mucosa<br>• Linea alba<br>• Leukoplakia<br>• Lichen planus<br>• Halitosis |

**PROCEDURE 13-1**  ORAL EXAMINATION *(CONTINUED)*

### Subgroup 2: Inspection of the Oral Cavity and Mucosal Surfaces

**1.** Oral cavity—preliminary visual inspection.

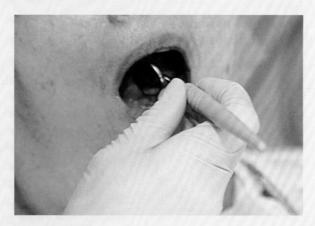

**Figure 13-18.**

• Visually inspect the entire oral cavity and oropharynx.
• Adjust the dental unit light so that the oral cavity is well illuminated.
• Use a dental mirror to look for any conditions that would cause the examination procedure to be modified or postponed. Examples include herpetic lesions or a red, inflamed throat.

*(continued)*

**PROCEDURE 13-1** ORAL EXAMINATION *(CONTINUED)*

### Subgroup 2: Inspection of the Oral Cavity and Mucosal Surfaces

2. Labial mucosa of the lower lip—visual inspection.

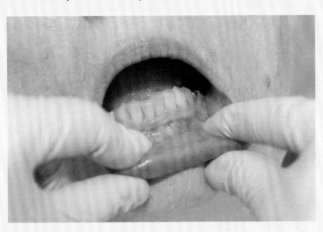

**Figure 13-19.**

- Visually inspect the labial mucosa of the lower lip. Place the ***index fingers of both hands on the inside*** with your ***thumbs on the outside of the lower lip.***
- **Tip: *Keep your index finger(s) inside the mouth and the thumb(s) outside the mouth while completing all the steps for examining the mucosal surfaces. This technique keeps your wet fingers inside the mouth while your dry fingers come in contact with the patient's face. Your patient will appreciate this courtesy.***
- Evert and retract the lip fully away from the teeth and alveolar ridge. Retract the lip completely so that you have a clear view of the entire labial mucosal surface and vestibule of the lower lip.

3. Labial mucosa of the upper lip—visual inspection.

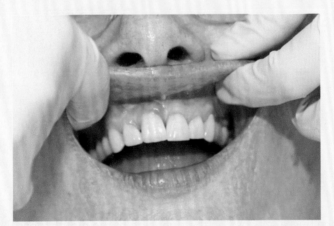

**Figure 13-20.**

- Examine the labial mucosa of the upper lip in a similar manner. Slide both **index fingers** upward to position them between the maxillary arch and the labial mucosa of the upper lip.
- Use your **thumbs** to evert and retract the upper lip.
- Stretch the tissue away from the dental arches. Visually examine the entire mucosal surface adjacent to the maxillary teeth as well as the tissue between the dental arches.

*(continued)*

**PROCEDURE 13-1** ORAL EXAMINATION *(CONTINUED)*

## Subgroup 2: Inspection of the Oral Cavity and Mucosal Surfaces

**4.** Buccal mucosa—visual inspection.

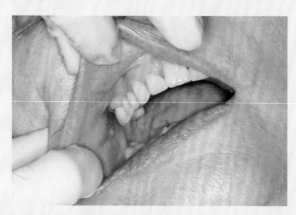

**Figure 13-21.**

- Begin with the buccal mucosa on the right side of the mouth, near the **maxillary arch**.
- Place the **index fingers of both hands on the inside** with the **thumbs on the outside** of the cheek. One hand and a mirror can also be used, taking care not to press the mirror rim against the soft tissue.
- Evert the cheek and stretch the tissue of the right cheek up and away from the maxillary teeth. Extend the tissue completely away from the teeth so that no folds remain to conceal a lesion or abnormality. *Proceed to Step 5 to examine the buccal mucosa adjacent to the mandibular arch on the right side of the mouth.*

**5.** Buccal mucosa—visual inspection.

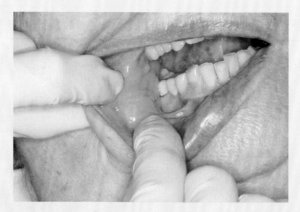

**Figure 13-22.**

- Next, inspect the buccal mucosa on the right side of the mouth, near the **mandibular arch**.
- Stretch the cheek down and **away from the mandibular arch** on the right side of the mouth.
- Extend the tissue completely away from the teeth so that no folds remain to conceal a lesion or abnormality.
- Visually inspect the buccal mucosa. *Repeat this process to examine the buccal mucosa on the left side of the mouth.*

*(continued)*

## SUBGROUP 3: UNDERLYING STRUCTURES OF THE LIPS AND CHEEKS

**Table 13-3** UNDERLYING STRUCTURES OF THE LIPS AND CHEEKS: WHAT CAN I EXPECT?

| Normal findings | • Firm tissue<br>• Moist tissue<br>• Intact tissue |
|---|---|
| Notable findings | • Swellings or nodules<br>• Changes in texture<br>• Tenderness upon palpation<br>• Minor salivary glands in the lips feel like small beads when palpated |

**PROCEDURE 13-1** ORAL EXAMINATION *(CONTINUED)*

### Subgroup 3: Palpation of the Underlying Structures of the Lips and Cheeks

**1.** Lower lip—palpate.

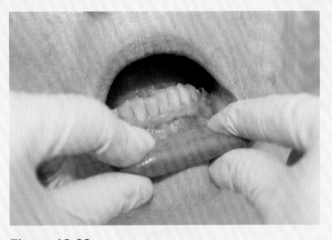

**Figure 13-23.**

• Palpate the lower lip by compressing the tissues between your index fingers and thumbs.

*(continued)*

**PROCEDURE 13-1** ORAL EXAMINATION *(CONTINUED)*

### Subgroup 3: Palpation of the Underlying Structures of the Lips and Cheeks

**2.** Right cheek—palpate.

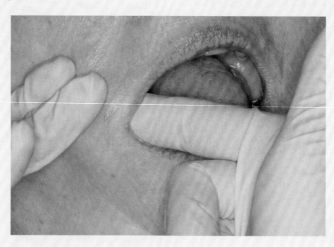

**Figure 13-24.**

- Reposition your *left hand with middle and ring fingers extraorally on the right cheek*. These fingers are not wet with saliva; your patient will appreciate this courtesy.
- Reposition *the index finger of your right hand so that it is opposite the fingers of your left hand*.
- Compress the tissues on the right cheek between your fingers.
- Palpate the entire length of the buccal mucosa.
- Continue with Step 3 to palpate the left buccal mucosa.

**3.** Upper lip—palpate.

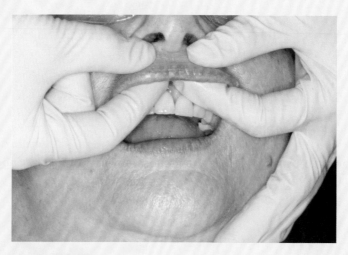

**Figure 13-25.**

- Compress the tissues of the upper lip between the index fingers and thumbs.
- Palpate from the right commissure of the mouth to the left.

*(continued)*

## SUBGROUP 4: FLOOR OF THE MOUTH

**Table 13-4** FLOOR OF MOUTH: WHAT CAN I EXPECT?

| | |
|---|---|
| **Normal findings** | • Sublingual frenum<br>• Sublingual caruncles on either side of frenum |
| **Notable findings** | • Changes in color or texture<br>• Lesions or other surface abnormalities<br>• Swelling, especially a unilateral swelling<br>• Mucocele or ranula (fluid-filled swelling caused by pooling of saliva within the tissues due to trauma to a salivary gland duct)<br>• Swelling due to salivary calculi or stones within a salivary gland or duct that obscure the flow of saliva and cause floor of mouth swelling<br>• Leukoplakia on floor of mouth<br>• Soft tissues should be palpated for hard areas or discomfort |

**PROCEDURE 13-1** ORAL EXAMINATION *(CONTINUED)*

### Subgroup 4: Floor of the Mouth

**1.** Anterior region of the floor of the mouth—visual inspection.

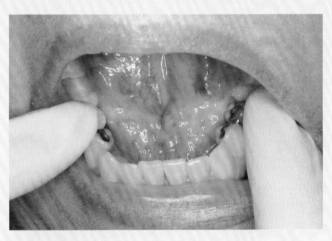

**Figure 13-26.**

• Ask the patient to touch the tip of the tongue to the roof of the mouth.
• Inspect the floor of the mouth. The inspection will be easier if the patient is in a chin-down position.
• With the floor of the mouth well illuminated, visually inspect the anterior portion.
• A mouth mirror may be helpful in providing indirect illumination.

*(continued)*

**PROCEDURE 13-1**    ORAL EXAMINATION *(CONTINUED)*

### Subgroup 4: Floor of the Mouth

**2.** Posterior region of the floor of the mouth—visual inspection.

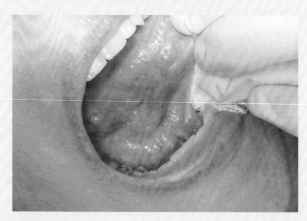

**Figure 13-27.**

- Instruct your patient to relax the tongue and protrude it slightly. Fold a damp gauze square in half and grasp the tip of the tongue between the sides of the gauze square.
- Use your ***right hand*** to pull the tongue gently to the left commissure of the lip.
- Using your ***left hand*** to apply gentle pressure upward against the submandibular gland will make it easier see the right posterior region of the floor of the mouth.
- Visually inspect the floor of the mouth. Repeat this procedure on the left side of the mouth.

**3.** Floor of the mouth—palpation.

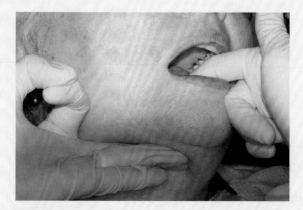

**Figure 13-28.**

- Place your ***right index finger on the floor of the mouth***.
- Place the ***middle and ring fingers of the left hand under the patient's chin*** on the right side of the head. Ask the patient to relax the tongue and close the mouth slightly. This maneuver relaxes the muscles in the floor of the mouth.
- Gently move the tongue out of the way with your index finger and touch the floor of the mouth. Palpate the floor of the mouth by pressing upward with your extraoral fingers and downward with your index finger as if you are "trying to make your fingers meet."
- Palpate from the right posterior region forward to the anterior region and then back to the left posterior region of the floor of the mouth.

*(continued)*

## SUBGROUP 5: SALIVARY GLAND FUNCTION

**Table 13-5** SALIVARY GLAND FUNCTION: WHAT CAN I EXPECT?

| Normal findings | • Normal flow of saliva |
|---|---|
| Notable findings | • Xerostomia<br>• Swellings in floor of mouth from blocked saliva glands or ducts or trauma |

**PROCEDURE 13-1** ORAL EXAMINATION *(CONTINUED)*

### Subgroup 5: Salivary Gland Function

**1.** Submandibular and sublingual ducts—examine.

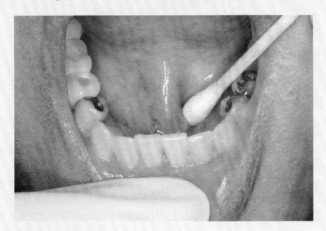

**Figure 13-29.**

- Ask the patient to raise his or her tongue toward the roof of the mouth.
- Use a gauze square to gently dry the area around the sublingual caruncles and sublingual fold.
- Press down gently with a cotton-tipped applicator in the region of the caruncles. A drop or stream of saliva should be evident.

*(continued)*

**PROCEDURE 13-1** ORAL EXAMINATION *(CONTINUED)*

## Subgroup 5: Salivary Gland Function

**1.** Parotid salivary ducts—examine.

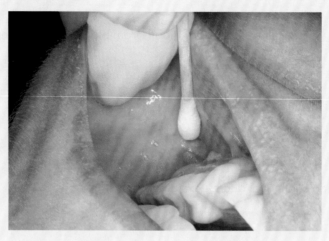

**Figure 13-30.**

- Ask your patient to open the mouth halfway so that the cheek is easy to retract.
- The purpose of this examination is to evaluate the functioning of the right parotid gland.
- Retract the right cheek and locate the parotid papilla on the buccal mucosa opposite to the maxillary right molars.
- Dry the papilla with a gauze square; it will be difficult to detect saliva flowing out of the papilla if the area is wet.
- Using the tip of a cotton-tipped applicator, press the area slightly above the parotid papilla. It may be helpful to roll the cotton-tipped applicator from an area slightly above the papilla down to the papilla while applying pressure. Repeat this rolling action several times as necessary.
- If the duct is functioning properly, a drop of saliva will be expressed from the papilla.
- Evaluate the parotid gland on the left side using the same procedure.

*(continued)*

## SUBGROUP 6: THE TONGUE

**Table 13-6** THE TONGUE: WHAT CAN I EXPECT?

| Normal findings | • Moist, pink, may have freckle-like pigmentation<br>• Papillae present<br>• Symmetrical appearance<br>• **Ventral surface**: Lingual veins are distinct, raised linear structures on ventral surface of the tongue; enlarged vessels relating to aging may result in lingual varicosities<br>• **Dorsal surface**: median groove, filiform, fungiform, circumvallate papillae; networks of grooves may be pronounced with advancing age<br>• **Lateral surface**: foliate papillae; scalloped outline from being pressed into the embrasure spaces |
|---|---|
| Notable findings | • Ulceration<br>• Lesions or swellings<br>• Nodules detectible upon palpation<br>• Variation in size, color, or texture<br>• Accumulated food debris may produce inflammation or malodor<br>• Asymmetrical shape<br>• Dry mouth<br>• Papillae absent<br>• Fissured or pebbly dorsal surface<br>• Geographic tongue<br>• Macroglossia<br>• Ankyloglossia<br>• Black hairy tongue with use of some antibiotics |

**PROCEDURE 13-1** ORAL EXAMINATION *(CONTINUED)*

### Subgroup 6: The Tongue

**1.** Ventral surface of the tongue—visual inspection.

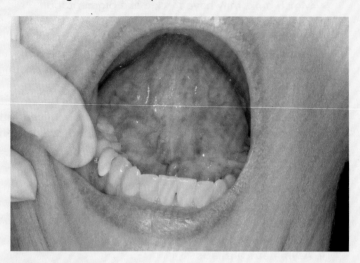

**Figure 13-31.**

- Ask the patient to open wide and touch the tip of the tongue to the roof of the mouth.
- Closely inspect the ventral surface of the tongue.
- Keep in mind that the tongue is a frequent site of oral cancer.

**2.** Dorsal surface of the tongue—visual inspection.

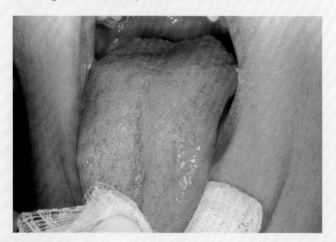

**Figure 13-32.**

- Ask the patient to relax the tongue and protrude it slightly from the mouth.
- Grasp the tongue with a damp gauze square. **Technique tip:** dry gauze may stick to the tongue, so use the air/water syringe to wet the gauze before use.
- Gently pull the tongue forward, being careful not to injure the lingual frenum on the incisal edges of the mandibular anterior teeth.
- Visually inspect the dorsal surface of the tongue. Use a mouth mirror, if it is helpful.
- Keep in mind that the tongue is a frequent site of oral cancer.

*(continued)*

**PROCEDURE 13-1** ORAL EXAMINATION *(CONTINUED)*

| Subgroup 6: The Tongue |
| :--- |

**3.** Lateral borders of the tongue—visual inspection.

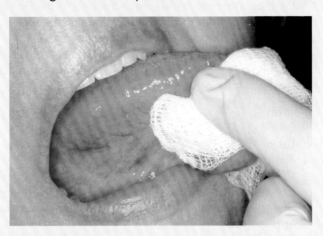

**Figure 13-33.**

- Gently pull the tongue to the left commissure and evert it slightly to obtain a clear view of the lateral surface and foliate papillae.
- Visually inspect the lateral surface of the tongue.
- Use a mirror to view the posterior portion of the lateral surface.
- Repeat this procedure to inspect the left border of the tongue.

**4.** Tongue—palpation.

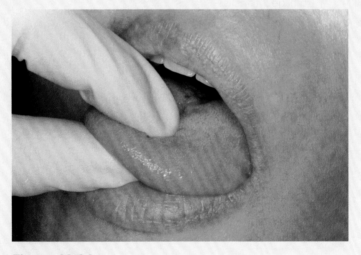

**Figure 13-34.**

- Palpate the body of the tongue between your index finger and thumb.
- Be alert for swellings or nodules.

*(continued)*

## SUBGROUP 7: PALATE, TONSILS, AND OROPHARYNX

**Table 13-7**  PALATE, TONSILS, AND OROPHARYNX: WHAT CAN I EXPECT?

| Normal findings | • Hard palate: mucosa is firmly attached to the bone; pale pink in color with a bluish hue to brown; palatine raphae and rugae; firm when palpated; common variation is palatine torus<br>• Soft palate: spongy in texture, firm but flexible; symmetrical elevation<br>• Tonsils: large in childhood, small or absent in adults<br>• Uvula: at midline |
|---|---|
| Notable findings | **Palate:**<br>• Swelling<br>• Lesions<br>• Tumors<br>• Cleft palate<br>• Changes in color (red, white, gray)<br>• Changes in texture are common in smokers, such as cobblestone appearance<br>• Snuff dipper's or tobacco chewer's patch<br>• Petechiae (discrete red spots on palate due to trauma)<br>• Ulcerations<br>• Trauma<br>• Paralysis will cause the soft palate to sag on the affected side of the face and the uvula to pull to the unaffected side<br><br>**Tonsils:**<br>• Inflamed tonsils<br>• Enlarged tonsils<br>• Areas of exudates (pus) evident<br><br>**Oropharynx:**<br>• Markedly reddened and inflamed<br>• Sore throat<br>• Discomfort when swallowing or eating<br><br>**Uvula**<br>• Deviates from midline |

**PROCEDURE 13-1** ORAL EXAMINATION *(CONTINUED)*

### Subgroup 7: Palate, Tonsils, and Oropharynx

**1.** Palate—preliminary visual inspection.

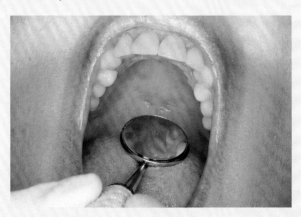

**Figure 13-35.**

- Visually inspect the hard and soft palate, uvula, oropharynx, and tonsils.

**2.** Hard and soft palate—palpate.

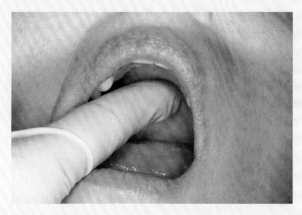

**Figure 13-36.**

- Use intermittent pressure with your index finger to palpate the hard and soft palate.
- **Technique tip:** Avoid sliding your finger across the palate because this technique may cause the patient to gag. Instead, lift your index finger away from the palate to reposition it. This technique facilitates palpation.

*(continued)*

**PROCEDURE 13-1** ORAL EXAMINATION *(CONTINUED)*

### Subgroup 7: Palate, Tonsils, and Oropharynx

**3.** Tonsils and oropharynx—visual inspection.

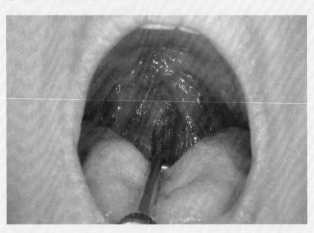

**Figure 13-37.**

- You will need a mirror to move the tongue out of your line of vision.
- Position the mouth mirror with the reflecting surface down.
- Ask the patient to say "ah" as you depress the back of the tongue downward and forward. Firm forward and downward pressure is needed to keep the tongue out of your line of vision.
- Visually inspect the tonsils and oropharynx.

**4.** Document. Document all notable findings from the oral examination in the patient chart or computerized record.

(continued)

# Ready References

## TOOLS FOR INTRODUCING THE ORAL EXAMINATION TO PATIENTS

### THE ORAL CANCER FOUNDATION'S DIALOGUE BUTTONS

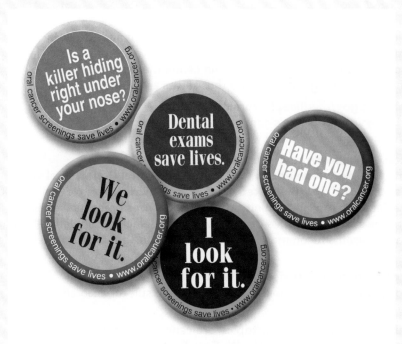

**Figure 13-38.  Examples of dialogue buttons from the Oral Cancer Foundation.**

An excellent way to make patients aware that an oral examination screening is available is to wear one of the oral exam dialogue buttons from The Oral Cancer Foundation. Seeing the "We look for it" button worn by a dental health care provider, patients inevitably ask, "What do you look for?" This provides an excellent opening to respond to patient questions with a statement such as, *"We look for oral cancer. Thirty thousand new patients will be diagnosed with this deadly disease this year. While you are here today, we can give you a thorough screening for oral cancer."* The "Dental exams saves lives" button usually creates a question in the patient's mind because few people associate dental exams with life-threatening events.

These buttons are available for purchase at the Oral Cancer Foundation website at http://oralcancerfoundation.org/products/dentist_products.htm

**READY REFERENCE 13-1** INTERNET RESOURCES FOR INFORMATION GATHERING

**http://www.nidcr.nih.gov/OralHealth/Topics/OralCancer/**
**National Institute of Dental and Craniofacial Research (NIDCR)** website resources:
- **Oral Cancer** (printer-friendly PDF version)
- **The Oral Cancer Exam** (printer-friendly PDF version). A step-by-step guide for patients on what to expect during an oral cancer exam.
- **What You Need to Know About Oral Cancer.** This brochure discusses possible causes, symptoms, diagnosis, and treatment of oral cancer. It also has information about rehabilitation and about sources of support to help patients cope with oral cancer.

**http://drc.hhs.gov/**
The NIDCR, in conjunction with the Division of Oral Health of the Centers for Disease Control and Prevention (CDC), has established a **Dental, Oral and Craniofacial Data Resource Center (DRC)**. This center is designed to facilitate use of available large-scale databases on oral health and related topics. The center makes relevant data in many areas available to a wide range of users and thus serves as a research resource.

**http://www.nlm.nih.gov/medlineplus/oralcancer.html**
The **National Library of Medicine's** compilation of links to government, professional, and nonprofit/voluntary organizations with information on oral cancer.

**http://www.cdc.gov/mmwr/preview/mmwrhtml/rr5021a1.htm**
**Promoting Oral Health: Interventions for Preventing Dental Caries, Oral and Pharyngeal Cancers, and Sports-Related Craniofacial Injuries.** This November 2001 report from the Task Force on Community Preventive Services presents the results of systematic reviews of the evidence of effectiveness of selected population-based interventions and presents recommendations for future interventions and intervention research.

**http://www.cdc.gov/mmwr/preview/mmwrhtml/rr5021a1.htm**
**NIDCR** links to resources about smokeless, chewing, and spit tobacco and the relationship to oral cancer.

**http://www.nidcr.nih.gov/oralhealth/topics/oralcancer/detectingoralcancer.htm**
**Detecting Oral Cancer: A Guide for Health Care Professionals** provided by the NIDCR and the National Institutes of Health.

**READY REFERENCE 13-2** INTERNET RESOURCES FOR ORAL CANCER EDUCATION

**http://www.oralcancerfoundation.org/products/dentist_products.htm**
The website of the **Oral Cancer Foundation** has resources to help dental health care providers make patients aware that oral cancer screenings are available in the dental setting. They suggest that dental clinicians wear a simple button as a way to begin dialogue with patients about the oral cancer screening examination in the dental office.

**http://www.spohnc.org/**
The **Support for People with Oral and Head and Neck Cancer (SPOHNC)** website. SPOHNC is a patient-directed, self-help organization dedicated to meeting the needs of oral and head and neck cancer patients. SPOHNC, founded in 1991 by an oral cancer survivor, addresses the broad emotional, physical, and humanistic needs of this population. This website includes many resources, including:

- **Eat Well—Stay Nourished**. A recipe and resource guide is a special cookbook that addresses the unique needs of oral and head and neck cancer patients.
- **We Have Walked in Your Shoes.** This new resource "packet" contains three sections of helpful information compiled by oral and head and neck cancer patients, survivors, and dental professionals. This valuable resource is presented in both English and Spanish and is a free download.
- **Oral Cancer and Head and Neck Awareness Bracelets.** SPOHNC offers an official oral and head and neck cancer awareness bracelet.

**READY REFERENCE 13-3** INTERNET RESOURCES FOR ORAL CANCER DETECTION

**http://www.oralcdx.com**
The website of **OralCDx**. This website has information on the use of a biopsy brush for early cancer detection.

**http://www.vizilite.com**
The website of **ViziLite**. This website has information about the use of a special light and oral solution for the identification of suspicious oral lesions.

## REFERENCES

1. U.S. Department of Health and Human Services. *Healthy People 2010 Midcourse Review.* Washington, DC: U.S. Department of Health and Human Services; 2007.
2. Healthy People. Healthy people 2020 topics and objectives index. http://www.healthypeople .gov/2020/topicsobjectives2020/default.aspx. Accessed October 5, 2011.
3. American Dental Hygienists' Association. *Standards for Clinical Dental Hygiene Practice.* Chicago, IL: American Dental Hygienists' Association; 2008. http://www.adha.org. Accessed October 5, 2011.
4. American Dental Hygienists' Association. *Policy Manual.* Chicago, IL: American Dental Hygienists' Association; 2011. http://www.adha.org. Accessed October 5, 2011.
5. National Cancer Institute. Oral cavity and pharynx cancer statistics fact sheet, surveillance, epidemiology, and end results (SEER) program. Bethesda, MD. http://www.seer.cancer.gov/statfacts/html/oralcav.html. Accessed October 5, 2011.
6. Oral Cancer Foundation. Oral cancer facts. http://oralcancerfoundation.org/facts/index.htm. Accessed October 5, 2011.
7. Rethman MP, Carpenter W, Cohen EE, et al. Evidence-based clinical recommendations regarding screening for oral squamous cell carcinomas. *J Am Dent Assoc.* 2010;141(5): 509–520.

## SUGGESTED READINGS

Langlais RP, Miller CS, Nield-Gehrig JS. Color atlas of common oral diseases. Philadelphia, PA: Lippincott Williams & Wilkins; 2009.

Margolis F. Oral pathology of tots and teens. The identification, etiology, and treatment of common oral lesions in infants, children, and adolescents. *Dimens Dent Hyg.* 2010;8(2):58–61.

Muzyka, BC. (2001). Assessing salivary gland hypofunction—Part One. *Pract Proced Aesthet Dent.* 13(9):688.

Muzyka, BC. (2002). Assessing salivary gland hypofunction—Part two. *Pract Proced Aesthet Dent.* 14(3):262.

# The Human Element

| BOX | |
|---|---|
| **13-2** | **Through the Eyes of a Student** |

*I so clearly remember the very first time that I did an intraoral exam. It was on my very first patient. Seeing my first patient was a day that I had dreamed about, but now that it was here, I was very nervous. The first part of the appointment went well, but then it was here—the time to do the oral examination. There seemed to be so much to check and I was worried that I would forget to check an area. Fortunately, my patient must have realized how nervous I was because she said, "Take your time, I am retired. I am in no hurry."*

*I started the exam and heard my instructor's voice in my mind saying that the key to any procedure is to work through it one step at a time. I concentrated on going step by step, and before I knew it, I had completed the exam. I remember my relief when I finished the exam. Suddenly it was over—the procedure that I had worried about all last night—and I felt like yelling, "I did it!" To this day, I don't think that I ever do an oral exam without remembering the first time I did this examination.*

*Joanne, R.D.H*
*Graduate, University of*
*North Carolina at Chapel Hill*

## PATIENT SCENARIO

You have been a dental hygienist for approximately 20 years and just started a new job as a nursing home hygienist. You provide prophylactic dental hygiene services to the residents in a variety of care facilities. Today, you are working with the founder of the company, Dr. Ari, and are seeing the patients on an Alzheimer floor. You complete the intraoral examination for your next patient, Florence, who is unresponsive and makes no eye contact. You notice three large white lesions in the back of Florence's throat. You check Florence's throat two additional times as best as you can as she is not very cooperative. Dr. Ari is very busy providing restorative care, but you ask him to check Florence's throat at his convenience. He states that you are probably mistaking the white lesions for "Cream of Wheat" that was served for breakfast. You examine Florence again and confirm that the lesions are **not** from a food source and again ask for Dr. Ari to examine Florence.

1. What ethical principles come into play here?
2. Why are you concerned about the white lesions in Florence's throat?
3. How should Florence's lesion be treated?

**Table 13-8   ENGLISH-TO-SPANISH PHRASE LIST FOR ORAL EXAMINATION**

| | |
|---|---|
| I am going to examine the soft tissues of your mouth. | Voy a examinar el tejido suave de la boca. |
| Please remove your partials or dentures. | Por favor saque las dentarudas. |
| I am going to recline the dental chair. | Voy a recliner la silla dental. |
| Please wear these safety glasses. | Por favor pongase estos espejuelos de seguridad. |
| Just relax. This examination is not painful and only takes a few minutes. | No tenga miedo. La examinación no duele, y solamente toma unos minutos. |
| At any time during the examination, please tell me if any area is tender. | A cualquier tiempo durante la examinación, por favor digame si tiene algun area que está sensible. |
| First, I will examine your lips and cheeks. | Primero voy a examiner los labios y las mejillas. |
| Please open wide. | Por favor abra la boca ancho. |
| Please close slightly. | Por favor cierre un poco. |
| Please tilt your head forward (back). | Por favor incline la cabeza hacia delante. Por favor incline la cabeza hacia atrás. |
| Please tilt your chin down. | Por favor incline la barbilla hacia abajo. |
| Please **turn** your head to the right (left). | Por favor vuelta la cabeza a la derecha. Por favor vuelta la cabeza a la izquierda. |
| Please **tilt** your head to the right (left). | Por favor incline la cabeza a la derecha. Por favor incline la cabeza a la izquierda. |
| Please look straight ahead. | Por favor mire al frente. |
| I am checking the floor of your mouth. | Estoy examinando el suelo de la boca. |
| I am checking your saliva ducts. | Estoy examinando la glandula de saliva. |
| Next, I will check your tongue. | Ahora voy a examiner la lengua. |
| Please press your tongue against the roof of your mouth. | Por favor aprete lau lengua contra el techo de la boca. |

*(continued)*

**Table 13-8**   ENGLISH-TO-SPANISH PHRASE LIST FOR ORAL EXAMINATION (*CONTINUED*)

| | |
|---|---|
| Please stick out your tongue. | Por favor protrude la lengua. |
| I am checking the roof of your mouth and throat. | Estoy examinando el techo de la boca y la garganta. |
| Everything looks (feels) fine. | Todo luce (parece) bien. |
| I am concerned about this area and would like to have it examined by a specialist. | Estoy preocupado sobre esta zona, y quiero que sea examinada por un médico/especialista. |
| Here are the names of several specialists in our area. | Aqui tiene nombres de varios médicos/especialistas en esta area. |
| I can set up an appointment with the specialist of your choice. | Yo le puedo hacer una cita con el especialista de su preferencia. |
| I will write a note to the specialist explaining my concerns. | Le voy a escribir una nota al especialista para explicarle la preocupación. |
| I am going to get my clinic instructor. | Voy a buscar mi instructor. |

## SECTION 5:
# Practical Focus—Fictitious Patient Cases

---

**DIRECTIONS:**

- The photographs in this section show the findings from the oral examination of fictitious patients A–E. Refer to previous modules to refresh your memory regarding each patient's health history and vital signs because there may be a connection between the patient's systemic health status or habits and the findings from the head and neck examination.

- If appropriate, use the **Lesion Descriptor Worksheet** to develop descriptions for the findings in this section.

- The pages in this section may be removed from the book for easier use by tearing along the perforated lines on each page.

- **Note:** The clinical photographs in a fictitious patient case are for illustrative purposes but are not necessarily from the same individual. The fictitious patient cases are designed to enhance the learning experiences associated with each case.

---

## SOURCES OF CLINICAL PHOTOGRAPHS

The author gratefully acknowledges the sources of the following clinical photographs in the "Practical Focus" section of this module.

- Figure 13-39. Dr. Richard Foster, Guilford Technical Community College, Jamestown, NC.
- Figure 13-41. From Fleisher GR, Ludwig W, Baskin MN. *Atlas of Pediatric Emergency Medicine*. Philadelphia, PA: Lippincott Williams & Wilkins; 2004.
- Figure 13-43. Dr. Richard Foster, Guilford Technical Community College, Jamestown, NC.
- Figure 13-44. Dr. Richard Foster, Guilford Technical Community College, Jamestown, NC.
- Figure 13-46. Dr. Richard Foster, Guilford Technical Community College, Jamestown, NC.
- Figure 13-48. Dr. John S. Dozier, Tallahassee, FL.

## FICTITIOUS PATIENT CASE A: MR. ALAN ASCARI

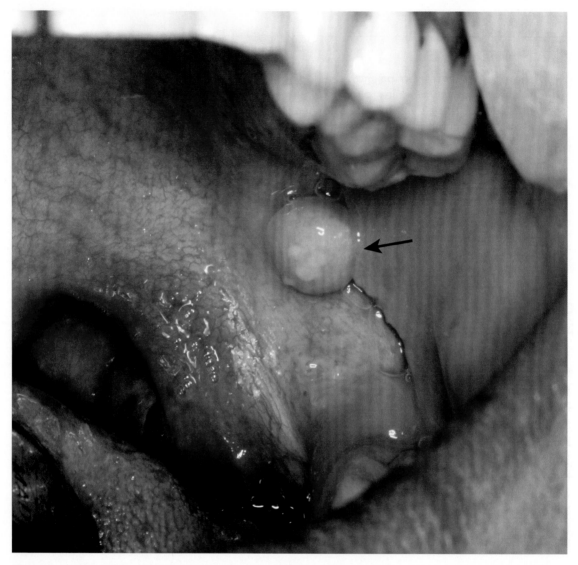

Figure 13-39.   Mr. Ascari: Finding on the left buccal mucosa.

# Lesion Descriptor Worksheet

*Directions: Highlight or circle the applicable descriptors*

| | |
|---|---|
| **Ⓐ Anatomic Location** | *Head*: Scalp, eye, ear, nose, cheek, chin, neck; right or left side<br>*Neck:* Midline, right, left; near certain anatomic structure<br>*Lip:* Upper, lower, commissure, vermillion border; labial mucosa<br>*Buccal mucosa:* Parotid papilla; mucobuccal fold; near tooth #<br>*Gingiva:* Free, attached; near tooth #<br>*Tongue:* Anterior third, middle third, posterior third; dorsal, ventral, right lateral, left lateral<br>*Floor of mouth:* Lingual frenum, sublingual folds, sublingual caruncle; near tooth #<br>*Palate:* Hard, soft; midline, incisive papilla; right side, left side<br>*Oropharynx:* Pillars, midline, uvula |
| **Ⓑ Border** | *Well demarcated:* Easy to see where lesion begins and ends<br>*Poorly demarcated:* Difficult to see where lesion begins and ends<br>*Regularly shaped:* Uniform border<br>*Irregularly shaped:* Border not uniform |
| **Ⓒ Color Change Configuration** | *Color:* Red, white, red and white, blue, yellow, brown, black<br>*Lesion pattern:* Single lesion or multiple lesions (discrete, grouped, confluent, linear) |
| **Ⓓ Diameter/ Dimension** | *If oblong or irregular in shape:* Length and width<br>*If circular or round in shape:* Diameter (measurement of a line running from one side of a circle through the center to the other side) |
| **Ⓣ T y p e** | |

| | | |
|---|---|---|
| | **Nonpalpable Flat Lesions** | *Macule* - Flat discolored spot, less than 1 cm in size<br>*Patch* - Flat discolored spot, larger than 1 cm in size |
| | **Palpable, Elevated, Solid Masses** | *Papule* - Solid raised lesion, less than 1 cm in diameter<br>*Plaque* - Superficial raised lesion, larger than 1 cm in diameter<br>*Nodule* - Marble-like lesion, larger than 1 cm in diameter<br>*Wheal* - Localized area of skin edema |
| | **Fluid-Filled Lesions** | *Vesicle* - Small blister filled with clear fluid, less than 1 cm in diameter<br>*Bulla* - Larger fluid-filled lesion, larger than 1 cm in diameter<br>*Pustule* - Small raised lesion filled with pus |
| | **Loss of Skin or Mucosal Surface** | *Erosion* - Loss of top layer of skin or mucosa<br>*Ulcer* - Craterlike lesion where top two layers of skin or mucosa are lost<br>*Fissure* - A linear crack |

**Figure 13-40A. Page 1 of Lesion Descriptor Worksheet for Mr. Ascari.**

# Lesion Descriptor Worksheet

*Directions:* Draw the lesion(s) on the appropriate illustration, showing the anatomic location, relative shape, and size.

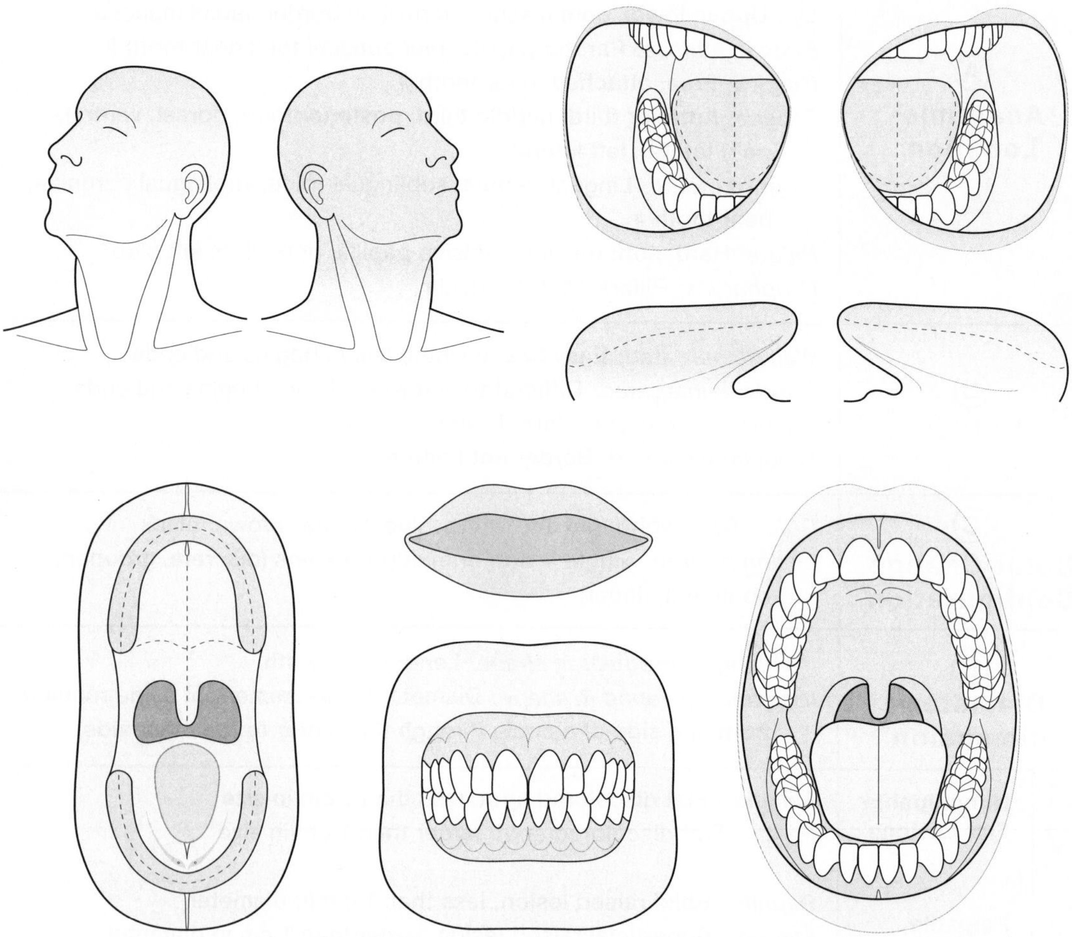

*Develop a chart entry:* Using each descriptor circled and the location indicated on this work-sheet, develop a written description of the lesion(s). After you have perfected the written description, enter it in the paper or computerized patient chart. Remember the A, B, C, D, T plan for formulating a description.

**Figure 13-40B.    Page 2 of Lesion Descriptor Worksheet for Mr. Ascari.**

# FICTITIOUS PATIENT CASE B: BETHANY BIDDLE

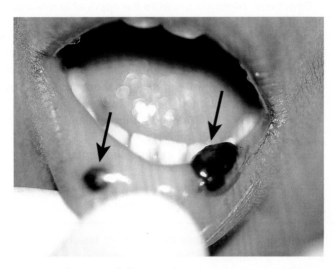

**Figure 13-41.** Bethany Biddle: Findings on mucosa of lower lip.

# Lesion Descriptor Worksheet

*Directions: Highlight or circle the applicable descriptors*

| | |
|---|---|
| **Ⓐ**<br>**Anatomic Location** | *Head:* Scalp, eye, ear, nose, cheek, chin, neck; right or left side<br>*Neck:* Midline, right, left; near certain anatomic structure<br>*Lip:* Upper, lower, commissure, vermillion border; labial mucosa<br>*Buccal mucosa:* Parotid papilla; mucobuccal fold; near tooth #<br>*Gingiva:* Free, attached; near tooth #<br>*Tongue:* Anterior third, middle third, posterior third; dorsal, ventral, right lateral, left lateral<br>*Floor of mouth:* Lingual frenum, sublingual folds, sublingual caruncle; near tooth #<br>*Palate:* Hard, soft; midline, incisive papilla; right side, left side<br>*Oropharynx:* Pillars, midline, uvula |
| **Ⓑ**<br>**Border** | *Well demarcated:* Easy to see where lesion begins and ends<br>*Poorly demarcated:* Difficult to see where lesion begins and ends<br>*Regularly shaped:* Uniform border<br>*Irregularly shaped:* Border not uniform |
| **Ⓒ**<br>**Color Change Configuration** | *Color:* Red, white, red and white, blue, yellow, brown, black<br>*Lesion pattern:* Single lesion or multiple lesions (discrete, grouped, confluent, linear) |
| **Ⓓ**<br>**Diameter/ Dimension** | *If oblong or irregular in shape:* Length and width<br>*If circular or round in shape:* Diameter (measurement of a line running from one side of a circle through the center to the other side) |
| **Ⓣ**<br>**T y p e** | **Nonpalpable Flat Lesions**<br><br>*Macule -* Flat discolored spot, less than 1 cm in size<br>*Patch -* Flat discolored spot, larger than 1 cm in size |
| | **Palpable, Elevated, Solid Masses**<br><br>*Papule -* Solid raised lesion, less than 1 cm in diameter<br>*Plaque -* Superficial raised lesion, larger than 1 cm in diameter<br>*Nodule -* Marble-like lesion, larger than 1 cm in diameter<br>*Wheal -* Localized area of skin edema |
| | **Fluid-Filled Lesions**<br><br>*Vesicle -* Small blister filled with clear fluid, less than 1 cm in diameter<br>*Bulla -* Larger fluid-filled lesion, larger than 1 cm in diameter<br>*Pustule -* Small raised lesion filled with pus |
| | **Loss of Skin or Mucosal Surface**<br><br>*Erosion -* Loss of top layer of skin or mucosa<br>*Ulcer -* Craterlike lesion where top two layers of skin or mucosa are lost<br>*Fissure -* A linear crack |

**Figure 13-42A. Page 1 of Lesion Descriptor Worksheet for Bethany Biddle.**

# Lesion Descriptor Worksheet

*Directions:* Draw the lesion(s) on the appropriate illustration, showing the anatomic location, relative shape, and size.

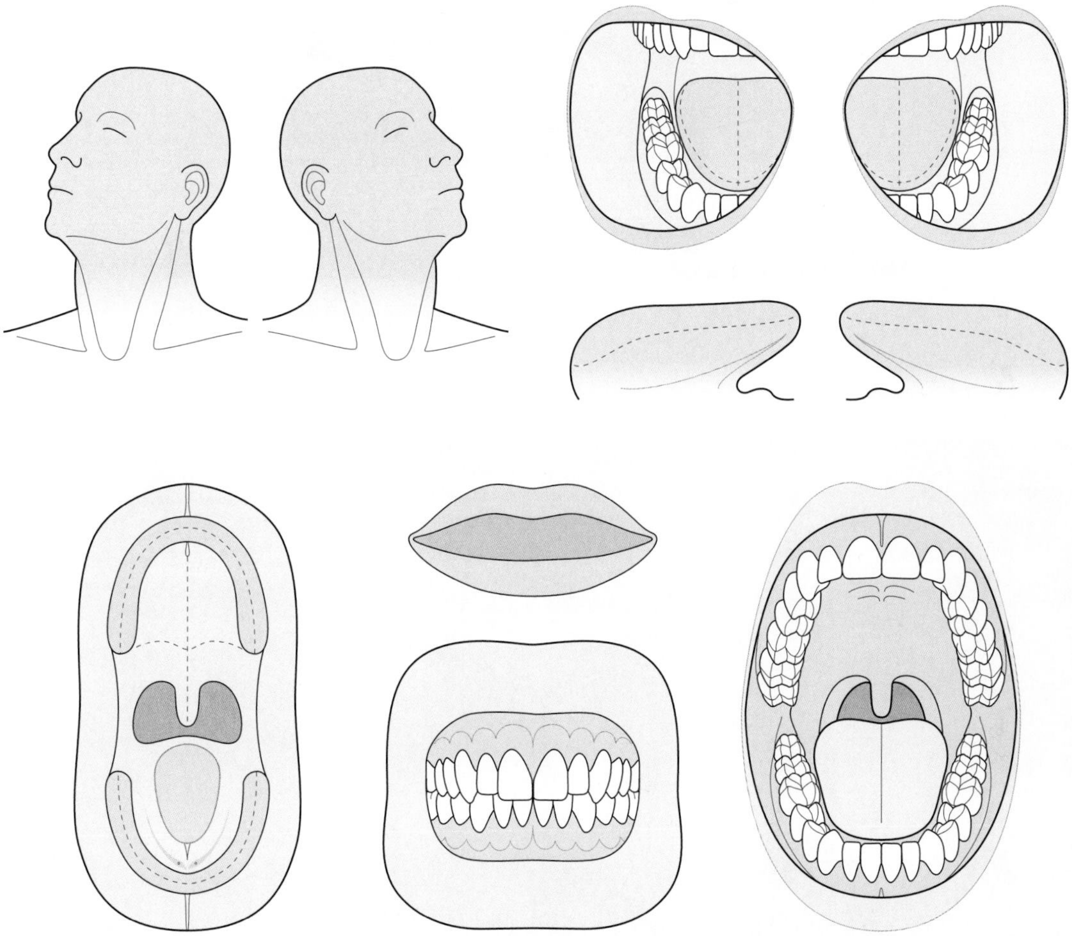

*Develop a chart entry:* Using each descriptor circled and the location indicated on this worksheet, develop a written description of the lesion(s). After you have perfected the written description, enter it in the paper or computerized patient chart. Remember the A, B, C, D, T plan for formulating a description.

**Figure 13-42B.   Page 2 of Lesion Descriptor Worksheet for Bethany Biddle.**

## FICTITIOUS PATIENT CASE C: MR. CARLOS CHAVEZ

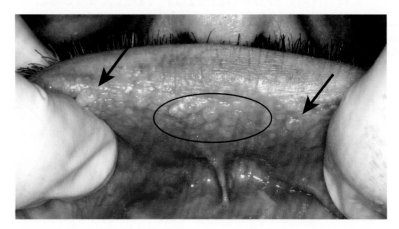

Figure 13-43. Mr. Chavez: Findings on mucosa of upper lip.

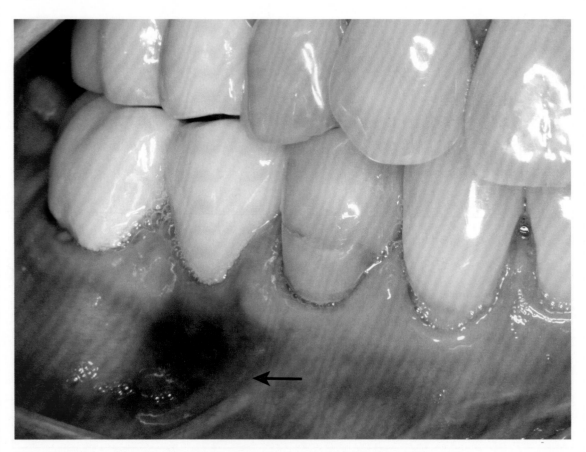

Figure 13-44. Mr. Chavez: Finding on tissue on mandibular right sextant.

# Lesion Descriptor Worksheet

*Directions: Highlight or circle the applicable descriptors*

| | |
|---|---|
| **Ⓐ** <br> **Anatomic Location** | *Head:* Scalp, eye, ear, nose, cheek, chin, neck; right or left side <br> *Neck:* Midline, right, left; near certain anatomic structure <br> *Lip:* Upper, lower, commissure, vermillion border; labial mucosa <br> *Buccal mucosa:* Parotid papilla; mucobuccal fold; near tooth # <br> *Gingiva:* Free, attached; near tooth # <br> *Tongue:* Anterior third, middle third, posterior third; dorsal, ventral, right lateral, left lateral <br> *Floor of mouth:* Lingual frenum, sublingual folds, sublingual caruncle; near tooth # <br> *Palate:* Hard, soft; midline, incisive papilla; right side, left side <br> *Oropharynx:* Pillars, midline, uvula |
| **Ⓑ** <br> **Border** | *Well demarcated:* Easy to see where lesion begins and ends <br> *Poorly demarcated:* Difficult to see where lesion begins and ends <br> *Regularly shaped:* Uniform border <br> *Irregularly shaped:* Border not uniform |
| **Ⓒ** <br> **Color Change Configuration** | *Color:* Red, white, red and white, blue, yellow, brown, black <br> *Lesion pattern:* Single lesion or multiple lesions (discrete, grouped, confluent, linear) |
| **Ⓓ** <br> **Diameter/ Dimension** | *If oblong or irregular in shape:* Length and width <br> *If circular or round in shape:* Diameter (measurement of a line running from one side of a circle through the center to the other side) |
| **Ⓣ** <br> **T y p e** | **Nonpalpable Flat Lesions** — *Macule* - Flat discolored spot, less than 1 cm in size <br> *Patch* - Flat discolored spot, larger than 1 cm in size <br><br> **Palpable, Elevated, Solid Masses** — *Papule* - Solid raised lesion, less than 1 cm in diameter <br> *Plaque* - Superficial raised lesion, larger than 1 cm in diameter <br> *Nodule* - Marble-like lesion, larger than 1 cm in diameter <br> *Wheal* - Localized area of skin edema <br><br> **Fluid-Filled Lesions** — *Vesicle* - Small blister filled with clear fluid, less than 1 cm in diameter <br> *Bulla* - Larger fluid-filled lesion, larger than 1 cm in diameter <br> *Pustule* - Small raised lesion filled with pus <br><br> **Loss of Skin or Mucosal Surface** — *Erosion* - Loss of top layer of skin or mucosa <br> *Ulcer* - Craterlike lesion where top two layers of skin or mucosa are lost <br> *Fissure* - A linear crack |

**Figure 13-45A.   Page 1 of Lesion Descriptor Worksheet for Mr. Chavez.**

# Lesion Descriptor Worksheet

*Directions:* Draw the lesion(s) on the appropriate illustration, showing the anatomic location, relative shape, and size.

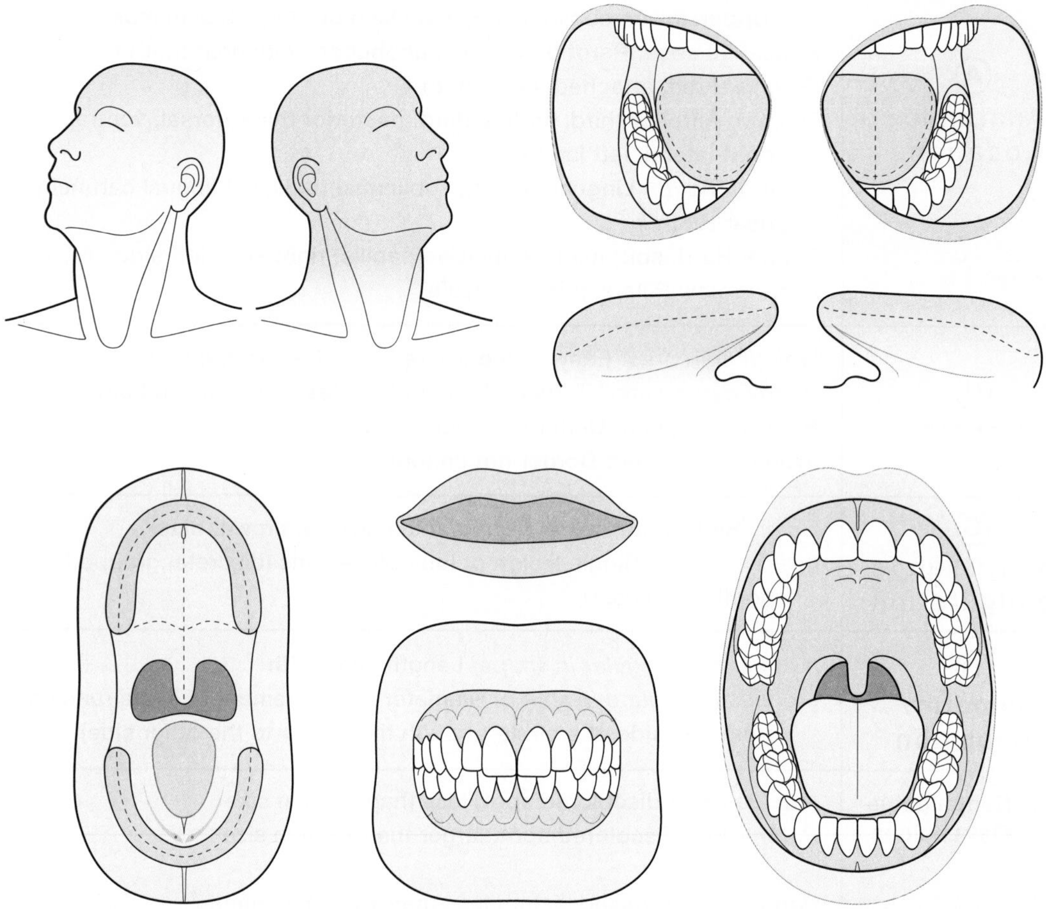

*Develop a chart entry:* Using each descriptor circled and the location indicated on this worksheet, develop a written description of the lesion(s). After you have perfected the written description, enter it in the paper or computerized patient chart. Remember the A, B, C, D, T plan for formulating a description.

_____

_____

_____

_____

**Figure 13-45B.  Page 2 of Lesion Descriptor Worksheet for Mr. Chavez.**

## FICTITIOUS PATIENT CASE D: MRS. DONNA DOI

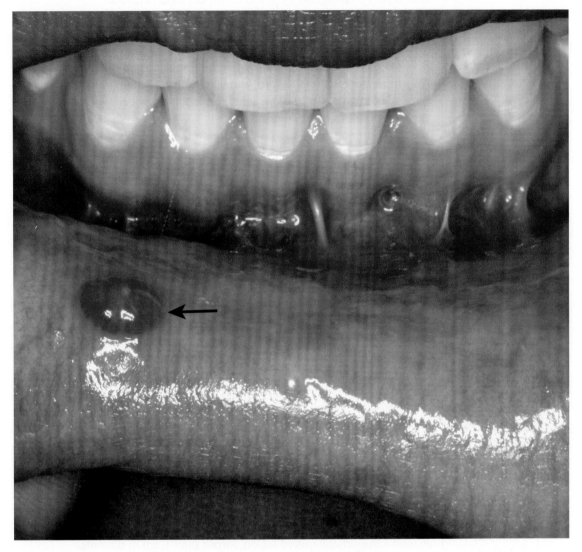

Figure 13-46.    Mrs. Doi: Finding on mucosa of lower lip.

# Lesion Descriptor Worksheet

*Directions: Highlight or circle the applicable descriptors*

| (A) Anatomic Location | *Head:* Scalp, eye, ear, nose, cheek, chin, neck; right or left side<br>*Neck:* Midline, right, left; near certain anatomic structure<br>*Lip:* Upper, lower, commissure, vermillion border; labial mucosa<br>*Buccal mucosa:* Parotid papilla; mucobuccal fold; near tooth #<br>*Gingiva:* Free, attached; near tooth #<br>*Tongue:* Anterior third, middle third, posterior third; dorsal, ventral, right lateral, left lateral<br>*Floor of mouth:* Lingual frenum, sublingual folds, sublingual caruncle; near tooth #<br>*Palate:* Hard, soft; midline, incisive papilla; right side, left side<br>*Oropharynx:* Pillars, midline, uvula |
|---|---|
| (B) Border | *Well demarcated:* Easy to see where lesion begins and ends<br>*Poorly demarcated:* Difficult to see where lesion begins and ends<br>*Regularly shaped:* Uniform border<br>*Irregularly shaped:* Border not uniform |
| (C) Color Change Configuration | *Color:* Red, white, red and white, blue, yellow, brown, black<br>*Lesion pattern:* Single lesion or multiple lesions (discrete, grouped, confluent, linear) |
| (D) Diameter/ Dimension | *If oblong or irregular in shape:* Length and width<br>*If circular or round in shape:* Diameter (measurement of a line running from one side of a circle through the center to the other side) |
| (T) Type | Nonpalpable Flat Lesions | *Macule* - Flat discolored spot, less than 1 cm in size<br>*Patch* - Flat discolored spot, larger than 1 cm in size |
| | Palpable, Elevated, Solid Masses | *Papule* - Solid raised lesion, less than 1 cm in diameter<br>*Plaque* - Superficial raised lesion, larger than 1 cm in diameter<br>*Nodule* - Marble-like lesion, larger than 1 cm in diameter<br>*Wheal* - Localized area of skin edema |
| | Fluid-Filled Lesions | *Vesicle* - Small blister filled with clear fluid, less than 1 cm in diameter<br>*Bulla* - Larger fluid-filled lesion, larger than 1 cm in diameter<br>*Pustule* - Small raised lesion filled with pus |
| | Loss of Skin or Mucosal Surface | *Erosion* - Loss of top layer of skin or mucosa<br>*Ulcer* - Craterlike lesion where top two layers of skin or mucosa are lost<br>*Fissure* - A linear crack |

**Figure 13-47A.　Page 1 of Lesion Descriptor Worksheet for Mrs. Doi.**

# Lesion Descriptor Worksheet

*Directions:* Draw the lesion(s) on the appropriate illustration, showing the anatomic location, relative shape, and size.

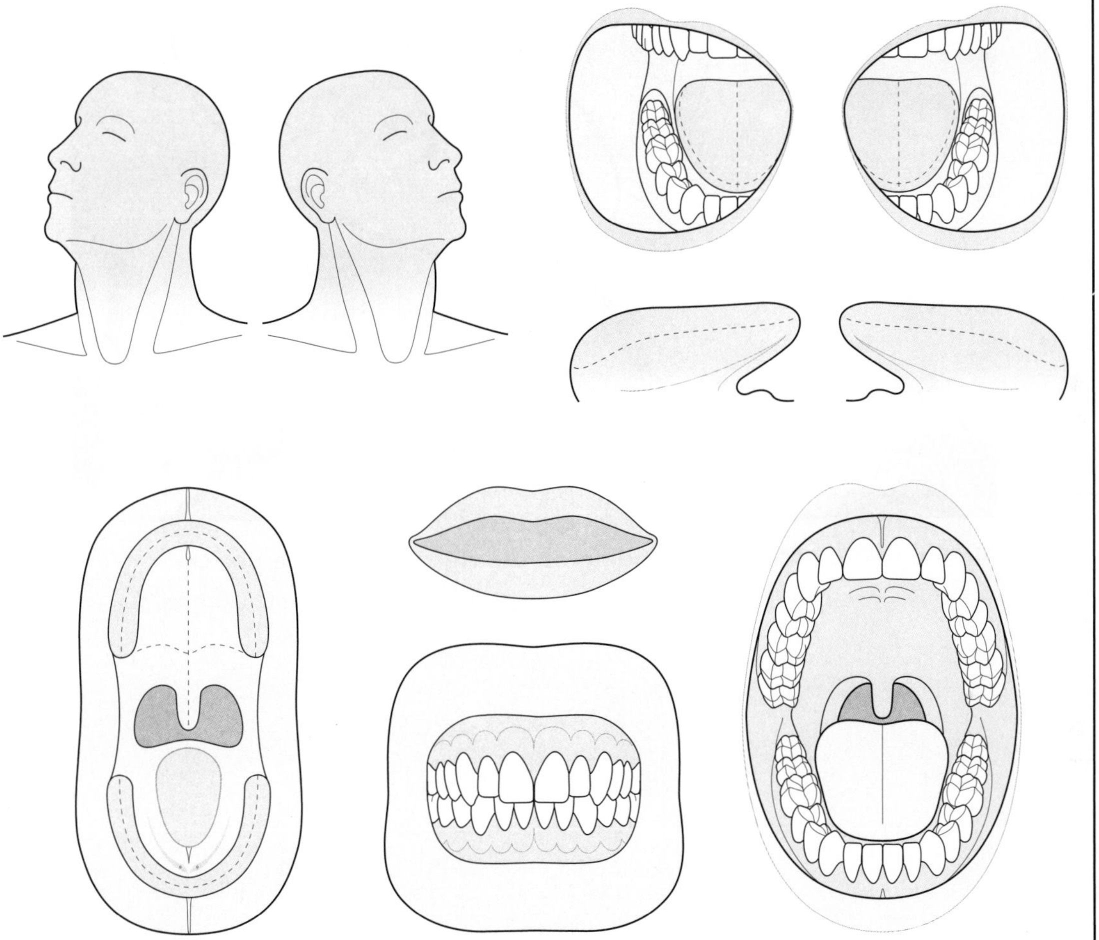

*Develop a chart entry:* Using each descriptor circled and the location indicated on this work-sheet, develop a written description of the lesion(s). After you have perfected the written description, enter it in the paper or computerized patient chart. Remember the A, B, C, D, T plan for formulating a description.

_____

_____

_____

_____

**Figure 13-47B.    Page 2 of Lesion Descriptor Worksheet for Mrs. Doi.**

## FICTITIOUS PATIENT CASE E: MS. ESTHER EADS

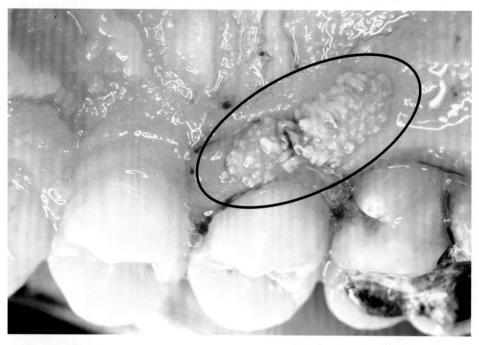

Figure 13-48.    Ms. Eads: Finding on the right side of the palate.

# Lesion Descriptor Worksheet

*Directions: Highlight or circle the applicable descriptors*

| | |
|---|---|
| **Ⓐ**<br>**Anatomic Location** | *Head*: Scalp, eye, ear, nose, cheek, chin, neck; right or left side<br>*Neck:* Midline, right, left; near certain anatomic structure<br>*Lip:* Upper, lower, commissure, vermillion border; labial mucosa<br>*Buccal mucosa:* Parotid papilla; mucobuccal fold; near tooth #<br>*Gingiva:* Free, attached; near tooth #<br>*Tongue:* Anterior third, middle third, posterior third; dorsal, ventral, right lateral, left lateral<br>*Floor of mouth:* Lingual frenum, sublingual folds, sublingual caruncle; near tooth #<br>*Palate:* Hard, soft; midline, incisive papilla; right side, left side<br>*Oropharynx:* Pillars, midline, uvula |
| **Ⓑ**<br>**Border** | *Well demarcated:* Easy to see where lesion begins and ends<br>*Poorly demarcated:* Difficult to see where lesion begins and ends<br>*Regularly shaped:* Uniform border<br>*Irregularly shaped:* Border not uniform |
| **Ⓒ**<br>**Color Change Configuration** | *Color:* Red, white, red and white, blue, yellow, brown, black<br>*Lesion pattern:* Single lesion or multiple lesions (discrete, grouped, confluent, linear) |
| **Ⓓ**<br>**Diameter/ Dimension** | *If oblong or irregular in shape:* Length and width<br>*If circular or round in shape:* Diameter (measurement of a line running from one side of a circle through the center to the other side) |
| **Ⓣ**<br>**T y p e** | **Nonpalpable Flat Lesions**<br>*Macule* - Flat discolored spot, less than 1 cm in size<br>*Patch* - Flat discolored spot, larger than 1 cm in size<br><br>**Palpable, Elevated, Solid Masses**<br>*Papule* - Solid raised lesion, less than 1 cm in diameter<br>*Plaque* - Superficial raised lesion, larger than 1 cm in diameter<br>*Nodule* - Marble-like lesion, larger than 1 cm in diameter<br>*Wheal* - Localized area of skin edema<br><br>**Fluid-Filled Lesions**<br>*Vesicle* - Small blister filled with clear fluid, less than 1cm in diameter<br>*Bulla* - Larger fluid-filled lesion, larger than 1cm in diameter<br>*Pustule* - Small raised lesion filled with pus<br><br>**Loss of Skin or Mucosal Surface**<br>*Erosion* - Loss of top layer of skin or mucosa<br>*Ulcer* - Craterlike lesion where top two layers of skin or mucosa are lost<br>*Fissure* - A linear crack |

**Figure 13-49A.   Page 1 of Lesion Descriptor Worksheet for Ms. Eads.**

# Lesion Descriptor Worksheet

*Directions:* Draw the lesion(s) on the appropriate illustration, showing the anatomic location, relative shape, and size.

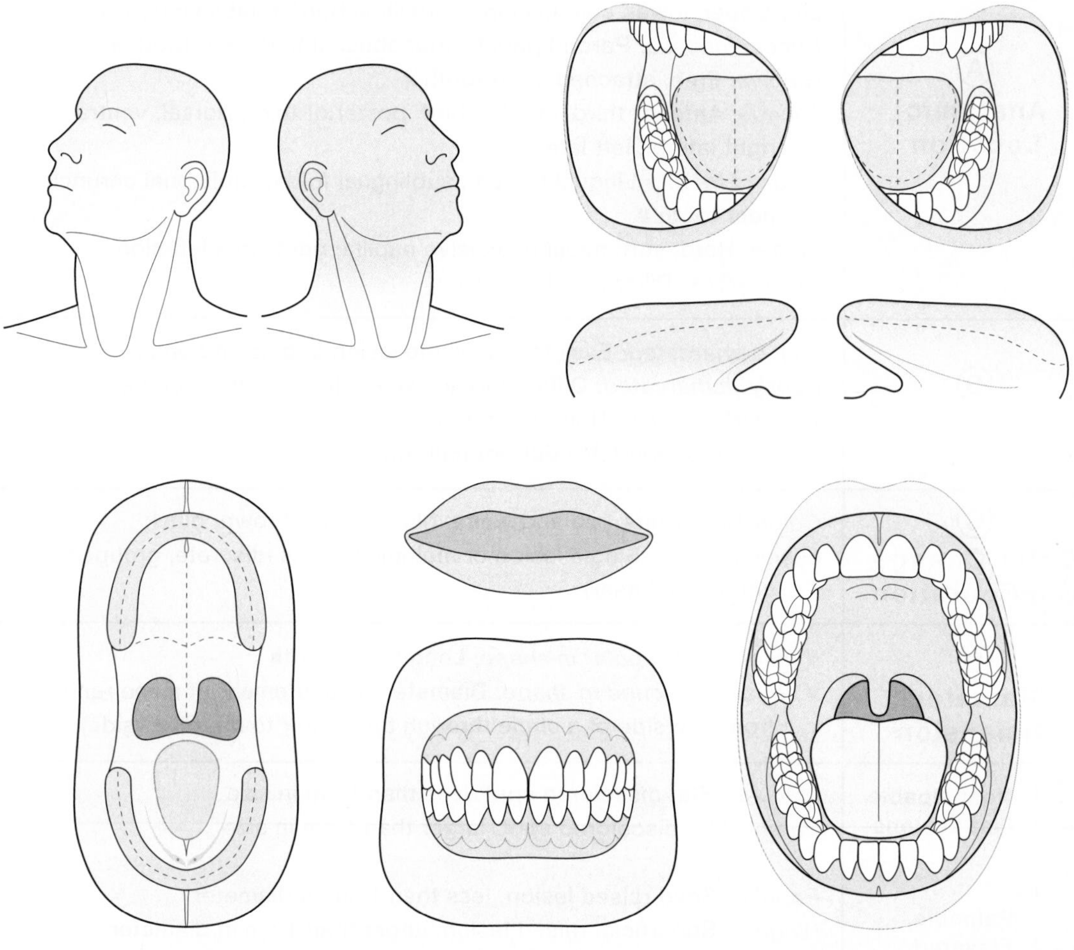

*Develop a chart entry:* Using each descriptor circled and the location indicated on this worksheet, develop a written description of the lesion(s). After you have perfected the written description, enter it in the paper or computerized patient chart. Remember the A, B, C, D, T plan for formulating a description.

_____

_____

_____

_____

**Figure 13-49B.   Page 2 of Lesion Descriptor Worksheet for Ms. Eads.**

## SECTION 6:
# Skill Check

**SKILL CHECKLIST:** ORAL EXAMINATION

Student: _____     Evaluator: _____

Date: _____

**DIRECTIONS FOR STUDENT:** Use **Column S**; evaluate your skill level as **S** (satisfactory) or **U** (unsatisfactory).

**DIRECTIONS FOR EVALUATOR:** Use **Column E**. Indicate **S** (satisfactory) or **U** (unsatisfactory). In the optional grade percentage calculation, and each **S** equals 1 point, and each **U** equals 0 points.

| CRITERIA | S | E |
| --- | --- | --- |
| Subgroup 1: Visual Inspection of the Lips and Vermillion Border | | |
| **Provides patient with safety glasses and positions patient in the supine position.** | | |
| **Dons gloves.** | | |
| **Visually inspects the lips and vermillion border.** | | |
| Subgroup 2: Inspection of the Oral Cavity and Mucosal Surfaces | | |
| **Adjusts the dental unit light so that the oral cavity is well illuminated.** | | |
| **Visually inspects the oral cavity and oropharynx. Identifies any condition that would cause the oral examination to be modified or postponed.** | | |
| **Visually inspects the upper and lower lips.** | | |
| **Visually inspects the buccal mucosa of both cheeks.** | | |
| Subgroup 3: Palpation of the Lips and Cheeks | | |
| **Palpates the upper and lower lips.** | | |
| **Palpates the buccal mucosa of both cheeks.** | | |
| Subgroup 4: Floor of the Mouth | | |
| **Inspects the anterior region of the mouth.** | | |
| **Retracts the tongue and inspects the posterior region of the floor of the mouth.** | | |
| **Palpates the floor of the mouth.** | | |
| Subgroup 5: Salivary Gland Function | | |
| **Examines the parotid salivary ducts in both sides of the mouth.** | | |
| **Examines the submandibular and sublingual ducts.** | | |

(continued)

**SKILL CHECKLIST:** ORAL EXAMINATION *(CONTINUED)*

| CRITERIA | S | E |
|---|---|---|
| **Subgroup 6: The Tongue**<br>**Inspects the ventral surface of the tongue.** | | |
| **Inspects the dorsal surface of the tongue.** | | |
| **Inspects the lateral surfaces of the tongue.** | | |
| **Palpates the tongue.** | | |
| **Subgroup 7: Palate, Tonsils, and Oropharynx**<br>**Visually inspects the palate.** | | |
| **Palpates the hard and soft palate.** | | |
| **Inspects the tonsils and oropharynx.** | | |
| **Documents notable findings in the patient chart or computerized record.** | | |

OPTIONAL GRADE PERCENTAGE CALCULATION

Each **S** equals 1 point, and each **U** equals 0 points. Using the **E** column, total the sum of the "**S**"s _____ divided by the total points possible (22) to calculate the percentage grade.

**COMMUNICATION SKILL CHECKLIST:** ORAL EXAMINATION

Student: _____     Evaluator: _____

Date: _____

> **Roles:**
> - Student 1 = Plays the role of a fictitious patient.
> - Student 2 = Plays the role of the clinician.
> - Student 3 or instructor = Plays the role of the clinic instructor near the end of the role-play.

**DIRECTIONS FOR STUDENT CLINICIAN:** Use **Column S**; evaluate your skill level as **S** (satisfactory) or **U** (unsatisfactory).

**DIRECTIONS FOR EVALUATOR:** Use **Column E** to record your evaluation of the student clinician's communication skills during the role-play. Indicate **S** (satisfactory) or **U** (unsatisfactory). In the optional grade percentage calculation, each **S** equals 1 point, and each **U** equals 0 points.

| CRITERIA | S | E |
|---|---|---|
| **Explains what is to be done.** | | |
| **Reports notable findings to the patient. As needed, makes referrals to a physician or dental specialist.** | | |
| **Encourages patient questions before and during the oral examination.** | | |
| **Answers the patient's questions fully and accurately.** | | |
| **Communicates with the patient at an appropriate level and avoids dental/medical terminology or jargon.** | | |
| **Accurately communicates the findings to the clinical instructor. Discusses the implications for dental treatment using correct medical and dental terminology.** | | |

OPTIONAL GRADE PERCENTAGE CALCULATION

Each **S** equals 1 point, and each **U** equals 0 points. Using the **E** column, total the sum of the "**S**"s _____ divided by the total points possible (6) to calculate the percentage grade.

# NOTES

MODULE

# 14 Gingival Description

## MODULE OVERVIEW

This module presents a systematic approach to describing the characteristics of the gingiva. The ability to formulate a concise, accurate, written or verbal description of the gingiva is an important component of patient assessment.

    This module covers the gingival description, including:

- Characteristics of the gingiva in health
- Changes in gingival characteristics in disease
- Formulating a description of gingival characteristics

## MODULE OUTLINE

## OBJECTIVES

- Describe gingival characteristics that are indicative of health and disease.
- Define the key terms used in this module:

| | |
|---|---|
| Papillary | Bulbous |
| Marginal | Blunted |
| Diffuse | Cratered |
| Enlarged | Nodular |
| Coronal to cementoenamel junction (CEJ) | Exudate |
| Apical to CEJ | |

- Provide information to the patient about gingival characteristics and any notable findings.
- Accurately communicate gingival characteristics to a clinical instructor. Discuss the implications of notable findings.
- Given an image of a sextant of the mouth, use the Gingival Descriptor Worksheet to identify characteristics of the gingiva.
- Demonstrate knowledge of gingival characteristics by applying information from this module to the fictitious patient cases A–E in this module.

**SECTION 1:**

# Learning to Look at the Gingiva

The ability to formulate a concise, accurate, written or verbal description of the gingiva is an important component of patient assessment process. The following characteristics of the gingiva should be assessed:
1. Color
2. Size
3. Position of margin
4. Shape of margins and papillae
5. Texture and consistency
6. Bleeding and/or exudate

## CHARACTERISTICS OF THE GINGIVA IN HEALTH

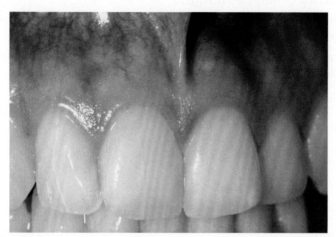

**Figure 14-1.  Healthy gingival tissues—facial aspect.** This gingival tissue exhibits all the signs of health: tissue that fits snugly around the tooth and tapers to meet the tooth at a fine edge; pointed papillae that completely fill the embrasure spaces; and firm, resilient tissue. (Courtesy of Dr. Don Rolfs, Periodontal Foundations, Wenatchee, WA.)

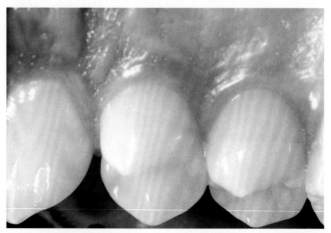

**Figure 14-2.  Healthy gingival tissues—lingual aspect.** This gingival tissue on the lingual aspect of the maxillary arch is an excellent example of health. (Courtesy of Dr. Don Rolfs, Periodontal Foundations, Wenatchee, WA.)

**TABLE 14-1** CHARACTERISTICS OF THE GINGIVA

| Characteristic | Healthy Tissue | Changes in Disease |
|---|---|---|
| Color | Uniform pink color<br>Pigmented | Bright red, bluish purple, white, or pale pink |
| Size | Fits snugly around the tooth | Enlarged |
| Position of margin | Near the cementoenamel junction (CEJ): 1–2 mm coronal to the CEJ | • More than 2 mm coronal to CEJ<br>• Apical to CEJ |
| Shape | Marginal gingiva: meets the tooth in a tapered or slightly rounded edge<br><br>Interdental papillae: flat, pointed papilla fills the embrasure space between two adjacent teeth | Marginal gingiva: meets the tooth in a rolled, thickened, or irregular edge<br><br>Interdental papillae: papilla may be bulbous, blunted, cratered, or missing |
| Texture | Normal<br>Stippled | • Smooth, shiny, no stippling<br>• Firm and nodular (fibrotic) |
| Consistency | Firm<br>Resilient under compression | • Soft, flaccid<br>• Spongy, puffy<br>• Leathery, not resilient |
| Bleeding/exudate | No bleeding<br>No exudate | • Spontaneous bleeding upon probing; heavy bleeding upon probing in acute gingivitis<br>• Exudate |

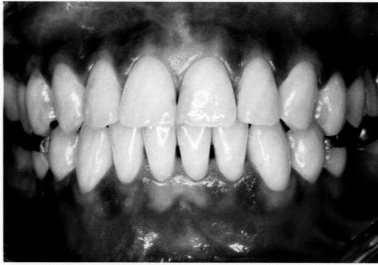

**Figure 14-3.   Color—normal variation.** Pigmented areas are commonly visible in the gingival tissues of dark-skinned individuals.

## CHANGES IN DISEASE

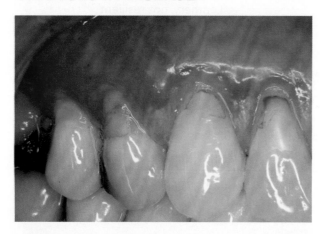

**Figure 14-4.   Change in color.** Red tissue. (Courtesy of Dr. Richard Foster, Guilford Technical Community College.)

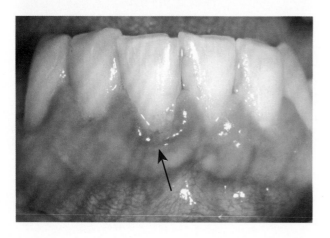

**Figure 14-5.   Change in color.** Red margin. (Courtesy of Dr. Don Rolfs.)

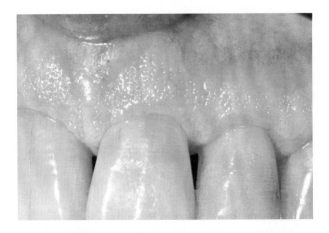

Figure 14-6. Change in color. Pale pink gingival tissue.

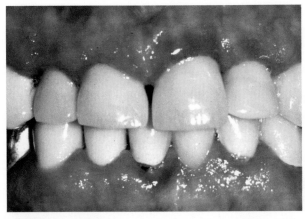

Figure 14-7. Change in size. Enlarged tissue.

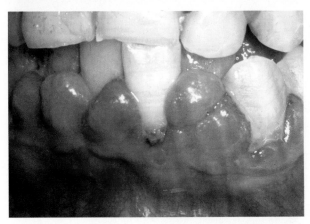

Figure 14-8. Change in size. Enlarged tissue.

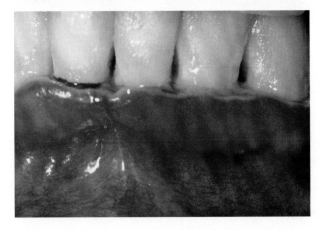

Figure 14-9. Change in position of margin. Gingival margin coronal to (above) the cementoenamel junction. (Clinical photographs on this page are courtesy of Dr. Don Rolfs.)

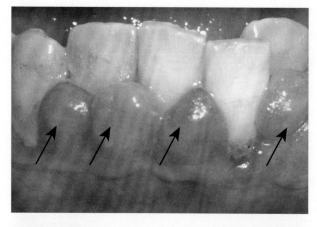

**Figure 14-10.   Change in position of margin.** Gingival margin coronal to (above) the cementoenamel junction.

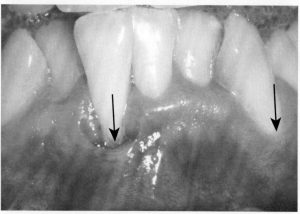

**Figure 14-11.   Change in position of margin.** Gingival margin apical to (below) the cementoenamel junction.

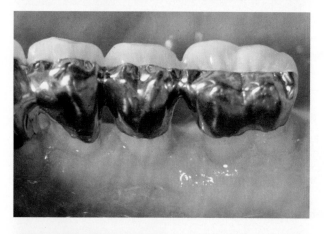

**Figure 14-12.   Change in position of margin.** Gingival margin apical to (below) the cementoenamel junction.

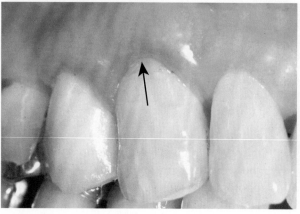

**Figure 14-13.   Change in shape of margin.** Gingival margin thickened and rolled. (Courtesy of Dr. Don Rolfs.)

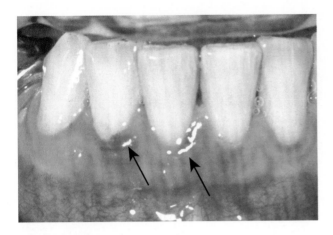

**Figure 14-14.   Change in shape of margin.** Gingival margin thickened and rolled.

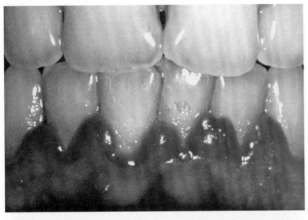

**Figure 14-15.   Change in shape of papilla.** Bulbous papillae.

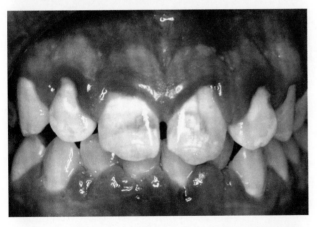

**Figure 14-16.   Change in shape of papilla.** Bulbous papilla.

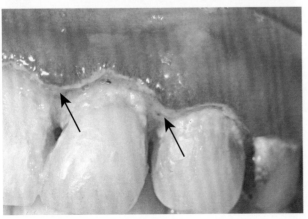

**Figure 14-17.   Change in shape of papilla.** Cratered papillae. (Courtesy of Dr. Don Rolfs.)

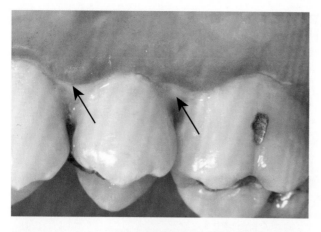

**Figure 14-18. Change in shape of papilla.** Cratered papillae.

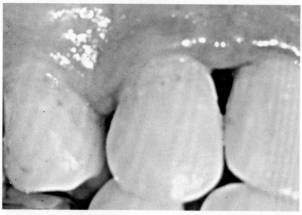

**Figure 14-19. Change in shape of papilla.** Missing and blunted papillae.

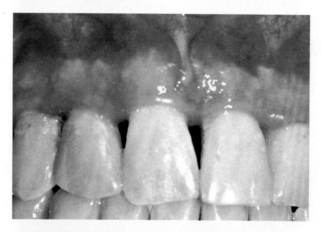

**Figure 14-20. Change in shape of papilla.** Missing, blunted papillae.

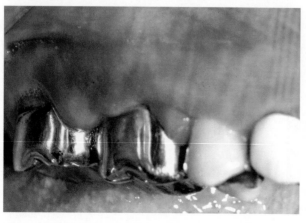

**Figure 14-21. Change in texture and consistency.** Tissue soft and flaccid (lacking firmness), spongy. (Courtesy of Dr. Don Rolfs.)

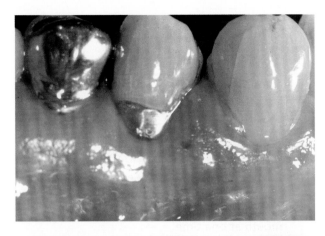

**Figure 14-22. Change in texture and consistency.** Smooth, shiny tissue.

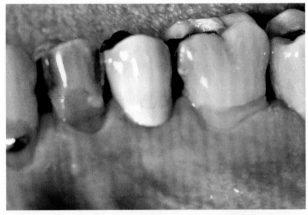

**Figure 14-23. Change in texture and consistency.** Smooth, shiny tissue.

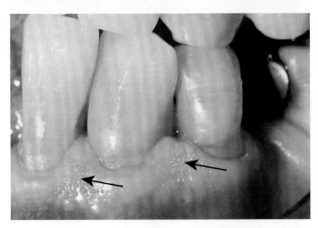

**Figure 14-24. Change in texture and consistency.** Nodular (fibrotic) tissue.

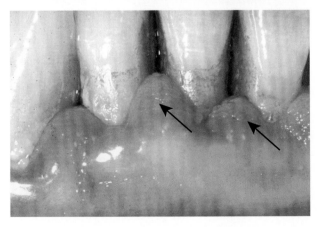

**Figure 14-25. Change in texture and consistency.** Nodular (fibrotic) tissue. (Courtesy of Dr. Don Rolfs.)

SECTION 2:

# Peak Procedure

**PROCEDURE 14-1**   DETERMINING GINGIVAL CHARACTERISTICS

| Action | Rationale |
|---|---|
| 1. **Choose sextant and aspect.** Select one sextant of the mouth for assessment; if applicable, choose the sextant that shows the most tissue changes. Select either the facial or lingual aspect of this sextant for examination. | • Focusing your attention on a specific aspect (facial or lingual) of one sextant is more efficient than trying to examine the entire mouth at one time. |
| 2. **Worksheet.** Use the **Gingival Descriptor Worksheet** from the "Ready References" section of this module. Circle or highlight the words that describe the facial or lingual aspect of the sextant.<br>A. Assess the color of the tissue. Changes in color may involve only the margin (**marginal**) or the papilla (**papillary**). Changes that involve both the marginal and papillary tissue are indicated as **diffuse** color changes.<br>B. Assess the size of the tissue.<br>C. Assess the position of the gingival margin.<br>D. Assess the shape of the margins and papillae in the sextant. | • The Gingival Descriptor Worksheet is helpful in identifying the gingival characteristics present in the sextant.<br>• Changes in gingival characteristics may be indicators of disease. |
| 3. **Examine.** Use compressed air and a periodontal probe to assess the texture and consistency, and enter your findings on the worksheet.<br>A. Healthy tissue is resilient when pressed lightly with the side (length) of a periodontal probe.<br>B. Soft, spongy tissue will retain the shape of the probe for several seconds.<br>C. Leathery, nodular tissue is very firm and not resilient when the tissue is pressed lightly with the probe. | • The texture and consistency of the tissue provides important clues about the health of the tissue. Normal tissue is very resilient. Soft, spongy tissue may be an indicator of gingivitis. Leathery, nodular tissue may be an indicator of periodontitis. |

(continued)

**PROCEDURE 14-1**   DETERMINING GINGIVAL CHARACTERISTICS *(CONTINUED)*

| Action | Rationale |
|---|---|
| **4. Observe.** Observe the sextant to check for any areas of spontaneous bleeding. Use a periodontal probe to check for bleeding upon probing and/or exudate. | • Bleeding and/or exudate are important indicators of inflammation. |
| **5. Chart.** Complete a **Gingival Characteristics Chart** from the "Ready References" section of this module. You will need a red/blue pencil and a yellow highlighter to complete this chart. You will be entering information for the same sextant and aspect selected for the Gingival Descriptor Worksheet.<br>A. Draw the location of the gingival margin on the chart.<br>B. Indicate areas of gingival recession with the yellow highlighter.<br>C. Enter gingival margin findings in red pencil at the root apices.<br>D. Enter papillae findings in blue pencil between the teeth near the root area. | • The Gingival Characteristics Chart is helpful in identifying the gingival characteristics present in the sextant.<br>• Changes in gingival characteristics may be indicators of disease. |

## SECTION 3:
# Ready References

## Gingival Descriptor Worksheet

*Directions:* Highlight or circle the applicable descriptors.

*In the last column, list your findings:*
- Indicate if a characteristic is localized or generalized.
- If localized, note
  - the tooth number or
  - the aspect, facial or lingual, of the sextant(s) or quadrant(s) exhibiting the characteristic.
- If bleeding is evident, indicate extent as light, moderate, or heavy.

| CHARACTERISTIC | NORMAL DESCRIPTORS | DISEASE DESCRIPTORS | | LIST FINDINGS |
|---|---|---|---|---|
| **Color** | Pink<br>Pigmented | Red<br>Bluish purple<br>White<br>Pale pink | *Distribution:*<br>Papillary<br>Marginal<br>Diffuse | |
| **Size** | Fits snugly around tooth | Enlarged | | |
| **Position of Margin** | Near the CEJ: 1–2 mm coronal to the CEJ | More than 2 mm coronal to the CEJ<br>Apical to the CEJ | | |
| **Shape of Margin** | Tapered or slightly rounded edge<br>Fits snugly around tooth | Thickened edge<br>Rolled edge<br>Irregular edge | | |
| **Shape of Papilla** | Flat, pointed papilla<br>Fills interproximal space | Bulbous papilla<br>Blunted papilla<br>Cratered papilla<br>Missing papilla | | |
| **Texture** | Normal<br>Stippled | Smooth and shiny<br>Nodular (fibrotic) | | |
| **Consistency** | Firm, resilient | Soft, flaccid<br>Spongy, puffy<br>Leathery, not resilient | | |
| **Bleeding, Exudate** | No bleeding<br>No exudate (pus) | Spontaneous bleeding<br>Bleeding on probing<br>Exudate | | |

Figure 14-26. Gingival Descriptor Worksheet.

# Gingival Characteristics Chart: Maxillary Arch

Case: _____     Aspect (circle):   Facial   Lingual

*Directions:* Use a red/blue pencil and a yellow highlighter to indicate the following:

With blue pencil, draw the location of the gingival margin

With yellow highlighter, show any areas of recession

| Key: Gingival Margins Findings | |
|---|---|
| Enter in red pencil at the root apex | |
| S | Snugly around tooth |
| E | Enlarged |
| T | Tapered or slightly rounded edge |
| R | Rolled, thickened edge |
| I | Irregular edge |
| N | Normal texture |
| S h | Shiny, smooth texture |
| N d | Nodular texture (fibrotic) |
| F | Firm, resilient |
| S o | Soft, spongy |
| L | Leathery, not resilient |

| Key: Papillae Findings | |
|---|---|
| Enter in blue pencil between the teeth near root area | |
| F | Fills the interproximal space |
| F l | Flat, pointed |
| B b | Bulbous |
| B l | Blunted |
| C | Cratered |
| M | Missing |

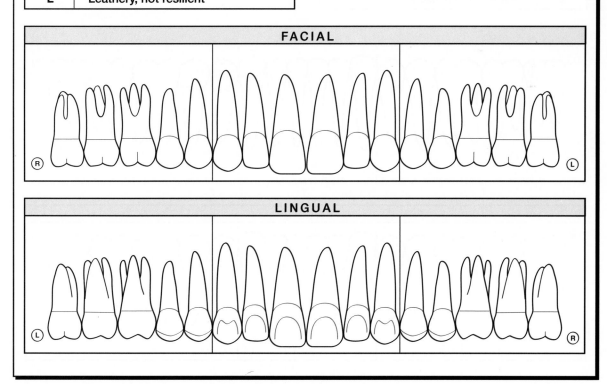

Figure 14-27.   Gingival Characteristics Chart: Maxillary Arch.

# Gingival Characteristics Chart: Mandibular Arch

**Case:** _____    **Aspect** (circle):    Facial    Lingual

*Directions:* Use a red/blue pencil and a yellow highlighter to indicate the following:

With blue pencil, draw the location of the gingival margin

With yellow highlighter, show any areas of recession

| Key: Gingival Margins Findings Enter in red pencil at the root apex ||
|---|---|
| S | Snugly around tooth |
| E | Enlarged |
| T | Tapered or slightly rounded edge |
| R | Rolled, thickened edge |
| I | Irregular edge |
| N | Normal texture |
| Sh | Shiny, smooth texture |
| Nd | Nodular texture (fibrotic) |
| F | Firm, resilient |
| So | Soft, spongy |
| L | Leathery, not resilient |

| Key: Papillae Findings Enter in blue pencil between the teeth near root area ||
|---|---|
| F | Fills the interproximal space |
| Fl | Flat, pointed |
| Bb | Bulbous |
| Bl | Blunted |
| C | Cratered |
| M | Missing |

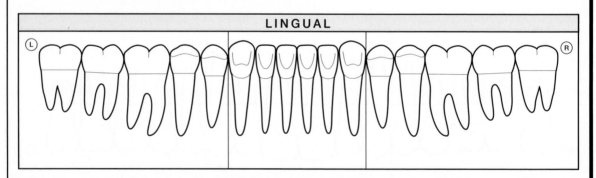

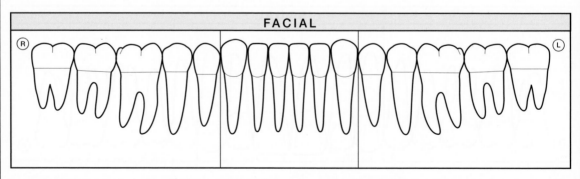

Figure 14-28.    Gingival Characteristics Chart: Mandibular Arch.

**READY REFERENCE 14-1** INTERNET RESOURCES

**http://www.perio.org/consumer/2a.html**
The website of the **American Academy of Periodontology** link to information about periodontal diseases.

**http://www.perio.org/consumer/gingivitis.htm**
The website of the **American Academy of Periodontology** link to information about gingivitis.

**http://www.bsperio.org/showpage.asp?id=patients**
Information for patients about periodontal disease on the website of the **British Society of Periodontology**.

**http://www.cap-acp.ca/en/index.html**
The website of the **Canadian Academy of Periodontology** has a wealth of information on the periodontium, gingivitis, periodontitis, the periodontal examination, and the link between systemic health and the periodontitis.

**http://www.nlm.nih.gov/medlineplus/ency/article/001056.htm**
Illustrations, causes, prevention, and treatment of gingivitis from the **National Library of Medicine**.

**SECTION 4:**

# The Human Element

BOX **14-1** **Through the Eyes of a Student**

*I was seeing Mr. L, a patient that I had seen 6 months ago. Before starting to write up a gingival description, I looked at the one I had done 6 months ago. Since the last time, we had covered gingival descriptors more in class. I realized that I now knew many more gingival descriptors, what they meant, and how to use them.*

*The gingival description from 6 months ago did not paint a very accurate picture of Mr. L's gingiva. I realized my description from last time would not be of any help today. Using the correct gingival descriptors, I wrote a description that really put into words what the gingival tissue looks like. At this moment, I realized for the first time how much I had learned in 6 months and how much better I understood the appearance of the gingiva. I really felt proud of myself at that moment.*

*Kim, student*
*South Florida Community College*

**PATIENT SCENARIO**

For the past 6 months, you have been working as a part-time dental hygienist for a dental group practice. Unfortunately, you have developed concerns about the quality of some of the dental care being delivered by the periodontist who is a member of the group practice. Your specific concerns about the quality of care center around apparent poor infection control procedures.

You have just finished seeing a new patient in the group practice, Mrs. Eliza Stuart. Mrs. Stuart is a 35-year-old homemaker who smokes one pack of cigarettes a day and has recently been diagnosed with type 2 diabetes. Mrs. Stuart has a 22-month-old daughter and has just found out that she is 8 weeks pregnant with her second child.

Although Mrs. Stuart denies any oral discomfort, her dental examination reveals many oral problems such as probing depths up to 7 mm, generalized alveolar bone loss on her posterior teeth, severe dental caries on several molar teeth, and multiple sites of moderate to severe gingival inflammation along with other signs of gingival inflammation including bleeding on probing. Based upon your clinical observations, you are convinced that Mrs. Stuart has chronic periodontitis.

Routine office policy dictates that Mrs. Stuart should be scheduled with the group practice periodontist. However, you are uncomfortable making the referral based on your concerns about infection control practices by the periodontist. You are conflicted about how to proceed with Eliza's treatment.

1. What ethical principles are in conflict in this dilemma?
2. How do you inform/educate Eliza about her oral/general health?
3. How should you handle future referrals to the periodontist in your office?

## TABLE 14-2   ENGLISH-TO-SPANISH PHRASE LIST FOR GINGIVAL DESCRIPTION

| | |
|---|---|
| Next, I will look at the color, contours, and texture of your gum tissue. | Voy a mirar el color, contorno, y textura de la tejida en su encia. |
| Just relax. This examination is not painful and only takes a few minutes. | No tenga miedo. La examinación no duele, y solamente toma unos minutos. |
| Please tilt your head forward (back). | Por favor incline la cabeza hacia delante. Por favor incline la cabeza hacia atrás. |
| Please **turn** your head to the right (left). | Por favor vuelta la cabeza a la derecha. Por favor vuelta la cabeza a la izquierda. |
| Please **tilt** your head to the right (left). | Por favor incline la cabeza a la derecha. Por favor incline la cabeza a la izquierda. |
| Please look straight ahead. | Por favor mire al frente. |
| There are several areas of gum tissue that I am concerned about. I will point them out to you. Please hold this mirror. | Hay varias areas de la tejida en la encia que me preocupan. Aguante este espejo, y se las voy a apuntar. |
| Healthy gum tissue is pink in color. | Tejida saludable es rosada en color. |
| Areas of pigmentation are normal on the gum tissues. | Areas de pigmentación son normal en las tejidas de la encia. |
| The tissue is _____ in this area. This is not normal. red blue purple swollen leathery | La tejida en _____ en esta area. Esto no es normal. rojo azul morado hinchado textura de cuero |
| You and I will work together as a team to improve the health of your gum tissues. | Vamos a trabajar juntos para mejorar la salud de las tejidas de las encias. |
| I am going to get my clinic instructor. | Voy a buscar mi instructor. |

**SECTION 5:**

# Practical Focus—Fictitious Patient Cases

**DIRECTIONS:**

- Use the steps outlined in Procedure 14-1, the Gingival Descriptor Worksheet, and the Gingival Characteristics Chart to develop descriptions for each of the patient cases. Examples of completed forms are shown on the following pages.

- In thinking about the health status of the gingival tissues in this module, you should take into account the health history and over-the-counter/prescription drug information that were revealed for each patient in previous modules. For each patient, answer the question, "Is there any connection between the gingival characteristics observed and the patient's health history or drug information?"

- The pages in this section may be removed from the book for easier use by tearing along the perforated lines on each page.

- Note: The clinical photographs in a fictitious patient case are for illustrative purposes but are not necessarily from the same individual. The fictitious patient cases are designed to enhance the learning experiences associated with each case.

## SOURCES OF CLINICAL PHOTOGRAPHS

The author gratefully acknowledges the sources of the following clinical photographs in the "Practical Focus" sections of this module.

- Figure 14-31. Courtesy of Dr. Don Rolfs, Periodontal Foundations, Wenatchee, WA.
- Figure 14-34. Dr. Richard Foster, Guilford Technical Community College, Jamestown, NC.
- Figure 14-37. Dr. Richard Foster, Guilford Technical Community College, Jamestown, NC.
- Figure 14-40. Dr. Richard Foster, Guilford Technical Community College, Jamestown, NC.
- Figure 14-43. Dr. Richard Foster, Guilford Technical Community College, Jamestown, NC.

# Gingival Descriptor Worksheet

*Directions:* Highlight or circle the applicable descriptors.

*In the last column, list your findings:*
- Indicate if a characteristic is localized or generalized.
- If localized, note
  - the tooth number or
  - the aspect, facial or lingual, of the sextant(s) or quadrant(s) exhibiting the characteristic.
- If bleeding is evident, indicate extent as light, moderate, or heavy.

| CHARACTERISTIC | NORMAL DESCRIPTORS | DISEASE DESCRIPTORS | LIST FINDINGS |
|---|---|---|---|
| **Color** | Pink<br>Pigmented | Red<br>Bluish purple<br>White<br>Pale pink | *Distribution:*<br>Papillary<br>Marginal<br>Diffuse | RED-MARGINAL: #9, 10<br>BLUISH-MARGINAL: 8<br>BLUISH-PAPILLARY: 8-7 |
| **Size** | Fits snugly around tooth | Enlarged | ENLARGED: ALL |
| **Position of Margin** | Near the CEJ:<br>1–2 mm coronal to the CEJ | More than 2 mm coronal to the CEJ<br>Apical to the CEJ | CORONAL TO CEJ: ALL |
| **Shape of Margin** | Tapered or slightly rounded edge<br>Fits snugly around tooth | Thickened edge<br>Rolled edge<br>Irregular edge | THICKENED/ROLLED: ALL |
| **Shape of Papilla** | Flat, pointed papilla<br>Fills interproximal space | Bulbous papilla<br>Blunted papilla<br>Cratered papilla<br>Missing papilla | BULBOUS: ALL |
| **Texture** | Normal<br>Stippled | Smooth and shiny<br>Nodular (fibrotic) | NODULAR: ALL |
| **Consistency** | Firm, resilient | Soft, flaccid<br>Spongy, puffy<br>Leathery, not resilient | LEATHERY: ALL |
| **Bleeding, Exudate** | No bleeding<br>No exudate (pus) | Spontaneous bleeding<br>Bleeding on probing<br>Exudate | SPONTANEOUS: #9 |

**Figure 14-29. Example of completed worksheet.** This example shows a completed Gingival Descriptor Worksheet for fictitious patient Z.

# Gingival Characteristics Chart: Maxillary Arch

**Case:** _EXAMPLE_  **Aspect** (circle): (Facial) Lingual

*Directions:* Use a red/blue pencil and a yellow highlighter to indicate the following:
With blue pencil, draw the location of the gingival margin
With yellow highlighter, show any areas of recession

| Key: Gingival Margins Findings | |
|---|---|
| Enter in red pencil at the root apex | |
| S | Snugly around tooth |
| E | Enlarged |
| T | Tapered or slightly rounded edge |
| R | Rolled, thickened edge |
| I | Irregular edge |
| N | Normal texture |
| S h | Shiny, smooth texture |
| N d | Nodular texture (fibrotic) |
| F | Firm, resilient |
| S o | Soft, spongy |
| L | Leathery, not resilient |

| Key: Papillae Findings | |
|---|---|
| Enter in blue pencil between the teeth near root area | |
| F | Fills the interproximal space |
| F l | Flat, pointed |
| B b | Bulbous |
| B l | Blunted |
| C | Cratered |
| M | Missing |

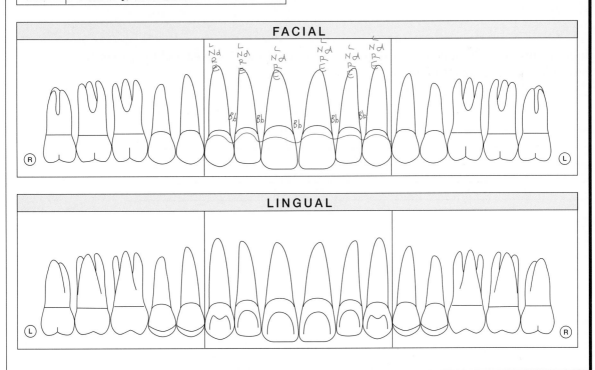

**Figure 14-30.   Example of completed chart.** This example shows a completed Gingival Characteristics Chart for fictitious patient Z.

## FICTITIOUS PATIENT CASE A: MR. ALAN ASCARI

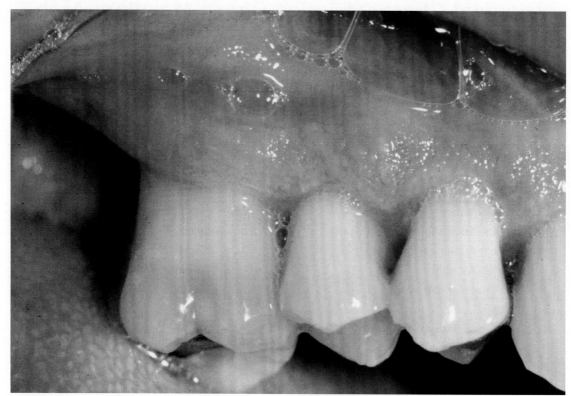

Figure 14-31.    Maxillary right posterior sextant, facial aspect for Mr. Ascari.

Indicate any connection between the gingival characteristics observed and the patient's health history or drug information:

_____

_____

_____

_____

_____

_____

_____

# Gingival Descriptor Worksheet

*Directions:* Highlight or circle the applicable descriptors.

*In the last column, list your findings:*
 • Indicate if a characteristic is localized or generalized.
 • If localized, note
   - the tooth number or
   - the aspect, facial or lingual, of the sextant(s) or quadrant(s) exhibiting the characteristic.
 • If bleeding is evident, indicate extent as light, moderate, or heavy.

| CHARACTERISTIC | NORMAL DESCRIPTORS | DISEASE DESCRIPTORS | | LIST FINDINGS |
|---|---|---|---|---|
| **Color** | Pink<br>Pigmented | Red<br>Bluish purple<br>White<br>Pale pink | *Distribution:*<br>Papillary<br>Marginal<br>Diffuse | |
| **Size** | Fits snugly around tooth | Enlarged | | |
| **Position of Margin** | Near the CEJ:<br>1–2 mm coronal to the CEJ | More than 2 mm coronal to the CEJ<br>Apical to the CEJ | | |
| **Shape of Margin** | Tapered or slightly rounded edge<br>Fits snugly around tooth | Thickened edge<br>Rolled edge<br>Irregular edge | | |
| **Shape of Papilla** | Flat, pointed papilla<br>Fills interproximal space | Bulbous papilla<br>Blunted papilla<br>Cratered papilla<br>Missing papilla | | |
| **Texture** | Normal<br>Stippled | Smooth and shiny<br>Nodular (fibrotic) | | |
| **Consistency** | Firm, resilient | Soft, flaccid<br>Spongy, puffy<br>Leathery, not resilient | | |
| **Bleeding, Exudate** | No bleeding<br>No exudate (pus) | Spontaneous bleeding<br>Bleeding on probing<br>Exudate | | |

**Figure 14-32.   Gingival Descriptor Worksheet for Mr. Ascari: Maxillary right posterior sextant, facial aspect.**

# Gingival Characteristics Chart: Maxillary Arch

Case: _____     **Aspect** (circle):   Facial   Lingual

*Directions:* Use a red/blue pencil and a yellow highlighter to indicate the following:

With blue pencil, draw the location of the gingival margin

With yellow highlighter, show any areas of recession

| Key: Gingival Margins Findings<br>Enter in red pencil at the root apex | |
|---|---|
| S | Snugly around tooth |
| E | Enlarged |
| T | Tapered or slightly rounded edge |
| R | Rolled, thickened edge |
| I | Irregular edge |
| N | Normal texture |
| S h | Shiny, smooth texture |
| N d | Nodular texture (fibrotic) |
| F | Firm, resilient |
| S o | Soft, spongy |
| L | Leathery, not resilient |

| Key: Papillae Findings<br>Enter in blue pencil between the teeth near root area | |
|---|---|
| F | Fills the interproximal space |
| F l | Flat, pointed |
| B b | Bulbous |
| B l | Blunted |
| C | Cratered |
| M | Missing |

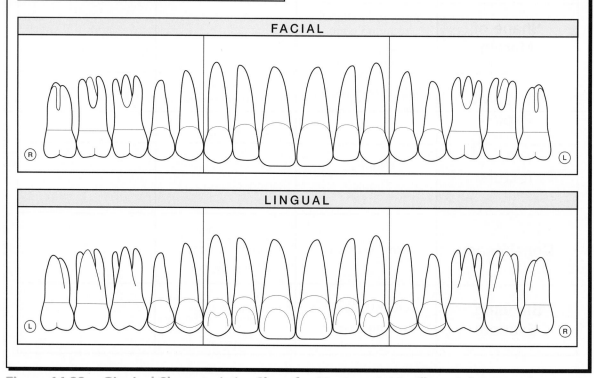

Figure 14-33.   Gingival Characteristics Chart for Mr. Ascari: Maxillary right posterior sextant, facial aspect.

## FICTITIOUS PATIENT CASE B: BETHANY BIDDLE

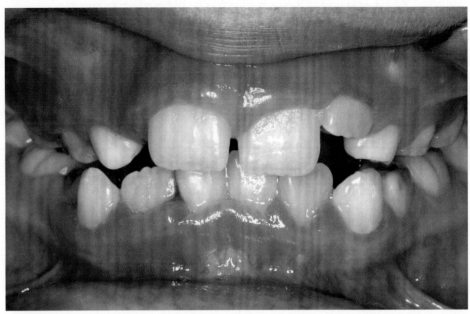

**Figure 14-34. Facial aspect of mandibular anterior sextant for Bethany Biddle.**

Indicate any connection between the gingival characteristics observed and the patient's health history or drug information:

_____
_____
_____
_____
_____
_____
_____

# Gingival Descriptor Worksheet

*Directions:* Highlight or circle the applicable descriptors.

*In the last column, list your findings:*
- Indicate if a characteristic is localized or generalized.
- If localized, note
  - the tooth number or
  - the aspect, facial or lingual, of the sextant(s) or quadrant(s) exhibiting the characteristic.
- If bleeding is evident, indicate extent as light, moderate, or heavy.

| CHARACTERISTIC | NORMAL DESCRIPTORS | DISEASE DESCRIPTORS | | LIST FINDINGS |
|---|---|---|---|---|
| **Color** | Pink<br>Pigmented | Red<br>Bluish purple<br>White<br>Pale pink | *Distribution:*<br>Papillary<br>Marginal<br>Diffuse | |
| **Size** | Fits snugly around tooth | Enlarged | | |
| **Position of Margin** | Near the CEJ:<br>1–2 mm coronal to the CEJ | More than 2 mm coronal to the CEJ<br>Apical to the CEJ | | |
| **Shape of Margin** | Tapered or slightly rounded edge<br>Fits snugly around tooth | Thickened edge<br>Rolled edge<br>Irregular edge | | |
| **Shape of Papilla** | Flat, pointed papilla<br>Fills interproximal space | Bulbous papilla<br>Blunted papilla<br>Cratered papilla<br>Missing papilla | | |
| **Texture** | Normal<br>Stippled | Smooth and shiny<br>Nodular (fibrotic) | | |
| **Consistency** | Firm, resilient | Soft, flaccid<br>Spongy, puffy<br>Leathery, not resilient | | |
| **Bleeding, Exudate** | No bleeding<br>No exudate (pus) | Spontaneous bleeding<br>Bleeding on probing<br>Exudate | | |

**Figure 14-35.   Gingival Descriptor Worksheet for Bethany Biddle: Mandibular anterior sextant, facial aspect.**

DIRECTIONS: *To use the Gingival Characteristics Chart for a patient with a mixed dentition, enter the letter of the primary tooth on the crown of the permanent tooth and cross out any missing teeth.*

# Gingival Characteristics Chart: Mandibular Arch

Case: _____      Aspect (circle):   Facial    Lingual

*Directions:* Use a red/blue pencil and a yellow highlighter to indicate the following:

With blue pencil, draw the location of the gingival margin

With yellow highlighter, show any areas of recession

| Key: Gingival Margins Findings<br>Enter in red pencil at the root apex | |
|---|---|
| S | Snugly around tooth |
| E | Enlarged |
| T | Tapered or slightly rounded edge |
| R | Rolled, thickened edge |
| I | Irregular edge |
| N | Normal texture |
| S h | Shiny, smooth texture |
| N d | Nodular texture (fibrotic) |
| F | Firm, resilient |
| S o | Soft, spongy |
| L | Leathery, not resilient |

| Key: Papillae Findings<br>Enter in blue pencil between the teeth near root area | |
|---|---|
| F | Fills the interproximal space |
| F l | Flat, pointed |
| B b | Bulbous |
| B l | Blunted |
| C | Cratered |
| M | Missing |

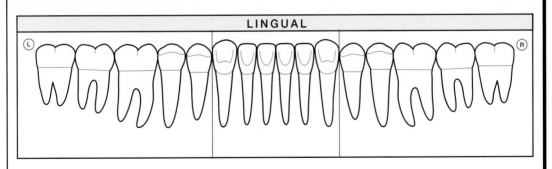

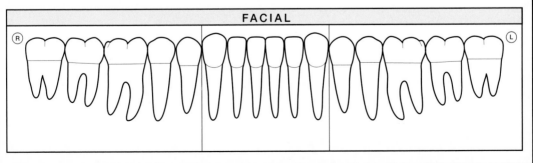

**Figure 14-36. Gingival Characteristics Chart for Bethany Biddle: Mandibular anterior sextant, facial aspect.**

# FICTITIOUS PATIENT CASE C: MR. CARLOS CHAVEZ

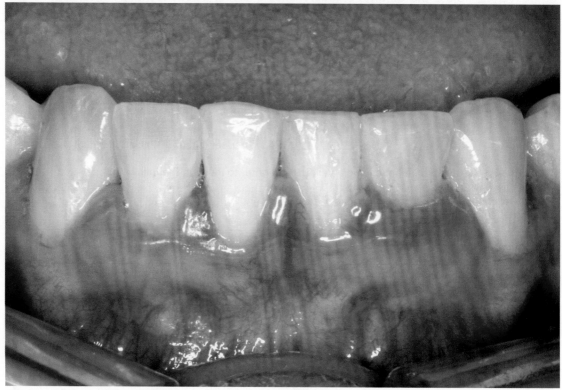

**Figure 14-37.   Facial aspect, mandibular anterior sextant for Mr. Chavez.**

Indicate any connection between the gingival characteristics observed and the patient's health history or drug information:

_____

_____

_____

_____

_____

_____

_____

# Gingival Descriptor Worksheet

*Directions:* Highlight or circle the applicable descriptors.

*In the last column, list your findings:*
  • Indicate if a characteristic is localized or generalized.
  • If localized, note
    - the tooth number or
    - the aspect, facial or lingual, of the sextant(s) or quadrant(s) exhibiting the characteristic.
  • If bleeding is evident, indicate extent as light, moderate, or heavy.

| CHARACTERISTIC | NORMAL DESCRIPTORS | DISEASE DESCRIPTORS | | LIST FINDINGS |
| --- | --- | --- | --- | --- |
| **Color** | Pink<br><br>Pigmented | Red<br>Bluish purple<br>White<br>Pale pink | *Distribution:*<br>Papillary<br>Marginal<br>Diffuse | |
| **Size** | Fits snugly around tooth | Enlarged | | |
| **Position of Margin** | Near the CEJ:<br>1–2 mm coronal to the CEJ | More than 2 mm coronal to the CEJ<br><br>Apical to the CEJ | | |
| **Shape of Margin** | Tapered or slightly rounded edge<br><br>Fits snugly around tooth | Thickened edge<br>Rolled edge<br>Irregular edge | | |
| **Shape of Papilla** | Flat, pointed papilla<br><br>Fills interproximal space | Bulbous papilla<br>Blunted papilla<br>Cratered papilla<br>Missing papilla | | |
| **Texture** | Normal<br>Stippled | Smooth and shiny<br>Nodular (fibrotic) | | |
| **Consistency** | Firm, resilient | Soft, flaccid<br>Spongy, puffy<br>Leathery, not resilient | | |
| **Bleeding, Exudate** | No bleeding<br>No exudate (pus) | Spontaneous bleeding<br>Bleeding on probing<br>Exudate | | |

**Figure 14-38.**  Gingival Descriptor Worksheet for Mr. Chavez: Mandibular anterior sextant, facial aspect.

# Gingival Characteristics Chart: Mandibular Arch

Case: _____   Aspect (circle):   Facial   Lingual

*Directions:* Use a red/blue pencil and a yellow highlighter to indicate the following:

With blue pencil, draw the location of the gingival margin

With yellow highlighter, show any areas of recession

| Key: Gingival Margins Findings | |
| --- | --- |
| Enter in red pencil at the root apex | |
| S | Snugly around tooth |
| E | Enlarged |
| T | Tapered or slightly rounded edge |
| R | Rolled, thickened edge |
| I | Irregular edge |
| N | Normal texture |
| S h | Shiny, smooth texture |
| N d | Nodular texture (fibrotic) |
| F | Firm, resilient |
| S o | Soft, spongy |
| L | Leathery, not resilient |

| Key: Papillae Findings | |
| --- | --- |
| Enter in blue pencil between the teeth near root area | |
| F | Fills the interproximal space |
| F l | Flat, pointed |
| B b | Bulbous |
| B l | Blunted |
| C | Cratered |
| M | Missing |

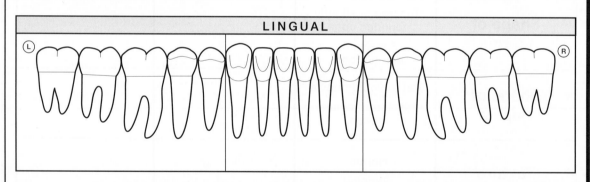

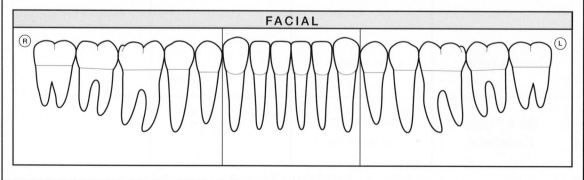

**Figure 14-39.**   Gingival Characteristic Chart for Mr. Chavez: Mandibular anterior sextant, facial aspect.

## FICTITIOUS PATIENT CASE D: MRS. DONNA DOI

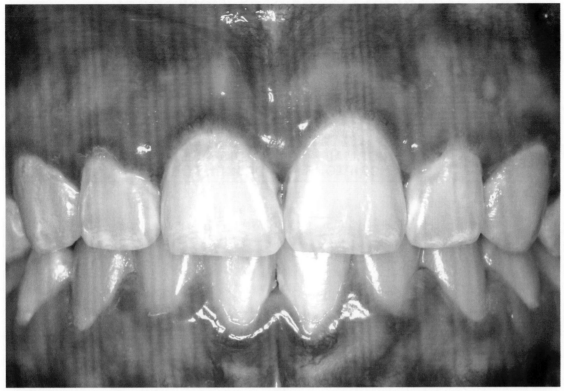

Figure 14-40. Facial aspect, maxillary anterior sextant for Mrs. Doi.

Indicate any connection between the gingival characteristics observed and the patient's health history or drug information:

_____

_____

_____

_____

_____

_____

_____

# Gingival Descriptor Worksheet

*Directions:* Highlight or circle the applicable descriptors.

*In the last column, list your findings:*
- Indicate if a characteristic is localized or generalized.
- If localized, note
  - the tooth number or
  - the aspect, facial or lingual, of the sextant(s) or quadrant(s) exhibiting the characteristic.
- If bleeding is evident, indicate extent as light, moderate, or heavy.

| CHARACTERISTIC | NORMAL DESCRIPTORS | DISEASE DESCRIPTORS | | LIST FINDINGS |
|---|---|---|---|---|
| **Color** | Pink<br>Pigmented | Red<br>Bluish purple<br>White<br>Pale pink | *Distribution:*<br>Papillary<br>Marginal<br>Diffuse | |
| **Size** | Fits snugly around tooth | Enlarged | | |
| **Position of Margin** | Near the CEJ:<br>1–2 mm coronal to the CEJ | More than 2 mm coronal to the CEJ<br>Apical to the CEJ | | |
| **Shape of Margin** | Tapered or slightly rounded edge<br>Fits snugly around tooth | Thickened edge<br>Rolled edge<br>Irregular edge | | |
| **Shape of Papilla** | Flat, pointed papilla<br>Fills interproximal space | Bulbous papilla<br>Blunted papilla<br>Cratered papilla<br>Missing papilla | | |
| **Texture** | Normal<br>Stippled | Smooth and shiny<br>Nodular (fibrotic) | | |
| **Consistency** | Firm, resilient | Soft, flaccid<br>Spongy, puffy<br>Leathery, not resilient | | |
| **Bleeding, Exudate** | No bleeding<br>No exudate (pus) | Spontaneous bleeding<br>Bleeding on probing<br>Exudate | | |

**Figure 14-41.    Gingival Descriptor Worksheet for Mrs. Doi: Maxillary anterior sextant, facial aspect.**

# Gingival Characteristics Chart: Maxillary Arch

Case: _____    **Aspect** (circle):   Facial   Lingual

*Directions:* Use a red/blue pencil and a yellow highlighter to indicate the following:

With blue pencil, draw the location of the gingival margin

With yellow highlighter, show any areas of recession

| Key: Gingival Margins Findings | |
|---|---|
| *Enter in red pencil at the root apex* | |
| S | Snugly around tooth |
| E | Enlarged |
| T | Tapered or slightly rounded edge |
| R | Rolled, thickened edge |
| I | Irregular edge |
| N | Normal texture |
| S h | Shiny, smooth texture |
| N d | Nodular texture (fibrotic) |
| F | Firm, resilient |
| S o | Soft, spongy |
| L | Leathery, not resilient |

| Key: Papillae Findings | |
|---|---|
| *Enter in blue pencil between the teeth near root area* | |
| F | Fills the interproximal space |
| F l | Flat, pointed |
| B b | Bulbous |
| B l | Blunted |
| C | Cratered |
| M | Missing |

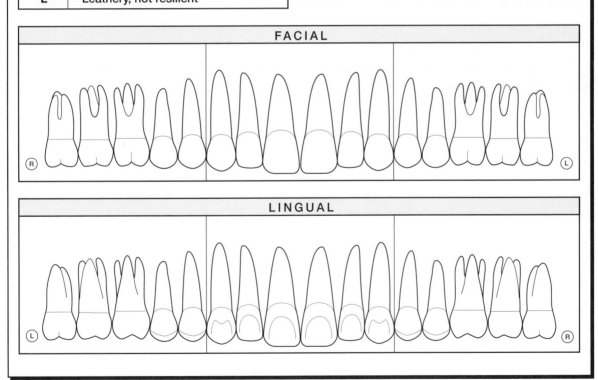

Figure 14-42.  Gingival Characteristics Chart for Mrs. Doi: Maxillary anterior sextant, facial aspect.

## FICTITIOUS PATIENT CASE E: MS. ESTHER EADS

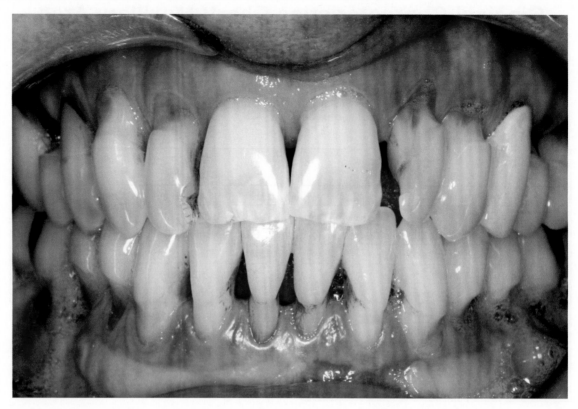

Figure 14-43.    Facial aspect, mandibular anterior sextant for Ms. Eads.

Indicate any connection between the gingival characteristics observed and the patient's health history or drug information:

_____
_____
_____
_____
_____
_____
_____

# Gingival Descriptor Worksheet

*Directions:* Highlight or circle the applicable descriptors.

*In the last column, list your findings:*
- Indicate if a characteristic is localized or generalized.
- If localized, note
  - the tooth number or
  - the aspect, facial or lingual, of the sextant(s) or quadrant(s) exhibiting the characteristic.
- If bleeding is evident, indicate extent as light, moderate, or heavy.

| CHARACTERISTIC | NORMAL DESCRIPTORS | DISEASE DESCRIPTORS | LIST FINDINGS |
|---|---|---|---|
| Color | Pink<br>Pigmented | Red, Bluish purple, White, Pale pink — Distribution: Papillary, Marginal, Diffuse | |
| Size | Fits snugly around tooth | Enlarged | |
| Position of Margin | Near the CEJ: 1–2 mm coronal to the CEJ | More than 2 mm coronal to the CEJ<br>Apical to the CEJ | |
| Shape of Margin | Tapered or slightly rounded edge<br>Fits snugly around tooth | Thickened edge<br>Rolled edge<br>Irregular edge | |
| Shape of Papilla | Flat, pointed papilla<br>Fills interproximal space | Bulbous papilla<br>Blunted papilla<br>Cratered papilla<br>Missing papilla | |
| Texture | Normal<br>Stippled | Smooth and shiny<br>Nodular (fibrotic) | |
| Consistency | Firm, resilient | Soft, flaccid<br>Spongy, puffy<br>Leathery, not resilient | |
| Bleeding, Exudate | No bleeding<br>No exudate (pus) | Spontaneous bleeding<br>Bleeding on probing<br>Exudate | |

**Figure 14-44. Gingival Descriptor Worksheet for Ms. Eads: Mandibular anterior sextant, facial aspect.**

# Gingival Characteristics Chart: Mandibular Arch

**Case:** _____     **Aspect** (circle):    Facial    Lingual

*Directions:* **Use a red/blue pencil and a yellow highlighter to indicate the following:**

With blue pencil, draw the location of the gingival margin
**With yellow highlighter, show any areas of recession**

| Key: Gingival Margins Findings | |
|---|---|
| *Enter in red pencil at the root apex* | |
| S | Snugly around tooth |
| E | Enlarged |
| T | Tapered or slightly rounded edge |
| R | Rolled, thickened edge |
| I | Irregular edge |
| N | Normal texture |
| S h | Shiny, smooth texture |
| N d | Nodular texture (fibrotic) |
| F | Firm, resilient |
| S o | Soft, spongy |
| L | Leathery, not resilient |

| Key: Papillae Findings | |
|---|---|
| *Enter in blue pencil between the teeth near root area* | |
| F | Fills the interproximal space |
| F l | Flat, pointed |
| B b | Bulbous |
| B l | Blunted |
| C | Cratered |
| M | Missing |

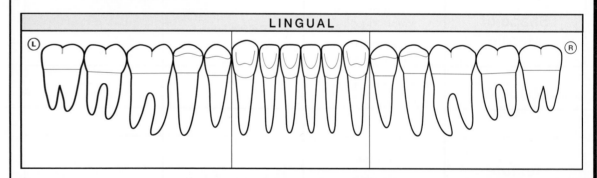

LINGUAL

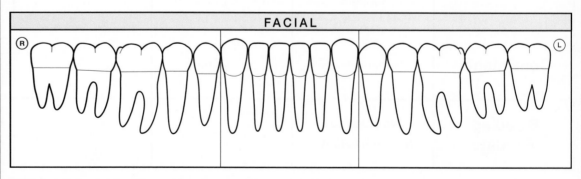

FACIAL

**Figure 14-45.    Gingival Characteristics Chart for Ms. Eads: Mandibular anterior sextant, facial aspect.**

**SECTION 6:**
# Skill Check

**SKILL CHECKLIST:** GINGIVAL DESCRIPTION

Student: _____ Evaluator: _____

Date: _____

**DIRECTIONS FOR STUDENT:** Use **Column S**; evaluate your skill level as **S** (satisfactory) or **U** (unsatisfactory).

**DIRECTIONS FOR EVALUATOR:** Use **Column E**. Indicate **S** (satisfactory) or **U** (unsatisfactory). Each **S** equals 1 point, and each **U** equals 0 points.

| CRITERIA | S | E |
|---|---|---|
| **Selects the facial or lingual aspect of a sextant that shows the most tissue changes and assesses this area.** | | |
| **For the selected area, accurately records the color of the gingival tissue on the Gingival Descriptor Worksheet.** | | |
| **Accurately records the size of the gingival tissue on the Gingival Descriptor Worksheet.** | | |
| **Accurately records the position of the gingival margin on the Gingival Descriptor Worksheet.** | | |
| **Accurately records the shape of the gingival margin on the Gingival Descriptor Worksheet.** | | |
| **Accurately records the shape of the papillae on the Gingival Descriptor Worksheet.** | | |
| **Accurately records the texture of the gingival tissue on the Gingival Descriptor Worksheet.** | | |
| **Accurately records the consistency of the tissue on the Gingival Descriptor Worksheet.** | | |
| **Checks for the presence or absence of bleeding and/or exudate. Notes bleeding and/or exudate, if applicable.** | | |
| **Accurately draws the position of the gingival margin in the selected area on the Gingival Characteristics Chart.** | | |
| **Indicates areas of recession with a yellow highlighter on the Gingival Characteristics Chart.** | | |
| **Enters gingival margin findings in red pencil at the root apices on the Gingival Characteristics Chart.** | | |
| **Enters findings for the papillae in blue pencil between the teeth on the Gingival Characteristics Chart.** | | |

OPTIONAL GRADE PERCENTAGE CALCULATION

Each **S** equals 1 point, and each **U** equals 0 points. Using the **E** column, total the sum of the "**S**"s _____ divided by the total points possible (13) to calculate the percentage grade.

## COMMUNICATION SKILL CHECKLIST: GINGIVAL DESCRIPTION

Student: _____    Evaluator: _____

Date: _____

> **Roles:**
> - Student 1 = Plays the role of a fictitious patient.
> - Student 2 = Plays the role of the clinician.
> - Student 3 or instructor = Plays the role of the clinic instructor near the end of the role-play.

**DIRECTIONS FOR STUDENT CLINICIAN:** Use **Column S**; evaluate your skill level as **S** (satisfactory) or **U** (unsatisfactory).

**DIRECTIONS FOR EVALUATOR:** Use **Column E** to record your evaluation of the student clinician's communication skills during the role-play. Indicate **S** (satisfactory) or **U** (unsatisfactory). Each **S** equals 1 point, and each **U** equals 0 points.

| CRITERIA | S | E |
|---|---|---|
| **Explains what is to be done.** | | |
| **Points out changes in gingival characteristics and explains their significance to the patient.** | | |
| **Encourages patient questions.** | | |
| **Answers the patient's questions fully and accurately.** | | |
| **Communicates with the patient at an appropriate level and avoids dental/medical terminology or jargon.** | | |
| **Accurately communicates the findings to the clinical instructor. Discusses the implications for dental treatment using correct dental terminology.** | | |

OPTIONAL GRADE PERCENTAGE CALCULATION

Each **S** equals 1 point, and each **U** equals 0 points. Using the **E** column, total the sum of the "**S**"s _____ divided by the total points possible (6) to calculate the percentage grade.

# 15 Mixed Dentition and Occlusion

## MODULE OVERVIEW

This module presents a systematic approach to identifying the teeth present in a mixed dentition and for classifying the occlusion.

This module covers:

- Mixed dentitions and how to recognize primary and permanent teeth in the mouth
- Angle's classification of occlusion and how to classify a patient's occlusion
- Additional characteristics of malocclusion and malpositions of individual teeth

Before beginning this module, you should have completed the chapters on the primary and permanent dentitions and Angle's classification of occlusion in a dental anatomy textbook.

## MODULE OUTLINE

## OBJECTIVES

- List the order of eruption of the permanent teeth.
- List the time ranges for permanent tooth eruption.
- In a clinical setting, distinguish the primary and permanent teeth in a mixed dentition.
- In a clinical setting, identify Angle's Class I, Class II, and Class III relationships.
- List and describe types of tooth malocclusions.
- Define the key terms used in this module:

| | |
|---|---|
| Mixed dentition | Open bite |
| Overbite | Edge to edge |
| Overjet | End-to-end |
| Angle's classification | Crossbite |
| Buccal groove of the mandibular first molar | Facioversion |
| | Linguoversion |
| Molar relation | Supraversion |
| Canine relation | Rotated |
| Class I, II, and III | |

- Provide information to a pediatric patient and his or her parent about the tooth eruption sequence.
- Provide information to a pediatric patient and his or her parent about the teeth present in the patient's mouth. Discuss the implications of notable findings.
- Provide information to a patient about occlusion, malocclusion, and any notable findings.
- Accurately communicate the findings to the clinical instructor. Discuss the implications of notable findings.
- Demonstrate knowledge of mixed dentitions by applying information from this module to the fictitious patient cases in this module.
- Given a patient case, establish the expected age of the individual by studying the mixed dentition.
- Demonstrate knowledge of occlusion and malocclusion by applying information from this module to the fictitious patient cases in this module.

**SECTION 1:**

# Sorting out a Mixed Dentition

The patient assessment includes examination of the dentition. As a child ages, the maxilla and mandible grow, making room for the eruption of the permanent teeth. For a period of several years, a child will have a **mixed dentition**. That is, the child will have a combination of some primary teeth and some permanent teeth. Determining which teeth are primary and which are permanent in a mixed dentition can be challenging. This section presents a review of tooth eruption patterns. Guides to these stages can be found in the "Ready References" section of this module.

## STAGES IN ERUPTION OF THE PRIMARY AND SECONDARY DENTITIONS

### Age 5 Years

The primary teeth usually erupt between ages 2 ½ and 5 ½ years; no permanent teeth are visible in the mouth (Fig. 15-1).

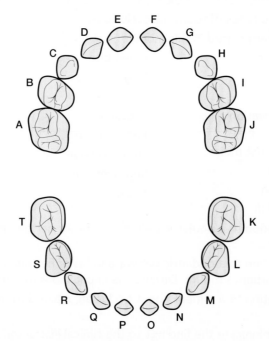

**Figure 15-1.  The primary dentition.** The incisors, canines, and molars present in the primary dentition of a 5-year-old child. Note that there are no primary premolars.

## Age 6 to 7 Years

As the maxilla and mandible grow, there is room for more teeth. From age 6 to 7 years, the permanent first molars erupt just distal to the second primary molars. No primary teeth are exfoliated to make room for these permanent molars. Eruption of the first molars is followed closely by the loss of the mandibular primary central incisors, which are quickly replaced by the permanent central incisors (Fig. 15-2).

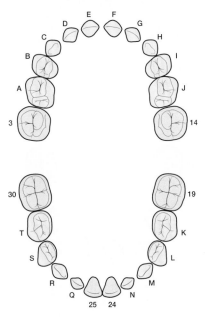

Figure 15-2.   Mixed dentition, age 6 to 7 years.

## Age 7 to 8 Years

By age 7 to 8 years, the permanent incisors have replaced the primary incisors (Fig. 15-3).

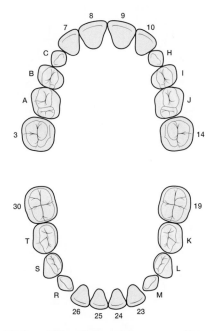

Figure 15-3.   Mixed dentition, age 7 to 8 years.

## Age 10 to 12 Years

All four mandibular premolars erupt into place, replacing the mandibular primary first molars and canines. On the maxillary arch, the permanent first premolars erupt and replace the primary first molars (Fig. 15-4).

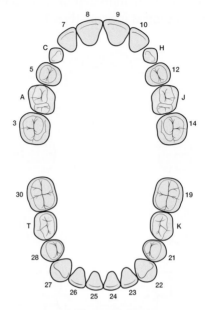

**Figure 15-4.   Mixed dentition, age 10 to 12 years.**

## Age 11 to 13 Years

The primary canines and the primary second molars are the last to exfoliate. Normally, all primary teeth are exfoliated by age 13 (Fig. 15-5).

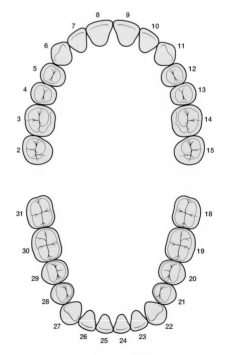

**Figure 15-5.   Permanent dentition, age 11 to 13 years.**

**SECTION 2:**
# Learning to Look at the Occlusion

## THE RELATIONSHIP OF THE MAXILLARY AND MANDIBULAR TEETH

The patient assessment includes an examination of the occlusion, the relationship of the teeth to each other when the incisal and occlusal surfaces of the mandibular arch contact those of the maxillary arch. The way that the teeth occlude during chewing and speaking is important for the appearance, comfort, and health of an individual.

The American Academy of Pediatric Dentistry defines malocclusion as the improper positioning of the teeth and jaws. Malocclusion is a variation of normal growth and development that can affect the bite, ability to maintain adequate plaque control, speech development, and appearance. A healthy occlusion normally exhibits overbite and overjet (Figs. 15-6 and 15-7). In addition, in a healthy occlusion, the maxillary teeth are positioned facial to the mandibular teeth (Fig. 15-8).

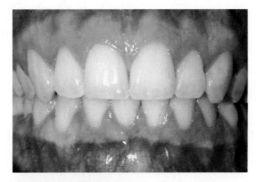

**Figure 15-6. Vertical overlap.** The maxillary incisors vertically overlap the mandibular incisors. The amount of vertical overlap is known as the overbite. (Courtesy of Dr. Don Rolfs, Periodontal Foundations, Wenatchee, WA.)

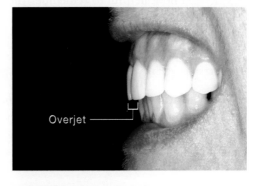

**Figure 15-7. Horizontal distance.** The maxillary incisors are labial to the mandibular incisors. The horizontal distance between the incisal edges of the maxillary teeth and the mandibular teeth is known as the overjet.

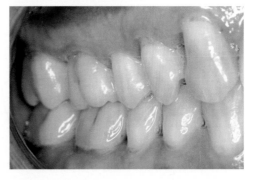

**Figure 15-8. Relationship of teeth.** The cusps of the maxillary teeth overlap the mandibular teeth. The maxillary teeth are facial to the mandibular teeth. (Courtesy of Dr. Richard Foster, Guilford Technical Community College.)

## ANGLE'S CLASSIFICATION

In 1887, Dr. Edward H. Angle developed a system for classifying the relationship of the mandibular teeth to the maxillary teeth. Angle's classification is still in widespread use today.

- Angle's classification system is based primarily on the relationship of the mandibular first molar to the maxillary first molar.
- According to Angle, there are three relationships that can exist between the first molars: Class I, Class II, or Class III.
- If the first molars are missing or malaligned, the relationship of the mandibular canine to the maxillary canine is used in determining the classification.
- *The key to understanding Angle's classification is **the position of the buccal groove of the mandibular permanent first molar** in relation to the maxillary teeth* (Fig. 15-9).

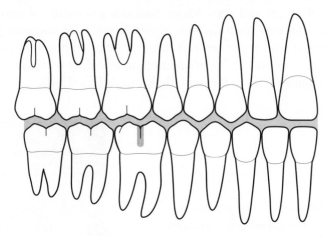

**Figure 15-9.  Angle's classification.** The key to understanding Angle's classification is the buccal groove of the mandibular first molar. In this illustration, the orange shading indicates the buccal groove. Many clinicians find it helpful to remember the phrase *"the mandibular groove moves"* when assessing occlusion.

## CLASS I: GROOVE IN THE NORMAL POSITION

- Molar relation: *The buccal groove of the mandibular first molar is directly in line with the mesiobuccal cusp of maxillary first molar* (Fig. 15-10).
- Canine relation: The maxillary permanent canine occludes with the distal half of the mandibular canine and the mesial half of the mandibular permanent premolar.

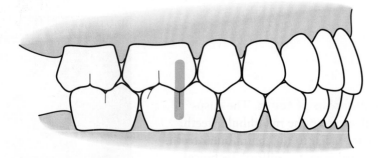

**Figure 15-10.  Angle's Class I occlusion.**

## CLASS II, DIVISION 1: GROOVE POSTERIOR TO THE NORMAL POSITION

- Molar relation: *The buccal groove of the mandibular first molar is distal to the mesiobuccal cusp of maxillary first molar by at least the width of a premolar* (Fig. 15-11).
- Canine relation: The distal surface of the mandibular canine is distal to the mesial surface of the maxillary canine by at least the width of a premolar.
- In Class II, Division 1, all four of the maxillary incisors are protruded.

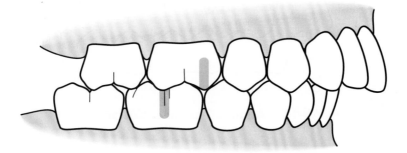

Figure 15-11.   Angle's Class II, Division 1 occlusion.

## CLASS II, DIVISION 2: GROOVE POSTERIOR TO THE NORMAL POSITION

- Molar relation: *The buccal groove of the mandibular first molar is distal to the mesiobuccal cusp of maxillary first molar by at least the width of a premolar* (Fig. 15-12).
- Canine relation: The distal surface of the mandibular canine is distal to the mesial surface of the maxillary canine by at least the width of a premolar.
- In Class II, Division 2, both maxillary lateral incisors protrude while both central incisors retrude.

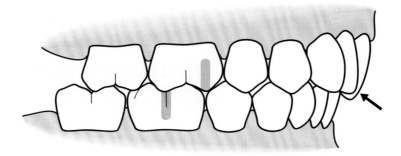

Figure 15-12.   Angle's Class II, Division 2 occlusion.

## CLASS III: GROOVE ANTERIOR TO THE NORMAL POSITION

- Molar relation: *The buccal groove of the mandibular first molar is mesial to the mesiobuccal cusp of maxillary first molar by at least the width of a premolar* (Fig. 15-13).
- Canine relation: The distal surface of the mandibular canine is mesial to the mesial surface of the maxillary canine by at least the width of a premolar.

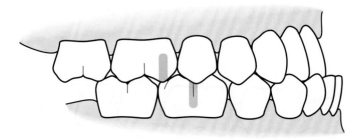

Figure 15-13.   Angle's Class III occlusion.

## OTHER CHARACTERISTICS OF MALOCCLUSION

Malocclusions may have many variations. Some of these variations are depicted in Figures 15-14 through 15-21.

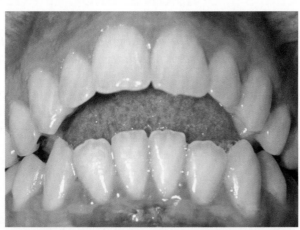

Figure 15-14.   Open bite. The maxillary anterior teeth do not overlap or contact the mandibular anterior teeth. (Courtesy of Dr. Don Rolfs, Periodontal Foundations, Wenatchee, WA.)

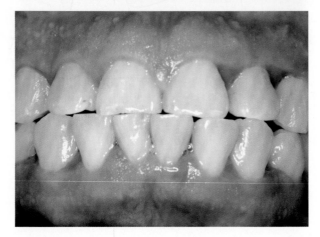

Figure 15-15.   Anterior edge-to-edge bite. The incisal surfaces on the maxillary and mandibular teeth occlude (meet). On posterior teeth, an end-to-end bite occurs when the cusps of the maxillary teeth occlude with the cusps of the opposing mandibular teeth. (Courtesy of Dr. Richard Foster, Guilford Technical Community College.)

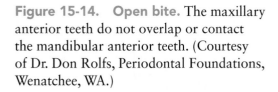

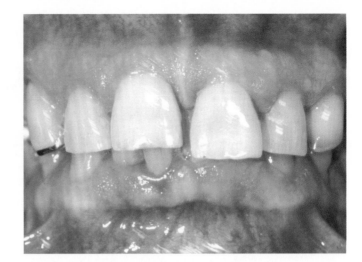

**Figure 15-16. Deep overbite.** The incisal edges of the maxillary anterior teeth are at a level of the cervical third of the mandibular anterior teeth. (Courtesy of Dr. Don Rolfs, Periodontal Foundations, Wenatchee, WA.)

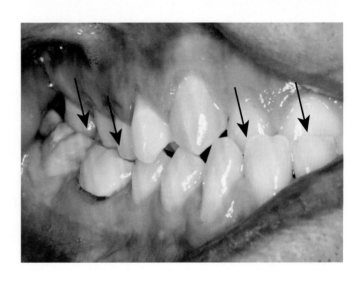

**Figure 15-17. Crossbite.** When one or more of the mandibular teeth are located facial to their maxillary counterparts. This photograph shows both an **anterior** and **posterior crossbite**. (Courtesy of Dr. Richard Foster, Guilford Technical Community College.)

## MALPOSITIONS OF INDIVIDUAL TEETH

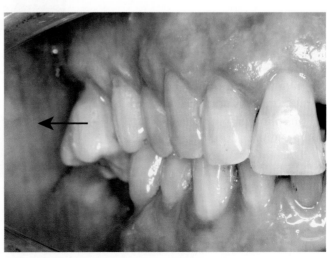

**Figure 15-18. Facioversion.** A tooth that is positioned facial to its normal position. In this photograph, the maxillary first molar is in facioversion. (Courtesy of Dr. Richard Foster, Guilford Technical Community College.)

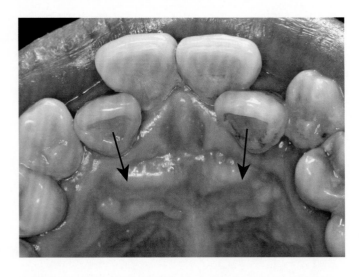

**Figure 15-19.   Linguoversion.** A tooth that is positioned lingual to its normal position. In this photograph, the maxillary lateral incisors are in linguoversion. (Courtesy of Dr. Richard Foster, Guilford Technical Community College.)

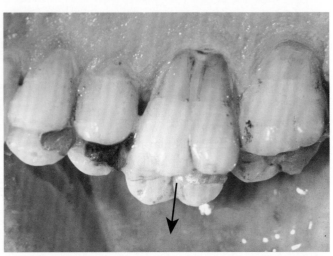

**Figure 15-20.   Supraversion.** A tooth that is positioned above the normal occlusal plane. In this photograph, the maxillary first molar is in supraversion. (Courtesy of Dr. Don Rolfs, Periodontal Foundations, Wenatchee, WA.)

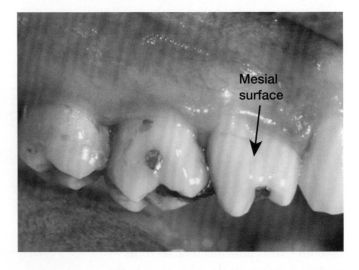

**Figure 15-21.   Rotated (torsiversion).** A tooth that is turned in relation to its normal position. In this photograph, the maxillary first premolar is rotated. (Courtesy of Dr. Don Rolfs, Periodontal Foundations, Wenatchee, WA.)

## SECTION 3:
# Peak Procedures

**PROCEDURE 15-1** IDENTIFYING TEETH IN A MIXED DENTITION

| Action | Rationale |
|---|---|
| 1. **Assemble resources.** Use the *Eruption Times* and the *Stages in Eruption* references from Section 4 of this module. | • These references will assist you in recognizing primary and permanent teeth. |
| 2. **Identify the primary teeth.** Circle the primary teeth present in red pencil on the *Mixed Dentition Worksheet* provided for each patient case. | • Focusing your attention on identifying the primary teeth will help you to sort out the mixture of primary and permanent teeth. |
| 3. **Identify the permanent teeth.** Circle the permanent teeth present in blue pencil on the *Mixed Dentition Worksheet*. | • Once you have identified the primary teeth, focus your attention on recognizing the permanent teeth present in the mouth. |
| 4. **Record.** Transfer the information from the *Mixed Dentition Worksheet* to the patient's chart or computerized record. | • Referring to the information entered on the *Mixed Dentition Worksheet* will facilitate the dental charting process. |

**PROCEDURE 15-2** OCCLUSION CLASSIFICATION AND CHARACTERISTICS

| Action | Rationale |
|---|---|
| 1. **Assemble resources.** Use the *Occlusion Classification: Molar Relationship* reference from Section 5 of this module. | • This reference will assist you in assessing the molar relationship.<br>• **NOTE:** If either the maxillary or mandibular molars are missing, the canines are used to classify the dentition. |
| 2. **Determine the molar relationship.** Enter your findings on the *Occlusion Worksheet* from the "Ready References" section of this module. | • The items listed on the worksheet will help you remember to check for all characteristics of malocclusion and tooth malpositions. |
| 3. **Record.** Transfer the information from the *Occlusion Worksheet* to the patient's chart or computerized record. | • Referring to the information entered on the *Occlusion Worksheet* will facilitate the documentation process. |

## SECTION 4:

# Ready References: Mixed Dentition

**NOTE:** The Ready References in this book may be removed from the book by tearing along the perforated lines on each page. Laminating or placing these pages in plastic protector sheets will allow them to be disinfected for use in a clinical setting.

## READY REFERENCE 15-1  ERUPTION TIMES: PRIMARY TEETH

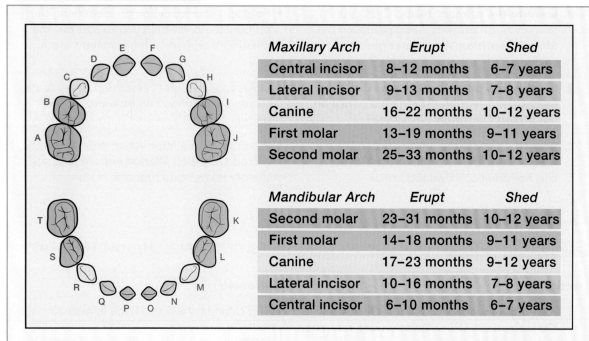

| Maxillary Arch | Erupt | Shed |
|---|---|---|
| Central incisor | 8–12 months | 6–7 years |
| Lateral incisor | 9–13 months | 7–8 years |
| Canine | 16–22 months | 10–12 years |
| First molar | 13–19 months | 9–11 years |
| Second molar | 25–33 months | 10–12 years |

| Mandibular Arch | Erupt | Shed |
|---|---|---|
| Second molar | 23–31 months | 10–12 years |
| First molar | 14–18 months | 9–11 years |
| Canine | 17–23 months | 9–12 years |
| Lateral incisor | 10–16 months | 7–8 years |
| Central incisor | 6–10 months | 6–7 years |

Figure 15-22.

**READY REFERENCE 15-2**    **ERUPTION TIMES: PERMANENT TEETH**

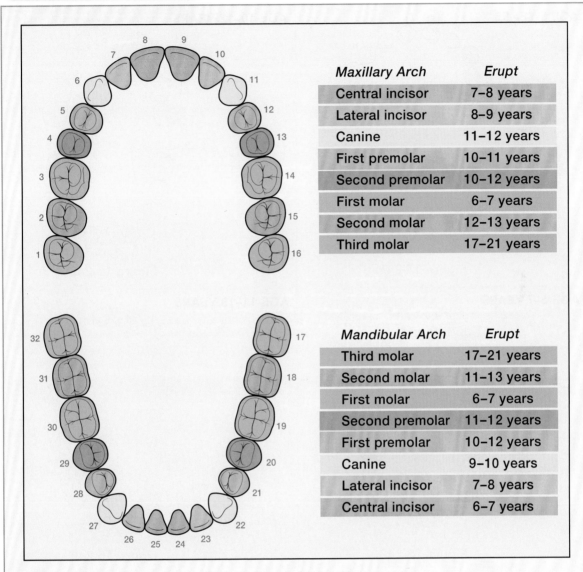

| Maxillary Arch | Erupt |
|---|---|
| Central incisor | 7–8 years |
| Lateral incisor | 8–9 years |
| Canine | 11–12 years |
| First premolar | 10–11 years |
| Second premolar | 10–12 years |
| First molar | 6–7 years |
| Second molar | 12–13 years |
| Third molar | 17–21 years |

| Mandibular Arch | Erupt |
|---|---|
| Third molar | 17–21 years |
| Second molar | 11–13 years |
| First molar | 6–7 years |
| Second premolar | 11–12 years |
| First premolar | 10–12 years |
| Canine | 9–10 years |
| Lateral incisor | 7–8 years |
| Central incisor | 6–7 years |

Figure 15-23.

## READY REFERENCE 15-3  STAGES IN ERUPTION

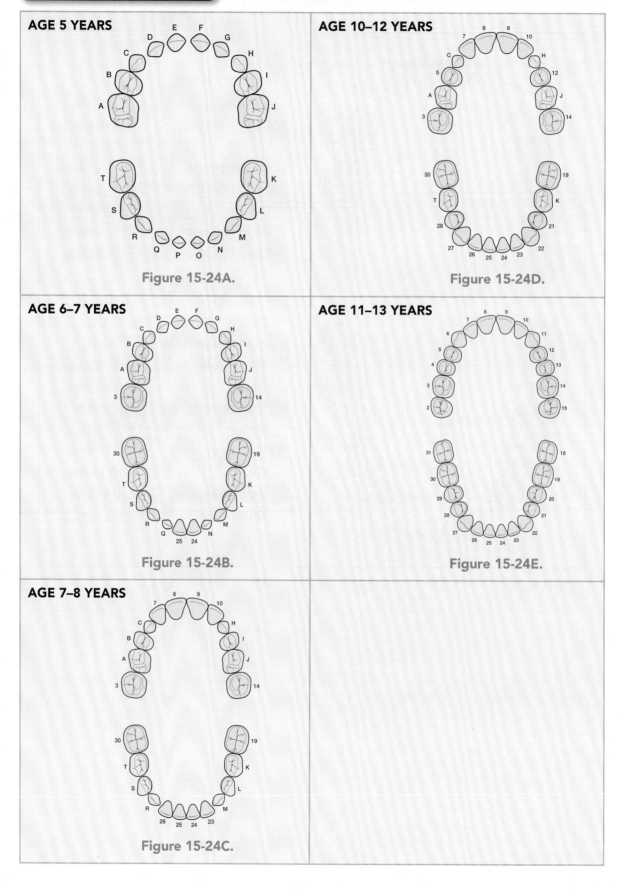

**AGE 5 YEARS**

Figure 15-24A.

**AGE 6–7 YEARS**

Figure 15-24B.

**AGE 7–8 YEARS**

Figure 15-24C.

**AGE 10–12 YEARS**

Figure 15-24D.

**AGE 11–13 YEARS**

Figure 15-24E.

**SECTION 5:**

# Ready References: Occlusion

The Ready References may be removed from the book by tearing along the perforated lines on each page. Laminating or placing these pages in plastic protector sheets will allow them to be disinfected for use in a clinical setting.

**READY REFERENCE 15-4** OCCLUSION CLASSIFICATION: MOLAR RELATIONSHIP

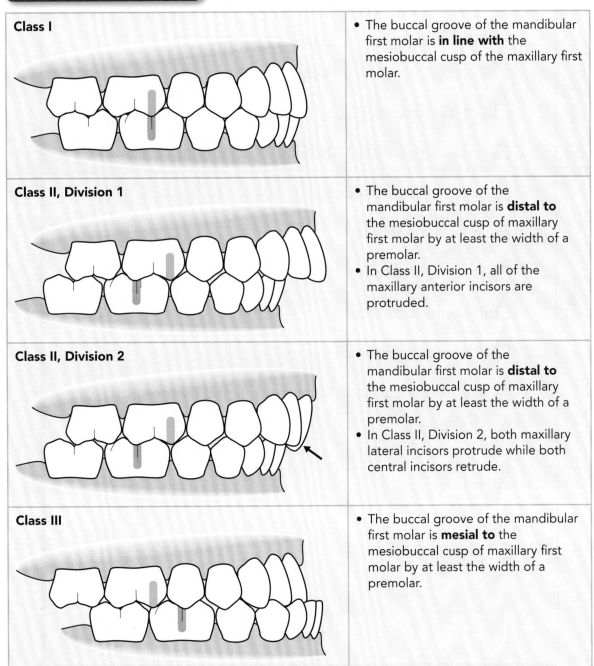

**Class I**

- The buccal groove of the mandibular first molar is **in line with** the mesiobuccal cusp of the maxillary first molar.

**Class II, Division 1**

- The buccal groove of the mandibular first molar is **distal to** the mesiobuccal cusp of maxillary first molar by at least the width of a premolar.
- In Class II, Division 1, all of the maxillary anterior incisors are protruded.

**Class II, Division 2**

- The buccal groove of the mandibular first molar is **distal to** the mesiobuccal cusp of maxillary first molar by at least the width of a premolar.
- In Class II, Division 2, both maxillary lateral incisors protrude while both central incisors retrude.

**Class III**

- The buccal groove of the mandibular first molar is **mesial to** the mesiobuccal cusp of maxillary first molar by at least the width of a premolar.

**READY REFERENCE 15-5**   **OCCLUSION WORKSHEET**

# Occlusion Worksheet

**Case** _____

☐ Canine relation:     Left:     I     II     III

                       Right:    I     II     III

☐ Molar relation:      Left:     I     II     III

                       Right:    I     II     III

☐ Anterior overjet: _____mm

☐ Anterior overbite:     Normal     Moderate     Severe

☐ Anterior edge to edge

☐ Anterior open bite

☐ Anterior crossbite

☐ Posterior end-to-end

☐ Posterior crossbite

☐ Malpositions of individual teeth, listed by tooth:

☐ Other findings:

**READY REFERENCE 15-6** INTERNET RESOURCES: MIXED DENTITION AND OCCLUSION

**Mixed Dentition**

**http://www.ada.org/public/topics/tooth_eruption.asp http://www.ada.org/2930.aspx**
Overview of tooth development and eruption on the website of the **American Dental Association.**

**http://www.uic.edu/classes/orla/orla312/dissected_skull_series.htm**
This **University of Illinois at Chicago** website has excellent images of dissected skulls showing dentitions at ages 2, 5, and 8.

**http://www.simplyteeth.com/category/sections/Adult/ToothGrowthEruption/**
**EruptionTeeth.asp?category=index&section=T&img=adult&page=13**
The **Simplyteeth** website has information on the eruption of the permanent teeth.

**Occlusion**

**http://health.allrefer.com/health/malocclusion-of-teeth-info.html**
Definitions and images related to the topic of occlusion are found on the **Health All Refer** website.

**http://www.merck.com/mrkshared/mmanual/section9/chapter106/106d.jsp**
Information on malocclusion on the **Merck Manual of Diagnosis and Therapy** website.

**http://www.aapd.org/publications/brochures/maloccl.asp**
Information on malocclusion on the **American Academy of Pediatric Dentistry** website.

**http://www.nlm.nih.gov/medlineplus/ency/article/001058.htm**
Information on malocclusion on the **MedlinePlus** website.

## SECTION 6:

# The Human Element

BOX **15-1**   **Through the Eyes of a Student**

*I had gotten pretty confident about charting a patient's teeth. I had seen several adult patients and one 16-year-old. But, then it happened. Sitting in my chair was my first patient with a mixed dentition. My palms began to sweat. As I looked in the mouth, I could not tell which teeth were permanent and which ones were primary. I really started to panic.*

*Then, I got out an eruption chart that I had laminated for clinic. I studied the chart to see which teeth were likely to be present in a child's mouth at age 11. I calmed down and thought about which primary teeth were likely to be present and which permanent teeth probably would have erupted by age 11.*

*I looked in the patient's mouth again and began marking the primary teeth that were present. Next, I crossed out the permanent teeth that were not present in the mouth. Before I knew it, I had prepared a chart of teeth present in my patient's mouth.*

*When my instructor reviewed my charting, she smiled and said, "Bravo, Skip!" I felt really proud of myself, but most important, I learned that I could handle new things when I just stay calm and stop to remember all the pieces of information in the puzzle (like primary dentition, adult dentition, and eruption patterns).*

*Skip, student*
*South Florida Community College*

**Table 15-1** ENGLISH-TO-SPANISH PHRASE LIST FOR MIXED DENTITION AND OCCLUSION

| | |
|---|---|
| This chart shows the age ranges when the baby teeth (primary teeth) erupt into the mouth. | Este grafico indica la edad cuando los dientes del bebe (dientes principales) eruptan en la boca. |
| This chart shows the age ranges when the permanent teeth erupt into the mouth. | Este grafico indica la edad cuando los dientes permanentes eruptan en la boca. |
| All of your baby teeth are in your mouth. | Todos los dientes principales están en la boca. |
| This is a permanent tooth. | Este es un diente permanente. |
| This is a baby tooth. | Este es un diente principal. |
| The baby teeth are needed to retain the space in the mouth for the eruption of the permanent teeth. | Los dientes principales son necesarios para retener el espacio en la boca para los dientes permanentes. |
| Your (your child's) teeth have an ideal bite. | Sus dientes (los dientes de su niño) tienen un mordisco ideal. |
| You (your child's) bite is not ideal. This bite could cause some dental problems in the future. | Sus dientes (los dientes de su niñ) no tienen un mordisco ideal. Esto puede provocar algunos problemas dentales en el futuro. |
| This tooth is out of alignment (position) with the other teeth in your mouth. | Este diente esta fuera de alineamento (posición) con los otros dientes en la boca. |
| The position of this tooth (these teeth) could cause dental problems in the future. | La posición de este diente (estos dientes) puede provocar problemas dentales en el futuro. |
| I would recommend seeing an orthodontist (dental specialist) about your (your child's) bite. | Yo le recomendo que consulte con un dentista especializando en orofacial sobre su mordisco (sobre el mordisco de su niño). |
| I am going to get my clinic instructor. | Voy a buscar mi instructor. |

**SECTION 7:**

# Practical Focus—Mixed Dentition

**DIRECTIONS:**

- Use the steps outlined in **Procedure 15-1** and the **Mixed Dentition Worksheet** to determine the primary and permanent teeth present for the three fictitious patient cases in this section. Bethany Biddle is a fictitious patient that you are familiar with from other modules in the book. The other two fictitious patients are unique to this module.

- Determine the expected age of each patient by studying his or her mixed dentition.

- The pages in this section may be removed from the book for easier use by tearing along the perforated lines on each page.

## SOURCES OF CLINICAL PHOTOGRAPHS

The author gratefully acknowledges the sources of the following clinical photographs in the Practical Focus sections of this module.

- Figure 15-26. Dr. Marci Marano Beck, Tallahassee, FL.
- Figure 15-27. Dr. Marci Marano Beck, Tallahassee, FL.
- Figure 15-29. Dr. Marci Marano Beck, Tallahassee, FL.
- Figure 15-30. Dr. Richard Foster, Guilford Technical Community College, Jamestown, NC.
- Figure 15-32. Dr. Don Rolfs, Periodontal Foundations, Wenatchee, WA.
- Figure 15-34. Dr. Richard Foster, Guilford Technical Community College, Jamestown, NC.
- Figure 15-35. Dr. Richard Foster, Guilford Technical Community College, Jamestown, NC.
- Figure 15-36. Dr. Richard Foster, Guilford Technical Community College, Jamestown, NC.
- Figure 15-37. Dr. Richard Foster, Guilford Technical Community College, Jamestown, NC.
- Figure 15-38. Dr. Don Rolfs, Periodontal Foundations, Wenatchee, WA.
- Figure 15-39. Dr. Don Rolfs, Periodontal Foundations, Wenatchee, WA.
- Figure 15-40. Dr. Don Rolfs, Periodontal Foundations, Wenatchee, WA.
- Figure 15-41. Dr. Richard Foster, Guilford Technical Community College, Jamestown, NC.
- Figure 15-42. Dr. Richard Foster, Guilford Technical Community College, Jamestown, NC.
- Figure 15-43. Dr. Don Rolfs, Periodontal Foundations, Wenatchee, WA.
- Figure 15-44. Dr. Richard Foster, Guilford Technical Community College, Jamestown, NC.
- Figure 15-45. Dr. Richard Foster, Guilford Technical Community College, Jamestown, NC.
- Figure 15-46. Dr. Richard Foster, Guilford Technical Community College, Jamestown, NC.

## FICTITIOUS PATIENT CASE B: Bethany Biddle

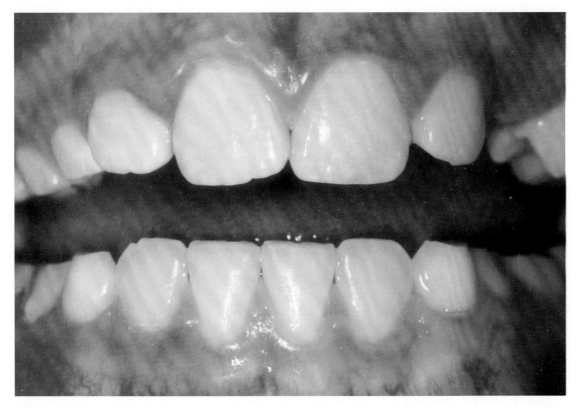

Figure 15-26.   Anterior view of Bethany's dentition.

## Directions for Case B:

- View the three photographs of Bethany's mouth on this and the following pages.
- Remove the **Mixed Dentition Worksheet** that follows the three photos of Bethany's mouth and indicate the primary and permanent teeth present.
- Indicate Bethany's expected age based on the primary and permanent teeth present in her mouth at this time: _____

## FICTITIOUS PATIENT CASE B: Bethany Biddle, *continued*

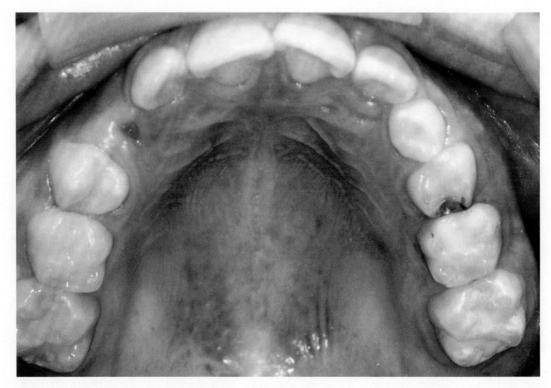

Figure 15-27.   Bethany's dentition: Maxillary arch.

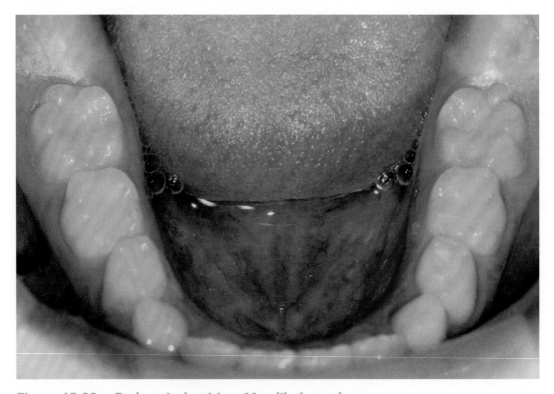

Figure 15-28.   Bethany's dentition: Mandibular arch.

# Mixed Dentition Worksheet

Case: _____

*Directions:* Use a red/blue pencil to indicate the following:
- Circle the primary teeth present in the mouth on the drawing of the primary dentition.
- Circle the permanent teeth present in the mouth on the drawing of the primary dentition.

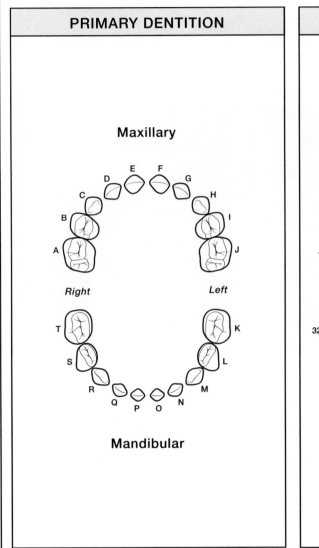

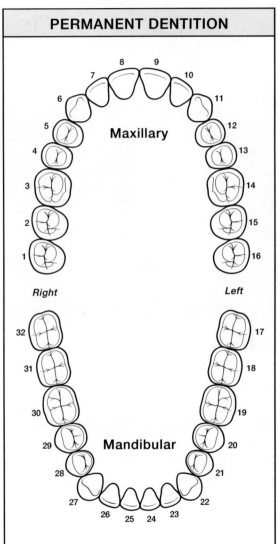

Figure 15-29. Mixed Dentition Worksheet for Bethany Biddle.

## FICTITIOUS PATIENT CASE: Lulu Lowe

Patient Case L is a pediatric patient with fixed orthodontic appliances and a mixed dentition.

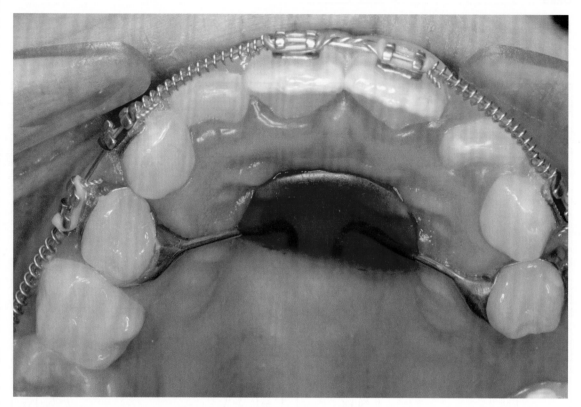

**Figure 15-30.   Lulu's dentition on the maxillary arch.**

### Directions for Case L:

- View the photograph of Lulu's mouth in Figure 15-30.
- Remove the **Mixed Dentition Worksheet** that follows and indicate the primary and permanent teeth present in Lulu's mouth.
- Indicate Lulu's expected age based on the primary and permanent teeth present in her mouth at this time: _____

# Mixed Dentition Worksheet

**Case:** _____

*Directions:* Use a red/blue pencil to indicate the following:
- Circle the primary teeth present in the mouth on the drawing of the primary dentition.
- Circle the permanent teeth present in the mouth on the drawing of the primary dentition.

| PRIMARY DENTITION | PERMANENT DENTITION |
|---|---|

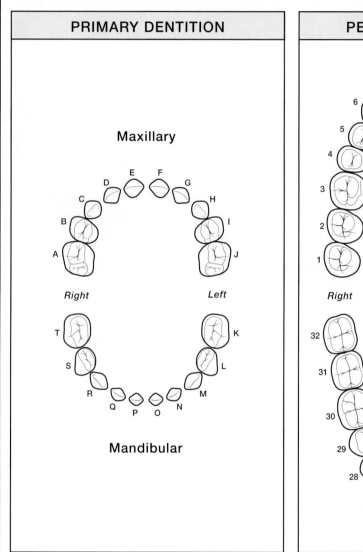

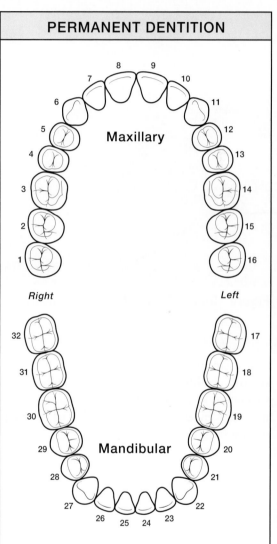

Figure 15-31. Mixed Dentition Worksheet for Lulu Lowe.

## FICTITIOUS PATIENT CASE: Kenneth Kole

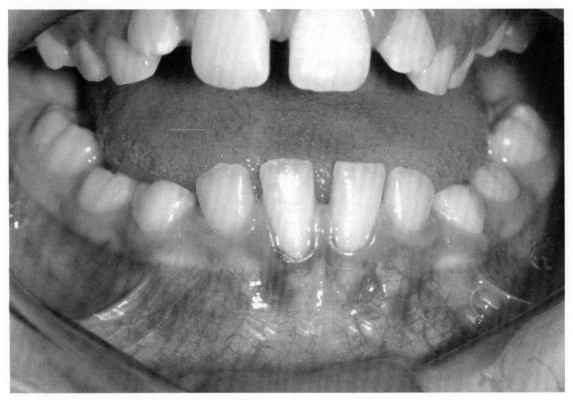

**Figure 15-32.   Kenneth Kole's dentition.**

## Directions for Case K:

- View the photograph of Kenneth's mouth in Figure 15-32.
- Remove the **Mixed Dentition Worksheet** that follows and indicate the primary and permanent teeth present in Kenneth's mouth.
- Indicate Kenneth's expected age based on the primary and permanent teeth present in his mouth at this time: _____

# Mixed Dentition Worksheet

**Case:** _____

*Directions:* **Use a red/blue pencil to indicate the following:**
- Circle the primary teeth present in the mouth on the drawing of the primary dentition.
- Circle the permanent teeth present in the mouth on the drawing of the primary dentition.

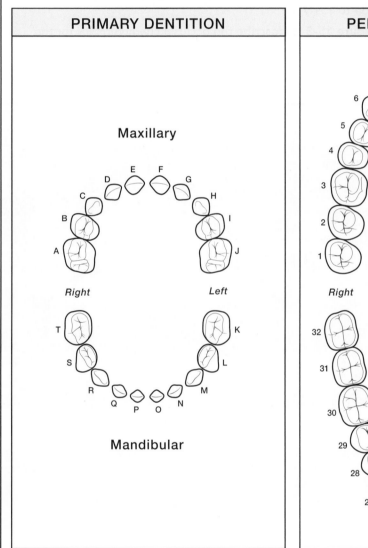

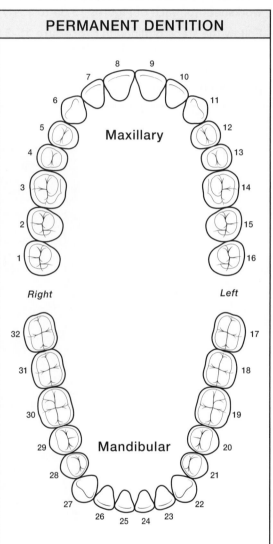

**Figure 15-33.**  **Mixed Dentition Worksheet for Kenneth Kole.**

## SECTION 8:

# Practical Focus—Occlusion

**DIRECTIONS:**

- Locate **Ready Reference 15-5,** the **Occlusion Worksheet,** in Section 5 of this module. Photocopy the **Occlusion Worksheet** or duplicate it on notebook paper so that you have a worksheet for each of Figures 15-34 to 15-47.

- Follow the steps outlined in **Procedure 15-2** to describe the occlusal characteristics for the fictitious patient cases shown in Figures 15-34 to 15-47.

- The pages in this section may be removed from the book for easier use by tearing along the perforated lines on each page.

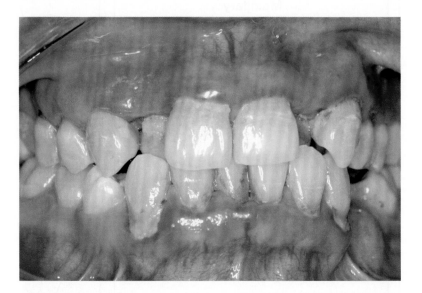

Figure 15-34.

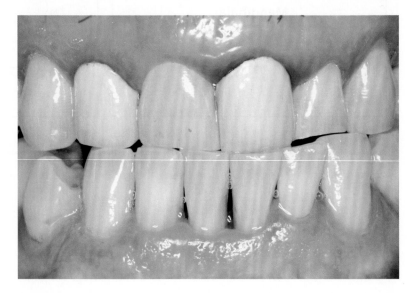

Figure 15-35.

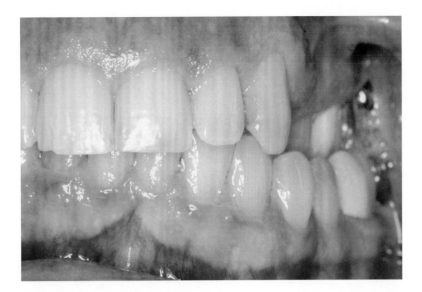

Figure 15-36.

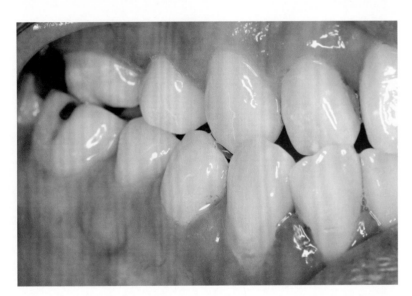

Figure 15-37.

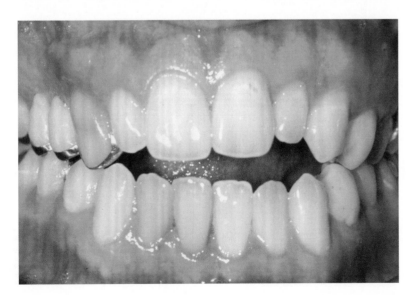

Figure 15-38.

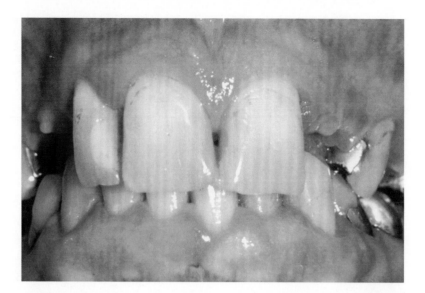

**Figure 15-39.**

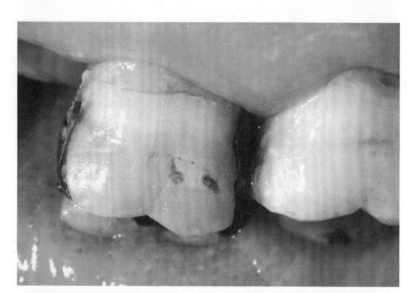

**Figure 15-40.**

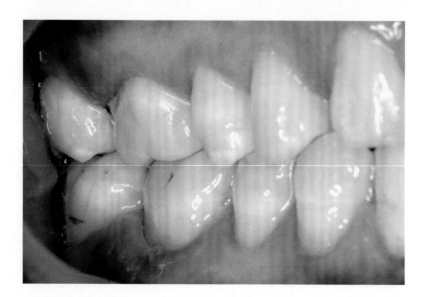

**Figure 15-41.**

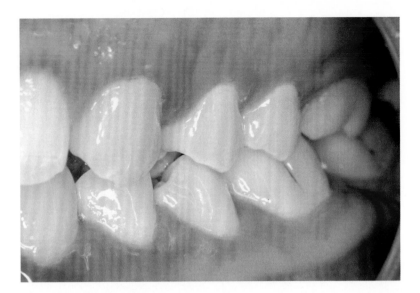

Figure 15-42.

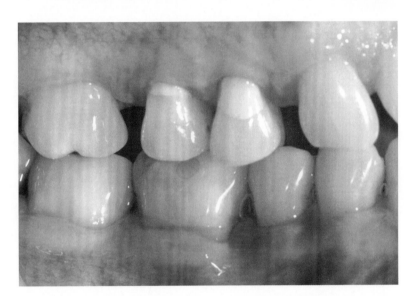

Figure 15-43.

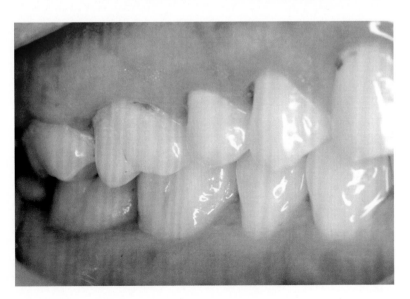

Figure 15-44.

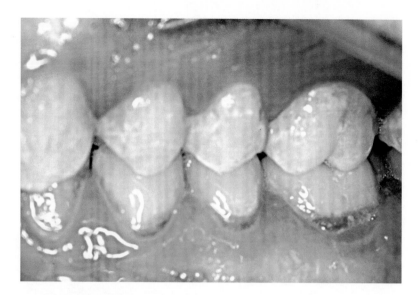

Figure 15-45.

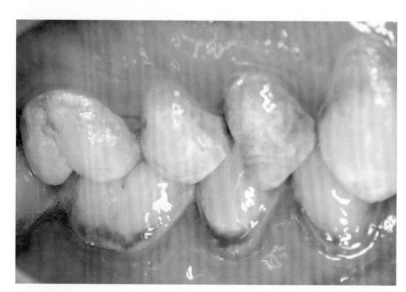

Figure 15-46.

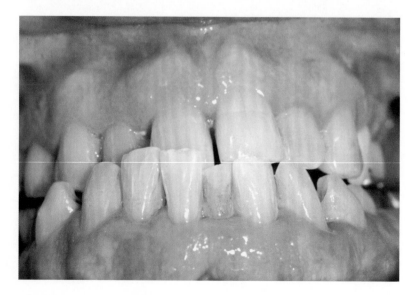

Figure 15-47.

## SECTION 9:
# Skill Check

### SKILL CHECKLIST:  MIXED DENTITION

Student: _____    Evaluator: _____

Date:      _____

**DIRECTIONS FOR STUDENT CLINICIAN:** Using **Column S**, evaluate your skill level as **S** (satisfactory) or **U** (unsatisfactory).

**DIRECTIONS FOR EVALUATOR:** Use **Column E**. Indicate **S** (satisfactory) or **U** (unsatisfactory). In the optional grade percentage calculation, each **S** equals 1 point and each **U** equals 0 points.

| CRITERIA | S | E |
|---|---|---|
| **Accurately identifies the primary teeth present in the dentition on the Mixed Dentition Worksheet.** | | |
| **Accurately identifies the permanent teeth present in the dentition on the Mixed Dentition Worksheet.** | | |
| **Accurately transfers the information to the patient chart or computerized record.** | | |

OPTIONAL GRADE PERCENTAGE CALCULATION

Using the entries in the **E** column, assign a point value of 1 for each **S** and 0 for each **U**. Add the total assigned as 1's _____ and divide by 3 to arrive at the percentage grade _____.

## SKILL CHECKLIST: OCCLUSION

Student: _____     Evaluator: _____

Date: _____

**DIRECTIONS FOR STUDENT CLINICIAN:** Using **Column S**, evaluate your skill level as **S** (satisfactory) or **U** (unsatisfactory).

**DIRECTIONS FOR EVALUATOR:** Use **Column E**. Indicate **S** (satisfactory) or **U** (unsatisfactory). In the optional grade percentage calculation, each **S** equals 1 point and each **U** equals 0 points.

| CRITERIA | S | E |
| --- | --- | --- |
| Accurately classifies the occlusion on the Occlusion Worksheet. | | |
| Accurately notes other characteristics of malocclusion or malpositions of individual teeth on the Occlusal Worksheet. | | |
| Accurately transfers the information to the patient chart or computerized record. | | |

OPTIONAL GRADE PERCENTAGE CALCULATION

Using the entries in the **E** column, assign a point value of 1 for each **S** and 0 for each **U**. Add the total assigned as 1's _____ and divide by 3 to arrive at the percentage grade _____.

**COMMUNICATION SKILL CHECKLIST:** MIXED DENTITION.

Student: _____   Evaluator: _____

Date: _____

---

**Roles:**

- Student 1 = Plays the role of the patient.
- Student 2 = Plays the role of the clinician.
- Student 3 or instructor = Plays the role of the clinic instructor near the end of the role-play.

---

**DIRECTIONS FOR STUDENT CLINICIAN:** Using **Column S**, evaluate your skill level as **S** (satisfactory) or **U** (unsatisfactory).

**DIRECTIONS FOR EVALUATOR:** Use **Column E**. Indicate **S** (satisfactory) or **U** (unsatisfactory). In the optional grade percentage calculation, each **S** equals 1 point and each **U** equals 0 points.

| CRITERIA | S | E |
|---|---|---|
| **Explains the eruption sequence of permanent teeth to the patient and/or parent.** | | |
| **Relates the eruption sequence to the teeth present in the patient's mouth.** | | |
| **Encourages patient questions.** | | |
| **Answers the patient's questions fully and accurately.** | | |
| **Communicates with the patient at an appropriate level and avoids dental/medical terminology or jargon.** | | |
| **Accurately communicates the findings to the clinical instructor. Discusses the implications for dental treatment using correct dental terminology.** | | |

OPTIONAL GRADE PERCENTAGE CALCULATION

Using the entries in the **E** column, assign a point value of 1 for each **S** and 0 for each **U**. Add the total assigned as 1's _____ and divide by 6 to arrive at the percentage grade _____.

## COMMUNICATION SKILL CHECKLIST: OCCLUSION

Student: _____    Evaluator: _____

Date: _____

> **Roles:**
> - Student 1 = Plays the role of the patient.
> - Student 2 = Plays the role of the clinician.
> - Student 3 or instructor = Plays the role of the clinic instructor near the end of the role-play.

**DIRECTIONS FOR STUDENT CLINICIAN:** Using **Column S**, evaluate your skill level as **S** (satisfactory) or **U** (unsatisfactory).

**DIRECTIONS FOR EVALUATOR:** Use **Column E**. Indicate **S** (satisfactory) or **U** (unsatisfactory). In the optional grade percentage calculation, each **S** equals 1 point and each **U** equals 0 points.

| CRITERIA | S | E |
|---|---|---|
| **Explains the role of occlusion in the health and appearance of the dentition.** | | |
| **Explains findings such as malocclusion or malpositions of individual teeth to the patient.** | | |
| **Encourages patient questions.** | | |
| **Answers the patient's questions fully and accurately.** | | |
| **Communicates with the patient at an appropriate level and avoids dental/medical terminology or jargon.** | | |
| **Accurately communicates the findings to the clinical instructor. Discusses the implications for dental treatment using correct dental terminology.** | | |

OPTIONAL GRADE PERCENTAGE CALCULATION

Using the entries in the **E** column, assign a point value of 1 for each **S** and 0 for each **U**. Add the total assigned as 1's _____ and divide by 6 to arrive at the percentage grade _____.

## MODULE OVERVIEW

Radiographic examination of patients provides valuable information related to the presence or absence of dentally related disease. However, radiographs should never be used as the sole source for diagnosis. It is only when the information derived from the radiographic assessment is combined with a careful review of the health history and periodontal charting of soft tissue findings that radiographic information becomes a powerful diagnostic aid.

This module covers the evaluation and assessment of radiographic information involving the recognition of normal anatomic structures and evaluation of the teeth and their supporting structures. It will require recognition and discernment of differences between normal and abnormal conditions, especially those relating to the assessment of the alveolar bone and periodontal structures.

If necessary, the normal radiographic anatomy and the radiographic manifestations of common dental diseases can be reviewed by referring to a dental radiology theory textbook before beginning this module.

## MODULE OUTLINE

## OBJECTIVES

- Identify the anatomic structures commonly visible on panoramic radiographs for fictitious patients.
- Explain radiographic technique and processing errors that could affect radiographic assessment.
- Given a set of radiographs, recognize and localize the location of each radiographically visible normal anatomic landmark.
- Describe the radiographic characteristics of normal and abnormal alveolar bone.
- Recognize and describe early radiographic evidence of periodontal disease.
- Classify the degree of alveolar bone loss as localized or generalized, slight, moderate, or severe/advanced.
- Explain the difference between vertical and horizontal alveolar bone loss and identify each type of bone loss on radiographs of simulated patients.
- Recognize potential etiologic agents for periodontal disease radiographically.
- Briefly and succinctly summarize radiographic findings on radiographs of simulated patients and relate them to pertinent elements from the health history, clinical charting, periodontal probing, etc.
- Gain practical experience in radiographic assessment by applying information from this module to the fictitious patient cases in this module.

## SECTION 1:
# Review of Radiographic Anatomy

Before attempting to interpret a set of radiographs, it is important to have an understanding of the anatomic structures visible on radiographs. This section presents a quick review of the anatomic structures readily and commonly visible on a panoramic radiograph (Figs. 16-1 and 16-2).

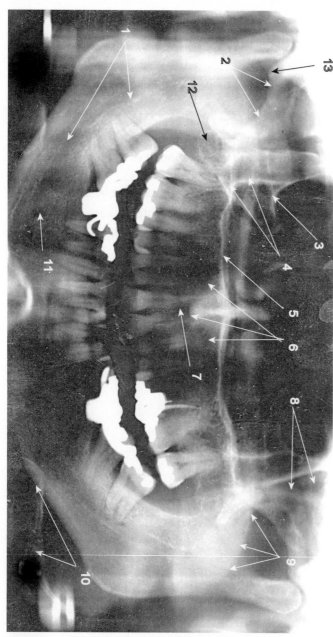

**Answers:**

1 – mandibular canal

2 – lower border of the zygomatic arch

3 – lower border of the orbit

4 – zygomatic process of the maxilla— also known as the "malar process"

5 – hard palate

6 – shadow of the nose

7 – incisive foramen

8 – pterygomaxillary fissure

9 – shadow of the soft palate

10 – hyoid bone (may be seen bilaterally)

11 – mental foramen

12 – tuberosity of the maxilla

13 – articular eminence

**Figure 16-1.   Panoramic radiograph of an adult patient.**

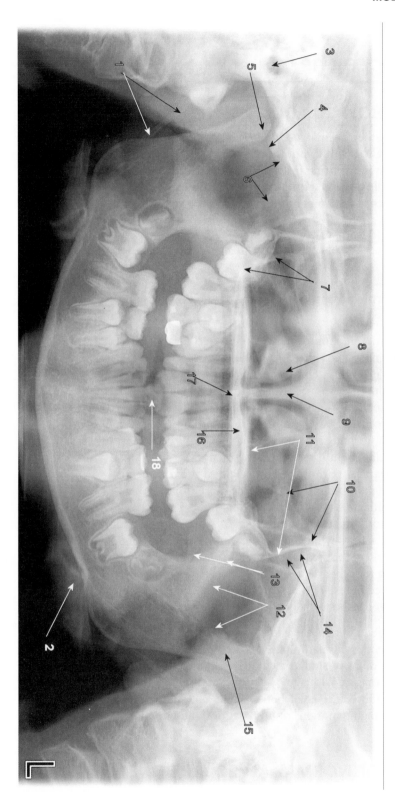

**Figure 16-2. Panoramic radiograph of a pedodontic patient.**

**Answers:**

1 – stylohyoid ligament

2 – hyoid bone

3 – external auditory meatus

4 – articular eminence

5 – head of the mandibular condyle

6 – lower border of the zygomatic arch

7 – zygomatic process of the maxilla/malar process

8 – inferior concha and turbinate

9 – nasal septum

10 – inferior orbital rim

11 – maxillary sinus

12 – mandibular notch

13 – coronoid process of the mandible

14 – pterygomaxillary fissure

15 – neck of the mandibular condyle

16 – hard palate

17 – anterior nasal spine

18 – bite guide of the panoramic unit

**SECTION 2:**

# Interpreting Radiographs

## WHAT TO LOOK FOR AND HOW TO LOOK FOR IT

When evaluating any radiograph—whether a single periapical, bitewing, or a complete mouth radiographic survey (CMRS)/full mouth x-ray (FMX)—perform the radiographic evaluation in a consistent, routine fashion from one time to the next. **When working with digital radiographs, remember that the information present and the interpretation process is the same as that for a conventional radiograph.** The order in which the evaluation is performed is not necessarily as critical as the consistency with which the clinician performs the task.

## FOUR-STEP ASSESSMENT

For convenience, the radiographic interpretative process can be divided into a series of steps:

- Step 1: Determine diagnostic value. Ask the question: "Do these radiographs exhibit the criteria for meeting minimal diagnostic acceptability?" **Refer to the "Ready References" section of this module for a brief definition of diagnostic acceptability.**
- Step 2: Recognize any significant technique or processing errors that will deter a clinician's ability to correctly evaluate all of the relevant dental structures.
- Step 3: Recognize the "normal" anatomic structures observable on the radiographs. **It is important to be able to distinguish normal structures from variations or deviations from normal. For example, the clinician should recognize the mental foramen as "normal anatomy" rather than "periapical pathology," especially if the foramen is anatomically close to the apex of the mandibular first or second premolar.**
- Step 4: Conduct a systematic and careful assessment of the teeth and their supporting tissues. **The clinician must be careful not to focus on only a single condition or deviation. For example, a dental hygienist will be naturally inclined to look at the alveolar bone first. Focusing on the alveolar bone early in the search process may distract the hygienist and cause him or her to stop searching for other dentally relevant deviations and variations from normal, such as calcified pulps, *dens in dente,* or periapical pathosis. To avoid this tendency to focus on the alveolar bone, he or she should look at the bone last.**

Regardless of his or her role in the dental team, the clinician should consistently examine radiographs for dental caries, periapical pathology, calcified pulps (indicators of possible prior trauma), asymmetry in pulps of similar teeth (an early loss of pulp vitality will produce a pulp that doesn't mature with age by getting smaller), changes in alveolar bone pattern from one area to another, alveolar bone height, and etiologic agents promoting dental disease, such as overhanging margins on restorations and crowns, calculus, or open contacts.

## RADIOGRAPHIC FEATURES OF NORMAL ALVEOLAR BONE

Normal alveolar bone height will vary slightly depending on the age of the patient. In general, normal alveolar bone height is 1.5 to 2 mm below and parallel to the cementoenamel junction (CEJ) of adjacent teeth (Fig. 16-3).

- The bone forming the alveolar crest should be smooth and intact with the radiolucent space adjacent to the root surface no wider than the width of the periodontal ligament space (PDLS).

- Many times, as in Figure 16-3, a distinct "crestal lamina dura" will be visible; in other words, the alveolar crest appears as a dense radiopaque line similar in density to the lamina dura surrounding the root of the tooth. The most important radiographic feature of the alveolar crest, however, is that it forms a smooth intact surface between adjacent teeth with only the width of the periodontal ligament (PDL) separating it from the adjacent tooth surface.

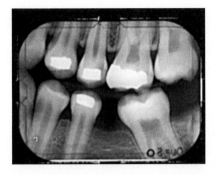

**Figure 16-3. Normal alveolar bone height.**
This radiograph shows a normal alveolar bone height that is 1.5 to 2 mm below and parallel to the cementoenamel junction. In this example, the alveolar crest is a dense radiopaque line similar in density to the lamina dura surrounding the root of the tooth.

> The most important radiographic feature of the alveolar crest is that it forms a smooth, intact surface between adjacent teeth with only the width of the PDL separating it from the adjacent root surface.

## RECOGNIZING EARLY EVIDENCE OF ALVEOLAR BONE LOSS

Early evidence of interproximal alveolar bone loss begins as a progressively increasing area of radiolucency where the alveolar crest and PDL meet.

1.  **Widening of periodontal ligament space.** Look for the earliest evidence of bone loss as a progressive widening of the PDLS as it approaches the alveolar crest (Fig. 16-4). This increasing area of radiolucency produces a triangular shape and is referred to as triangulation.
    - **Triangulation** is the widening of the PDLS caused by the resorption of bone along either the mesial or distal aspect of the interdental (interseptal) crestal bone (Fig. 16-4).
    - Depending on the patient's self care (oral hygiene) and other factors, this increased widening of the PDLS may be seen on the mesial or distal of a single tooth or on multiple teeth.
2.  **Loss of integrity of crestal lamina dura.** An additional early radiographic sign of alveolar bone loss is a loss of the integrity of the crestal lamina dura between adjacent teeth.

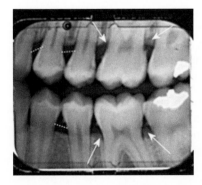

**Figure 16-4. Early evidence of alveolar bone loss.**
The crestal bone on this radiograph demonstrates triangulation, a pointed, triangular appearance that indicates a widening of the periodontal ligament space due to bone loss.

## SECTION 3:
# Peak Procedure

**PROCEDURE 16-1**   ASSESING RADIOGRAPHS

| Action | Rationale |
|---|---|
| **1.** Determine if the radiographs are diagnostically acceptable. Ask the question, "Do these radiographs exhibit the criteria for meeting minimal diagnostic acceptability?" | • A complete mouth radiographic survey/ full mouth x-ray (CMRS/FMX) should exhibit sufficient radiographic information to provide the dentist with an adequate amount of information to determine the patient's specific treatment needs.<br>• Usually, this means that the CMRS/FMX should show each interproximal space at least once without overlap and each root apex at least once. |
| **2.** Look for technique or processing errors. Ask the questions:<br>• "Are there any significant technique or processing errors that will influence my ability to correctly evaluate all of the relevant dental structures?"<br>• "What would I do to correct these errors next time?" | • Any significant technique and/or processing errors will negatively impact the clinician's ability to evaluate all of the relevant dental structures. |
| **3.** Recognize normal structures. | • It is important to distinguish normal anatomic structures from variations or deviations from normal. |
| **4.** Conduct a systemic assessment of the teeth and their supporting tissues. | • Conducting the assessment in a consistent and thorough manner will assure that all aspects of the CMRS/FMX are evaluated.<br>• A systematic assessment should include identification of:<br>  o Teeth present/absent in the dentition<br>  o Dental caries<br>  o Periapical pathology or calcified pulps<br>  o Asymmetry in pulps of similar teeth<br>  o Changes in alveolar bone pattern from one area to another<br>  o Alveolar bone height<br>  o Etiologic agents promoting dental disease, such as overhanging margins on restorations and crowns, calculus deposits, and open contacts |
| **5.** Place radiographs in the patient chart or computerized record for use at all appointments. | • At the start of each appointment, place the radiographs on a chairside view box or display them on a computer screen.<br>• Radiographs provide useful information during treatment and patient education. |

# Cone Beam Computed Tomography

One amazing new dental radiographic technology is called **cone beam computed tomography** (CBCT) or **cone beam volume tomography** (CBVT). These very sophisticated imaging systems ultimately may completely replace the need for intraoral, panoramic, or other extraoral radiographic imaging techniques. With this technology or advances in this current technology, individuals reading this paragraph will witness a time in the not-too-distant future when all that will be necessary to diagnostically image a patient will be to have him or her sit in a chair, stabilize his or her head in some minimal way, and activate the unit, similar to exposing a panoramic radiograph today. Image capture will take less than 20 seconds and show up on our computer screen within 2 to 4 minutes. The software will automatically create a three-dimensional view of the patient from any desired angle. The details of the images will surpass any of our current extraoral imaging systems and be approximately equivalent to or better than our intraoral radiographs.

Space does not permit a detailed explanation of CBCT principles, but in its simplest form, the CBCT unit produces an adjustable beam of radiation and exposes an area of the patient's head as small as 4 cm × 4 cm up to 15 cm × 15 cm (essentially the whole head). In less than 20 seconds, the unit uses a pulsed radiation exposure to expose the patient's head in a 360-degree circle. During its rotation around the patient's head, the unit will expose more than 500 individual images of the patient's head; these individual images are called "basis images." Computer software takes these 500+ images and creates small, discrete image volumes, called "voxels," that the software can reassemble into sagittal, coronal, and axial images of the patient's head. The voxels vary in size from 0.09 to 0.45 mm and will determine the overall resolution of the image we are viewing.

Currently, CBCT units designed specifically for dental purposes may seem expensive; however, when compared to the cost of medical CBCT and CT units, they are relatively inexpensive and provide truly amazing detail not available in any other dental imaging system. Examples of CBCT volumes are shown in Figures 16-5 to 16-10.

Figures 16-5A–E represent the detail associated with a "small-volume" CBCT unit with a voxel size of 0.125 mm. Observe the exquisite bony detail depicted in this case of cementifying fibroma. Even though these are motionless images, the software permits moving the section we view in increments of 0.25 to 1 mm (Figs. 16-5C–E) or more in any direction within a three-dimensional space in real time. The thicknesses of the section below are 1 mm thick.

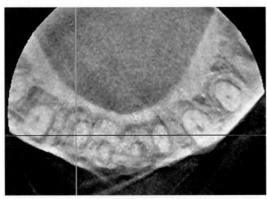

Figure 16-5A.

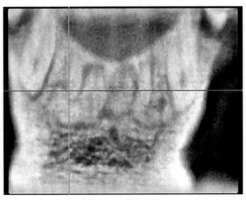

Figure 16-5B.

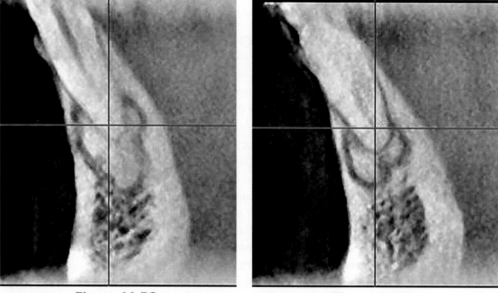

Figure 16-5C.                         Figure 16-5D.

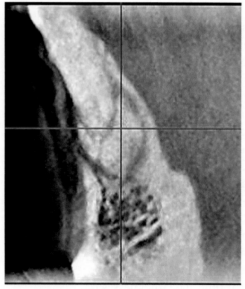

Figure 16-5E.

One of the major benefits of CBCT is their use in precisely identifying the quality and thickness of bone in prospective implant sites as well as clearly identifying and delineating areas of pathology. The technology also provides uncompromised detail for evaluating potential root fractures; potential complications associated with symptomatic endodontically treated teeth; or pre-surgical evaluation of impacted third molars and their relationship to adjacent teeth, the maxillary sinus, or the mandibular canal.

The sections shown below in Figures 16-6A–C illustrate a small odontoma located between and lingual to the canine and first premolar.

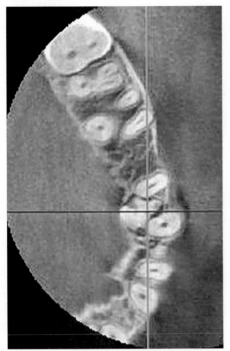

Figure 16-6A.

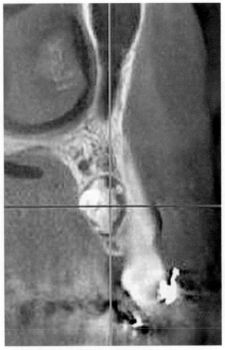

Figure 16-6B.

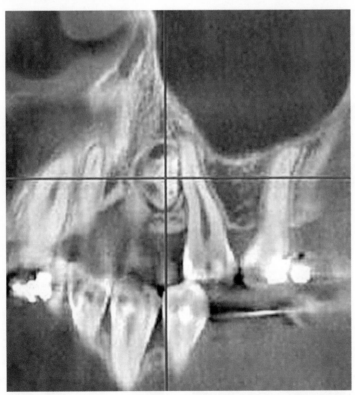

Figure 16-6C.

Figures 16-7A–B are examples of an acute maxillary sinusitis; note the small bubbles in the fluid filling the sinus.

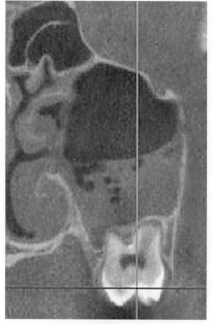

**Figure 16-7A.**

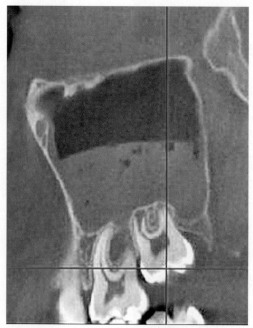

**Figure 16-7B.**

Figures 16-8A–B show how clearly endodontic problems are depicted in the CBCT images; note the resorption of the root apex of the second premolar.

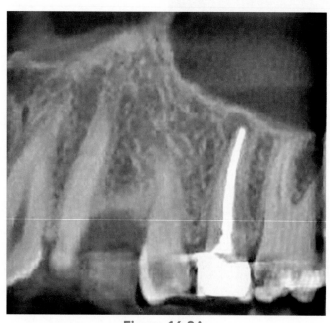

**Figure 16-8A.**

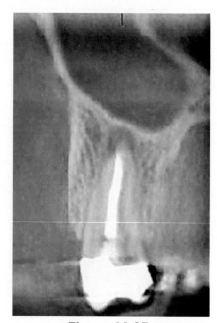

**Figure 16-8B.**

Figure 16-9 shows a recent extraction with bone graft material in the extraction socket. Distal to the extraction socket is a well-circumscribed "mixed" lesion [combination of radiolucent and radiopaque features] indicative of some type of residual pathology; the inferior portion of the lesion has eroded the superior border of the mandibular canal.

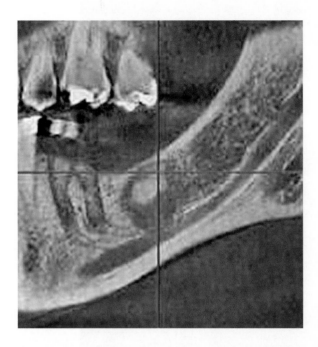

Figure 16-9. Recent extraction.

Figures 16-10A–C illustrate an example of a "large-volume" CBCT unit that can be used to evaluate the entire oral–maxillofacial complex. Large-volume CBCT images may be used in a three-dimensional analysis of the maxillofacial complex in pretreatment and posttreatment planning for orthognathic surgery and orthodontic treatment, as well as multiple implant site planning.

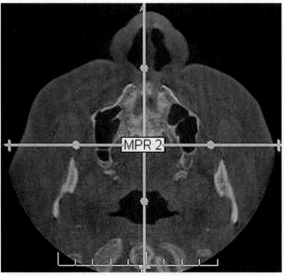

Figure 16-10A.

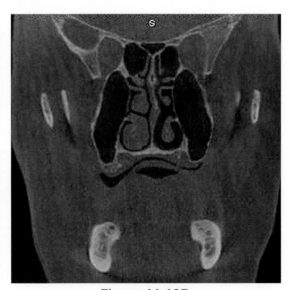

Figure 16-10B.

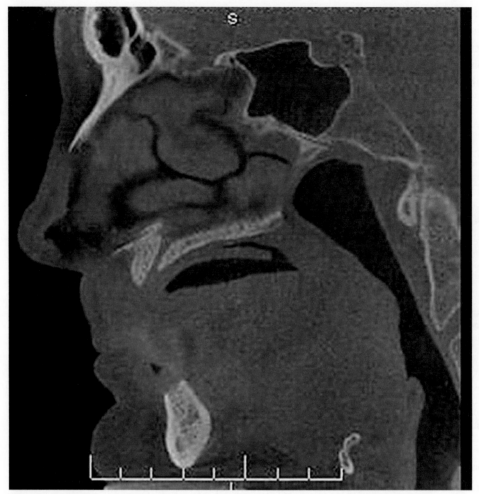

**Figure 16-10C. Image from a large-volume cone beam computed tomography unit.** An example of a CBCT image used to evaluate the entire oral–maxillofacial complex.

## SECTION 5:
# Ready References

**NOTE:** The Ready References in this book may be removed from the book by tearing along the perforated lines on each page. Laminating or placing these pages in plastic protector sheets will allow them to be disinfected for use in a clinical setting.

### READY REFERENCE 16-1 HELPFUL CONCEPTS IN RADIOLOGY

**Minimally diagnostically acceptable**—with reference to a CMRS/FMX, at the very least, each interproximal space should be visible somewhere without significant overlap, and each root apex should be visible. **Significant overlap** is an overlap that is more than one-half the width of the enamel or obscures the dentinoenamel junction (DEJ).

**Rule of symmetry**—or right side/left side check—is based upon the principle that most human beings are symmetrical in appearance; that is, the right side looks like the left side.
- **EXAMPLE: Assessing for periapical pathology:**
  o When assessing for the presence of periapical pathology, the clinician should first look at the apex of the right first molar and then immediately compare it to the apex of the left first molar.
  o When evaluating symmetry, the question the clinician should ask is, "Does the right root look like the left?"
  o If the answer is "yes, they both look alike," then the roots are probably normal.
  o If the answer is "no," then the question becomes "why not?" The clinician's task is to identify what makes one root apex different from the one on the opposite side of the mouth.
- Continue assessing the right and left sides in this manner. For example, if you see caries on the mesial surface of the right maxillary second premolar, immediately look at the mesial surface of the left maxillary second premolar. This technique really works, and you will be amazed at how many deviations and variations you will find if you persist in using this strategy.

**Thorough assessment**—a thorough assessment involves looking for more than caries and periodontal disease.
- A quick glance at any pathology textbook or the relevant sections of your radiology textbook will reveal a vast array of conditions that can manifest in the oral cavity in a many subtle and not-so-subtle ways.
- It is appropriate that your radiographic assessment be sufficiently sensitive and thorough such that you can identify deviations and variations from normal.
- The rule of symmetry method of evaluating individual teeth and/or areas of the jaw is a highly effective strategy.

# Radiographic Evaluation Worksheet

*Directions:* Complete the four steps listed below.
Attach additional sheets to this form as needed.

1. *Diagnostic acceptability*: Do these radiographs exhibit the criteria for meeting minimal diagnostic acceptability? If not, why?

2. *Technique*: List any significant technique or processing errors that will influence your ability to correctly evaluate all of the relevant dental structures.

3. *Normal anatomic structures*: List the "normal" anatomic structures observable on the radiographs.

4. *Systematic assessment*: Conduct a thorough assessment of the teeth and supporting structures and provide a written summary of your findings.

**Figure 16-11.   Radiographic Evaluation Worksheet.**

**READY REFERENCE 16-2**   RADIOGRAPHIC EVIDENCE OF BONE LOSS

### Radiographic Evidence of the Extent of Bone Loss

- **Slight**—the crest of the alveolar bone is approximately 3–4 mm apical to the cementoenamel junction (CEJ).
- **Moderate**—crest of the alveolar bone is approximately 4–5 mm apical to the CEJ.
- **Severe/advanced**—crest of the alveolar bone is more than 5 mm apical to the CEJ or the bone covers less than one-half of the anatomic root length as measured from the CEJ to the root apex.

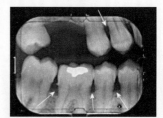

**Figure 16-12A.   Slight bone loss.**

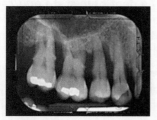

**Figure 16-12B.   Severe bone loss.**

### Radiographic Evidence of the Distribution of Bone Loss

- **Generalized**—bone loss involving more than 50% of the erupted teeth in one arch.
- **Localized**—bone loss involving fewer than 50% of the erupted teeth in one arch.
- When noting such conditions in the patient's record, it is appropriate to identify where the localized lesions occur—such as "mandibular R & L central and lateral incisor region."

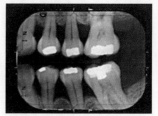

**Figure 16-12C.   Generalized bone loss.**

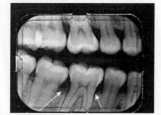

**Figure 16-12D.   Localized bone loss.**

### Radiographic Evidence of the Patterns of Bone Loss

- **Horizontal pattern of bone loss**—a fairly uniform reduction in the height of the bone radiographically throughout an arch or quadrant.
- **Vertical pattern of bone loss**—an uneven pattern of bone loss that typically involves a single tooth; this uneven pattern of bone loss leaves a trench-like area of missing bone alongside the root.

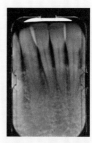

**Figure 16-12E.   Horizontal pattern.**

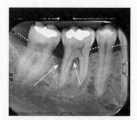

**Figure 16-12F.   Vertical pattern.**

## READY REFERENCE 16-3   INTERNET RESOURCES: DENTAL RADIOGRAPHS

**http://www.ada.org/prof/resources/topics/radiography.asp**
**American Dental Association (ADA) (and U.S. Food and Drug Administration [FDA])**
**Guide to Patient Selection for Dental Radiographs** on the website of the **ADA**.

**http://www.e-radiography.net/technique/dental/Kodak%20Dental%20**
**Prescribing%20dental%20radiogphs%20.pdf**
A PDF booklet, **Guidelines for Prescribing Radiographs**, is available for download from
this **Kodak Dental Systems** website.

**http://www.dent.ohio-state.edu/radiologycarie/tips.htm**
An excellent self-instructional module on **Interpretation Tips** on the website of the
**College of Dentistry, Ohio State University**. This module allows the viewer to select a
radiograph by number, evaluate it, and click to read the answer.

**http://www.ada.org/public/topics/xrays_faq.asp**
Information for patients on how x-rays work and other common questions about
radiographs on the website of the **ADA**.

**http://www.cda.org/page/patient_education_tools**
Patient education tools on the website of the **California Dental Association**. Scroll
down for education materials in English, Spanish, and several other languages.

**http://www.eapd.eu/12A5AECC.en.aspx**
Guidelines for the use of dental radiographs in children from the **European Association**
**of Pediatric Dentistry.**

**http://www.ada.org/2760.aspx#ifpregnant**
Patient education information for pregnant women on dental radiographs on the
website of the ADA. Scroll down page to locate this section.

**SECTION 6:**
# The Human Element

BOX **16-1**   **Tips from an Experienced Clinician**

## Limitations of Radiographs

Keep in mind the fact that periapical and interproximal/bitewing radiographs are two-dimensional representations of a three-dimensional object, and the changes in alveolar bone facial or lingual to the tooth may be obscured by the superimposition of the tooth and the overlying alveolar bone. In addition, alveolar bone height will vary depending upon the radiographic technique used to capture the image; in general, bisecting-angle radiographs will produce more distortion of the tooth and alveolar bone compared to radiographs obtained using the paralleling principle.

## Key Features of Radiographic Accuracy

Key features of radiographic accuracy to look for prior to attempting any interpretation, especially of alveolar bone height, are:

- Radiographic superimposition of the buccal and lingual cusp tips on posterior teeth
- Absence of interproximal overlap potentially obscuring the cementoenamel junction (CEJ)
- Radiographs of sufficient density [darkness] to permit identification of the CEJ

## Using Radiographs in Patient Education

**NOTE:** The radiographs on patient A can be extremely useful in educating the patient regarding the extent and severity of his or her existing disease. For example, the big, easily discerned chunks of calculus on the interproximal spaces can be useful in explaining the "inflammatory" nature of the periodontal disease process—if you have patients, consider the relationship of a splinter in their finger with the subsequent reddening and potential infection should the splinter not be removed in a timely fashion. Similarly, calculus can be portrayed as causing a similar effect in the gum tissues as that of a splinter. The patient should be able to recognize bone loss in the posterior areas of the maxilla if you identify the CEJ as the level where the bone level should be "normally."

## Mastering Radiographic Interpretation

As a beginning student of radiographic interpretation, it is easy to feel overwhelmed by the importance of recognizing sometimes very subtle changes in bony architecture that can have important consequences in terms of patient care and treatment. As with any skill development, it will take time and patience. Develop a systematic approach to analyzing your radiographs so that you know you are covering all of the essential elements. You may wish to start by developing a checklist of normal anatomic structures and another list of deviations and variations from normal that have clinical implications: caries, calculus, calcified pulps, *dens in dente*, periapical radiolucencies/radiopacities, and so forth, simply as a reminder to look for each of these things. With repetition and implementation of the rule of symmetry, you will find that your radiographic assessment skills will increase significantly.

**TABLE 16-1** ENGLISH-TO-SPANISH PHRASE LIST FOR RADIOGRAPHS

| | |
|---|---|
| X-rays (radiographs) help us to better understand your dental needs. | Las radiografías nos ayudan entender sus necesidades dentales. |
| Let me show you some things that I found on your x-rays (radiographs). | Le voy a enseñar unas cosas que he encontrado en sus radiografías. |
| The x-rays show us that you have a cavity/decay. (Clinician points to relevant area.) | Las radiografías nos enseñan que usted tiene un carie/caries. |
| Cavities show up as black, dark gray areas on your teeth. | Caries se mostran como areas negras o gris en los dientes. |
| The x-ray shows us that you may have an infected tooth (abscess). See the dark area around the root of this tooth? (Clinician can compare this to a tooth that has normal bone, so patient can see the difference.) | Las radiografías indican que puede tener un diente infectado (absceso). ¿Nota el area oscura alrededor de la raíz de este diente? |
| The x-rays show us bone loss around these teeth. (Clinician points to relevant areas.) | Las radiografías indican perdida de hueso alrededor de estos dientes. |
| The normal bone level should be here. | El nivel de hueso normal debe estar aqui. |
| Your bone level is here. | Su nivel de hueso está aqui. |
| Do you have any questions about x-rays? | ¿Tiene alguna pregunta sobre sus radiografías? |
| I am going to get my clinic instructor. | Voy a buscar mi instructor. |

## SECTION 7:

# Practical Focus—Fictitious Patient Cases

**DIRECTIONS:**

• This section shows the radiographs for four fictitious patients A, C, D, and E.

• The first patient, Donna Doi, has radiographs that provide an example of a thorough evaluation using the steps outlined in Peak Procedure 16-1 in this module. Use Peak Procedure 16-1 and the Radiograph Evaluation Worksheet to assess the radiographs for the remaining fictitious patient cases, patients A, C, and E.

• The pages in this section may be removed from the book for easier use by tearing along the perforated lines on each page.

• Note: The clinical photographs and radiographs in a fictitious patient case are for illustrative purposes but not necessarily from the same individual. The fictitious patient cases are designed to enhance the learning experiences associated with each case.

# EXAMPLE: FICTITIOUS PATIENT CASE D: MRS. DONNA DOI

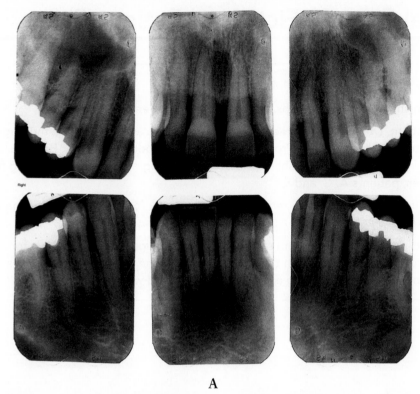

A

**Right**                                                                                                          **Left**

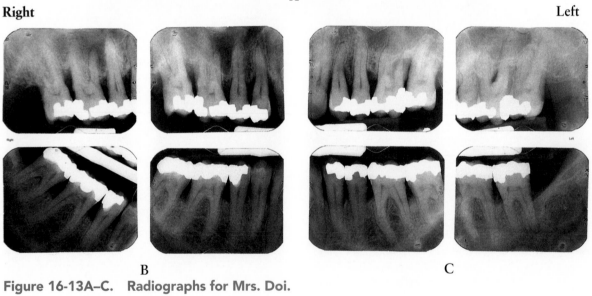

B                                                                          C

**Figure 16-13A–C.    Radiographs for Mrs. Doi.**

# EXAMPLE: RADIOGRAPHIC EVALUATION FOR PATIENT CASE D

1. **Diagnostic Acceptability. Ask the question, "Do these radiographs exhibit the criteria for meeting minimal diagnostic acceptability?" If not, why not?**
   - This series of radiographs consists of 14 periapical radiographs. There are no interproximal/bitewing radiographs available.
   - The paralleling principle was used, and there is good superimposition of the cusp tips suggesting minimal image distortion.
   - Each interproximal space may be seen at least once—somewhere. However, each root apex is not visible at least once; the distal root of the right mandibular second molar is not visible.
   - **Conclusion: No, the set of radiographs does not exhibit minimal diagnostic acceptability.** We would need to retake the mandibular right molar periapical radiograph. Note: several of the individual radiographs exhibit rather severe horizontal overlapping of interproximal spaces; you might feel that the interproximal space of the maxillary left first and second molar is not adequately open, but the chapter author considers this to be "minimally" acceptable but not ideal.

2. **Technique. Ask the question, "Are there any significant technique or processing errors that will influence my ability to correctly evaluate all of the relevant dental structures?"**
   - There are no obvious processing errors, but several of the periapical radiographs exhibit less than optimal film placement: for example, the maxillary and mandibular right and left canine regions do not center the canines well; the maxillary central incisor radiograph is slightly off center, but this doesn't affect the diagnostic value, only the "esthetic" value of the radiograph.
   - The mandibular right molar periapical is tipped cutting off the apices of the premolars; however, these apices are visible on the premolar radiograph.
   - The maxillary left molar periapical exhibits severe overlap of all interproximal spaces.

   **Problem Solving**: Is the overlap of the maxillary left molar radiograph due to excessive horizontal angulation from the mesial or distal? How can you tell? (Hint: look up "Clark's technique/shift-shot/buccal object rule" in your textbook if you don't know.)

3. **Normal Anatomic Structures. Recognize the "normal" anatomic structures observable on the radiographs.** Radiographically visible "normal" anatomic structures on each of the radiographs include:
   - Maxillary right molar: maxillary sinus, lower border of the maxillary sinus, tuberosity of the maxilla
   - Maxillary right premolar: maxillary sinus, anterior and lower border of the maxillary sinus
   - Maxillary right canine: large portion of the maxillary sinus and anterior border of the maxillary sinus; a small portion of the lower border of the nasal fossa may be seen along the upper mesial corner of the radiograph.
   - Maxillary central incisor: incisive foramen is easily seen between the two central incisors, tiny bit of the anterior nasal spine; the nasal fossa and the lower border of the nasal fossa are not easily discerned; a faint radiopacity corresponding to the tip of the nose may also be seen. The lip line is discernable along the central and lateral incisal edges.
   - Maxillary left canine: anterior portion and border of the maxillary sinus
   - Maxillary left premolar: maxillary sinus, lower and anterior border of the maxillary sinus

- Maxillary left molar: maxillary sinus, lower border of the maxillary sinus, tuberosity of the maxilla, coronoid process of the mandible
- Mandibular right molar: external oblique line (distal to second molar); a small portion of the submandibular fossa is visible along the lower distal corner of the radiograph.
- Mandibular right premolar: none noted
- Mandibular right canine: the submandibular fossa may be slightly visible due to angulation at the lower distal edge of the radiograph; no other anatomic structures noted
- Mandibular central incisor: genial tubercles are barely visible at the bottom of the radiograph. Nutrient canals are visible as thin, vertical, radiolucent lines.
- Mandibular left canine: The mental foramen is visible between the apex of the second premolar and first molar.
- Mandibular left premolar: none noted, possibly the submandibular fossa along the lower distal edge of the film
- Mandibular left molar: external oblique line, mandibular canal

4. **Systematic Assessment. Conduct a thorough assessment of the teeth and supporting structures and provide a written summary of your findings.** There were no significant deviations or variations in the symmetry of pulp chambers, no periapical radiolucencies were noted, restorations appear to be clinically acceptable, and there were no open contacts or significantly rotated teeth. Heavy calculus deposits were noted in all four quadrants, and there is generalized moderate-to-severe alveolar bone loss throughout the mandible and maxilla. Bone loss is especially severe around the distal buccal roots of the maxillary right and left first molars. Increased radiolucency in the trifurcations of the maxillary first molars and maxillary right second molar; the bifurcation of the mandibular right second molar exhibits an increased radiolucency and the PDL in the bifurcation area is radiographically more prominent when compared to the other mandibular molar teeth (rule of symmetry).

*Problem-Solving Answer:* *If you identified the excessive horizontal overlap of the interproximal spaces as due to excessive horizontal angulation due to positioning the central ray of the x-ray unit too far from the* **distal***, you are correct. According to Clark's rule, objects on the lingual move in the direction of tube shift. If you look closely at the position of the first molar root apices, the lingual and distal-buccal roots are superimposed. Excessive angulation from the mesial would cause the mesial-buccal and lingual roots to overlap.*

# FICTITIOUS PATIENT CASE A: MR. ALAN ASCARI

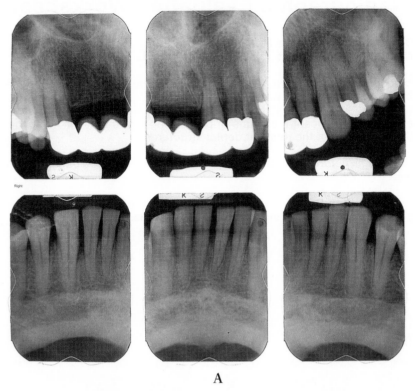

A

Right                                                                                    Left

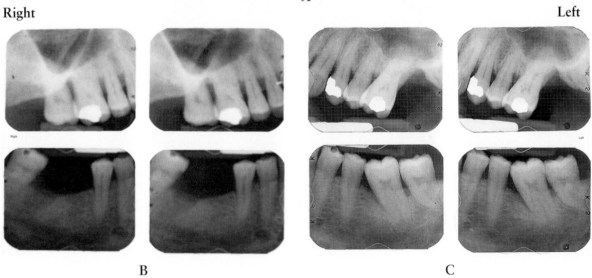

B                                                                C

**Figure 16-14A–C.   Radiographs for Mr. Ascari.**

# Radiographic Evaluation Worksheet

*Directions:* Complete the four steps listed below.
Attach additional sheets to this form as needed.

1. *Diagnostic acceptability*: Do these radiographs exhibit the criteria for meeting minimal diagnostic acceptability? If not, why?

2. *Technique*: List any significant technique or processing errors that will influence your ability to correctly evaluate all of the relevant dental structures.

3. *Normal anatomic structures*: List the "normal" anatomic structures observable on the radiographs.

4. *Systematic assessment*: Conduct a thorough assessment of the teeth and supporting structures and provide a written summary of your findings.

**Figure 16-15. Radiographic Evaluation Worksheet for Mr. Ascari.**

# FICTITIOUS PATIENT CASE C: CARLOS CHAVEZ

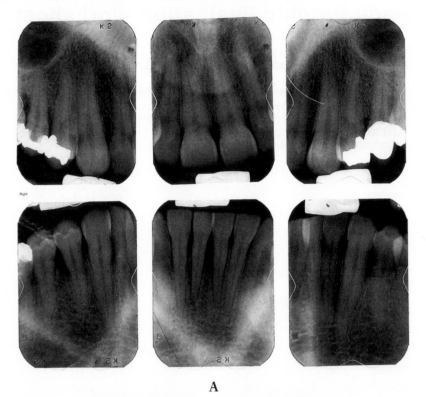

**A**

Right                                                                                                    Left

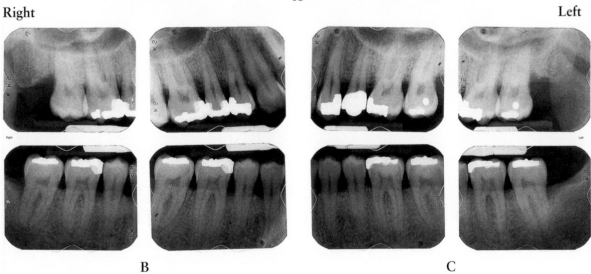

**B**                                                         **C**

**Figure 16-16A–C.** Radiographs for Mr. Chavez.

# Radiographic Evaluation Worksheet

*Directions:* Complete the four steps listed below.
Attach additional sheets to this form as needed.

1. *Diagnostic acceptability*: Do these radiographs exhibit the criteria for meeting minimal diagnostic acceptability? If not, why?

2. *Technique*: List any significant technique or processing errors that will influence your ability to correctly evaluate all of the relevant dental structures.

3. *Normal anatomic structures*: List the "normal" anatomic structures observable on the radiographs.

4. *Systematic assessment*: Conduct a thorough assessment of the teeth and supporting structures and provide a written summary of your findings.

**Figure 16-17.   Radiographic Evaluation Worksheet for Mr. Chavez.**

# FICTITIOUS PATIENT CASE E: MS. ESTHER EADS

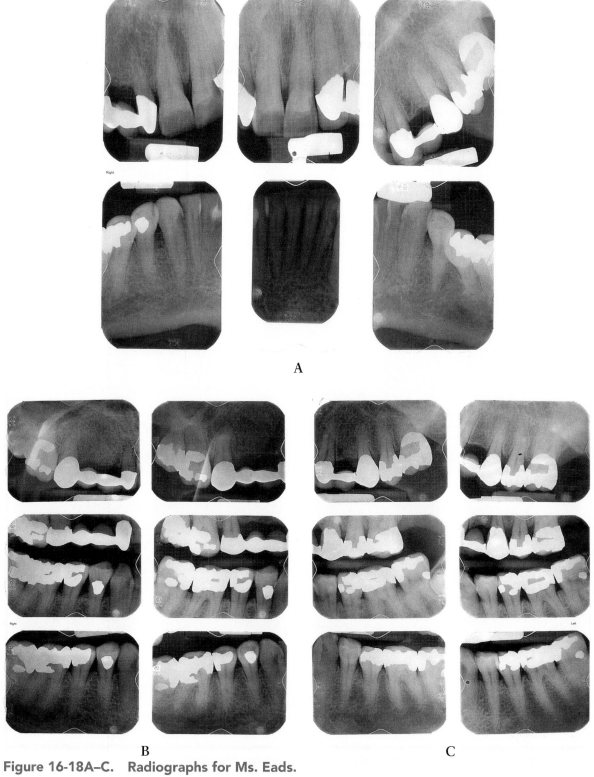

**Figure 16-18A–C.** **Radiographs for Ms. Eads.**

# Radiographic Evaluation Worksheet

*Directions:* Complete the four steps listed below.
Attach additional sheets to this form as needed.

1. *Diagnostic acceptability*: Do these radiographs exhibit the criteria for meeting minimal diagnostic acceptability? If not, why?

2. *Technique*: List any significant technique or processing errors that will influence your ability to correctly evaluate all of the relevant dental structures.

3. *Normal anatomic structures*: List the "normal" anatomic structures observable on the radiographs.

4. *Systematic assessment*: Conduct a thorough assessment of the teeth and supporting structures and provide a written summary of your findings.

**Figure 16-19.  Radiographic Evaluation Worksheet for Ms. Eads.**

**SECTION 8:**
# Practical Focus—Panoramic Radiographs

**DIRECTIONS:**

- This section has six panoramic radiographs for interpretation.

- Please provide a brief description of the radiographic findings to include, but not to be limited to, the following, if present, for each panoramic radiograph:

  ○ Missing teeth

  ○ General description of alveolar bone height in each arch

  ○ Presence or absence of calculus, caries, periapical pathology (if any)

  ○ Dental restorative materials

  ○ Any radiographic "deviations" from normal

- The pages in this section may be removed from the book for easier use by tearing along the perforated lines on each page.

## PANORAMIC RADIOGRAPH 1

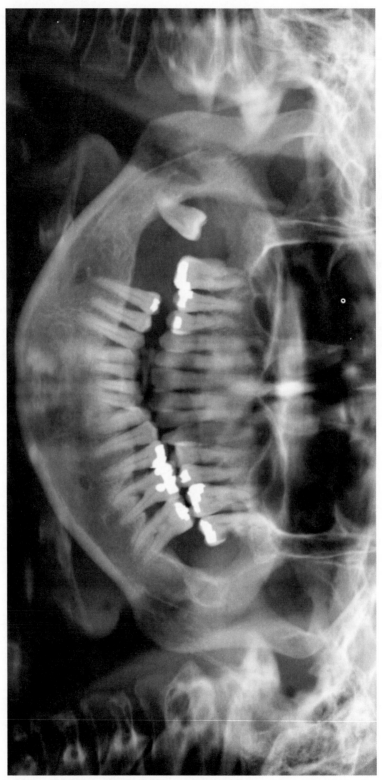

**Figure 16-20. Panoramic radiograph 1.**

# PANORAMIC RADIOGRAPH 2

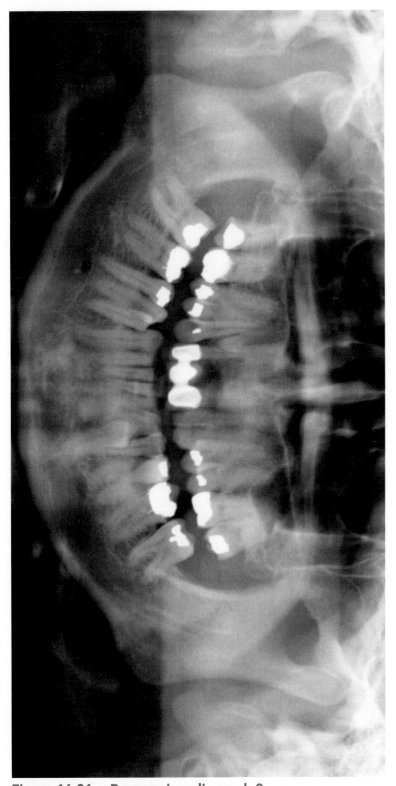

**Figure 16-21. Panoramic radiograph 2.**

## PANORAMIC RADIOGRAPH 3

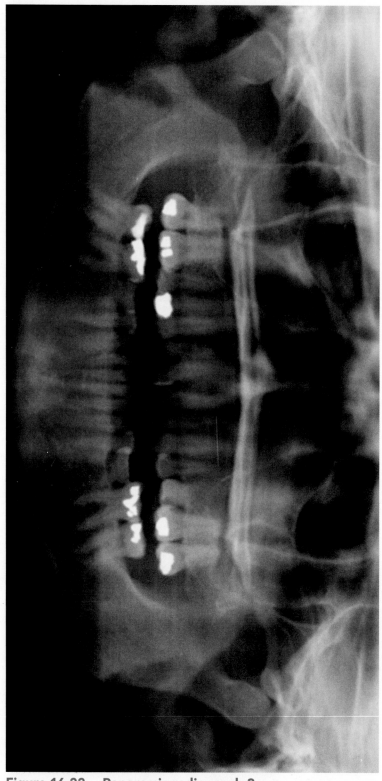

**Figure 16-22.** Panoramic radiograph 3.

# PANORAMIC RADIOGRAPH 4

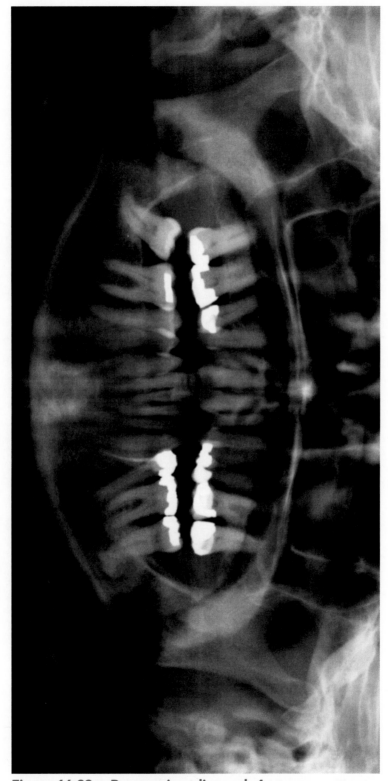

**Figure 16-23.   Panoramic radiograph 4.**

## PANORAMIC RADIOGRAPH 5

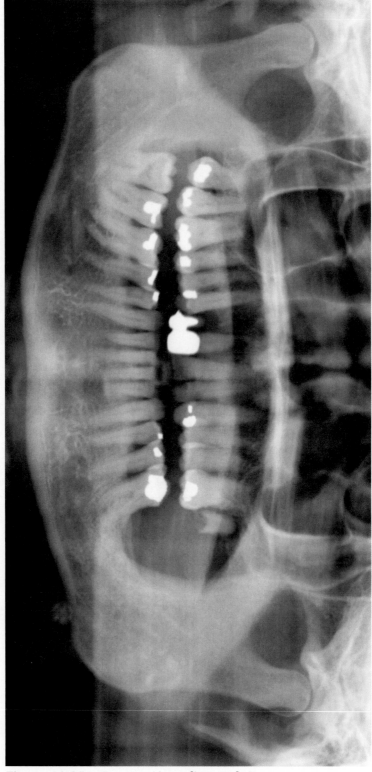

**Figure 16-24.   Panoramic radiograph 5.**

# PANORAMIC RADIOGRAPH 6

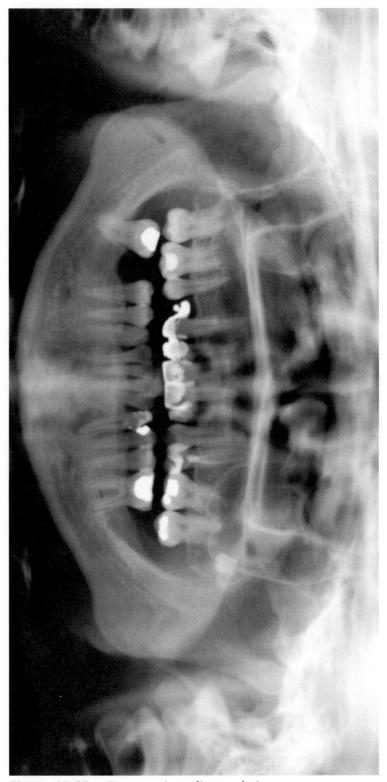

**Figure 16-25. Panoramic radiograph 6.**

SECTION 9:
# Skill Check

**SKILL CHECKLIST:** DENTAL RADIOGRAPHS

Student: _____     Evaluator: _____

Date: _____

**DIRECTIONS FOR STUDENT CLINICIAN:** Using **Column S**, evaluate your skill level as **S** (satisfactory) or **U** (unsatisfactory).

**DIRECTIONS FOR EVALUATOR:** Use **Column E**. Indicate **S** (satisfactory) or **U** (unsatisfactory). In the optional grade percentage calculation, each **S** equals 1 point, and each **U** equals 0 points.

| CRITERIA | S | E |
|---|---|---|
| **Defines the term minimal diagnostic acceptability.** | | |
| **Given a set of CMRS/FMX, determines if the radiographs exhibit the criteria for meeting minimal diagnostic acceptability.** | | |
| **Recognizes and lists in writing any significant technique or processing errors that would influence a clinician's ability to correctly evaluate all the relevant dental structures on the radiographs.** | | |
| **Lists in writing the "normal" anatomic structures observable on the radiographs.** | | |
| **Conducts a thorough assessment of the teeth and supporting structures and provides a written summary of his or her findings.** | | |

OPTIONAL: SATISFACTORY PERFORMANCE CRITERIA
Student written assessment is in 80% agreement with the evaluator's assessment.

## COMMUNICATION SKILL CHECKLIST: DENTAL RADIOGRAPHS

Student: _____     Evaluator: _____

Date: _____

> **Roles:**
> - Student 1 = Plays the role of the patient.
> - Student 2 = Plays the role of the clinician.
> - Student 3 or instructor = Plays the role of the clinic instructor near the end of the role-play.

**DIRECTIONS FOR STUDENT CLINICIAN:** Using **Column S**, evaluate your skill level as **S** (satisfactory) or **U** (unsatisfactory).

**DIRECTIONS FOR EVALUATOR:** Use **Column E**. Indicate **S** (satisfactory) or **U** (unsatisfactory). In the optional grade percentage calculation, each **S** equals 1 point, and each **U** equals 0 points.

| CRITERIA | S | E |
|---|---|---|
| **Explains to the patient how radiographs help clinicians to better understand a patient's dental needs.** | | |
| **Points out and explains findings on the radiographs to the patient.** | | |
| **Encourages patient questions.** | | |
| **Answers the patient's questions fully and accurately.** | | |
| **Communicates with the patient at an appropriate level and avoids dental/medical terminology or jargon.** | | |
| **Accurately communicates the findings to the clinical instructor. Discusses the implications for dental treatment using correct medical and dental terminology.** | | |

OPTIONAL GRADE PERCENTAGE CALCULATION

Using the entries in the **E** column, assign a point value of 1 for each **S** and 0 for each **U**. Add the total assigned as 1's _____ and divide by 6 to arrive at the percentage grade. _____

# 17 Comprehensive Patient Cases F–K

## MODULE OVERVIEW

Module 17 presents six fictitious patient cases, patients F–K. The fictitious patient cases in this module provide opportunities to practice interpreting and communicating assessment information.

## MODULE OUTLINE

## OBJECTIVES

- Demonstrate knowledge of information gathering and evaluation by applying concepts from the modules in this book to fictitious comprehensive patient cases F–K.
- During a role-play, provide information to each patient about his or her assessment findings.
- During a role-play, accurately communicate the assessment findings to the clinical instructor. Discuss the implications for dental treatment using correct medical and dental terminology.

## SOURCES OF CLINICAL PHOTOGRAPHS

The authors gratefully acknowledge the sources of the clinical photographs in this module.

### Case F

- Figure 17-4. Image provided by Stedman's Medical Dictionary.
- Figure 17-5. Dr. Richard Foster, Guilford Technical Community College, Jamestown, NC.
- Figure 17-6. Dr. Richard Foster, Guilford Technical Community College, Jamestown, NC.
- Figure 17-7. Dr. Don Rolfs, Periodontal Foundations, Wenatchee, WA.

### Case G

- Figure 17-12. From Langlais RP, Miller CS, Nield-Gehrig JS. *Color Atlas of Common Oral Diseases*. 4th ed. Philadelphia, PA: Lippincott Williams & Wilkins; 2009.
- Figure 17-13. Dr. Richard Foster, Guilford Technical Community College, Jamestown, NC.
- Figure 17-14. Dr. Richard Foster, Guilford Technical Community College, Jamestown, NC.

### Case H

- Figure 17-19. Dr. Richard Foster, Guilford Technical Community College, Jamestown, NC.
- Figure 17-20. Dr. Richard Foster, Guilford Technical Community College, Jamestown, NC.
- Figure 17-21. Dr. Richard Foster, Guilford Technical Community College, Jamestown, NC.

### Case I

- Figure 17-26. Centers for Disease Control and Prevention Public Health Image Library (PHIL).
- Figure 17-27. Dr. Richard Foster, Guilford Technical Community College, Jamestown, NC.
- Figure 17-28. Dr. Richard Foster, Guilford Technical Community College, Jamestown, NC.

### Case J

- Figure 17-33. Dr. Charles Goldberg, University of California San Diego School of Medicine.
- Figure 17-34. Image provided by Stedman's Medical Dictionary.
- Figure 17-35. Dr. Richard Foster, Guilford Technical Community College, Jamestown, NC.
- Figure 17-36. Dr. Richard Foster, Guilford Technical Community College, Jamestown, NC.
- Figure 17-37. Dr. Richard Foster, Guilford Technical Community College, Jamestown, NC.
- Figure 17-38. Catherine Ranson, George Brown College, Toronto.
- Figure 17-39. Catherine Ranson, George Brown College, Toronto.

### Case K

- Figure 17-42. From Goodheart HP. *Goodheart's Photoguide of Common Skin Disorders*. 2nd ed. Philadelphia, PA: Lippincott Williams & Wilkins; 2003.
- Figure 17-43. Dr. Richard Foster, Guilford Technical Community College, Jamestown, NC.
- Figure 17-44. Dr. Richard Foster, Guilford Technical Community College, Jamestown, NC.

DIRECTIONS FOR COMPLETING THE FICTITIOUS PATIENT CASES:

1. Compile and analyze findings. Follow the Peak Procedures outlined in Modules 4–16 to assess the patient findings.

2. Create a summary statement. Use notebook paper to create a summary worksheet for each patient. List the significant findings for each assessment category and explain how each finding will impact the dental hygiene care plan.

3. Complete the communication role-play in Section 7 of this module. Clearly and accurately communicate assessment findings to each patient. Present assessment findings to your clinical instructor and discuss the implications of these findings for patient care.

Note: The clinical photographs and radiographs in this module are for illustrative purposes but are not necessarily from the same individual. The components of a fictitious patient case were selected to enhance the learning experiences associated with the case.

## SECTION 1:

# Patient F, Mr. Frasier Fairhall

MetLife                                                                                                                        University of the Pacific

### HEALTH HISTORY - English

Patient Name: _Fairhall, Frasier F._                    Patient Identification Number: _F-345680_

Birth Date: _57 years_

### I. CIRCLE APPROPRIATE ANSWER (leave BLANK if you do not understand question):

1. (Yes)  No    Is your general health good?
2. Yes  (No)   Has there been a change in your health within the last year?
3. Yes  (No)   Have you been hospitalized or had a serious illness in the last three years?
              If YES, why? _____
4. Yes  (No)   Are you being treated by a physician now? For what? _____

Date of last medical exam? _10 years ago_        Date of last dental exam? _5 years_
5. Yes  (No)   Have you had problems with prior dental treatment?
6. Yes  (No)   Are you in pain now?

### II. HAVE YOU EXPERIENCED:

| | | |
|---|---|---|
| 7. Yes (No) | Chest pain (angina)? | 18. Yes (No) Dizziness? |
| 8. Yes (No) | Swollen ankles? | 19. Yes (No) Ringing in ears? |
| 9. Yes (No) | Shortness of breath? | 20. Yes (No) Headaches? |
| 10. Yes (No) | Recent weight loss, fever, night sweats? | 21. Yes (No) Fainting spells? |
| 11. (Yes) No | Persistent cough, coughing up blood? | 22. Yes (No) Blurred vision? |
| 12. (Yes) No | Bleeding problems, bruising easily? _gums bleed when_ | 23. Yes (No) Seizures? |
| 13. Yes (No) | Sinus problems? _I brush_ | 24. Yes (No) Excessive thirst? |
| 14. Yes (No) | Difficulty swallowing? | 25. Yes (No) Frequent urination? |
| 15. Yes (No) | Diarrhea, constipation, blood in stools? | 26. (Yes) No Dry mouth? |
| 16. Yes (No) | Frequent vomiting, nausea? | 27. Yes (No) Jaundice? |
| 17. Yes (No) | Difficulty urinating, blood in urine? | 28. Yes (No) Joint pain? |

### III. DO YOU HAVE OR HAVE YOU HAD:

| | | |
|---|---|---|
| 29. Yes (No) | Heart disease? | 40. Yes (No) AIDS? |
| 30. Yes (No) | Heart attack, heart defects? | 41. Yes (No) Tumors, cancer? |
| 31. Yes (No) | Heart murmurs? | 42. Yes (No) Arthritis, rheumatism? |
| 32. Yes (No) | Rheumatic fever? | 43. Yes (No) Eye diseases? |
| 33. Yes (No) | Stroke, hardening of arteries? | 44. Yes (No) Skin deases? |
| 34. Yes (No) | High blood pressure? | 45. Yes (No) Anemia? |
| 35. Yes (No) | Asthma, TB, emphysema, other lung disease? | 46. Yes (No) VD (syphilis or gonorrhea)? |
| 36. (Yes) No | Hepatitis, other liver disease? _2 years ago_ | 47. Yes (No) Herpes? |
| 37. Yes (No) | Stomach problems, ulcers? _Iodine, ragweed,_ | 48. Yes (No) Kidney, bladder disease? |
| 38. (Yes) No | Allergies to: drugs, foods, medications, latex? _and cats_ | 49. Yes (No) Thyroid, adrenal disease? |
| 39. Yes (No) | Family history of diabetes, heart problems, tumors? | 50. Yes (No) Diabetes? |

### IV. DO YOU HAVE OR HAVE YOU HAD:

| | | |
|---|---|---|
| 51. Yes (No) | Psychiatric care? | 56. Yes (No) Hospitalization? |
| 52. Yes (No) | Radiation treatments? | 57. Yes (No) Blood transfusions? |
| 53. Yes (No) | Chemotherapy? | 58. Yes (No) Surgeries? |
| 54. Yes (No) | Prosthetic heart valve? | 59. Yes (No) Pacemaker? |
| 55. Yes (No) | Artificial joint? | 60. Yes (No) Contact lenses? |

### V. ARE YOU TAKING:

| | | |
|---|---|---|
| 61. Yes (No) | Recreational drugs? | 63. (Yes) No Tobacco in any form? _cigarettes,_ |
| 62. (Yes) No | Drugs, medications, over-the-counter medicines (including Aspirin), natural remedies? | 64. (Yes) No Alcohol? _3 packs/day_ |
| | | _4 cocktails/day_ |

Please list: _See Medication List_

### VI. WOMEN ONLY:

65. Yes  (No)   Are you or could you be pregnant or nursing?          63. Yes  (No)   Taking birth control pills?

### VII. ALL PATIENTS:

64. (Yes)  No    Do you have or have you had anyother diseases or medical problems NOT listed on this form?
If so, please explain: _have trouble sleeping; get sores in my mouth often_

_To the best of my knowledge, I have answered every question completely and accurately. I will inform my dentist of any change in my health and/or medication._

Patient's signature: _Frasier Fairhall_                                                        Date: _1-15-20XX_

### RECALL REVIEW:

1. Patient's signature: _____ Date: _____

2. Patient's signature: _____ Date: _____

3. Patient's signature: _____ Date: _____

The Health History is created and maintained by the University of Pacific School of Dentistry, San Francisco, California.
Support for the translation and dissemination of the Health Histories comes from MetLife Dental Care.

Figure 17-1. Medical history for fictitious patient F.

# Medication List

Patient ___FRASIER FAIRHALL___          Date ___2/05/XX___

| PRESCRIBED |
|---|
| NONE |

| OVER-THE-COUNTER |
|---|
| NYTOL SLEEPING PILL - ONE EACH NIGHT |

| VITAMINS, HERBS, DIET SUPPLEMENTS |
|---|
| NONE |

Figure 17-2.  Medication list for fictitious patient F.

# Smoking History

Patient ___FRASIER FAIRHALL___ Date ___2/05/XX___

1. At what age did you begin to smoke? ___13___

2. How many cigarettes do you smoke per day now? ___3 PACKS___
   Per day at your heaviest? ___3 PACKS___

3. How many times have you tried to stop smoking? ___5___
   ☐ Never tried to stop

4. What is the longest period of time you have gone without smoking? ___5 DAYS___

5. What forms of tobacco are you currently using? *(Please check all that apply.)*
   ☒ Cigarettes          ☐ Chewing tobacco
   ☐ Pipes               ☐ Snuff
   ☐ Cigars              ☐ Other

6. Do your ☐ family members, ☒ friends, ☒ co-workers smoke? *(Please check all that apply. Circle if you live with any of these smokers.)*

7. What smoking cessation methods have you tried? *(Please check all that apply.)*
   ☐ None                ☐ Self-help programs
   ☒ Cold turkey         ☐ Gradual reduction
   ☐ Hypnosis            ☐ Laser
   ☐ Acupuncture         ☒ Other ___NICOTINE GUM___

8. Are you being ☒ encouraged, or ☐ discouraged to stop smoking by any of the following? *(Please check all that apply.)*
   ☐ Spouse or significant other    ☐ Friend
   ☒ Child                          ☐ Co-worker
   ☐ Other family member

9. Who do you turn to for support? *(Please check all that apply.)*
   ☒ Spouse or significant other    ☐ Counselor
   ☐ Parent                         ☐ Healthcare provider
   ☐ Sibling                        ☐ Friend
   ☒ Other family member            ☐ Co-worker
   ☐ Clergy/rabbi/priest

Please rank the following on a scale of 1 (strongly disagree) to 5 (strongly agree):
   I am ready to stop smoking at this time:        1 ② 3 4 5
   I am concerned about weight gain:               ① 2 3 4 5
   I am concerned about dealing with stress:       1 2 3 4 ⑤

*Frasier Fairhall*                    *Esther Manheim, DH2*
_____           _____
Patient Signature                     Reviewed by

Figure 17-3.   Smoking history for fictitious patient F.

## Vital Signs

Name _FRASIER FAIRHALL_    Date _2/05/XX_

Temperature _98.2°F (36.77°C)_    Pulse _80_

Respiratory Rate _20_    Blood Pressure _158/100_

Tobacco Use:    ☐ Never    ☐ Former

☒ Cigarettes _3_ packs/day    ☐ Pipe    ☐ Smokeless tobacco

Figure 17-4.    Vital signs findings for fictitious patient F.

**Finding:**

Location: left side of face

Size: two raised lesions; each lesion is 1 cm in diameter

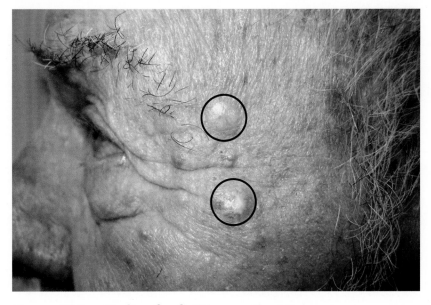

Figure 17-5.    Finding for fictitious patient F.

**Finding:**

Location: floor of the mouth

Size: 1 cm in anterior-posterior length;

0.5 cm in superior-inferior width

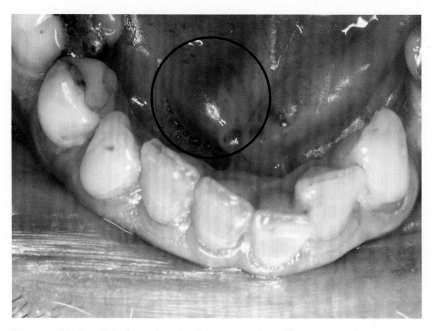

Figure 17-6.   Finding for fictitious patient F.

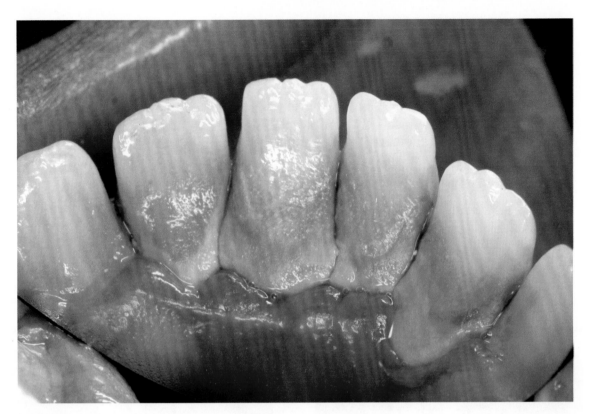

Figure 17-7. Fictitious patient F: Mandibular anterior sextant, lingual aspect.

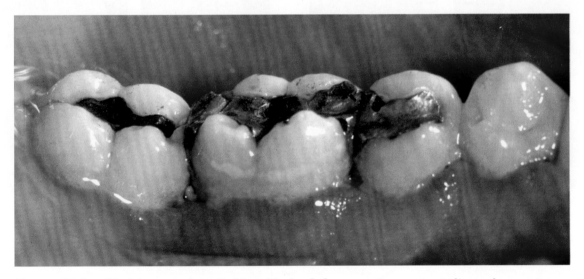

Figure 17-8. Fictitious patient F: Mandibular left posterior sextant, lingual aspect.

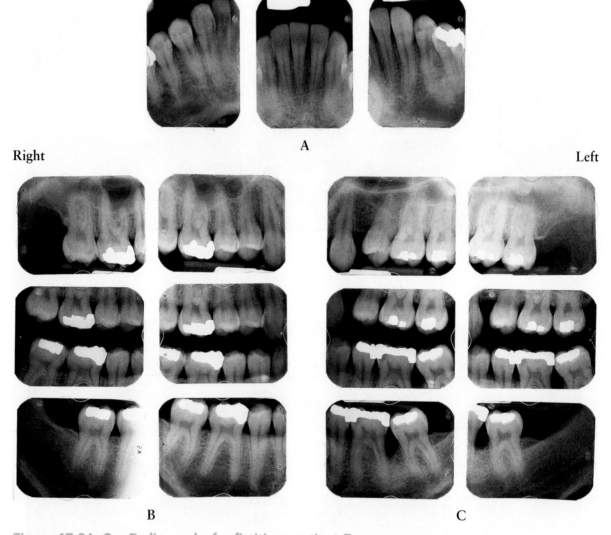

**Right**

**Left**

A

B

C

**Figure 17-9A–C. Radiographs for fictitious patient F.**

## SECTION 2:

# Patient G, Mr. Gumercindo de la Garza

MetLife                                                                        University of the Pacific

### HISTORIA MÉDICA - Spanish

Nombre del paciente: _De La Garza, Gumersindo_          No. de Ident. del Paciente: _G-369221_

Fecha de nacimiento: _16 years_

#### I. MARQUE CON UN CÍRCULO LA RESPUESTA CORRECTA (Deje en BLANCO si no entiende la pregunta):

1. (Sí)  No    ¿Está en buena salud general?
2. Sí  (No)   ¿Han habido cambios en su salud durante el último año?
3. Sí  (No)   ¿Ha estado hospitalizado/a o ha tenido de una enfermedad grave en los últimos tres años?
   ¿Si Sí, por qué?_____
4. (Sí)  No    ¿Se encuentra actualmente bajo tratamiento médico? ¿Para qué? _Type I diabetes_

   Fecha de su último examen médico: _4 months ago_           Fecha de su última cita dental: _1 year ago_
5. (Sí)  No    ¿Ha tenido problemas con algún tratamiento dental en el pasado? _gums bleed when I brush_
6. Sí  (No)   ¿Tiene algún dolor ahora?

#### II. HA NOTADO:

7. Sí  (No)   ¿Dolor de pecho (angina)?
8. Sí  (No)   ¿Los tobillos hinchados?
9. Sí  (No)   ¿Falta de aliento?
10. Sí  (No)  ¿Reciente pérdida de peso, fiebre, sudor en la noche?
11. Sí  (No)  ¿Tos persistente o tos con sangre?
12. Sí  (No)  ¿Problemas de sangramiento, moretes?
13. Sí  (No)  ¿Problemas nasales (sinusitis)?
14. Sí  (No)  ¿Dificultad al tragar?
15. Sí  (No)  ¿Diarrea, estreñimiento, sangre en las heces?
16. Sí  (No)  ¿Vómitos con frecuencia, náuseas?
17. Sí  (No)  ¿Difucltad al orinar, sangre en la orina?

18. Sí  (No)  ¿Mareos?
19. Sí  (No)  ¿Ruidos o zumbidos en los oídos?
20. Sí  (No)  ¿Dolores de cabeza?
21. Sí  (No)  ¿Desmayos?
22. Sí  (No)  ¿Vista borrosa?
23. Sí  (No)  ¿Convulsiones?
24. Sí  (No)  ¿Sed excesiva?
25. Sí  (No)  ¿Orina con frecuencia?
26. Sí  (No)  ¿Boca seca?
27. Sí  (No)  ¿Ictericia?
28. Sí  (No)  ¿Dolor o rigidez en las articulaciones?

#### III. TIENE O HA TENIDO:

29. Sí  (No)  ¿Enfermedades del corazón?
30. Sí  (No)  ¿Infarto de corazón, defectos en el corazón?
31. Sí  (No)  ¿Soplos en el corazón?
32. Sí  (No)  ¿Fiebre reumática?
33. Sí  (No)  ¿Apoplejía, endurecimiento de las arterias?
34. Sí  (No)  ¿Presión sanguínea alta?
35. Sí  (No)  ¿Asma, tuberculosis, enfisema, otras enfermedades pulmonares?
36. Sí  (No)  ¿Hepatitis, otras enfermedades del hígado?
37. (Sí)  No   ¿Problemas del estómago, úlceras?  _Aspirin causes_
38. (Sí)  No   ¿Alergias a remedios, comidas, medicamentos látex?  _hives_
39. Sí  (No)  ¿Familiares con diabetes, problemas de corazón, tumores?

40. Sí  (No)  ¿SIDA?
41. Sí  (No)  ¿Tumores, cáncer?
42. Sí  (No)  ¿Artritis, reuma?
43. Sí  (No)  ¿Enfermedades de los ojos?
44. Sí  (No)  ¿Enfermedades de la piel?
45. Sí  (No)  ¿Anemia?
46. Sí  (No)  ¿Enfermedades venéreas (sífilis o gonorrea)?
47. Sí  (No)  ¿Herpes?
48. Sí  (No)  ¿Enfermedades renales (riñón), vejiga?
49. Sí  (No)  ¿Enfermedades de tiroides o glándulas suprarrenales?
50. (Sí)  No   ¿Diabetes?

#### IV. TIENE O HA TENIDO:

51. Sí  (No)  ¿Tratamiento psiquiátrico?
52. Sí  (No)  ¿Tratamientos de radiación?
53. Sí  (No)  ¿Quimioterapia?
54. Sí  (No)  ¿Válvula artificial del corazón?
55. Sí  (No)  ¿Articulación articial?

56. Sí  (No)  ¿Hospitalizaciones?
57. Sí  (No)  ¿Transfusiones de sangre?
58. Sí  (No)  ¿Circugías?
59. Sí  (No)  ¿Marcapasos?
60. Sí  (No)  ¿Lentes de contacto?

#### V. ESTÁ TOMANDO:

61. Sí  (No)  ¿Drogas de uso recreativo?
62. (Sí)  No   ¿Remedios, medicamentos, medicamentos sin receta (incluyendo aspirina)?

63. Sí  (No)  ¿Tabaco de cualquier tipo?
64. Sí  (No)  ¿Alcohol (bebidas alcohólicas)?

Liste por favor: _See Medication List_

#### VI. SÓLO PARA MUJERES:

65. Sí  (No)  ¿Está o podría estar embarazada o dando pecho?        63. Sí  No    ¿Está tomando pastillas anticonceptivas?

#### VII. PARA TODOS LOS PACIENTES:

64. Sí  (No)  ¿Tiene o ha tenido alguna otra enfermedad o problema médico que NO está en este cuestionario?
Si la respuesta es afirmativa, explique:_____

Que yo sepa, he respondido completamente y correctamente todas las preguntas. Informaré a mi dentista si hay algún cambio en mi salud y/o en los medicamentos que tomo.
Firma del Paciente: _Gumersindo De La Garza_                    Fecha: _1-15-20XX_

#### REVISIÓN SUPLEMENTARIA:

1. Firma del Paciente: _June Ricard (guardian: Gumersindo is an exchange student living with us for 6 months)_    Fecha: _1-15-20XX_
2. Firma del Paciente: _____    Fecha: _____
3. Firma del Paciente: _____    Fecha: _____

The Health History is created and maintined by the University of Pacific School of Dentistry, San Francisco, California.
Support for the translation and dissemination of the Health Histories comes from MetLife Dental Care.

**Figure 17-10.   Medical history for fictitious patient G.**

## Medication List

Patient _GUMERCINDO DE LA GARZA_    Date _____ **2/05/XX** _____

| PRESCRIBED |
| --- |
| HUMULIN N INSULIN INJECTION SC B.I.D. |

| OVER-THE-COUNTER |
| --- |
| NONE |

| VITAMINS, HERBS, DIET SUPPLEMENTS |
| --- |

**Figure 17-11.   Medication list for fictitious patient G.**

## Vital Signs

Name _GUMERCINDO DE LA GARZA_ Date _2/05/XX_

Temperature _96.8°F  (36°C)_ Pulse _60_

Respiratory Rate _16_ Blood Pressure _110/70_

Tobacco Use:    ☒ Never        ☐ Former

☐ Cigarettes ___packs/day      ☐ Pipe      ☐ Smokeless tobacco

Figure 17-12.   Vital signs findings for fictitious patient G.

**Finding:**

Location: lower lip
Size: 0.5 cm in diameter

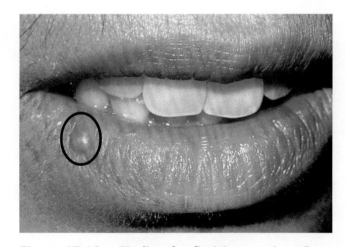

Figure 17-13.   Finding for fictitious patient G.

**Finding:**

Location: ventral surface of tongue

Size: 2.5 cm in anterior-posterior length; 1.5 cm in width

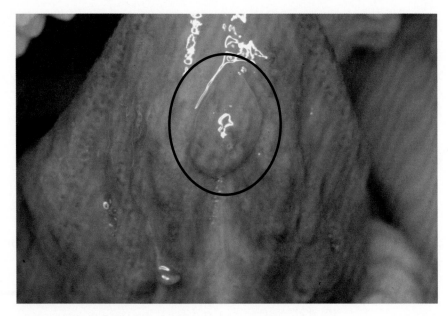

Figure 17-14.   Finding for fictitious patient G.

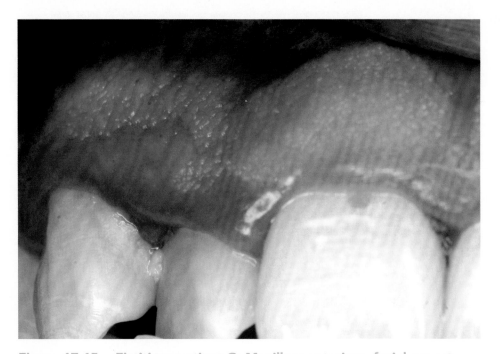

Figure 17-15.   Fictitious patient G: Maxillary anteriors, facial aspect.

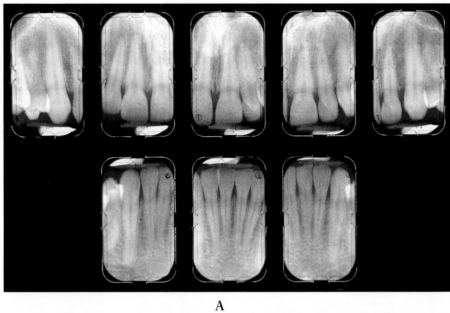

A

Right                                                                                                    Left

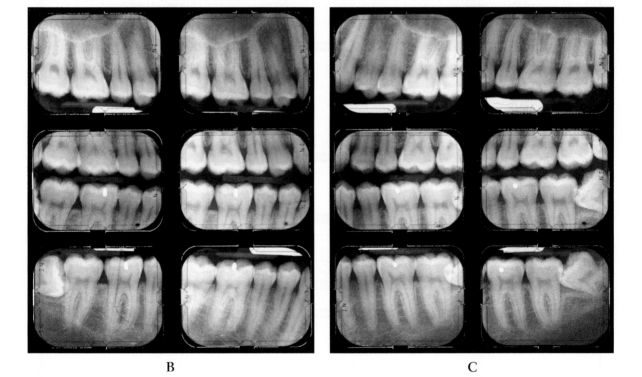

B                                                      C

Figure 17-16A–C.   Radiographs for fictitious patient G.

## SECTION 3:

# Patient H, Mr. Harry Haversmith

| MetLife | | University of the Pacific |
|---|---|---|

**HEALTH HISTORY - English**

Patient Name: _Haversmith, Harry H._      Patient Identification Number: _H-789441_

Birth Date: _32 years_

**I. CIRCLE APPROPRIATE ANSWER (leave BLANK if you do not understand question):**

1. (Yes)  No   Is your general health good?
2. Yes  (No)   Has there been a change in your health within the last year?
3. (Yes)  No   Have you been hospitalized or had a serious illness in the last three years?
   If YES, why? _chest pain_
4. (Yes)  No   Are you being treated by a physician now? For what? _regular checkups by cardiologist_
   Date of last medical exam? _3 months ago_      Date of last dental exam? _2 years ago_
5. Yes  (No)   Have you had problems with prior dental treatment?
6. Yes  (No)   Are you in pain now?

**II. HAVE YOU EXPERIENCED:**

| | | | | | | |
|---|---|---|---|---|---|---|
| 7. | (Yes) | No | Chest pain (angina)? | 18. Yes | (No) | Dizziness? |
| 8. | Yes | (No) | Swollen ankles? | 19. Yes | (No) | Ringing in ears? |
| 9. | Yes | (No) | Shortness of breath? | 20. Yes | (No) | Headaches? |
| 10. | Yes | (No) | Recent weight loss, fever, night sweats? | 21. Yes | (No) | Fainting spells? |
| 11. | Yes | (No) | Persistent cough, coughing up blood? | 22. Yes | (No) | Blurred vision? |
| 12. | Yes | (No) | Bleeding problems, bruising easily? | 23. Yes | (No) | Seizures? |
| 13. | Yes | (No) | Sinus problems? | 24. Yes | (No) | Excessive thirst? |
| 14. | Yes | (No) | Difficulty swallowing? | 25. Yes | (No) | Frequent urination? |
| 15. | Yes | (No) | Diarrhea, constipation, blood in stools? | 26. Yes | (No) | Dry mouth? |
| 16. | Yes | (No) | Frequent vomiting, nausea? | 27. Yes | (No) | Jaundice? |
| 17. | Yes | (No) | Difficulty urinating, blood in urine? | 28. Yes | (No) | Joint pain? |

**III. DO YOU HAVE OR HAVE YOU HAD:**

| | | | | | | |
|---|---|---|---|---|---|---|
| 29. | Yes | (No) | Heart disease? | 40. Yes | (No) | AIDS? |
| 30. | (Yes) | No | Heart attack, heart defects? | 41. Yes | (No) | Tumors, cancer? |
| 31. | Yes | (No) | Heart murmurs? | 42. Yes | (No) | Arthritis, rheumatism? |
| 32. | Yes | (No) | Rheumatic fever? | 43. Yes | (No) | Eye diseases? |
| 33. | Yes | (No) | Stroke, hardening of arteries? | 44. Yes | (No) | Skin deases? |
| 34. | (Yes) | No | High blood pressure? | 45. Yes | (No) | Anemia? |
| 35. | Yes | (No) | Asthma, TB, emphysema, other lung disease? | 46. Yes | (No) | VD (syphilis or gonorrhea)? |
| 36. | Yes | No | Hepatitis, other liver disease? | 47. Yes | (No) | Herpes? |
| 37. | Yes | (No) | Stomach problems, ulcers? | 48. Yes | (No) | Kidney, bladder disease? |
| 38. | (Yes) | No | Allergies to: drugs, foods, medications, latex? _Penicllin_ | 49. Yes | (No) | Thyroid, adrenal disease? |
| 39. | Yes | (No) | Family history of diabetes, heart problems, tumors? | 50. Yes | (No) | Diabetes? |

**IV. DO YOU HAVE OR HAVE YOU HAD:**

| | | | | | | |
|---|---|---|---|---|---|---|
| 51. | Yes | (No) | Psychiatric care? | 56. Yes | (No) | Hospitalization? |
| 52. | Yes | (No) | Radiation treatments? | 57. Yes | (No) | Blood transfusions? |
| 53. | Yes | (No) | Chemotherapy? | 58. Yes | (No) | Surgeries? |
| 54. | Yes | (No) | Prosthetic heart valve? | 59. Yes | (No) | Pacemaker? |
| 55. | Yes | (No) | Artificial joint? | 60. Yes | (No) | Contact lenses? |

**V. ARE YOU TAKING:**

| | | | | | | |
|---|---|---|---|---|---|---|
| 61. | Yes | (No) | Recreational drugs? | 63. (Yes) | No | Tobacco in any form? |
| 62. | (Yes) | No | Drugs, medications, over-the-counter medicines (including Aspirin), natural remedies? | 64. (Yes) | No | Alcohol? _one glass of wine about 3x a week_ |

Please list: _See Medication List_

**VI. WOMEN ONLY:**

| | | | | | | |
|---|---|---|---|---|---|---|
| 65. | Yes | (No) | Are you or could you be pregnant or nursing? | 63. Yes | (No) | Taking birth control pills? |

**VII. ALL PATIENTS:**

64. Yes  (No)   Do you have or have you had anyother diseases or medical problems NOT listed on this form?
If so, please explain: _____

_To the best of my knowledge, I have answered every question completely and accurately. I will inform my dentist of any change in my health and/or medication._

Patient's signature: _Harry H. Haversmith_      Date: _1-15-20XX_

**RECALL REVIEW:**

1. Patient's signature: _____   Date: _____
2. Patient's signature: _____   Date: _____
3. Patient's signature: _____   Date: _____

The Health History is created and maintained by the University of Pacific School of Dentistry, San Francisco, California.
Support for the translation and dissemination of the Health Histories comes from MetLife Dental Care.

Figure 17-17.   Medical history for fictitious patient H.

# Medication List

Patient ___HARRY HAVERSMITH___     Date ___2/05/XX___

| PRESCRIBED |
| --- |

NITRO - DUR PATCH

TENORMIN    25MG/DAY

VASOTEC    10MG/DAY

| OVER-THE-COUNTER |
| --- |

COUGH DROPS FOR COUGH

| VITAMINS, HERBS, DIET SUPPLEMENTS |
| --- |

ONE MULTIVITAMIN/DAY

Figure 17-18.   Medication list for fictitious patient H.

## Vital Signs

Name __HARRY HAVERSMITH__   Date __2/05/XX__

Temperature __99.6°F (37.55°C)__ Pulse __100__

Respiratory Rate __20__   Blood Pressure __130/88__

Tobacco Use:   ☒ Never      ☐ Former

☐ Cigarettes ___packs/day   ☐ Pipe   ☐ Smokeless tobacco

Figure 17-19.   Vital signs findings for fictitious patient H.

**Finding:**

Location: left side of neck below border of the mandible

Size: 8 cm in superior-inferior length; 4 cm in width

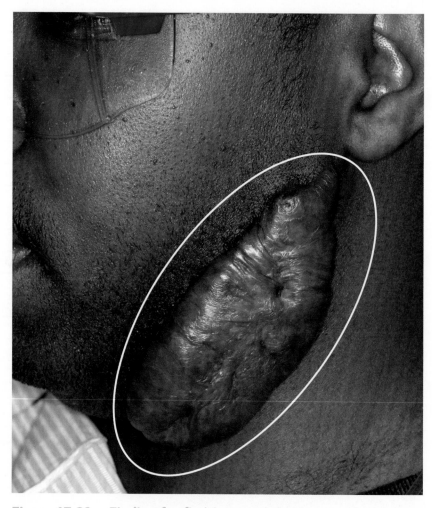

Figure 17-20.   Finding for fictitious patient H.

**Finding:**

Location: raised lesion on
          dorsal surface
          of tongue

Size: 0.5 mm in diameter

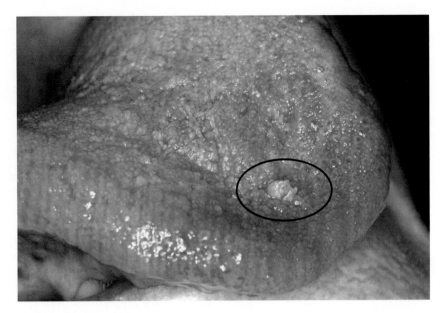

Figure 17-21.   Finding for fictitious patient H.

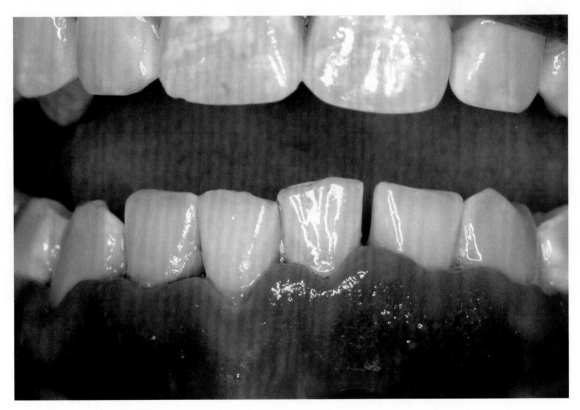

Figure 17-22.   Fictitious patient H: Mandibular anterior sextant, facial aspect.

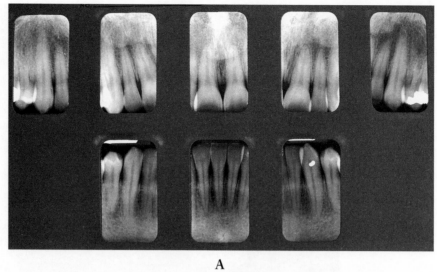

A

Right                                                                                                    Left

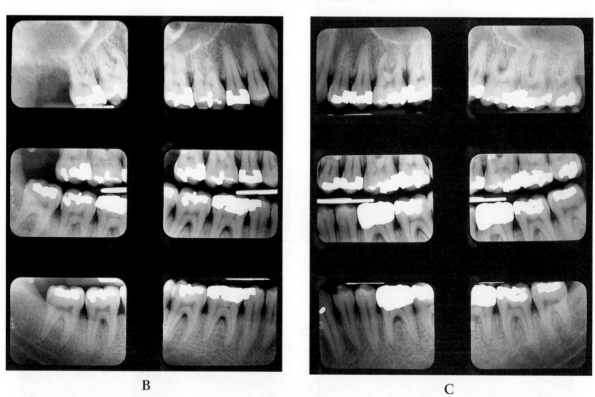

B                                                    C

Figure 17-23A–C.   Radiographs for fictitious patient H.

## SECTION 4:

# Patient I, Ms. Ida Iannuzzi

MetLife                                                                                                    University of the Pacific

| HEALTH HISTORY - English |
|---|

Patient Name: _Iannuzzi, Ida I._     Patient Identification Number: _I-041288_

Birth Date: _82 years_

### I. CIRCLE APPROPRIATE ANSWER (leave BLANK if you do not understand question):

1. (Yes) No — Is your general health good?
2. Yes (No) — Has there been a change in your health within the last year?
3. Yes (No) — Have you been hospitalized or had a serious illness in the last three years?
   If YES, why? _____
4. (Yes) No — Are you being treated by a physician now? For what? _arthritis and glaucoma_
   Date of last medical exam? _1 year ago_     Date of last dental exam? _6 months ago_
5. (Yes) No — Have you had problems with prior dental treatment?
6. Yes (No) — Are you in pain now? _(joint pain, no dental pain)_

### II. HAVE YOU EXPERIENCED:

7. Yes (No) — Chest pain (angina)?
8. Yes (No) — Swollen ankles?
9. Yes (No) — Shortness of breath?
10. Yes (No) — Recent weight loss, fever, night sweats?
11. Yes (No) — Persistent cough, coughing up blood?
12. Yes (No) — Bleeding problems, bruising easily?
13. Yes (No) — Sinus problems?
14. Yes (No) — Difficulty swallowing?
15. Yes (No) — Diarrhea, constipation, blood in stools?
16. Yes (No) — Frequent vomiting, nausea?
17. Yes (No) — Difficulty urinating, blood in urine?
18. Yes (No) — Dizziness?
19. Yes (No) — Ringing in ears?
20. Yes (No) — Headaches?
21. Yes (No) — Fainting spells?
22. (Yes) No — Blurred vision? _Glaucoma_
23. Yes (No) — Seizures?
24. Yes (No) — Excessive thirst?
25. Yes (No) — Frequent urination?
26. (Yes) No — Dry mouth?
27. Yes (No) — Jaundice?
28. (Yes) No — Joint pain?

### III. DO YOU HAVE OR HAVE YOU HAD:

29. Yes (No) — Heart disease?
30. Yes (No) — Heart attack, heart defects?
31. Yes (No) — Heart murmurs?
32. Yes (No) — Rheumatic fever?
33. Yes (No) — Stroke, hardening of arteries?
34. Yes (No) — High blood pressure?
35. Yes (No) — Asthma, TB, emphysema, other lung disease?
36. Yes (No) — Hepatitis, other liver disease?
37. Yes (No) — Stomach problems, ulcers?
38. Yes (No) — Allergies to: drugs, foods, medications, latex?
39. Yes (No) — Family history of diabetes, heart problems, tumors?
40. Yes (No) — AIDS?
41. Yes (No) — Tumors, cancer?
42. (Yes) No — (Arthritis, rheumatism?)
43. Yes (No) — Eye diseases?
44. Yes (No) — Skin deases?
45. Yes (No) — Anemia?
46. Yes (No) — VD (syphilis or gonorrhea)?
47. Yes (No) — Herpes?
48. Yes (No) — Kidney, bladder disease?
49. Yes (No) — Thyroid, adrenal disease?
50. Yes (No) — Diabetes?

### IV. DO YOU HAVE OR HAVE YOU HAD:

51. Yes (No) — Psychiatric care?
52. Yes (No) — Radiation treatments?
53. Yes (No) — Chemotherapy?
54. Yes (No) — Prosthetic heart valve?
55. (Yes) No — Artificial joint? _knee replacement about 20 years ago_
56. Yes (No) — Hospitalization?
57. Yes (No) — Blood transfusions?
58. Yes (No) — Surgeries?
59. Yes (No) — Pacemaker?
60. Yes (No) — Contact lenses?

### V. ARE YOU TAKING:

61. Yes (No) — Recreational drugs?
62. (Yes) No — Drugs, medications, over-the-counter medicines (including Aspirin), natural remedies?
63. Yes (No) — Tobacco in any form?
64. Yes (No) — Alcohol?

Please list: _See Medication List_

### VI. WOMEN ONLY:

65. Yes (No) — Are you or could you be pregnant or nursing?
63. Yes (No) — Taking birth control pills?

### VII. ALL PATIENTS:

64. Yes (No) — Do you have or have you had anyother diseases or medical problems NOT listed on this form?
If so, please explain: _____

_To the best of my knowledge, I have answered every question completely and accurately. I will inform my dentist of any change in my health and/or medication._

Patient's signature: _Ida I. Iannuzzi_     Date: _1-15-20XX_

### RECALL REVIEW:

1. Patient's signature: _____     Date: _____
2. Patient's signature: _____     Date: _____
3. Patient's signature: _____     Date: _____

The Health History is created and maintained by the University of Pacific School of Dentistry, San Francisco, California.
Support for the translation and dissemination of the Health Histories comes from MetLife Dental Care.

**Figure 17-24.** Medical history for fictitious patient I.

# Medication List

Patient ___IDA IANNUZZI___                    Date ___2/05/XX___

## PRESCRIBED

REMERON   30MG/DAY

ALPHAGEN   1 DROP IN EYES T.I.D.

## OVER-THE-COUNTER

NONE

## VITAMINS, HERBS, DIET SUPPLEMENTS

DRINK ONE CAN OF ENSURE
EACH DAY

Figure 17-25.   Medication list for fictitious patient I.

## Vital Signs

Name __IDA IANNUZZI__          Date __2/05/XX__

Temperature __96°F  (35.55°C)__   Pulse __60__

Respiratory Rate __16__          Blood Pressure __110/76__

Tobacco Use:   ☒ Never      ☐ Former

☐ Cigarettes ___packs/day    ☐ Pipe    ☐ Smokeless tobacco

Figure 17-26.   Vital signs findings for fictitious patient I.

**Finding:**

Location: corners of the lips

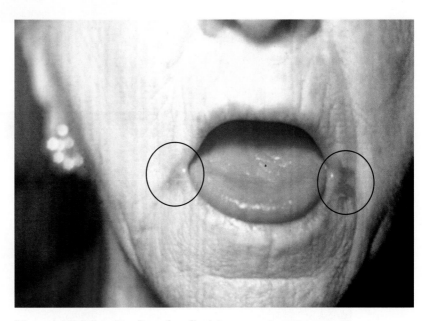

Figure 17-27.   Finding for fictitious patient I.

**Finding:**

Location: right buccal
      mucosa

Size: 1 cm in superior-
      inferior length;
      5 mm in anterior-
      posterior width

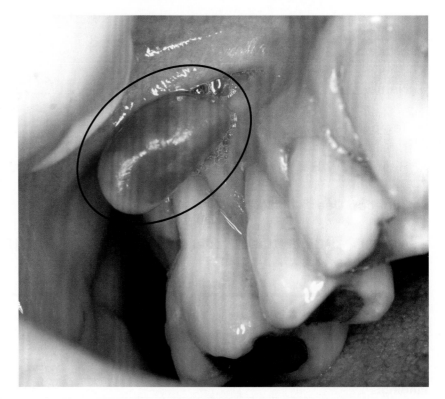

Figure 17-28.    Finding for fictitious patient I.

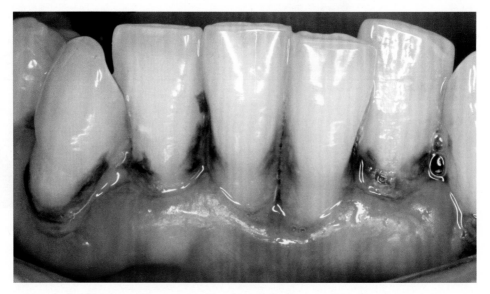

Figure 17-29.    Fictitious patient I: Mandibular anterior sextant,
facial aspect.

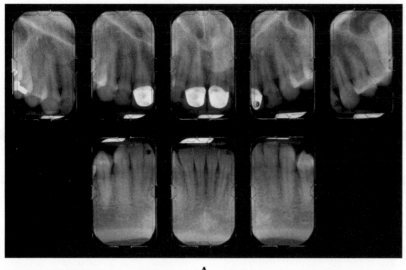

A

Right                                                                                                          Left

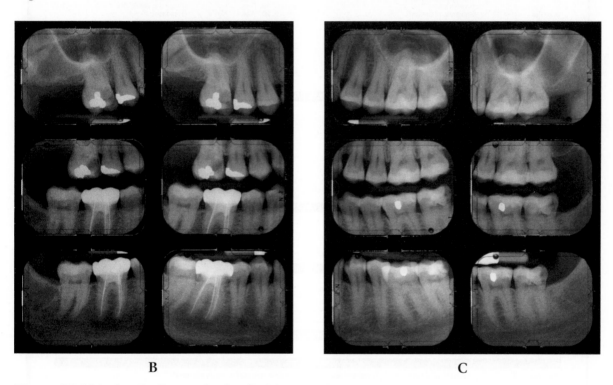

B                                                                                    C

Figure 17-30A–C.   Radiographs for fictitious patient I.

## SECTION 5:

# Patient J, Mr. John Jolicoeur

---

MetLife                                                   University of the Pacific

**HEALTH HISTORY - English**

Patient Name: _Jolicoeur, John J._        Patient Identification Number: _J-915432_

Birth Date: _69 years_

**I. CIRCLE APPROPRIATE ANSWER (leave BLANK if you do not understand question):**

1. (Yes) No — Is your general health good?
2. Yes (No) — Has there been a change in your health within the last year?
3. Yes (No) — Have you been hospitalized or had a serious illness in the last three years?
   If YES, why? _____
4. Yes (No) — Are you being treated by a physician now? For what? _____
   Date of last medical exam? _about 10 years ago_    Date of last dental exam? _Cannot remember_
5. Yes (No) — Have you had problems with prior dental treatment?
6. (Yes) No — Are you in pain now? _(toothache)_

**II. HAVE YOU EXPERIENCED:**

| | | |
|---|---|---|
| 7. Yes (No) | Chest pain (angina)? | 18. Yes (No) Dizziness? |
| 8. Yes (No) | Swollen ankles? | 19. (Yes) No Ringing in ears? _hard of hearing_ |
| 9. Yes (No) | Shortness of breath? | 20. Yes (No) Headaches? |
| 10. Yes (No) | Recent weight loss, fever, night sweats? | 21. Yes (No) Fainting spells? |
| 11. Yes (No) | Persistent cough, coughing up blood? | 22. Yes (No) Blurred vision? |
| 12. Yes (No) | Bleeding problems, bruising easily? | 23. Yes (No) Seizures? |
| 13. Yes (No) | Sinus problems? | 24. Yes (No) Excessive thirst? |
| 14. Yes (No) | Difficulty swallowing? | 25. Yes (No) Frequent urination? |
| 15. Yes (No) | Diarrhea, constipation, blood in stools? | 26. Yes (No) Dry mouth? |
| 16. Yes (No) | Frequent vomiting, nausea? | 27. Yes (No) Jaundice? |
| 17. Yes (No) | Difficulty urinating, blood in urine? | 28. Yes (No) Joint pain? |

**III. DO YOU HAVE OR HAVE YOU HAD:**

| | | |
|---|---|---|
| 29. Yes (No) | Heart disease? | 40. Yes (No) AIDS? |
| 30. Yes (No) | Heart attack, heart defects? | 41. Yes (No) Tumors, cancer? |
| 31. Yes (No) | Heart murmurs? | 42. Yes (No) Arthritis, rheumatism? |
| 32. Yes (No) | Rheumatic fever? | 43. Yes (No) Eye diseases? |
| 33. Yes (No) | Stroke, hardening of arteries? | 44. Yes (No) Skin deases? |
| 34. Yes (No) | High blood pressure? | 45. Yes (No) Anemia? |
| 35. Yes (No) | Asthma, TB, emphysema, other lung disease? | 46. Yes (No) VD (syphilis or gonorrhea)? |
| 36. Yes (No) | Hepatitis, other liver disease? | 47. Yes (No) Herpes? |
| 37. Yes (No) | Stomach problems, ulcers? | 48. Yes (No) Kidney, bladder disease? |
| 38. Yes (No) | Allergies to: drugs, foods, medications, latex? | 49. Yes (No) Thyroid, adrenal disease? |
| 39. Yes (No) | Family history of diabetes, heart problems, tumors? | 50. Yes (No) Diabetes? |

**IV. DO YOU HAVE OR HAVE YOU HAD:**

| | | |
|---|---|---|
| 51. Yes (No) | Psychiatric care? | 56. Yes (No) Hospitalization? |
| 52. Yes (No) | Radiation treatments? | 57. Yes (No) Blood transfusions? |
| 53. Yes (No) | Chemotherapy? | 58. Yes (No) Surgeries? |
| 54. Yes (No) | Prosthetic heart valve? | 59. Yes (No) Pacemaker? |
| 55. (Yes) No | Artificial joint? _knee replacement about 20 years ago_ | 60. Yes (No) Contact lenses? |

**V. ARE YOU TAKING:**

| | | |
|---|---|---|
| 61. Yes (No) | Recreational drugs? | 63. (Yes) No Tobacco in any form? _cigarettes,_ |
| 62. Yes (No) | Drugs, medications, over-the-counter medicines (including Aspirin), natural remedies? | 64. (Yes) No Alcohol? _2 packs/day_ _several beers/day_ |

Please list: _____

**VI. WOMEN ONLY:**

| | | |
|---|---|---|
| 65. Yes (No) | Are you or could you be pregnant or nursing? | 63. Yes (No) Taking birth control pills? |

**VII. ALL PATIENTS:**

64. Yes (No) — Do you have or have you had anyother diseases or medical problems NOT listed on this form?
If so, please explain: _____

_To the best of my knowledge, I have answered every question completely and accurately. I will inform my dentist of any change in my health and/or medication._

Patient's signature: _John Jolicoeur_        Date: _1-15-20XX_

**RECALL REVIEW:**

1. Patient's signature: _____ Date: _____

2. Patient's signature: _____ Date: _____

3. Patient's signature: _____ Date: _____

The Health History is created and maintained by the University of Pacific School of Dentistry, San Francisco, California.
Support for the translation and dissemination of the Health Histories comes from MetLife Dental Care.

**Figure 17-31. Medical history for fictitious patient J.**

# Medication List

Patient ___JOHN JOLICOEUR___     Date ___2/05/XX___

| PRESCRIBED |
| --- |
| NONE |

| OVER-THE-COUNTER |
| --- |
| ASPIRIN |

| VITAMINS, HERBS, DIET SUPPLEMENTS |
| --- |
| NONE |

Figure 17-32. Medication list for fictitious patient J.

# Smoking History

Patient ___JOHN JOLICOEUR___     Date ___2/05/XX___

1. At what age did you begin to smoke? ___13 YRS___

2. How many cigarettes do you smoke per day now? ___2 PACKS___
   Per day at your heaviest? ___2 PACKS___

3. How many times have you tried to stop smoking? _____
   ☒ Never tried to stop

4. What is the longest period of time you have gone without smoking? ___N/A___

5. What forms of tobacco are you currently using? *(Please check all that apply.)*
   ☒ Cigarettes      ☐ Chewing tobacco
   ☐ Pipes      ☒ Snuff
   ☐ Cigars      ☐ Other

6. Do your ☒ family members, ☒ friends, ☐ co-workers smoke? *(Please check all that apply. Circle if you live with any of these smokers.)*

7. What smoking cessation methods have you tried? *(Please check all that apply.)*
   ☒ None      ☐ Self-help programs
   ☐ Cold turkey      ☐ Gradual reduction
   ☐ Hypnosis      ☐ Laser
   ☐ Acupuncture      ☐ Other _____

8. Are you being ☐ encouraged, or ☐ discouraged to stop smoking by any of the following? *(Please check all that apply.)*
   ☐ Spouse or significant other      ☐ Friend
   ☐ Child      ☐ Co-worker
   ☐ Other family member

9. Who do you turn to for support? *(Please check all that apply.)*
   ☐ Spouse or significant other      ☐ Counselor
   ☐ Parent      ☐ Healthcare provider
   ☒ Sibling      ☐ Friend
   ☐ Other family member      ☐ Co-worker
   ☒ Clergy/rabbi/priest

Please rank the following on a scale of 1 (strongly disagree) to 5 (strongly agree):
I am ready to stop smoking at this time:      1   2   3   ④   5
I am concerned about weight gain:      ①   2   3   4   5
I am concerned about dealing with stress:      ①   2   3   4   5

_____John Jolicoeur_____      _____Miccala Smith, DHI_____
Patient Signature          Reviewed by

**Figure 17-33.** Smoking history for fictitious patient J.

## Vital Signs

Name _____JOHN JOLICOEUR_____     Date _____2/05/XX_____

Temperature ___98.4°F (36.88°C)___ Pulse ___90___

Respiratory Rate ___18___     Blood Pressure ___180/110___

Tobacco Use:     ☐ Never          ☐ Former

☒ Cigarettes _2_ packs/day     ☐ Pipe     ☐ Smokeless tobacco

Figure 17-34.   Vital signs findings for fictitious patient J.

**Finding:**

Location: right side of neck

Size: 5 cm in diameter

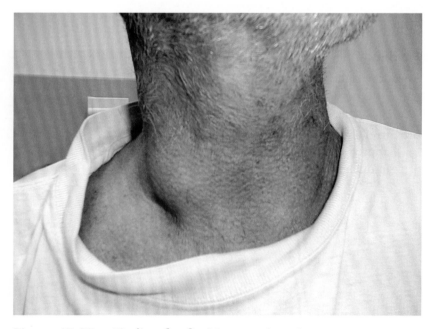

Figure 17-35.   Finding for fictitious patient J.

**Finding:**

Location: left side of nose

Size: 6 mm in superior-
inferior height at
midline of lesion;
17 mm in width

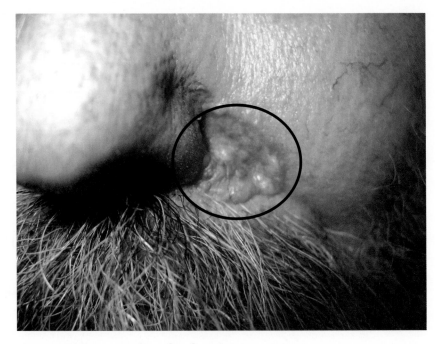

Figure 17-36.   Finding for fictitious patient J.

**Finding:**

Location: right, lateral
border of
tongue

Size: irregular border,
approximately 1 cm
in diameter

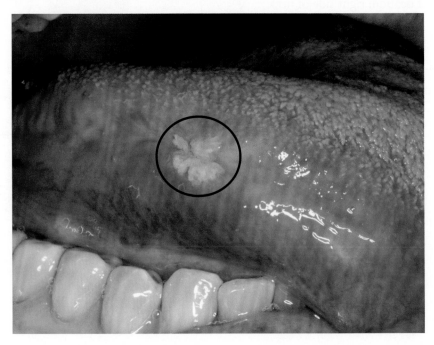

Figure 17-37.   Finding for fictitious patient J.

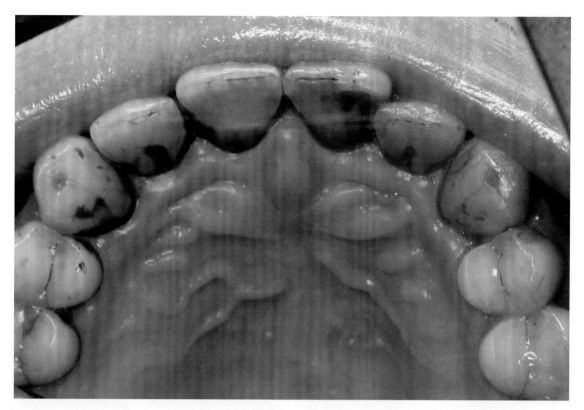

Figure 17-38. Fictitious patient J: Maxillary anterior sextant, lingual aspect.

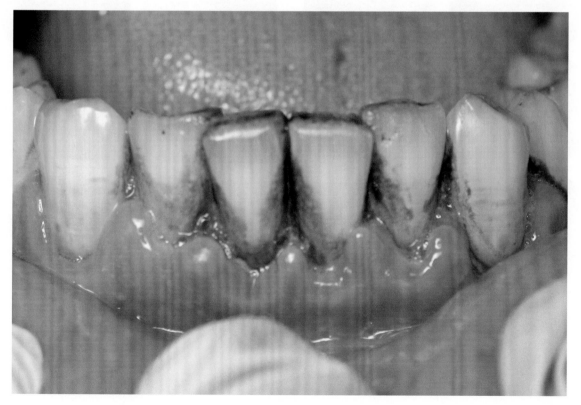

Figure 17-39. Fictitious patient J: Mandibular anterior sextant, facial aspect.

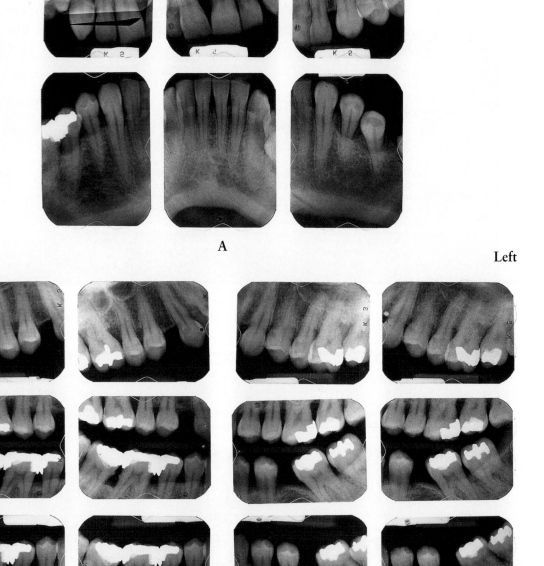

**Right**                                                                                                    **Left**

A

B                                              C

Figure 17-40A–C.   Radiographs for fictitious patient J.

## SECTION 6:

# Patient K, Mr. Kwan Kang

MetLife                                                                                   University of the Pacific

**HEALTH HISTORY - English**

Patient Name: _Kang, Kwan K._          Patient Identification Number: _K-515926_

Birth Date: _75 years_

**I. CIRCLE APPROPRIATE ANSWER (leave BLANK if you do not understand question):**

1. Yes (No)   Is your general health good?
2. Yes (No)   Has there been a change in your health within the last year?
3. (Yes) No   Have you been hospitalized or had a serious illness in the last three years?
            If YES, why? _emphysema_
4. Yes (No)   Are you being treated by a physician now? For what? _emphysema_

Date of last medical exam? _2 weeks ago_          Date of last dental exam? _5 years ago_

5. Yes (No)   Have you had problems with prior dental treatment?
6. (Yes) No   Are you in pain now? _(toothache)_

**II. HAVE YOU EXPERIENCED:**

| | | | | | |
|---|---|---|---|---|---|
| 7. Yes (No) | Chest pain (angina)? | | 18. (No) Yes | Dizziness? |
| 8. Yes (No) | Swollen ankles? | | 19. Yes (No) | Ringing in ears? |
| 9. (Yes) No | Shortness of breath? | | 20. Yes (No) | Headaches? |
| 10. (Yes) No | Recent weight loss, fever, night sweats? | | 21. Yes (No) | Fainting spells? |
| 11. Yes (No) | Persistent cough, coughing up blood? | | 22. Yes (No) | Blurred vision? |
| 12. Yes (No) | Bleeding problems, bruising easily? | | 23. Yes (No) | Seizures? |
| 13. Yes (No) | Sinus problems? | | 24. Yes (No) | Excessive thirst? |
| 14. Yes (No) | Difficulty swallowing? | | 25. Yes (No) | Frequent urination? |
| 15. Yes (No) | Diarrhea, constipation, blood in stools? | | 26. (Yes) No | Dry mouth? |
| 16. Yes (No) | Frequent vomiting, nausea? | | 27. Yes (No) | Jaundice? |
| 17. Yes (No) | Difficulty urinating, blood in urine? | | 28. Yes (No) | Joint pain? |

**III. DO YOU HAVE OR HAVE YOU HAD:**

| | | | | | |
|---|---|---|---|---|---|
| 29. Yes (No) | Heart disease? | | 40. Yes (No) | AIDS? |
| 30. Yes (No) | Heart attack, heart defects? | | 41. Yes (No) | Tumors, cancer? |
| 31. Yes (No) | Heart murmurs? | | 42. Yes (No) | Arthritis, rheumatism? |
| 32. Yes (No) | Rheumatic fever? | | 43. Yes (No) | Eye diseases? |
| 33. Yes (No) | Stroke, hardening of arteries? | | 44. Yes (No) | Skin deases? |
| 34. Yes (No) | High blood pressure? | | 45. Yes (No) | Anemia? |
| 35. (Yes) No | Asthma, TB, (emphysema,) other lung disease? | | 46. Yes (No) | VD (syphilis or gonorrhea)? |
| 36. Yes (No) | Hepatitis, other liver disease? | | 47. Yes (No) | Herpes? |
| 37. Yes (No) | Stomach problems, ulcers? | | 48. Yes (No) | Kidney, bladder disease? |
| 38. Yes (No) | Allergies to: drugs, foods, medications, latex? | | 49. Yes (No) | Thyroid, adrenal disease? |
| 39. Yes (No) | Family history of diabetes, heart problems, tumors? | | 50. Yes (No) | Diabetes? |

**IV. DO YOU HAVE OR HAVE YOU HAD:**

| | | | | | |
|---|---|---|---|---|---|
| 51. Yes (No) | Psychiatric care? | | 56. Yes (No) | Hospitalization? |
| 52. Yes (No) | Radiation treatments? | | 57. Yes (No) | Blood transfusions? |
| 53. Yes (No) | Chemotherapy? | | 58. Yes (No) | Surgeries? |
| 54. Yes (No) | Prosthetic heart valve? | | 59. Yes (No) | Pacemaker? |
| 55. Yes (No) | Artificial joint? | | 60. Yes (No) | Contact lenses? |

**V. ARE YOU TAKING:**

| | | | | | |
|---|---|---|---|---|---|
| 61. Yes (No) | Recreational drugs? | | 63. (Yes) No | Tobacco in any form? _Quit 6 months ago_ |
| 62. (Yes) No | Drugs, medications, over-the-counter medicines (including Aspirin), natural remedies? | | 64. Yes (No) | Alcohol? |

Please list: _See Medication List_

**VI. WOMEN ONLY:**

65. Yes (No)   Are you or could you be pregnant or nursing?          63. Yes (No)   Taking birth control pills?

**VII. ALL PATIENTS:**

64. Yes (No)   Do you have or have you had anyother diseases or medical problems NOT listed on this form?
If so, please explain: _____

_To the best of my knowledge, I have answered every question completely and accurately. I will inform my dentist of any change in my health and/or medication._

Patient's signature: _Kwan Kang_                                    Date: _1-15-20XX_

**RECALL REVIEW:**

1. Patient's signature: _____   Date: _____

2. Patient's signature: _____   Date: _____

3. Patient's signature: _____   Date: _____

The Health History is created and maintained by the University of Pacific School of Dentistry, San Francisco, California.
Support for the translation and dissemination of the Health Histories comes from MetLife Dental Care.

**Figure 17-41.   Medical history for fictitious patient K.**

# Medication List

Patient _____KWAN KANG_____          Date _____2/05/XX_____

## PRESCRIBED

SUPPLEMENTAL OXYGEN

MUCOMYST   2ML OF 10% SOLUTION
EVERY 4 HOURS

ATROVENT   2 PUFFS Q.I.D.

## OVER-THE-COUNTER

NONE

## VITAMINS, HERBS, DIET SUPPLEMENTS

NONE

Figure 17-42.   Medication list for fictitious patient K.

## Vital Signs

Name __KWAN KANG__          Date __2/05/XX__

Temperature __96.8°F (36°C)__   Pulse __90__

Respiratory Rate __20__        Blood Pressure __118/80__

Tobacco Use:   ☐ Never      ☒ Former

   ☒ Cigarettes __3__ packs/day   ☐ Pipe   ☐ Smokeless tobacco
   ↘ NO LONGER SMOKES

Figure 17-43.   Vital signs findings for fictitious patient K.

**Finding:**

Location: left temporal
        region

Size: 1 cm in diameter

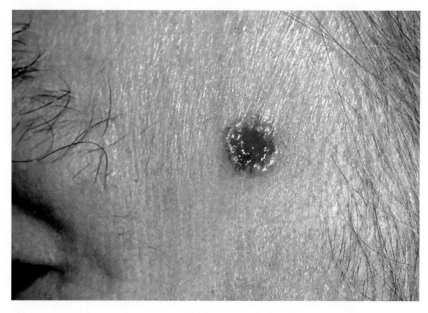

Figure 17-44.   Finding for fictitious patient K.

**Finding:**

Location: ventral surface
              of tongue, to
              right of midline

Size: 6 mm in diameter

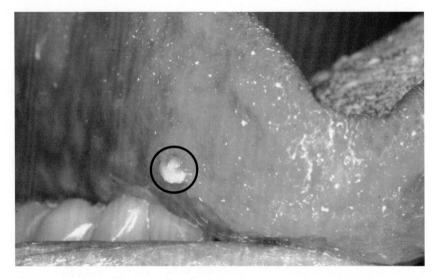

Figure 17-45.   Finding for fictitious patient K.

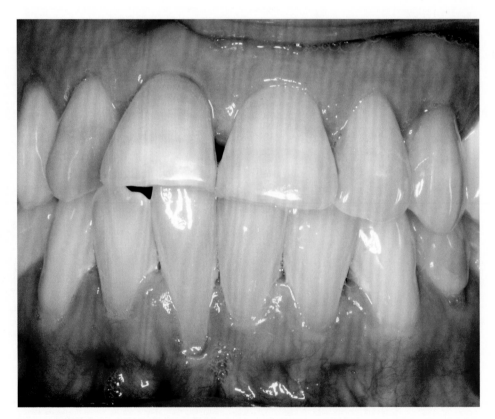

Figure 17-46.   Finding for fictitious patient K.

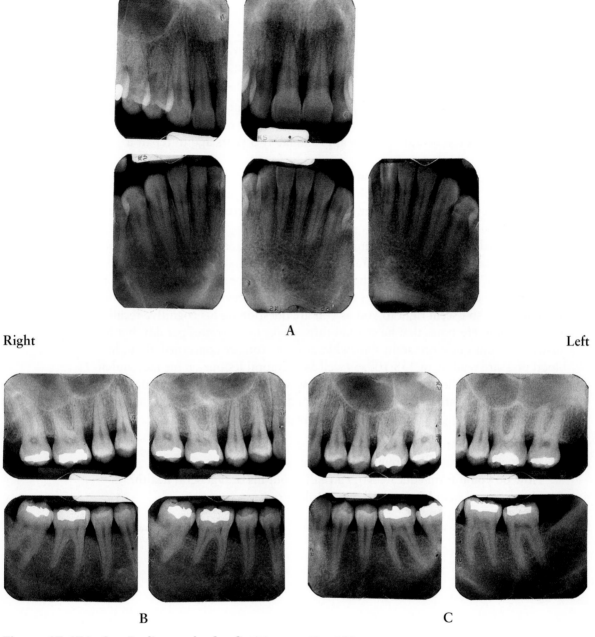

A

Right                                                                                                    Left

B                                                                    C

Figure 17-47A–C.  Radiographs for fictitious patient K.

## SECTION 7:

# The Human Element

---

### PATIENT SCENARIO: MR. FRASIER FAIRHALL

You have just seated Frasier Fairhall, who is a new patient in your group practice. Mr. Fairhall is a 57-year-old male with a chief complaint of "bleeding gums." He states that his last dental visit was approximately 5 years ago to repair a broken filling.

The first thing you notice as you review Mr. Fairhall's medical history responses is the apparent strong smell of alcohol on his breath. As you observe the patient during the discussion, you note that his face is red, his breathing is heavy, and he seems a bit disoriented.

Mr. Fairhall's last physical examination was approximately 10 years ago, although he states that he was treated for hepatitis 2 years ago. Although he answered "no" to question 61 on the written health history form, he admits to the occasional use of recreational drugs during your verbal review of his medical history. Something doesn't seem right to you as you are questioning his cognitive recall for accurate dates. He states that he smokes three packs of cigarettes per day, but his answers to your questions seem somewhat evasive. You are concerned about his blood pressure reading of 158/100, as well as extraoral lesions on his face and an intraoral lesion in the floor of his mouth. However, you are most concerned about his sobriety and treating him in his present condition and are fearful of his getting into a car and driving following the appointment.

1. Do you have to treat Mr. Fairhall today?
2. What ethical principles are involved in this scenario?
3. How do you inform/educate Mr. Fairhall about his oral/general health?
4. How can you help Mr. Fairhall quit smoking?

## SECTION 8:
# Skill Check

**SKILL CHECKLIST:**   COMMUNICATIONS ROLE-PLAY

Student: _____   Evaluator: _____

Date: _____

### DIRECTIONS:

Play the role of the clinician in one or more role-plays selected by your instructor.

> **Roles:**
> - Student 1 = Plays the role of the patient.
> - Student 2 = Plays the role of the clinician.
> - Student 3 or instructor = Plays the role of the clinic instructor near the end of the role-play.

**DIRECTIONS FOR STUDENT CLINICIAN:** Using **Column S**, evaluate your skill level as **S** (satisfactory) or **U** (unsatisfactory).

**DIRECTIONS FOR EVALUATOR:** Use **Column E**. Indicate **S** (satisfactory) or **U** (unsatisfactory). In the optional grade percentage calculation, each **S** equals 1 point and each **U** equals 0 points.

| CRITERIA | S | E |
|---|---|---|
| **Uses appropriate nonverbal behavior such as maintaining eye contact, sitting at the same level as the patient, nodding head when listening to patient, etc.** | | |
| **Interacts with the patient as a peer, avoids a condescending approach. Collaborates with the patient and provides advice. Gains the patient's trust and cooperation.** | | |
| **Reports all notable findings to the patient and explains whether the findings are normal or outside the normal range and the significance of these findings. Communicates using common, everyday words. Avoids dental terminology.** | | |
| **Listens attentively to the patient's comments. Respects the patient's point of view.** | | |
| **Listens attentively to the patient's questions. Encourages patient questions. Clarifies for understanding, when necessary.** | | |
| **Answers the patient's questions fully and accurately. Checks for understanding by the patient. Clarifies information.** | | |
| **Accurately communicates the findings to the clinical instructor. Discusses the implications for dental treatment. Uses correct medical and dental terminology.** | | |

OPTIONAL GRADE PERCENTAGE CALCULATION

Each **S** equals 1 point, and each U equals 0 points.  Using the **E** column, total the sum of the "**S**"s _____ divided by Total Points Possible (7) equals the Percentage Grade _____.

# NOTES

# GLOSSARY

## A

**Abdominal aortic aneurysm**—occurs when part of the aorta—the main artery of the body—becomes weakened. If left untreated the aorta can burst.

**Addiction**—a chronic dependence on a substance, such as smoking, despite adverse consequences.

**Aneroid manometer**—a round dial-type gauge to indicate pressure readings.

**Angle's classification**—a system for classifying the relationship of the mandibular teeth to the maxillary teeth.

**Antecubital fossa**—the hollow or depressed area in the underside of the arm at the bend of the elbow.

**Aphasia**—a disorder that results from damage to language centers of the brain. It can result in a reduced ability to understand what others are saying, to express ideas, or to be understood.

**Ask. Advise. Refer. (AAR)**—the ADHA's national Smoking Cessation Initiative (SCI) designed to promote cessation intervention by dental hygienists.

**Asymptomatic**—a condition or disease that has no symptoms that are detectable to the patient; an example of a asymptomatic condition is hypertension.

**Attention Deficit Hyperactivity Disorder (ADHD)**—a developmental disorder believed to be caused primarily by genetic factors. Patients with ADHD may experience problems such as difficulty with sustained attention, excessive activity, and increased distractibility.

**Auscultation**—the act of listening for sounds within the body to evaluate the condition of the heart, blood vessels, lungs, or other organs.

**Auscultatory gap**—a period of abnormal silence that occurs between the Korotkoff phases that are heard during the measurement of blood pressure.

## B

**Bidis**—small, often flavored, hand-rolled cigarettes.

**Blood pressure**—pressure exerted against the blood vessel walls as blood flows through them. *Also see: systolic pressure and diastolic pressure.*

**Blood pressure cuff**—an airtight, flat, inflatable bladder covered by a cloth sheath that is used when measuring blood pressure.

**Brachial artery**—the main artery of the upper arm; it divides into the radial and ulnar arteries at the elbow. The brachial artery is used when taking blood pressure.

**Bulla**—a large blister filled with clear fluid; usually over 1 cm in diameter; commonly seen in burns.

## C

**Cancer**—a term for diseases in which abnormal cells divide without control. Cancer cells can invade nearby tissues and spread through the bloodstream and lymphatic system to other parts of the body. *Also see head and neck cancer.*

**Capacity for consent**—the ability of a patient to fully understand the proposed treatment, possible risks, unanticipated outcomes and alternative treatments—takes into account the patient's age, mental capacity and language comprehension.

**Carcinogen**—a chemical or other substance that causes cancer.

**Celsius temperature scale**—the temperature scale used in most countries for measuring body temperature. *Also see fahrenheit temperature scale.*

**Chewing tobacco**—also known as spit tobacco, chew, dip, and chaw—is tobacco cut for chewing. *Also see smokeless tobacco and snuff.*

**Chronic obstructive pulmonary disease (COPD)**—a lung disease in which the airways in the lungs produce excess mucus resulting in frequent coughing. Smoking accounts for 80% to 90% of the risk for developing COPD.

**Clinical Practice Guideline for Treating Tobacco Use and Dependence**—guidelines published by the United States Department of Health and Human Services is considered the benchmark for cessation techniques and treatment delivery strategies. The Clinical Practice Guideline may be downloaded at http://www. surgeongeneral
.gov/tobacco/treating_tobacco_use.pdf.

**Circumvallate papillae**—the 8 to 12 large papillae that form a V-shaped row on the tongue.

**Closed questions**—questions that can be answered with a yes or no, or a one- or two-word response, and do not provide an opportunity for the patient to elaborate.

**Communication**—the exchange of information between individuals.

**Coronary artery disease (CAD)**—a thickening of the coronary arteries—is the most common type of heart disease. CAD results in a narrowing of the arteries so that the supply of blood and oxygen to the heart is restricted or blocked. Smoking is the major risk factor for CAD.

**Cuff**—*see blood pressure cuff*

**Cultural awareness**—the development of sensitivity and cross-cultural understanding.

**Cultural blindness**—occurs when a person ignores differences and proceeds as though the differences did not exist (e.g., *"There is no reason to change how we do things, as long we are nice to our patients, that is enough."*).

**Cultural competency**—the application of cultural knowledge, behaviors, and interpersonal and clinical skills to enhance a dental health care provider's effectiveness in managing patient care.

**Cultural imposition**—is the belief that everyone should conform to the majority (e.g., *"Why should we have to translate our forms, if they can't read English they can just go elsewhere."*).

**Culture**—a pattern of learned behavior, values, and beliefs exhibited by a group that shares history and geographic proximity. Culture determines health attitudes, roles, and behaviors of providers and patients.

**Culture, low contact**—cultures prefer 4 to 12 feet of body space during personal interaction and little, if any, physical contact.

**Culture, high contact**—cultures that prefer 1 inch to 4 feet of body space during personal interaction and much contact between people.

# D

**Dental health history**—a record of the patient's past and present dental experiences.

**Diaphragm endpiece**—the amplifying device of a stethoscope that is used to hear loud sounds like the blood rushing thorough the arteries.

**Diastolic pressure**—the pressure exerted against the vessel walls when the heart relaxes.

**Diplomacy**—the art of treating people with tact and genuine concern.

**Discrimination**—the differential treatment of an individual due to minority status (e.g., "*We just are not equipped to care for people like that.*").

**Dysarthria**—speech problems that are caused by the muscles involved with speaking or the nerves controlling them. Individuals with dysarthria have difficulty expressing certain words or sounds.

# E

**Empathy**—identifying with the feelings or thoughts of another person; an essential factor in effective communication.

**Environmental tobacco smoke (ETS)**—occurs when nonsmokers inhale a mixture of smoke from a burning cigarette, pipe, or cigar and the smoke exhaled by the smoker. Also known as secondhand smoke or passive smoking.

**Estimated systolic pressure**—an estimation of the actual systolic blood pressure that is determined by palpating the brachial artery pulse and inflating the cuff until the pulsation disappears. This point at which the pulsation disappears is the estimated systolic pressure.

**Ethnic competence**—the development of skills that assist a person to behave in a culturally appropriate way to meet the expectations and behaviors of a given group.

**Ethnicity and culture**—qualities of human groups, including language, diet, attire, religions, customs, beliefs, worldviews, kinship systems, and historical or territorial identity.

**Ethnocentrism**—the inability to accept another cultures' worldview (e.g., "*My way is best*").

**Extraoral examination**—*See head and neck examination*

# F

**Fahrenheit temperature scale**—the temperature scale used in most countries for measuring body temperature. *Also see celsius temperature scale.*

**Filiform papillae**—the long, thin, gray, hairlike papillae that cover the anterior two thirds of the dorsal surface of the tongue.

**Fissure**—a linear crack in the top two layers of the skin or mucosa.

**Follate papillae**—the 3 to 5 large, red, leaflike projections on the lateral border of the posterior third of the tongue.

**Fungiform papillae**—the broad, round, red, mushroom-shaped papillae of the tongue.

# G

**Galinstan**—the most common alternative to a mercury thermometer.

**Glass thermometer**—a small glass tube with a bulb at the end containing mercury that is used to take an oral temperature. When the thermometer bulb is warmed, the mercury moves up the glass tube.

**Goiter**—an enlarged thyroid gland.

# H

**Head and neck cancer**—cancer that arises in the head or neck region (in the nasal cavity, sinuses, lip, mouth, salivary glands, throat, or larynx [voice box]).

**Head and neck examination**—a physical examination technique consisting of a systematic visual inspection of the skin of the head and neck combined with palpation of the lymph nodes, salivary glands, thyroid gland, and temporomandibular joint.

**Health literacy**—the ability of an individual to understand and act on health information and advice.

**Hookah**—a large water pipe with a hose used to smoke flavored tobacco.

**Hypertension**—high blood pressure; blood pressure that stays at or above 140/90.

**Hypertensive**—an individual with abnormally high blood pressure.

**Hypotensive**—an individual with abnormally low blood pressure.

# I

**Idiom**—a distinctive, often colorful expression in which the meaning cannot be understood from the combined of its individual words (e.g., the phrase "to kill two birds with one stone.").

**Informed consent**—involves providing complete and comprehensive information about patient assessment procedures and planned dental hygiene treatments so that the patient can make a well-informed decision about either accepting or rejecting the proposed treatment. Informed consent not only involves informing the patient about the expected successful outcomes of assessment procedures, but the possible risks, unanticipated outcomes and alternative treatments as well. The patient also should be made aware of the costs for each of the options involved, which may influence the patient's ultimate decision. *Also see: capacity for consent and informed refusal.*

**Informed refusal**—the patient's right to refuse one or more of the recommended assessment or treatment procedures.

**Inspection**—the systematic visual examination of a patient's general appearance, skin, or a part of the body to observe its condition.

**Intraoral examination**—*see oral examination.*

# K

**Korotkoff sounds**—the series of sounds that is heard as the pressure in the sphygmomanometer cuff is released during the measurement of arterial blood pressure.

# L

**Laryngectomy**—the surgical removal of the voice box due to cancer; affects approximately 9,000 individuals each year, most are older adults.

**Lesion of the soft tissue**—an area of abnormal appearing skin or mucosa that does not resemble the soft tissue surrounding it; such as a variation in color, texture, or form of an area of skin or mucosa.

**Literacy:** *See health literacy*

**Lymph**—a clear fluid that carries nutrients and waste materials between the body tissues and the bloodstream.

**Lymphadenopathy**—the term for enlarged lymph nodes.

**Lymphatic system**—a network of lymph nodes connected by lymphatic vessels that plays an important part in the body's defense against infection.

**Lymph nodes**—small bean-shaped structures that filter out bacteria, fungi, viruses, and other unwanted substances to eliminate them from the body.

## M

**Macule**—a small, flat, discolored spot on the skin or mucosa that does not include a change in skin texture or thickness; less than 1 cm in size; the discoloration can be brown, black, red, or lighter than the surrounding skin.

**Malocclusion**—the improper positioning of the teeth and jaws.

**Manometer**—a gauge that measures the air pressure in millimeters used when measuring blood pressure. *Also see aneroid manometer and mercury manometer*

**Medical alert box**—a specified area (such as a box) on the patient chart or computerized record in which medical conditions/diseases or medications that necessitate modifications or special precautions for treatment are clearly marked.

**Mercury manometer**—a device with a column of mercury to indicate pressure readings.

**Metastasis**—the spread of cancer from the original tumor site to other parts of the body by tiny clumps of cells transported by the blood or lymphatic system.

**Mixed dentition**—a combination of primary and permanent teeth in a dentition.

**Multilanguage Health History Project**—an initiative of the University of the Pacific Dental School (UOP) to address the needs of patients and dental health care providers who do not speak the same language.

## N

**Nicotine replacement therapy (NRT)**—nicotine-containing medications used for smoking cessation.

**Nodule**—a raised, marblelike lesion detectable by touch, usually 1 cm or more in diameter; it can be felt as a hard mass distinct from the tissue surrounding it.

**Nonverbal communication**—the transfer of information between persons without using spoken, written, or sign language.

## O

**Occlusion**—the relationship of the teeth to each other when the incisal and occlusal surfaces of the mandibular arch contact those of the maxillary arch.

**Open-ended questions**—questions that require more than a one-word response and allow the patient to express ideas, feelings, and opinions.

**Oral examination**—a physical examination technique consisting of the systemic inspection of the oral structures.

**Overbite**—the amount of vertical overlap that occurs when the maxillary incisors vertically overlap the mandibular incisors.

**Overjet**—the horizontal distance between the incisal edges of the maxillary teeth and the mandibular teeth.

## P

**Palpation**—the examination of a part of the body by using the fingertips to move or compress a structure against the underlying tissue. The most sensitive part of the hand—the fingertips—should be used for palpation.

**Papillae**—the taste sensitive structures of the tongue. *Also see filiform, fungiform, follate, and circumvallate papilla.*

**Papule**—a solid raised lesion that is usually less than 1 cm in diameter; may be any color.

**Parotid glands**—the largest of the salivary glands; each gland is located between the ear and the jaw.

**Passive smoking**—*see environmental tobacco smoke*

**Patch**—a flat, discolored spot on the skin or mucosa; larger than 1 cm in size.

**Patient-centered care**—an approach to health care that emphasizes respecting the patient as a whole, unique individual. A patient centered approach to patient care recognizes that there are two experts present during the interaction between a health care provider and patient. One expert is the health care provider who has clinical knowledge. The second expert is the patient who brings experience, beliefs, and values to the dental treatment planning process.

**Peripheral vascular disease (PVD)**—a vascular disease that occurs when fat and cholesterol build up on the walls of the arteries blocking the supply blood to the arms and legs.

**Personal filters**—when involved in the act of communication, factors in a person's life, such as his or her life experiences, age, gender, and cultural diversity, that act as filters to incoming information.

For this reason, the message received may not be the message sent. Normal human biases or personalized filters create major barriers to effective communication.

**Personal space**—the physical distance maintained between persons; a powerful concept that we use in determining the meaning of messages conveyed by another person.

**Pharmacotherapy**—the treatment of a medical condition using one or more medications.

**Plaque**—a superficial raised lesion often formed by the coalescence (joining) of closely grouped papules; more than 1 cm in diameter; a plaque differs from a nodule in its height, a plaque is flattened and a nodule is a bump.

**Presbycusis**—the loss of hearing that gradually occurs in most individuals as they grow old.

**Proxemics**—the study of the distance an individual maintains from other persons and how this separation relates to environmental and cultural factors.

**Pulse points**—the sites on the surface of the body where rhythmic beats of an artery can be easily felt.

**Pulse rate**—an indication of an individual's heart rate. Pulse rate is measured by counting the number of rhythmic beats that can be felt over an artery in 1 minute.

**Pustule**—a small, raised lesion filled with pus.

## Q

**Quitlines**—toll-free telephone centers staffed by trained smoking cessation experts.

# R

**Racial group**—a group of people who share socially constructed differences based on visible characteristics or regional linkages.

**Radial artery**—a branch of the brachial artery beginning below the elbow and extending down the forearm on the thumb-side of the wrist and into the hand.

**Reflection**—the act of repeating something that someone has just said.

**Respiratory rate**—is measured by counting the number of times that a patient's chest rises in one minute.

**Risk factors**—are conditions that increase a person's chances of getting a disease (such as cancer).

# S

**Secondhand smoke**—occurs when nonsmokers inhale a mixture of smoke from a burning cigarette, pipe, or cigar and the smoke exhaled by the smoker. *Also see environmental tobacco smoke.*

**Service animal**—any guide dog or other animal that is trained to provide assistance to a person with a disability.

**Smoker's cough**—the chronic cough experienced by smokers because smoking impairs the lung's ability to clean out harmful material. Coughing is the body's way of trying to get rid of the harmful material in the lungs.

**Smokeless tobacco**—is tobacco that is not smoked but used in another form. Snuff and chewing tobacco are the two main forms of smokeless tobacco in use in the United States and Canada. *Also see chewing tobacco and snuff.*

**Snuff**—a smokeless tobacco in the form of a powder that is placed between the gingiva and the lip, or cheek or inhaled into the nose. *Also see smokeless tobacco and snuff.*

**Soft tissue lesion**—*see lesion of the soft tissue.*

**Sphygmomanometer**—a device used to measure blood pressure consisting of a cuff with an inflatable bladder, a hand bulb with a valve used to inflate and deflate the bladder, and a pressure gauge.

**Sphygmomanometer C=cuff**—*see blood pressure cuff*

**Stereotype**—an oversimplified, standardized image that one individual uses to categorize other individuals or groups.

**Sternomastoid muscle**—a long, thick, superficial muscle on each side of the head with its origin on the mastoid process and insertion on the sternum and clavicle (also called the sternocleidomastoid muscle).

**Stethoscope**—a device that makes sound louder and transfers it to the clinician's ears.

**Sublingual glands**—the smallest of the three glands salivary glands; located in the anterior floor of the mouth next to the mandibular canines.

**Submandibular glands**—the salivary glands located below the jaw toward the back of the mouth.

**Systolic pressure**—the pressure created by the blood as it presses through and against the vessel walls. *Also see estimated systolic pressure.*

# T

**Temperature**—the measurement of the degree of heat in a living body.

**Temporomandibular joint (TMJ)**—the joint that connects the mandible to the temporal bone at the side of the head. One of the most complicated joints in the body, it allows the jaw to open and close, move forward and backward, and from side to side.

**Territory**—the space we consider as belonging to us. The way that people handle space is largely determined by their culture. *Also see: culture, low-contact and culture, high-culture.*

**Thermometer**—*see glass thermometer.*

**Thyroid gland**—one of the endocrine glands, secretes thyroid hormone that controls the body's metabolic rate; located in the middle of the lower neck.

**Triangulation**—the widening of the periodontal ligament space (PDLS) caused by the resorption of bone along either the mesial or distal aspect of the interdental (interseptal) crestal bone as observed on a radiograph.

## U

**Ulcer**—a craterlike lesion of the skin or mucosa where the top two layers of the skin are lost.

## V

**Verbal communication**—the use of spoken, written, or sign language to exchange information between individuals.

**Vesicle**—a small blister filled with a clear fluid; usually 1 cm or less in diameter.

**Vital signs**—a person's temperature, pulse, respiration, and blood pressure.

## W

**Wheal**—a raised, somewhat irregular area of localized edema; often itchy, lasting 24 hours or less; usually due to an allergic reaction, such as to a drug or insect bite.

**White-coat (or office) hypertension**—blood pressure that rises above its usual level when it is measured in a health care setting (such as a medical or dental office, where a health care provider may be wearing a white laboratory coat).

**Withdrawal symptoms**—the unpleasant symptoms experienced by a smoker when trying to quit smoking, such as craving for nicotine, irritability, anger, anxiety, fatigue, depressed mood, difficulty concentrating, restlessness, and sleep disturbance.